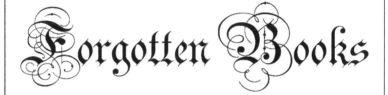

ISBN 978-1-331-10829-0
PIBN 10145866

1 MONTH OF
FREE
READING

at

www.ForgottenBooks.com

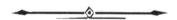

By purchasing this book you are eligible for one month membership to ForgottenBooks.com, giving you unlimited access to our entire collection of over 1,000,000 titles via our web site and mobile apps.

To claim your free month visit:
www.forgottenbooks.com/free145866

OXFORD MEDICAL PUBLICATIONS

DISEASES OF THE HEART

MACKENZIE

PUBLISHED BY THE JOINT COMMITTEE OF
HENRY FROWDE AND HODDER & STOUGHTON
AT THE OXFORD PRESS WAREHOUSE
FALCON SQUARE, LONDON, E.C.

OXFORD MEDICAL PUBLICATIONS

DISEASES OF THE HEART

BY

Sir) JAMES MACKENZIE, M.D., F.R.C.P.

LL.D. Ab. & Ed. F.R.C.P.I. (Hon.)

PHYSICIAN TO THE LONDON HOSPITAL (IN CHARGE OF THE CARDIAC DEPARTMENT),
CONSULTING PHYSICIAN TO THE VICTORIA HOSPITAL, BURNLEY

THIRD EDITION

LONDON

HENRY FROWDE   HODDER & STOUGHTON

OXFORD UNIVERSITY PRESS   WARWICK SQUARE, E.C.

1913

OXFORD: HORACE HART
PRINTER TO THE UNIVERSITY

PREFACE TO THE THIRD EDITION

THE advances that have been made in the knowledge of the heart since the last edition of this book was published (1910) have necessitated the re-writing of the greater portion of this work. These advances have been mainly along three lines: First, the clearer differentiation of the signs of disease. For this purpose the introduction of the electrocardiogram has been of the greatest service. Second, the bearing of heart manifestations on the question of heart failure, present or remote. Third, the basing of treatment on sound and scientific principles. The study of cardiac physiology and therapy has hitherto been based on what happens to normal hearts with normal rhythm. These later investigations have shown that in hearts affected by disease the reaction of the heart to stimulation is profoundly altered; in consequence, it is necessary that the physiology of diseased hearts, and especially of those with abnormal rhythm, should be carefully studied. So far some progress has been made, and we can now treat such conditions as auricular fibrillation and auricular flutter in an intelligent manner. Moreover, later investigations have also shown how helpless we are in the face of many conditions, and the recognition of our helplessness provides an object to which investigation should be directed.

To give practical proof of the views expressed in the text I have added many illustrative cases in the Appendix.

J. M.

133 HARLEY STREET,
August, 1913.

PREFACE TO THE SECOND EDITION

THE speedy exhaustion of the first edition of this book, and the demand for its translation into a number of languages, is an evidence of the interest taken in the more recent methods of studying diseases of the heart. It is extremely gratifying to find many investigators entering a field full of promise of new and original observations, embracing every aspect of the circulatory system.

I wish to point out that, in setting forth my own experiences, I desire to keep the record of facts apart from their interpretation. For this reason the numerous figures in the text represent the actual facts as recorded by the movements of the heart and blood-vessels, and are therefore far more trustworthy than a verbal description. The interpretation of these tracings represents the present state of my knowledge. These interpretations may ultimately be proved to be incorrect, but the recorded movements will continue to serve for other and more fitting explanations.

A vast amount of clinical and experimental work still remains to be done to explain the variable changes in the heart's action due to disease, and my explanations can, consequently, only be tentative. Should other investigators prove these interpretations wrong by the discovery of new facts, I shall rejoice with them, for they will have shed fresh light, and will have reached a plane higher than I have been able to attain.

A valuable addition to the methods for clinical and experimental observation has been made by the recording of the electrical changes caused by the contraction of the heart chambers. I am indebted to my friend, Dr. Lewis, for kindly writing a short appendix on this subject.

J. M.

January, 1910.

PREFACE TO THE FIRST EDITION

In the following pages are given the results of observations on affections of the heart, made during an active practice of over a quarter of a century. As the nature of the heart affection can only be inferred from the presence of one or more symptoms, my special object has been to ascertain the mechanism by which the symptoms are produced, to find out their relationship to organic changes in the heart, to ascertain their prognostic significance, and, finally, to employ them as a guide for treatment.

This line of observation has revealed many new and unexpected features, and has necessitated the employment of special methods and the watching of individual cases for many years.

To make the results of use in practice it has been found necessary to enter into considerable detail, and it has been difficult to make the account at the same time succinct and intelligible. A certain amount of detail is necessary, yet too much would be wearisome and perhaps confusing, hence controversy has been avoided and the observations have been given with the explanation that seems most reasonable.

Many methods of examination that occupy prominent places in text-books have been briefly dealt with or even ignored, not because I do not recognize their usefulness in certain cases, but because my object has been to deal with matters of practical value in the every-day examination of patients. It may appear that an unnecessary amount of attention has been devoted to details, many of which can only be recognized by special apparatus. But to bring conviction proof had to be elaborated. Many of the seemingly trivial signs, such as the minute differences in the size of a pulse-beat, or a slight delay between the auricular and ventricular systoles, are really of vital importance in revealing changes which have been proved to be due to very definite affections of the heart. In the same manner the study of irregularities is of the greatest service, as their presence is easily detected and their significance has never been properly understood. A close study of irregularities throws an unexpected light upon the functional derangements of the heart, and affords grounds for an intelligent diagnosis upon which a rational treatment and prognosis can be based.

The main purpose of all my work has been to obtain a guide for treatment, and my readers may be disappointed at the seeming barrenness of my work in this respect. A careful search has been made for the essential principles that should govern a rational treatment, and if only few drugs and suggestions are given, it is because the treatment of cardiac disease at present in vogue requires careful revision in the light of the more accurate diagnosis now made possible by means of the graphic method of examination.

In routine practice it is not usually necessary to take graphic records. If one is trained to make careful and minute observations by the ordinary methods, and to have these checked by graphic records, one can ultimately acquire the power of recognizing the majority of movements of the circulation without graphic records. In regard to the tracings given in this book, a selection has been made from an enormous number of observations, and are rarely exceptional, but are types of the commoner forms. The interpretation of these records may prove to be faulty, and an endeavour has therefore been made to keep the actual observation separate from the interpretation, so that if the latter be erroneous, the recorded movements may at least remain available for future workers in this field.

It was originally intended to give a more complete account of the morbid anatomy of the heart, and for that purpose Professor Keith has investigated a great number of hearts, of which I have kept careful clinical records, but the investigation, so far, has brought to both of us the conviction that before the pathology of the heart can be put on a satisfactory basis a more thorough and minute examination of the post-mortem appearances in correlation with the clinical symptoms is necessary. The post-mortem aspect of heart disease is therefore dealt with very briefly, and my observations in this respect are intended to be suggestive rather than conclusive.

I had intended to give the means of judging the state of the heart in cases apart from those directly due to affections of the heart, as in fevers, pregnancy, surgical diseases, diseases of other organs, the administration of chloroform. This has only been carried out to a limited extent, because, when the results came to be analysed, I did not see my way clear in all cases to give satisfactory guides, so that many observations have been omitted. I hesitated to include my observations on chloroform administration, because the matter is still very vague. I feel convinced that the reason chloroform is attended with so much danger will never be solved until prolonged and painstaking investigation is made during its administration along the lines of observation detailed in this book, and I leave my remarks in this unsatisfactory state in the hope that others may solve the question.

What a tool is to a workman, so should a text-book be to the busy practitioner. In cases of heart affection one or two symptoms are usually most prominent, and by giving clear definitions of the terms employed, and by arranging the index and the discussion in the text, an endeavour has been made to facilitate the rapid inquiry into the meaning of any given symptom.

J. M.

LONDON, W.
September, 1908.

CONTENTS

PAGE

DEFINITION OF TERMS xxi

CHAPTER I

THE APPRECIATION OF AFFECTIONS OF THE HEART

The object of the physician's examination. Methods adopted in describing affections of the heart. Causes of confused diagnosis. The relative importance of symptoms. The essential symptoms of heart failure. Inadequacy of the methods usually employed to estimate the heart's efficiency 1

CHAPTER II

THE PATHOLOGY OF HEART FAILURE

What is heart failure ? The back-pressure theory of heart failure. Compensation. The origin of these views. Evil done by the back-pressure theory. Heart failure and pathological changes. Functional impairment of the heart. The evidences of impaired function 5

CHAPTER III

THE PRINCIPLES UNDERLYING THE PRODUCTION OF HEART FAILURE

The purpose of the circulation and how it is attained. The importance of the heart muscle. The meaning of heart failure. The two forces of the heart muscle. The reserve force of the heart muscle. How heart failure begins. The relation between exhaustion and restoration of the reserve force of the heart. Conditions exhausting the reserve force 10

CHAPTER IV

EXHAUSTION OF THE HEART MUSCLE

Importance of the exhaustion of the reserve force. Effect of exhaustion in the individual beat of the heart. Exhaustion and restoration of the reserve force. Estimation of the amount of reserve force. Evidences of exhaustion. Practical value of estimating the cardiac condition by the degrees of exhaustion. The restoration of the exhausted heart : 14

CHAPTER V

DETERMINATION OF THE VALUE OF SYMPTOMS

The necessity for appreciating the meaning of symptoms. How the significance of symptoms is acquired. Discrimination of the significance of symptoms. Signs of exhaustion of the reserve force 18

CHAPTER VI

THE PRODUCTION AND SIGNIFICANCE OF SYMPTOMS

PAGE

Definition of the term symptom. The significance of physical signs. The production of the symptoms of heart failure. Abnormal rhythms. Objective sign of heart failure. Principles governing the production of symptoms . . 23

CHAPTER VII

FUNDAMENTAL FUNCTIONS OF THE HEART MUSCLE-CELLS

Myogenic doctrine. Stimulus production. Excitability. Conductivity. Contractility. Tonicity. Co-ordination of functions. Characteristics of the functions of the heart muscle-fibres 27

CHAPTER VIII

DEVELOPMENT, ANATOMY, AND PHYSIOLOGY OF THE HEART

The primitive cardiac tube. The functions of the primitive cardiac tube. The remains of the primitive cardiac tube in the mammalian heart. Functions of the sino-auricular node, the pacemaker of the heart. Functions of the auriculo-ventricular node and bundle. Functional anatomy of the heart. The nerve supply of the heart: Afferent fibres; cardiac ganglion cells 32

CHAPTER IX

THE EXAMINATION OF THE PATIENT

The importance of the patient's statement. The patient's aspect. The patient's sensations. The condition of other organs. The patient's history. The field of cardiac response. The chief complaints: Breathlessness; the sense of exhaustion; pain: a constriction of the chest; a persistent aching. The patient's consciousness of the heart's action. Cerebral symptoms: Dizziness or giddiness; loss of consciousness; Adams-Stokes syndrome; effect of a failing heart on the cerebral functions 43

CHAPTER X

RESPIRATORY SYMPTOMS

Breathlessness, or air-hunger. The sense of suffocation. Inability to stop breathing. Quiet, rapid breathing, free from distress. Continuous laboured breathing. Laboured breathing brought on by exertion. Attacks of breathlessness (cardiac asthma). Cheyne-Stokes respiration. Slow respiration. Pulmonary haemorrhage. Acute suffocative oedema of the lungs 51

CHAPTER XI

REFLEX OR PROTECTIVE PHENOMENA

Classification of symptoms in visceral disease. Insensitiveness of the viscera to ordinary stimuli. The mechanism by which pain and other reflex phenomena are produced in visceral disease (the viscero-sensory reflex). The purpose of visceral reflexes. Why pain is referred to regions remote from the organ . . 57

CHAPTER XII

THE RELATION OF THE HEART TO CEREBRO-SPINAL NERVES

PAGE

The relationship of the heart to sensory nerves. Cutaneous distribution of the cervical and upper dorsal nerves. Herpes zoster and sensory disorders. Areas in which pain and hyperalgesia are felt in affections of the heart. Hyperalgesia in acute dilatation of the heart and liver. Symptoms in the head and neck (vagal reflexes). The pain of angina pectoris as a viscero-sensory reflex. The viscero-motor reflex 63

CHAPTER XIII

SENSORY DISORDERS AS A RESULT OF HEART AFFECTION

Conditions in which angina pectoris is induced. Conditions giving rise to attacks of angina pectoris. Conditions predisposing to an attack. Association of angina pectoris with exhaustion of the muscle of the heart. Cardiac exhaustion and the susceptibility to nerve stimulation. The sensory phenomena produced by over-exertion in healthy hearts. Sensory disturbances in weakened hearts. The significance of sensory disturbances 71

CHAPTER XIV

ANGINA PECTORIS

Mechanism by which the symptoms of angina pectoris are provoked. Conditions inducing an attack. Character and duration of an attack. The symptoms present during an attack of angina pectoris: Pain ; constriction of the chest ; feeling of impending dissolution. The state of the heart and arteries. Symptoms of an attack. Establishment of a tendency to recurrence of the attacks. Prognosis. Treatment: Improvement of the condition of the heart ; treatment during an attack 76

CHAPTER XV

HEART AFFECTIONS AND A HYPER-SENSITIVE NERVOUS SYSTEM

Reaction of visceral disease on the central nervous system. Pseudo-angina pectoris, a useless and misleading term. Exaggerated sensory phenomena with and without valvular disease. Exaggerated sensory phenomena, with pathological changes in the heart. Characteristics of the sensory phenomena. Air suction. Prognosis in cases with exaggerated sensory symptoms. Treatment 87

CHAPTER XVI

VASO-MOTOR SYMPTOMS

The vaso-motor nerves. Origin and distribution. Function of the vaso-motor nerves. Agents influencing the vaso-motor nervous system. The sense of exhaustion and syncope. Vaso-motor angina pectoris. The circulatory symptoms in the X disease. The cause of the X complaint. Treatment 96

CONTENTS

CHAPTER XVII

INSTRUMENTAL METHODS OF EXAMINATION

PAGE

The sphygmograph. The polygraph. The clinical polygraph. The ink polygraph. The electrocardiograph · · · · · · · · · · · · 104

CHAPTER XVIII

THE POSITION AND MOVEMENTS OF THE HEART

The position of the heart. The standards for recognizing the events in a cardiac revolution. Conditions of the chest-wall permitting the recognition of certain movements of the heart. The nature of the movements graphically recorded. The apex beat. Interpretation of a tracing of an apex beat due to the systole of the left ventricle. The auricular wave. Retraction of yielding structures in the neighbourhood of the heart during ventricular systole. Liver movement due to cardiac aspiration. Epigastric pulsation. The apex beat due to the right ventricle. Significance of the inverted cardiogram. Alteration of the apex beat due to retraction of the lung. The shock due to the ventricular systole · · · 112

CHAPTER XIX

EXAMINATION OF THE ARTERIAL PULSE

Superiority of the digital examination. What is the pulse ? Inspection of the arteries. Digital examination of the arteries : The condition of the walls ; the size of the artery ; character of the pulse ; the pulse-rate ; the size of the pulse-wave ; the impact of the pulse-wave on the finger ; the rhythm of the pulse ; the two radial pulses compared. The value of a sphygmogram. Definition of a sphygmogram. Events occurring during a cardiac revolution revealed by the sphygmogram. Features of the sphygmogram due to instrumental defect · · · · · 129

CHAPTER XX

ARTERIAL PRESSURE

The cause of arterial pressure. Methods of measuring the blood-pressure. Increased blood-pressure. Hyperpiesis. Effect on the heart of increased peripheral resistance. Increased arterial pressure and heart failure. Prognosis of high blood-pressure. Treatment of high arterial pressure · · · · · · · 137

CHAPTER XXI

THE VENOUS PULSE

What the venous pulse shows. Inspection of the jugular pulse. Methods of recording the jugular pulse. The recognition of the events in a jugular pulse. Description of the events in a cardiac cycle. The causes of the variation of pressure in the auricle and in the jugular vein. Standards for interpreting a jugular tracing. The carotid wave. The notch on the ventricular wave. The diastolic wave. Changes due to variation in the rate of the heart. Method of analysing a tracing. The ventricular form of the venous pulse. Anomalous forms of the venous pulse. Conditions giving rise to a venous pulse · · · · · · · · · 145

CHAPTER XXII

ENLARGEMENT AND PULSATION OF THE LIVER

PAGE

Reflex or protective symptoms. Signs of enlargement of the liver. Pulsation of the liver. Conditions producing enlargement and pulsation of the liver. Jaundice. Different forms of the liver movement. Differential diagnosis of liver enlargement. Prognosis. Treatment 161

CHAPTER XXIII

INCREASED FREQUENCY OF THE HEART'S ACTION

The normal rate. Classification of cases of increased frequency. Those cases in which the heart is suddenly stimulated to increased rate by mental excitement. Cases which respond to a call upon the heart's energy by increased frequency. Cases in which the heart's rate is continuously increased. Cases in which the increased frequency of the heart occurs in irregular paroxysmal attacks. The cause of increased frequency of the heart's action. Prognosis 168

CHAPTER XXIV

DIMINISHED FREQUENCY OF THE HEART'S ACTION

Definition of the term 'bradycardia'. Normal bradycardia 177

CHAPTER XXV

THE IRREGULAR ACTION OF THE HEART

Significance of irregular action of the heart. Places where the heart's contraction may start. Classification of irregularities: Irregularities arising in the sino-auricular node (sinus irregularities); extra-systoles; the irregularity due to auricular fibrillation; irregularities due to auricular flutter; irregularities due to failure of the conducting power of the auriculo-ventricular bundle; the pulsus alternans 180

CHAPTER XXVI

SINUS IRREGULARITIES (THE YOUTHFUL TYPE OF IRREGULARITY)

Character of the irregularity. Ætiology. Symptoms. Associated symptoms. Diagnostic significance of the youthful type of irregularity. Treatment . . . 183

CHAPTER XXVII

THE EXTRA-SYSTOLE

Definition of the term 'extra-systole'. The character of the irregularity. Recognition of the extra-systole. The different forms of extra-systole. The ventricular extra-systole. The interpolated extra-systole. Simultaneous occurrence of the normal auricular systole and of the ventricular extra-systole. The auricular extra-systole. The extra-systoles arising in the auriculo-ventricular node (nodal extra-systole). Conditions inducing extra-systoles. Sensations produced by extra-systoles. Prognosis in cases with extra-systoles. Treatment 188

CHAPTER XXVIII

SOME RARE FORMS OF CARDIAC IRREGULARITY

PAGE

Sino-auricular block. Blocked auricular extra-systoles. Escaped ventricular beats and nodal beats. Multiple extra-systoles of auricular origin. Multiple extra-systoles of ventricular origin. Causes of multiple extra-systoles. Prognosis . . . 203

CHAPTER XXIX

ABNORMAL RHYTHMS

The cause of abnormal rhythms. Result of onset or offset of an abnormal rhythm. The bearing of abnormal rhythms on the efficiency of the heart and their reaction to stimuli and drugs 209

CHAPTER XXX

AURICULAR FIBRILLATION

The importance of recognizing auricular fibrillation. Type of case showing auricular fibrillation. Personal experiences in the recognition of auricular fibrillation. What is auricular fibrillation ? Conditions inducing auricular fibrillation. Duration of auricular fibrillation. Effect on the ventricles : Rate ; rhythm. The size of the heart. The jugular pulse in auricular fibrillation. Fibrillation waves. The electrocardiogram in auricular fibrillation. Changes in the heart's murmurs. Auricular fibrillation and digitalis. Effect on the heart's efficiency. Causes of heart failure in auricular fibrillation. Clinical characteristics : The patient's history ; the patient's sensations ; character of the pulse. Symptoms of heart failure. Auricular fibrillation and angina pectoris. Prognosis. Treatment : General ; the use of digitalis : method of administration ; danger in the administration of digitalis 211

CHAPTER XXXI

AURICULAR FLUTTER

Definition of the term 'auricular flutter'. Auricular flutter as a common clinical condition. Conditions giving rise to auricular flutter. The symptomatology of auricular flutter. Jugular pulse with auricular flutter. Radial pulse in auricular flutter. Auricular flutter and fibrillation. Auricular flutter and paroxysmal tachycardia. Auricular flutter and digitalis. Prognosis. Treatment . . . 237

CHAPTER XXXII

PAROXYSMAL TACHYCARDIA

Definition. Symptoms. Prognosis. Treatment 251

CHAPTER XXXIII

THE PULSUS ALTERNANS

Different forms of alternation. Conditions producing the pulsus alternans. Cause of the pulsus alternans. Differential diagnosis. Prognosis. Treatment . . 255

CHAPTER XXXIV

AFFECTIONS OF THE CONDUCTING FUNCTIONS OF THE AURICULO-VENTRICULAR
BUNDLE (HEART-BLOCK, ADAMS-STOKES DISEASE, VENTRICULAR RHYTHM)

PAGE

Definition. Methods of recognizing depression of conductivity. The intersystolic
period (*a–c* interval). Depression of conductivity without arrhythmia. Missed
beats due to depression of conductivity. Independent ventricular rhythm due to
heart-block. Effect of the auricular contraction on the radial pulse. Ætiology.
Significance of the milder forms of depression of conductivity. Symptoms
associated with heart-block. Prognosis. Treatment 261

CHAPTER XXXV

ACUTE FEBRILE AFFECTIONS OF THE HEART

Manner in which the heart is affected in fever. The febrile heart. Acute febrile
affections of the heart. Symptoms in myocarditis. Symptoms in endocarditis.
Symptoms in pericarditis. The heart in rheumatic fever. The heart in pneumonia.
The heart in diphtheria. Septic infections. Prognosis. Treatment . . . 277

CHAPTER XXXVI

POISONED HEARTS

Symptoms. Associated symptoms. Prognosis. Treatment 291

CHAPTER XXXVII

AFFECTIONS OF THE MYOCARDIUM

Introduction. Evidences of the impairment of the myocardium. Acute affections
of the myocardium. Subacute affections of the myocardium. Progress of
myocardial disease 295

CHAPTER XXXVIII

AFFECTIONS OF THE MYOCARDIUM (*continued*)
DILATATION OF THE HEART

The cause of dilatation of the heart. The function of tonicity. The symptoms of
depression of tonicity. Evidence of dilatation of the heart. Functional murmurs
and dilatation of the heart. The effects of dilatation of the heart, and how they are
brought about. Dropsy. Dropsy and dilatation of the heart. Enlargement of
the liver. Œdema of the lungs. Urinary symptoms. Prognosis. Treatment . 300

CHAPTER XXXIX

THE SENILE HEART

Introduction. Conditions inducing degenerative changes in the arterial system.
Obliteration of the capillaries. Symptoms. Prognosis. Treatment . . . 313

CHAPTER XL

SOUNDS AND MURMURS, NORMAL AND ABNORMAL

PAGE

Introduction. The attitude of the profession to abnormal sounds. Variations in the sounds of the heart. The cause of functional murmurs. The quantity of blood thrown back to cause a murmur. The differentiation of functional and organic murmurs. The significance of functional murmurs. The significance of organic murmurs 321

CHAPTER XLI

VALVULAR DEFECTS

The manner of heart failure with valvular defects. Mitral stenosis: Conditions inducing heart failure in mitral stenosis; the murmurs present in mitral stenosis; progress and symptoms in mitral stenosis; occasional symptoms. Mitral regurgitation: Murmurs due to mitral regurgitation: conditions inducing heart failure in mitral regurgitation 329

CHAPTER XLII

VALVULAR DEFECTS (continued)

Affections of the tricuspid valves: Tricuspid incompetence; tricuspid stenosis. Disease of the aortic valves: Ætiology; aortic stenosis; aortic regurgitation. Prognosis in valvular affections. Treatment 336

CHAPTER XLIII

ADHESIVE MEDIASTINO-PERICARDITIS

Ætiology. Symptoms. Prognosis. Treatment 343

CHAPTER XLIV

CONGENITAL AFFECTIONS OF THE HEART

Ætiology. Symptoms. Prognosis. Treatment 346

CHAPTER XLV

PROGNOSIS

Responsibility of the medical profession. Basis for prognosis 347

CHAPTER XLVI

TREATMENT

What to treat. Difficulty in estimating the effects of remedies. Principles of treatment. Remedial measures. Rest. Diet. Exercises. Massage. Venesection. Baths. Spa treatment. The Nauheim baths. Cause of the efficacy of the spa treatment 351

CHAPTER XLVII

TREATMENT (*continued*)

PAGE

Drugs. Digitalis. Preparation and method of administration. Strophanthus. Squills. The nitrites. Iodide of potassium. Sedatives. Oxygen. Aconite. Atropine. Other drugs 370

APPENDIX

CASES 386

INDEX 471

DEFINITION OF TERMS

ALTHOUGH I have endeavoured in the text to explain clearly what I mean by any term, yet many terms will be employed before the reader reaches the places where they are explained. For that reason I give here a brief description of the more important terms that have been lately introduced or are not found in current literature, or which I have employed to describe conditions that have not been hitherto recognized.

a–c interval is the time between the beginning of the auricular and carotid waves in tracings of the jugular pulse. (Intersystolic period.)

Arterial degeneration is the term used to cover all forms of arterial disease. As I deal with arterial disease only so far as it embarrasses the work of the heart, I use this to avoid the more specific terms concerning which there is still so much difference of opinion.

Auricular fibrillation. A condition in which the fibres of the auricle, in place of contracting in a systematic and co-ordinate manner, contract independently of one another, with the result that the auricle ceases to be a contracting chamber. The stimulus from the fibrillating auricle produces an irregular action of the ventricle. sometimes with a great increase in rate. Auricular fibrillation may last for varying periods of time, and many cases of paroxysmal tachycardia, with an irregular rhythm, are due to this condition.

Auricular flutter. A term used by MacWilliam to describe the great increase in the rate of auricular contractions, resulting from the application of a weak electrical stimulus to the auricular wall. A similar condition occurs in man as a result of disease, when the auricular contractions, in place of starting at the auriculo-ventricular node (q. v.), start at some other place in the auricular wall. The rate of the auricle may exceed 300 per minute. In the majority of cases the ventricle fails to respond to each auricular beat, and irregularities of a very diverse kind may be found in the arterial pulse. Auricular flutter may last for periods of varying duration, and many cases of paroxysmal tachycardia, with a regular rhythm, are due to this condition.

Auricular venous pulse is the form of jugular pulsation where the wave due to the auricle is found preceding the ventricular contraction in contradistinction to the ventricular venous pulse (q. v.). Sometimes called also the normal or negative venous pulse.

Auriculo-ventricular bundle (a.-v. bundle, Gaskell's bridge, Kent's or His's bundle). The bundle of tissue which passes from the auriculo-ventricular node to the right and left ventricles (Fig. 2 and 3).

Auriculo-ventricular node (a.-v. node, Knoten of Tawara) is the enlargement of the remains of the primitive cardiac tissue found in the wall of the right auricle, from which the auriculo-ventricular bundle arises (Fig. 2).

Cardio-sclerosis. Fibrous changes affecting the endocardium and myocardium are found in the majority of cases in two groups of people, those with a history of an acute febrile affection — most commonly rheumatic fever — and those with evidences of arterial degeneration. The symptoms resulting from both conditions have a great similarity, but there are circumstances, such as age and response to treatment, that sharply separate them; the term cardio-sclerosis, unless qualified, will always refer to the group with arterial degeneration. Fatty changes are frequently present in cardio-sclerosis, but they cannot be distinguished by clinical methods.

Conductivity is the term used by Gaskell to describe that function of the fibres of the heart muscle which conveys the stimulus from fibre to fibre. It is usually studied by observing the time between the systole of the auricles and ventricles.

Contractility is Gaskell's term for the power of contracting possessed by the muscle.

Extra-systole is the premature contraction of the auricle (auricular extra-systole) or of the ventricle (ventricular extra-systole), or both chambers together (nodal extra-systole), while the fundamental or sinus rhythm is maintained. Usually the extra-systole is followed by a long pause (compensatory pause). Rarely the premature contraction occurs between two normal beats (interpolated extra-systole). Two or more premature contractions of the auricle or ventricle may follow one another (multiple extra-systoles).

Heart-block is the term used by Gaskell to signify the stoppage or blocking of the stimulus for contraction in its passage from the auricles to the ventricles.

Hyperalgesia. An abnormal sensitiveness to pain, shown by a painful response to such stimulation as would not normally produce pain, e.g. lightly pressing the skin (cutaneous hyperalgesia) or muscles (muscular hyperalgesia) between the thumb and forefinger.

Myogenic theory. The view that the heart muscle-fibres possess in themselves the power of originating and conveying the stimulus for the contraction of the heart, as opposed to the neurogenic theory, where it is held that the heart acts only in response to nerve stimulation.

Nodal rhythm. A rare action of the heart, in which auricles and ventricles contract simultaneously (Fig. 114). (In the previous editions of this book, the condition called Auricular Fibrillation was described under the term 'nodal rhythm'.)

Palpitation is used in a twofold sense, to describe (a) attacks of increased frequency of the heart's action, (b) the sensation by which a patient is conscious of the excited and usually increased frequent action of the heart.

Paroxysmal tachycardia is applied to a sudden increase in the heart's rate, usually followed by an equally sudden reversion to the normal. It is due to the starting of the heart's contraction at some part other than the normal. (See Auricular Fibrillation and Auricular Flutter.)

Pulsus alternans means that form of abnormal rhythm where the radial pulse is perfectly regular, but where there is an alternation in the size of the beats. It is frequent in tachycardias of auricular origin. When it occurs with the normal rhythm, it indicates profound exhaustion of the heart muscle.

Pulsus bigeminus is applied to that form of pulse irregularity where every second beat is an extra-systole, and is usually smaller than the preceding normal beat. The smaller beat is invariably followed by a pause longer than the pause preceding it.

Sino-auricular node (s.-a. node). The term given by Keith and Flack to a small bundle of tissue representing the remains of the primitive cardiac tube (portion of the sinus venosus) near the mouth of the superior vena cava.

Tonicity is the term applied to that function of the heart muscle which keeps the heart during diastole in a state of slight contraction. Depression of this function results in dilatation of the heart and of the auriculo-ventricular orifices.

Ventricular rhythm. This term is applied to the ventricular contractions in cases of complete heart-block. As this occurs when a lesion severs the auriculo-ventricular bundle, it is assumed that the remaining fibres of the auriculo-ventricular bundle in the ventricles start the ventricular contractions,—the rate being very slow, rarely above thirty-two beats per minute. (In some of my earlier writings I employed this term to describe the condition given under Auricular Fibrillation.)

Ventricular venous pulse is that form of jugular pulsation in which the auricular wave disappears or coincides with the period of ventricular systole, there being no sign of the auricular wave at the normal period of the cardiac cycle. Sometimes called the positive or pathological venous pulse.

Viscero-motor reflex. The term used to describe the contraction of muscles of the external body-wall in response to a stimulation from a diseased viscus.

Viscero-sensory reflex. The sensory symptoms (pain and hyperalgesia) evoked by the stimulation from a diseased viscus of a sensory nerve in its passage from its peripheral distribution in the external body-wall to the brain.

DISEASES OF THE HEART

CHAPTER I

THE APPRECIATION OF AFFECTIONS OF THE HEART

The object of the physician's examination.
Methods adopted in describing affections of the heart.
Causes of confused diagnosis.
The relative importance of symptoms.
The essential symptoms of heart failure.
Inadequacy of the methods usually employed to estimate the heart's efficiency.

The object of the physician's examination.—When a physician examines a patient, his object is to ascertain the nature and significance of certain signs and symptoms. When this investigation is applied to the organs of the circulation, the main purpose of the physician is to determine what bearing such signs or symptoms have on the efficiency of the circulation, whether they foreshadow heart failure or indicate its presence. The essential question in all cases being the ability of the heart to maintain an efficient circulation, it is necessary to comprehend clearly what is meant by heart failure and what evidences are provoked by its presence.

Before this question can be answered satisfactorily, it is necessary first to appreciate the general principles which govern the efficiency of the circulation and how their modification impairs the circulation. When these principles are grasped, the manner in which their infringement produces heart failure will become clear, and we shall be placed in a position to understand the nature and meaning of the symptoms by which we can recognize heart failure. From the knowledge thus acquired, we gain the measure by which we can estimate the clinical significance of any sign, whether or not we understand the mechanism of its production.

Methods adopted in describing affections of the heart. Before entering upon the consideration of heart failure, it is necessary to clear away many misconceptions widely held by physicians as to the significance of many normal and abnormal signs produced by the heart. These misconceptions, handed down from one generation to another, have not only hampered investigation, but have prejudiced the mind as to the nature and significance of many obscure phenomena. These misconceptions have been fostered to a great extent by the attempt of authorities to deal with diseases of the heart by taking each separate lesion and endeavouring to describe the symptoms which arise in consequence of this lesion. But although this method is one that seems at first sight to be both logical and practical, it is impossible in our present state of knowledge. Not only are the lesions imperfectly recognized, but the symptoms of heart failure which we detect are themselves usually not the outcome of the organic lesion, but are often the result of the embarrassment of the heart muscle, induced, it may be, by the lesion. Thus the symptoms of heart failure with valvular disease are usually attributed to the diseased valve, and the nature of the complaint is described as ' mitral disease ' or ' aortic disease ', according to the orifice at which an abnormal sound is produced. As a matter of fact, the heart failure is usually not the outcome of the valve lesion. No doubt in some cases the heart failure may be precipitated by the inability of the heart muscle to overcome the difficulties created by a damaged valve, but it is more frequently brought about by coincident changes in the heart muscle. These changes are sometimes due to a demonstrable lesion of the heart muscle ; at other times they are so subtle that no evidence can be found by our present methods. As heart failure is often due to a modification of the special functions of the heart muscle, and as the functional pathology of the heart is only beginning to be understood, it is not surprising that a large class of symptoms have been either misinterpreted or overlooked. As it is sometimes one function which gives way and sometimes another, we get a great variety of symptoms, corresponding to the exhaustion of different functions. But these functions may become exhausted, with and without gross lesions of the muscle or valves, and as a consequence similar symptoms may be induced not only by organic lesions of great variety and extent, but may be present with no perceptible lesion of the heart. Acute affections of the heart, for instance, are often described as ' endocarditis ' or ' pericarditis ', because there happens to be a murmur or a pericardial friction sound. But in addition to these sounds there may be present a great number of symptoms, such as inefficiency of the heart muscle, dilatation of the heart, irregular action of the heart, and so forth, and these are given as being the symptoms of the endocarditis or the pericarditis, while as a matter of fact these symptoms are not the outcome of the endocarditis or the pericarditis, but of a myocardial affection. This myocardial affection may be the outcome of a microbic invasion of the heart muscle which can be detected post-mortem, or it may be due to a poisoning, depressing the functions of the heart muscle, and baffling the attempt to detect it post-mortem. Hitherto, the attempt to give a precise description of the symptoms pertaining to each organic lesion has led writers to ascribe phenomena to lesions with which they have no connexion, and this accounts for the confused and contradictory symptomatology of heart affections at the present time.

Causes of confused diagnosis.—In searching for a reason for this confusion, I am inclined to attribute it to the fact that the human mind attaches the greatest importance to that class of phenomena which most strongly affects the senses. Many of the really vital and all-important symptoms are so subtle and so slight that the most careful methods are required for their detection, whereas a roaring murmur or an irregular pulse thrusts itself upon our attention. The result is that the subtle signs are ignored and too much stress laid upon the murmur or the irregularity. Murmurs and irregularities have, therefore, come to occupy a place in the cardiac symptomatology which is not in accordance with their true significance. If any one will seriously search in literature for the origin of the present-day conception of such obvious phenomena, he will find that this conception arose when the nature of the phenomena was not understood, and opinions were formed of their significance before any one attempted to follow the life-history of individuals presenting them. Generation after generation has been content to adopt the traditions without taking the trouble to investigate their truth.

The relative importance of symptoms.—These considerations have led me to adopt a method of description which seeks to place symptoms in a proper perspective. By recognizing the fact that the first consideration of the physician is the possibility of heart failure, and that the attention of the physician or the patient is drawn to the heart by the appearance of one or more symptoms, and that it is only by the recognition of the symptoms that the disease can be inferred, each symptom is defined and differentiated as clearly as our present knowledge permits, both in regard to the mechanism by which it is produced and its relation to the efficiency of the heart's power. Then the various pathological conditions with which it may be associated are described. After clearly differentiating the various phenomena, their bearing on the heart's efficiency has to be determined. For this purpose associated symptoms must be sought for. Certain individuals may show apparently identical phenomena, as a murmur or an irregularity ; some of these may drift and die, others may lead strenuous lives and show no sign of heart failure. The recognition of the difference in these individuals cannot be determined by the presence of one abnormal sign, but by the presence or absence of associated symptoms. The significance of any given symptom can only be appreciated by the careful watching of individuals through many years. By such methods alone can it be hoped to get an opinion based on trustworthy grounds.

The essential symptoms of heart failure.—While it is necessary in every case to recognize the evidence afforded by a careful physical examination, supplemented when necessary by the use of mechanical aids, it must be borne in mind that the facts when revealed do not give the information which is essential to the physician. I have said that the essential question for the physician to decide is whether the symptoms indicate the presence of heart failure or the likelihood of its occurrence. A satisfactory answer to this question can only be obtained by appreciating how the heart comports itself in doing its work. This knowledge can only be acquired by understanding what happens when the individual is engaged in some occupation that calls for some effort on the part of the heart. Hence all means of observation employed when the body is at rest can only yield very incomplete evidence. The kind of evidence which is essential in both acute and chronic affections of the heart is to be sought for in the symptoms evoked when effort is made, frequently only evoked then, as well as in symptoms of functional inefficiency when the body is at rest. These symptoms are often so elusive and so insignificant that they readily escape attention, while it is often difficult to appraise their value when detected. As our knowledge of what is meant by heart failure increases, the real significance of such symptoms will be revealed.

Inadequacy of the methods usually employed to estimate the heart's efficiency.—As the bearing of any sign or symptom on the heart's efficiency is the essential question, there have been many attempts to find some method which could estimate the integrity of the heart. Attempts have been made by counting the heart-beats after a short period of exertion, more or less violent, a method which is of little use except in rare cases, and is full of fallacies and liable to mislead. Instrumental methods appeal so strongly to the imagination that we have attempted methods of valuation which are based entirely on a misconception of what it is they should reveal. We have elaborate blood-pressure instruments, supposed to show the co-efficiency of the heart's strength in the terms of a mathematical formula. We have graphic records and even the electrocardiograph. I am the last to decry the use of these methods, for they all have a very important sphere of usefulness, but I have little hesitation in saying that, as a means of estimating the heart's integrity and capacity, and elucidating the significance of symptoms, they can only supply very limited information.

CHAPTER II

THE PATHOLOGY OF HEART FAILURE

What is heart failure ?
The back-pressure theory of heart failure.
Compensation.
The origin of these views.
Evil done by the back-pressure theory.
Heart failure and pathological changes.
Functional impairment of the heart.
The evidences of impaired function.

What is heart failure?—Seeing that the essential question in all cases is whether heart failure is present or likely to arise, it is necessary to grasp fully the meaning of heart failure. Heart failure may be defined as the condition in which the heart is unable to maintain an efficient circulation when called upon to meet the efforts necessary to the daily life of the individual. This definition is purposely made wide to embrace cases of advanced failure, and those in which there is but slight evidence of inefficiency when an extreme effort is made. It is needful to insist upon this, as the absence of a clear conception of what constitutes heart failure has led to the neglect of some of the really essential symptoms which indicate its presence, and to the magnifying of the importance of certain obvious signs (as murmurs and irregularities) which often have no relation to or bearing on heart failure.

The back-pressure theory of heart failure.—When we consider what are the pathological conditions which induce heart failure, we are at once faced with a subject of great complexity which our present knowledge fails to explain fully. Hitherto the view most commonly held has been that the heart failure results from the inability of the left ventricle to throw sufficient blood into the arterial system, with the result that the ventricle dilates and sends a regurgitant stream back into the auricle. This traditional view is set out with great detail in a recent book, and as it represents the opinion universally held by the medical profession, I give a brief *résumé* of the view. The author, wishing to show the steps by which heart failure arises, selects for illustration a case of pure incompetence of the aortic valves. On account of the regurgitation, the left ventricle increases in size during diastole. An increase in rate is a favourable sign, as it shortens the diastole. After a time there is hypertrophy as well as dilatation of the left ventricle. The next step is the stasis and increase in pressure in the left auricle, and after this there is an embarrassment of the pulmonary circulation and the right ventricle. The lung is then injured (œdematous, infarcts, tendency to bronchitis, hæmorrhage), and the patient becomes cyanotic and dyspnœic. With this there sets in an irregular action of the heart, a disturbance of the muscular mechanism, and the patient becomes like one with mitral disease. Finally, the distress of the right heart becomes so great that tricuspid incompetence takes place, and the last and extreme stage of heart failure sets in with distension of the venous system.

Compensation.—Arising out of this conception of heart failure from backward pressure is the idea that the prevention of heart failure in cases of valvular disease is due to the muscle of the heart hypertrophying and becoming stronger to meet the embarrassment caused by the valve defect in its work. Hence when the valve defects are detected and there is no sign of heart failure, we are told that 'compensation is good', and when heart failure sets in, 'compensation has given way' or 'decompensation' has set in. If the patient recovers, 'compensation is restored.'

Unfortunately writers never give sufficient detail to convey a clear idea of what they have in view when they speak of compensation. In practice it will be found that authorities take up a curious position. We shall find people with perfectly normal and efficient hearts, in whom a systolic murmur may be detected, spoken of as having mitral regurgitation with good compensation. The same language is used where there is some valvular disease, as in aortic disease, in the absence of engorgement of the lung or dropsy or the so-called signs of backward pressure. Even in cases where the exhaustion may be so extreme that death impends from heart failure, the heart is spoken of as having good compensation, because none of the 'back-pressure' symptoms are present.

The origin of these views.—These views are the outcome of the discovery of auscultation. Shortly after its discovery, before the meaning of the heart sounds, normal and abnormal, had been understood, bruits were found associated with extreme heart failure. This association was at once assumed to be of vital significance, and in later years, when a better knowledge of these murmurs permitted the recognition of their causation as being due to defects of certain orifices, their importance as the origin of heart failure was supposed to be established, and gradually the back-pressure theory was evolved to explain heart failure. It may be remarked that this back-pressure view did not arise from careful observation of individual cases passing through the different stages, but from attempts to describe the progress of the failure by reasoning backwards from the evidence present in advanced conditions. That is to say, cases with histories of damaged valves have been found with all the evidences of heart failure, and with the changes in the heart and lungs. The physician has then filled in the gaps of the history by assuming that the events happened as required by the theory. The reason I say this is because no one has ever described the stages as they occur from actual observation, and because, when I have watched the progress of heart failure, other circumstances, such as the sudden inception of a new rhythm, have arisen which were not suspected to exist, while in the great number of cases of grave heart failure so-called signs of back pressure are entirely absent. There is no doubt that certain facts seem to conform with this view. In aortic regurgitation we get an enlarged left ventricle, and in mitral stenosis we find pulmonary stasis and hypertrophy of the right ventricle.

Evil done by back-pressure theory.—The combating of this theory might be considered unnecessary and superfluous were it not for the fact of the grievous mischief it has done to individual patients, and the hampering effect it has had upon the advance of medical science. It is questionable whether the discovery of auscultation so far has done more harm than good. Human nature is so constituted that the evil is usually associated with what is mysterious. This particularly applies to noises and sounds whose cause is unknown. The modification of the sounds which are perfectly consistent with a healthy heart has never been thoroughly understood, and in consequence a false standard has been set up of what is normal and what is pathological. As a result we find a great many perfectly healthy people looked upon as diseased, and treated as suffering from a serious complaint, and their future life restricted, because of the presence of some sign, as a murmur or an irregularity, which owing to an imperfect knowledge of the real nature of the sign, and a confused conception of what constituted heart failure, had misled the physician in estimating its significance.

Heart failure and pathological changes.—It is practically a hopeless matter in the present state of our knowledge to correlate the various forms of heart failure with gross changes found post-mortem, either with the naked eye or the microscope. We can recognize, during life, many signs provoked by organic changes in the heart, such as the murmurs peculiar to disease at the various orifices, and different forms of irregular action, such as those induced by damage done to the auriculo-ventricular bundle, and those due to a damaged auricle starting an abnormal rhythm, but these are not signs of heart failure. The symptoms provoked by a failing heart are so varied in character that we do not yet fully understand the mechanism by which they are produced, nor the laws which govern their production. Even when we get a series of well-defined symptoms, such as those shown by orthopnœa, dyspnœa, dropsy, enlargement of the liver, or those shown by attacks of angina pectoris, we shall find the pathological changes in the heart so varied that it is impossible to attribute the symptoms with assurance to any given pathological condition. This becomes all the more impressive when we find fatal heart failure associated with no perceptible lesions of the structures of the heart sufficient to account for the heart failure. No doubt a pathological process may play a considerable part in impairing the functional efficiency of the heart, but the fact that the heart may fail to do its work when there is abundance of seemingly healthy muscle present forces us to the conclusion that the heart failure is really the outcome of the impairment of the functions of the heart muscle itself, while the seemingly healthy muscle is the seat of changes too subtle for our present methods to detect.

Functional impairment of the heart.—The view that functional impairment is the essential cause of heart failure, gives a direction to the lines on which heart failure needs to be studied. Hitherto the presence of some organic lesion, as a damaged valve or a sclerosed coronary artery, has been looked upon as the cause of heart failure, and the physician has been content with the finding of such gross changes. But if we would understand the action of any organ, we must not look merely to its post-mortem appearances, but seek for the modified functions that occur during life. There is naturally a disposition to seek to correlate the symptoms during life with lesions found post-mortem, but a due regard must be given to the mechanism by which the symptoms are produced. Thus a diseased coronary artery or aorta is found in individuals who suffered during life from angina pectoris. One attributes the angina pectoris to the coronary artery and another to the aortic disease, not realizing that neither the coronary artery nor the aorta is the actual agent provoking the heart failure, of which the anginal symptom is but an expression. In like manner, dyspnœa and dropsy are not the outcome of the diseased valve found post-mortem or recognized during life. Practically every one who has systematically studied this subject recognizes that the symptoms of heart failure during life may be identical with a great variety of organic lesions. From this we can but conclude that the symptoms cannot be the direct outcome of the lesion, and that some condition common to all must be the cause of the symptoms. As the common cause can only be an interference with the function of the heart muscle, it behoves us to study these functions with greater care if we would seek to understand the pathology of heart failure.

The evidences of impaired function.—Perhaps no organ of the body gives better evidence of its functional integrity and impairment than the heart. It exhibits its evidences in so many ways, directly by its own action, and indirectly by influencing the functions of organs and tissues remote from it. It is necessary, however, to understand what are the evidences of impairment, and what are the signs exhibited by a normal healthy heart. A murmur may be the outcome of a disease process or of a functional impairment, yet it may be an expression of a perfectly normal heart. An irregular heart may be evidence of a profound and fatal exhaustion, of an impaired organ, or it may be a perfectly normal sign. In like manner, breathlessness may be a sign of great gravity, of an impaired organ, or it may occur with a normal heart. That is to say, if we deal with such phenomena in a loose and general way we fail to appreciate their significance. If, however, we study more closely their mechanism we shall find that murmurs, irregularities, and breathlessness are capable of being separated into very distinct and definite groups, and this differentiation enables us to ascertain their true significance. Of late years enormous advance has taken place in the detection of the phenomena exhibited by the action of the heart muscle. Abnormal signs (as modified sounds, abnormal rhythms, changes in size and shape) may result from a limited lesion or a depressed function of some part of the heart muscle, and then their analysis and the recognition of other symptoms associated with them may throw a flood of light upon the nature of the disease process and of the functions of the heart muscle. Abnormal rhythms are of importance as they give a clue to the nature of the changes going on in the heart muscle which may induce heart failure. Apart from these direct evidences of the interferences with the function of the heart, there are the great groups of subjective signs which are essential to the recognition of the very earliest signs of impairment of the heart's efficiency, and their careful appreciation gives us the knowledge of the degree of impairment, and provides the clue for obtaining the necessary information.

CHAPTER III

THE PRINCIPLES UNDERLYING THE PRODUCTION OF HEART FAILURE

The purpose of the circulation and how it is attained.
The importance of the heart muscle.
The meaning of heart failure.
The two forces of the heart muscle.
The reserve force of the heart muscle.
How heart failure begins.
The relation between exhaustion and restoration of the reserve force of the heart.
Conditions exhausting the reserve force.

The purpose of the circulation and how it is attained.—The purpose of the circulation is the supply of a constant stream of material capable of nourishing the tissues, and the removal of such waste products as are capable of entering the circulatory channels. In order to facilitate the exchange of products between the blood and the tissues, a certain degree of slowing of the flow takes place as the blood passes through the capillaries. As a continuous pressure is required to force the blood onwards, the intermittent pressure conveyed to the blood-stream by the heart is converted by the resiliency of the arterial walls into a constant pressure at the periphery of the arterial system. The maintenance of the arterial pressure is the outcome of the force exerted by the ventricles and of the resistance of the smaller arteries and capillaries. The full force of the ventricular contraction is not spent on the blood-current merely during the period of systole. In throwing the blood into the arterial system, it does so with such force that it distends to a slight extent the larger arteries. The elastic coats of the arteries, as soon as the ventricular systole is over, compress the column of blood within them, and in this manner maintain a degree of arterial pressure during the period that the ventricle is not acting. The ventricular force is thus stored up by the distension of the elastic coats of the arteries, and liberated during the ventricular diastole.

The importance of the heart muscle.—The heart muscle supplies the force which maintains the circulation. In the normal condition, the various parts of the mechanism of the circulation are so adjusted that all parts combine to facilitate the work of the heart and to attain the object of the circulation. Any disturbance of that adjustment must at once entail more work upon the heart muscle, inasmuch as a departure from the normal means the embarrassment of the heart in maintaining its capacity to meet the requirements of the body. So long as the heart can overcome the impediment, and maintain the circulation in a normal manner, no symptoms are evoked, but if the heart is no longer able to carry on the circulation efficiently, then certain phenomena at once arise, and these phenomena we call ' symptoms of heart failure '.

The meaning of heart failure.—From this consideration it will be realized that heart failure is simply inability of the heart muscle to maintain the circulation, and that this failure of the heart muscle is due to too great a strain being put upon it. This may arise from overwork when the circulatory organs are healthy, or by a disturbance of the normal adjustment of the various factors concerned in the circulation. This disturbance may arise in a great many ways, but the final result is the same, that is to say, embarrassment of the heart muscle and its final exhaustion. The heart muscle, therefore, is of such prime importance in what we call heart failure that a close and intimate study of its properties is essential. This will be dealt with later on in some detail ; here I want to insist upon features of the heart muscle which are essential in the consideration of every form of heart failure, namely, the nature of the forces by which the heart maintains an efficient circulation.

The two forces of the heart muscle.—As the heart possesses the power, not only of maintaining an efficient circulation when the body is at rest, but of varying its activity according to the bodily requirements, the force inherent in the heart muscle may be considered, for practical purposes, to be composed of two parts, that is to say, a part which is employed to maintain an efficient circulation when the body is at rest, and which therefore may be called the ' rest force ', and a part which is called into action when effort is made, and which might be termed the ' reserve force '. The rest force is the minimal force which the heart can exert to maintain the circulation at a level consistent with life. The impairment of this rest force produces those evidences of heart failure which persist when the body is at rest, such as dropsy, dyspnœa, and the continuance of such impairment eventually leads to a fatal issue.

The reserve force of the heart muscle.—The second part of the heart's force is that which is called upon when the body makes some effort. While the body is at rest this potential force is not exercised, but its possession enables us to undertake with ease all forms of effort. Inasmuch as this part of the heart's force is only used when exertion is made, it may appropriately be called the ' reserve force ' of the heart. Although we recognize what the reserve force is, it is not very easy to define it in words. Physiologists do not seem to have given it that study which its importance demands. Although difficult to define, its existence is proved in every movement of the body, and in every effort which is made, as it is by the possession of this faculty that we are able with ease to undertake all forms of effort.

The functional efficiency of the heart depends on the amount of this reserve force, and it is by estimating the amount of this reserve force that we recognize the presence and degree of heart failure, and the bearing of any sign or symptom on the heart's efficiency, which is the essential matter in the study of all forms of affections of the heart.

How heart failure begins.—If we bear in mind the division that I have given of the heart's power, it will be found that heart failure invariably starts, in the first instance, by exhaustion of the reserve force. The exhaustion is slight at first, but by the persistence of the causal factors it proceeds apace, until after a period, long or short, this exhaustion induces such distress as to compel attention, or the rest force is encroached upon, and with the exhaustion of the rest force a point of danger to the life of the individual is reached.

The relation between exhaustion and restoration of the reserve force of the heart.—From this conception of the exhaustion of the heart's strength, we can perceive the manner in which heart failure arises. The daily routine of a man accustomed to bodily labour shows a period of rest and a period of work, the one balancing the other, the period of exhaustion of the reserve force requiring a sufficient period of repose for its restoration. The life of man is so marked out that each day's work is roughly estimated by what a healthy man can do. If an individual has to do the work of a healthy man, but is hampered by some inherent defect, his reserve force is more speedily exhausted, and he requires a longer period of recuperation. If this is not obtained, then, in course of time, exhaustion increases and the period of rest becomes insufficient and heart failure sets in. In the first instance, then, heart failure is no more than the inability of the heart to regain sufficient reserve force during its period of rest. The rate at which heart failure progresses depends upon the unequal relation between the bodily exertion and the amount of rest. The agents embarrassing the heart in its work need not necessarily be cardiac in origin ; it may be the blood-vessels that are at fault, or diseases of other systems. When it is a heart lesion which embarrasses the heart in its work, the failure should not necessarily be considered as due to the heart lesion, but due to the individual's attempt to do the work of a healthy man, handicapped by his defect. In the recognition of these facts we get the clue, not only to the cause of the heart failure, but also a reasonable suggestion as to its rational therapy.

Conditions exhausting the reserve force.—I have already remarked that, in the normal condition, the adjustment of all parts concerned in carrying on the circulation is essential to efficiency. Any disturbance of the adjustment at once calls for an increased effort on the part of the heart muscle. Such calls are made first on the reserve force, and, if persisted in, lead sooner or later to its exhaustion. The causes are extraordinarily varied in character, and may arise from a disturbance of the factors on which the normal circulation depends. It is from this standpoint that diseases of the heart should be considered, inasmuch as it is only by looking at the matter in this light that a proper perspective is obtained in regard to the significance of any abnormality. Thus, irregular action of the heart will be described from the point of view of its effect upon the efficient performance of the heart, as well as the condition producing it. Valvular defects will be studied, not as a specific affection to be considered in themselves, but rather as a source of embarrassment to the heart muscle in its work, or as indicating the presence of a lesion that may have extended to the muscular wall. In the same manner, arterial degeneration and high blood-pressure will be considered as conditions which upset the normal adjustment of the factors which carry on the circulation. Inherent defects of the muscular wall itself will also be viewed in their bearing on the heart's efficiency. The relative efficiency of independent functions of the muscle-fibres will be kept constantly in view, inasmuch as organic lesions act deleteriously through disturbing the normal harmony of these functions. Depressions of the individual functions may arise without any gross organic lesions, and lead to serious embarrassment of the circulation. While I am far from comprehending the full effect of functional depression, for the study of functional pathology is in its infancy, yet I hope the facts I detail may help forward a line of observation which promises much for future investigation.

CHAPTER IV

EXHAUSTION OF THE HEART MUSCLE

Importance of the exhaustion of the reserve force.
Effect of exhaustion in the individual beat of the heart.
Exhaustion and restoration of the reserve force.
Estimation of the amount of reserve force.
Evidences of exhaustion.
Practical value of estimating the cardiac condition by the degrees of exhaustion.
The restoration of the exhausted heart.

Importance of the exhaustion of the reserve force.—The view that heart failure first sets in by exhaustion of the reserve force of the heart muscle is so reasonable that it needs but to be stated to be accepted. But though widely accepted, it is rarely employed in a systematic manner for estimating the degree of heart failure or for determining the actual damage of the heart. For these purposes, the condition of the reserve force is the only reliable standard by which we can estimate the significance of any sign or symptom, or gain an idea to what extent any given lesion has affected the functional efficiency of the heart. The due appreciation of what is meant by exhaustion gives us, then, not only a true conception of what heart failure is, but supplies us with the only principles on which a reliable opinion can be based. Seeing the importance of exhaustion and its applicability to every case of heart affection, even when we are unable to explain the nature of the changes which weaken the heart, it is necessary to consider very fully the functions of the heart muscle in their relation to the exhaustion and restoration of the reserve force.

Effect of exhaustion in the individual beat of the heart.—The effect of exhaustion can be studied in two ways : firstly, in the individual contraction of the heart, and secondly, in the reserve force of the heart. From the researches into the functions of the heart muscle (see p. 30), it is found that after the exercise of any given function, it is necessary for its efficient performance that a sufficient rest should follow before it is again exercised. When the function of contraction is exercised, the muscle contracts with all the energy it possesses at the time. After such a contraction the exhaustion is so complete that the muscle, for the time being, is incapable of further contraction until an interval elapses, during which the power of contraction is gradually restored. The reason for this is that the expenditure of energy represented by the contraction has utilized the specific material which was stored up in the muscle-cells. Before another contraction can take place, the material has to be renewed, and this requires not only time but also a supply of suitable material. If the muscle be made to contract before the restoration is complete, the resultant contraction is feebler and less efficient. It is necessary, then, that for the full efficiency of a beat, a period of repose and a sufficient supply of nutriment should precede a contraction.

The various functions of the heart muscle are normally so co-ordinated that the periods of contraction occur at such times when all the functions are equally and efficiently restored. In disease, certain of these functions may be injuriously affected, so that the harmony of their action is interfered with. When this happens, an irregularity or inequality in the beats of the heart is produced.

Exhaustion and restoration of the reserve force.—While it is essential for the efficiency of the individual contraction of the heart that a period of sufficient rest should follow each contraction, it is also essential for the efficiency of the reserve force that a period of rest should follow its exercise. If these periods of rest are insufficient, then, inevitably, exhaustion sets in. This results whether the heart is healthy or affected by some lesion. In the former case it may take a long time before the exhaustion is perceived, but the evidence will none the less surely arise. When there is an affection of the heart which impairs its functional efficiency, or embarrasses the heart in its work (as valvular and arterial disease), exhaustion is the more speedily induced. Individuals with hearts encumbered usually attempt to lead lives similar to those led by healthy persons, so that their hearts are forced to do the work of healthy hearts. The heart being hampered by a defect, a greater burden is thrown upon the heart muscle, and longer periods of rest are necessary for the restoration of the spent reserve force. Such people, in their attempt to keep up with their fellows, do not get a sufficient period of rest, with the result that heart failure supervenes.

Estimation of the amount of reserve force.—I have endeavoured to find some standard by which the amount of reserve force and its exhaustion could be expressed in terms of precision. I have, however, failed to find any definite standard, and when one reflects it will be realized that it is not possible that a measure of such definite precision, as to be applicable to all cases, should be attainable. Seeing that the ability to undertake effort is due to the possession of a reserve force, we recognize that in healthy people, the amount of reserve force is subject to great variations. In trained athletes there are some capable of much greater endurance than others, and the terms short-winded and long-winded imply really different amounts of reserve force. The term 'training' used in athletics implies amongst other things the acquisition of an increased amount of reserve force. This is due to the power possessed by the heart of increasing the efficiency of its functions by their systematic and judicious exercise. Conversely, the neglect to exercise the reserve force leads to a diminution of its amount, as witnessed in the speedy exhaustion of healthy people who lead sedentary lives. This latter fact is of importance when the amount of reserve force is limited in people who may present some abnormal cardiac condition. In such people the limitation of the field of cardiac response may be due to the lack of exercise of the reserve force.

The standard, therefore, by which we can estimate the amount of the reserve force is in the main personal, each individual unconsciously acquiring the knowledge of what he can do. So long as he exercises the heart within the limits of his powers, no symptoms arise, but as soon as the reserve force is exhausted, and the effort is persisted in, distress and discomfort are experienced. Thus it will be seen that the evidence of exhaustion is common to sound and impaired hearts, varying only in the ease with which it is provoked.

Evidences of exhaustion.—Evidences of exhaustion are of two kinds, those due to the organ itself, and those due to other organs on account of the inefficient circulation. Organs that are capable of being stimulated to exertion by the will are apt to be exhausted by the calls made upon them. So long as such calls do not induce exhaustion, the organs respond with little consciousness of effort, but when forced to work beyond their normal capacity, or when exhaustion sets in, then the individual becomes conscious of distress and discomfort, which may at first be slight, but ultimately may become so severe as to call imperatively for a cessation of the cause of distress. The means by which this distress arises is due to a mechanism with which all such muscular organs are provided, and which is protective in its purpose. While the symptoms evoked by this protective mechanism, as regards the heart, will be dealt with later in detail, here it is only necessary to point out that symptoms that arise in this way, and those that are due to an inefficient blood-supply to other organs, are in the early stages of exhaustion entirely subjective. Being subjective, it is not easy to appreciate them, as individual peculiarities so frequently modify their character, while a description of their nature is dependent entirely upon the sufferer, for each one embodies in his description qualities peculiar to himself. When the exhaustion becomes more advanced, objective evidences of heart failure, such as dropsy, enlargement of the liver, may appear; but it is to be borne in mind that exhaustion has gone far before these signs become perceptible, and that extreme and grave exhaustion may occur without such objective evidences.

Practical value of estimating the cardiac condition by the degrees of exhaustion.—So far it will be seen that the physician has to consider in every case the efficiency of the heart, and this can only be done by testing its functional capacity, and the functional capacity can only be appreciated by understanding how the heart responds to effort. Here we get the only method of estimating the significance of any abnormal sign. When we come to deal with the cases which show signs of organic disease, however instructive these signs may be, their significance cannot be estimated until their bearing on the functional capacity of the heart is appreciated. When this is done, we have some reasonable grounds for basing an intelligent prognosis.

Recognizing that heart failure depends on exhaustion of the heart muscle, and that the value of any abnormal cardiac sign depends on whether it is an evidence of a condition that predisposes to exhaustion, we are able to appreciate the extent of the damage done to the heart and to base a treatment on sound and scientific principles. The view that exhaustion is the cause of heart failure, and it is the exhaustion we have to treat, seems so simple that it scarce needs to be remarked. Yet this essential and self-evident aspect is so frequently overlooked and ignored that I consider it necessary to insist on its importance, and later I will demonstrate how it helps us in the treatment of our patients.

The restoration of the exhausted heart.—If we grasp the significance of exhaustion, we can appreciate the dangers associated with it and the manner in which these dangers can be avoided, so that an individual with a heart lesion may be enabled to lead a life free from suffering. The perception of the conditions which lead to exhaustion, also leads us to realize how exhaustion is recovered from. As the heart failure has been induced by the periods of rest being too short to restore the reserve force, so the recovery from heart failure takes place when the heart is placed under circumstances which call for less effort than the enfeebled heart is capable of undertaking. Under such circumstances the progressive failure is stayed, and imperceptibly the heart gathers strength by accumulating more and more power, and, with the return of the reserve force, the symptoms of heart failure disappear. The recognition of these facts is of the first importance in connexion with both the subject of recovery from heart failure and the principles on which a scientific therapy can be based. The practical application of this view and its great importance will be demonstrated when the subject of treatment is discussed (Chap. XLVI).

CHAPTER V

DETERMINATION OF THE VALUE OF SYMPTOMS

The necessity for appreciating the meaning of symptoms.
How the significance of symptoms is acquired.
Discrimination of the significance of symptoms.
Signs of exhaustion of the reserve force.

The necessity for appreciating the meaning of symptoms.—The idea put forth here that heart failure results from exhaustion of the heart muscle is so evident that it might not be considered necessary to dwell upon it at much length. Seeing, however, that the recognition of the degree of exhaustion is of the first importance in every instance, this aspect of the subject cannot be too strongly insisted upon nor too carefully investigated.

It is one of the curious matters in medicine that the commonplace and self-evident are the things which are the most frequently ignored. I am repeatedly told by experienced physicians that the views here expressed are ' common knowledge ', and that every one knows all about them. But if justification were needed for insisting upon this line of observation, we have but to observe how the profession employs this ' common knowledge '. One has but to turn to the writings of authorities and ask how an abnormal sign, such as a murmur or an irregular action of the heart, should be estimated, to find that the matter is never dealt with in such a manner as to bring out its bearing on the heart's efficiency. I have before me the certificates of a number of insurance companies, to be filled in by the medical examiners. In none of them is there any inquiry to bring out this essential information. In one form an inquiry is made as to the presence of an abnormal sign. If an abnormal sign, such as an irregularity or a murmur, is present, another special certificate has to be filled in, in which there are no fewer than fifteen questions asked, not one of which has reference to this essential matter of the exhaustion of the heart muscle. I have come across several cases where lives have been insured for large sums and death has ensued within a few months of the medical examination for life insurance. The lives had been passed as good because they revealed no objective symptoms, whereas an inquiry into the functional efficiency of the organ would have revealed symptoms which would have indicated a grave state of exhaustion of the heart. On the other hand, I am continually seeing people who are rejected for life insurance, or for entrance into the services, who exhibit some simple sign, indicative neither of heart disease nor heart failure, and which the medical examiner has totally misinterpreted and for which he has rejected the candidate.

In like manner, individuals with some supposed abnormal sign are frequently subjected to courses of treatment, which would have been recognized as unnecessary had the essential question of the bearing of the sign on the heart's efficiency been appreciated. These futile attempts at treatment were not the acts of inexperienced practitioners, but were prescribed by the highest authorities, such as teachers in large schools. This being so, it will be understood how the students from such schools pass into the world with wrong ideas as to the nature of many phenomena.

How the significance of symptoms is acquired.—The chief reason for this lack of appreciation of the essential matter in cardiac symptomatology is that symptoms have not been investigated in such a way as to bring out their real nature. The knowledge of the significance of symptoms can only be acquired after patiently observing individuals exhibiting them for long periods of years, and noticing how they meet the exigencies of life. Hitherto teachers and others who have influenced the profession in such matters, have not had the opportunity of watching a sufficient number of individuals to find out for themselves the meaning of many cardiac signs, and have been content to fall back on the surmises of their predecessors. In this way the significance of many phenomena is based upon tradition, the tradition arising at a time when its exponents were profoundly ignorant of the nature of the symptoms. For that reason the significance of cardiac phenomena has been described from such imperfect data that the conception of the meaning of many phenomena is little more than guesswork.

In order to determine the value of any given symptom in affections of the heart, a long and patient inquiry is needed. To begin with, a thorough knowledge of the symptom itself as it presents itself to us, and its differentiation from others which it may resemble, whether it is a murmur, an irregularity, or an objective sensation, must be acquired. Then all attendant circumstances, as the presence of other evidence of the heart's condition, and particularly the state of the heart's efficiency, as shown by the response to effort, must be carefully noted, as well as the presence of affections of other organs and the history of past illnesses, the environment of the individual, and the nature of his work. After this, patient observations must be made at various periods of the individual's life, and advantage taken of untoward circumstances, as periods of hard bodily labour, pregnancy, and parturition, and such illnesses as typhoid, pneumonia, or influenza.

It is evident that such observations can only be undertaken by a physician who is likely to see individual patients during all these circumstances, and that can only be done by the general practitioner. Such a line of observation

I have attempted, and I warn those who would follow this line of research that it is no primrose path. The investigators in hospital wards and laboratories have little idea of the difficulties the general practitioner has to encounter. He must ever be on the alert, prepared to make an observation at any hour of the day or night, and may have to spend many hours in a wretched hovel watching the changes in a woman during labour. Attacks of illness, which may arise suddenly during day and night, must find him prepared to take advantage of his opportunities. The little I have been able to do in this respect, has but opened my eyes to the extraordinarily rich field for investigation that lies before the general practitioner.

Though I have been able to find the significance of some phenomena, there are many others of whose significance I have yet only a dim perception. It was necessary to recognize and to distinguish the peculiar features of many phenomena, before it was possible to watch individuals possessing them. This of itself has taken many years, so that one has to be content to describe some of these phenomena, leaving it to others to watch the individual cases and find out the bearing of these phenomena on the patient's future.

In order to obtain a method by which may be shown the bearing of signs, normal and abnormal, on the individual's future, I gradually evolved the plan here described. This method, though at first sight so simple and self-evident, is, when thoroughly understood, not difficult to apply, but the power of using it can only come after a long personal investigation into a large number of cases. Although I may be able to communicate a certain amount of my experience, yet the reader, if he seeks to understand what heart failure is, will have himself to search and wait, for I am quite conscious that my knowledge is extremely limited. Notwithstanding my limitations, I have tested the method sufficiently to know that this line of inquiry is the one which will ultimately yield the most satisfactory results.

Discrimination of the significance of symptoms.—One of the most difficult subjects is to appreciate the full meaning of any symptom. A great help to this end will be found if the principle is adhered to that an opinion should never be based on the presence of one sign alone, however abnormal the physician may deem it. The search for other signs should be carefully undertaken, and it may be put down as an axiom, that any sign which is indicative of heart failure, is always accompanied by other symptoms. The converse is equally true, that any sign, unaccompanied by abnormal phenomena, may be taken to be of little or no significance, so far as the functional efficiency of the heart is concerned.

The accompanying signs may be revealed by careful physical examination, but the most important are those revealed by the patient's sensations. In fact, the latter class of symptoms is the essential. We may find many associated phenomena, such as increase in the size of the heart, murmurs, irregularities, yet the patient's power of response to effort so good that these associated phenomena have only a slight practical significance, so far as the essential question is concerned.

Signs of exhaustion of the reserve force.—I have already dwelt on the fact that exhaustion of the reserve force is made evident in the first instance only by subjective sensations. There are so many subjective sensations provoked by the different parts of the circulation, that it is not always easy to determine whether a symptom is cardiac in origin or whether the heart is only secondarily affected. Thus symptoms of exhaustion and syncope are often attributed to cardiac weakness, and while it may be true that the heart is concerned in their production, yet the heart is rarely the source of the trouble. Syncope may arise from a mental impression, as by the sight of blood, and though the syncope is due to the temporary enfeeblement of the heart, yet properly speaking the syncope is not an evidence of cardiac weakness, but merely shows the sensitiveness of the heart to vagal stimulation. In like manner the sense of exhaustion which seems to affect the whole body in some people is not primarily cardiac but vaso-motor, due to the accumulation of blood in certain areas (as in the abdominal veins) and a depletion of other areas (as the brain).

The chief symptom which shows a limitation of the field of cardiac response is the distress or discomfort, referable mainly to the region of the chest and throat. This included the sensations of breathlessness, suffocation, tightness or oppression across the chest, and the consciousness of violent or disagreeable action of the heart itself. While many of these sensations may be provoked by a healthy heart when forced to work after its store of reserve force is exhausted, it is the too ready production of them which indicates the abnormal limitations of the heart. As I have said, the standard by which we can distinguish the healthy from the weakened heart is not rigid and fixed, but depends on each individual's peculiarity, and this is but one of the many difficulties with which we meet in estimating the value of signs in different people. When we find a case of limited response, the most thorough inquiry should be made into the patient's response to effort when at his best. It may be that we get a history of breathlessness readily induced at all times, and we may then suspect that the patient is a normally short-winded individual. In such people we may find that they can undertake other forms of effort for as long a period as others who are ' long-winded ', and by this means we can discriminate between a normally short-winded person and one with some heart lesion. Again, the condition which may have produced the limitation may not be due to a direct cardiac affection, but may arise from conditions which impair the heart's efficiency, as in individuals who are anæmic or lead sedentary lives and have not sufficiently exercised the heart's functions. In all cases it is necessary to find out what is the patient's power of response when at his best, as by ascertaining how far he can walk with comfort, and to find out when the limitation began, whether it was gradual or rapid, and all the antecedent and attendant circumstances which might have had a part in its production.

When the limitation is due to a heart lesion, its nature has to be carefully worked out. A physical examination may reveal certain abnormal signs, such as increase in the size of the heart, murmurs, or irregularities. The cause of these abnormal signs must be sought for, for they may be the outcome of some functional disturbance, of some organic lesion, of some toxic condition, as alcohol, arsenic, infection, fever, or of some slowly progressive lesion left by a previous infection, such as rheumatic fever, influenza. As I shall show later, the significance of such lesions as disease of the valves depends on whether the lesion is stationary or associated with changes in the heart muscle or arteries.

In chronic affections of the heart, like those which give rise to pain, it is imperative in all cases to ascertain the extent of the damage done to the heart. The easy production of pain by exertion may be influenced by two conditions, an extreme degree of exhaustion of the heart muscle and a very susceptible nervous system. In such cases as the latter, the individual as a whole has to be studied. In cases of degenerative changes in the heart, it is also necessary to know the extent of the damage. The most severe exhaustion and extensive degeneration may be present and yield no physical sign. If the heart's strength is tested, the response to effort will help greatly. Thus if the pain is invariably induced by a slight effort and persists after a period of rest, then we know that the heart lesion is very advanced and there is but a small amount of healthy heart muscle. If, on the other hand, it is readily induced at one time, but at other times the individual is capable of a good deal of effort, perhaps can walk three or four miles in comfort, we can then recognize that there is still left a fair amount of good functioning heart muscle, and that the pain is partly induced by some additional provocative agent at the times when a little effort induces it. In all cases it is necessary to find out how much effort the patient can undertake under the most favourable circumstances, for it will be found that, in this way, the best idea is obtained of the amount of healthy muscle.

However extreme the exhaustion may be, it is wise never to hazard an opinion as to the outcome of the illness until a period of treatment, and particularly of complete rest, has been tried. In the great majority of cases the exhaustion has been brought about by the individual doing more than his heart was capable of undertaking, and consequently a great deal of his suffering has come about because he has not had sufficient rest. A period of rest, therefore, will restore the heart's powers to a certain extent, and it is only by waiting to see what power is regained that we get the data on which to base an estimate of the functional efficiency of the heart.

CHAPTER VI

THE PRODUCTION AND SIGNIFICANCE OF SYMPTOMS

Definition of the term symptom.
The significance of physical signs.
The production of the symptoms of heart failure.
Abnormal rhythms.
Objective signs of heart failure.
Principles governing the production of symptoms.

Definition of the term symptom.—The meaning of the term symptom as employed here embraces all manifestations due to or exhibited by the organs of the circulation. It is not possible to limit the term to merely abnormal manifestations, because, on examination, we shall find manifestations, of the same nature in every respect, at one time evidences of impairment, at another time of a condition quite in accord with health. Thus, breathlessness may be an expression of exhaustion due to disease, or an expression of the transient exhaustion of a healthy heart. Again, a systolic mitral murmur may be a sign of impairment or a manifestation of a healthy heart; for it is wrong to assume that a heart to be healthy should necessarily be free from murmurs.

The significance of physical signs.—The manifestations which are revealed by a physical examination rarely yield the information which it is essential for the examining physician to acquire. The presence of a murmur or irregularity, or increase in the size of the heart, may reveal to us the nature of some disease process, but it does not tell us what bearing it may have on the heart's power to maintain an efficient circulation. Thus the recognition of the symptoms which indicate the presence of auricular fibrillation does not supply us with the information which enables us to recognize the ability of the heart to do its work, hampered by the presence of this abnormal rhythm. The perception of some marked abnormality may be of great use in indicating the nature of a disease, and from experience we may learn the probable course of the disease; if steps are not taken to modify its effect on the heart's efficiency. We must therefore seek for other evidence to appreciate the heart's power. This information is to be found, as I have already stated, in gaining a knowledge of the manner in which the heart does its work.

The production of the symptoms of heart failure.—As the invariable question is, What is the bearing of any given condition on the patient's future? it is necessary to have a clear understanding not only of what heart failure is, but the manner in which it is manifested. The best way to find out what are the symptoms produced by heart failure, is to study the effects of exhaustion on the healthy subject. As I have already pointed out, no sign of exhaustion is produced in health until the heart fails to supply sufficient blood to some organ, whether the organ is the heart itself or some remote part, as the feet or the brain.

The earliest symptom, then, will be produced by that organ which first fails to get sufficient supply of material for its due functioning. In the vast majority of cases, the most sensitive centre in this respect is the respiratory centre in the brain. When the heart fails to send sufficient blood to supply this centre with enough oxygen, or fails to remove from it the products of exhaustion, breathlessness is at once set up; and it is for this reason that breathlessness is so frequently the earliest sign of exhaustion of the reserve force.

The failure of the heart to supply blood to itself or to its nervous mechanism calls forth symptoms sometimes at an early stage of its exhaustion. These symptoms are varied in character, the most common being a disagreeable consciousness of the heart's action. In health this is shown usually by violence or rapidity in its action; in disease by sensations due to the abnormal action of the heart, as fluttering sensations and the sensation produced by irregular action. It is probable that these sensations, with the altered action of the heart, are the outcome of nervous stimulation, or of a stimulation of the more excitable structures in and about the auricle, for we have the curious fact that in complete heart-block, where the ventricle beats independently of the auricle, effort, however violent, has no effect upon its rate.

The more common form of cerebral symptom in heart failure is the weariness that comes on with prolonged mental effort and an impairment of the memory for recent events. The effect of an inefficient circulation on the brain affords an excellent opportunity for this study of heart failure. Giddiness is a symptom frequently present and usually of a very transient nature. Its real cause seems to be a deficient supply of blood to the brain, and may therefore arise from a vascular disturbance as well as from a cardiac. So far as it is cardiac, it is interesting to note the progressive phenomena induced by a cessation of the heart's action in those conditions where the ventricle may cease to contract for a brief period, or when the contractions are insufficient to send enough blood to the brain. In certain cases of heart-block, giddiness may arise during effort, because the ventricular rate does not increase; consequently the output of the heart is insufficient to supply the brain as well as the muscular system. When the ventricle pauses, we find th first symptom is slight giddiness, speedily recovered from if the ventricular standstill is brief, but if the standstill is longer, then the giddiness is followed by loss of consciousness. If the standstill be still more prolonged, convulsive movements of the skeletal muscles are produced.

Under certain circumstances all these stages may be found in the history of one individual.

Various forms of dyspnœa may arise from an inefficient supply of blood to the brain. Notwithstanding that the exact conditions which induce Cheyne-Stokes respiration are still obscure, it is so frequently present with evidence of circulatory enfeeblement, that it may be a symptom of inefficient blood-supply to the respiratory centre. Notably is this the case in advanced degenerative changes in the heart muscle; but its frequent sudden appearance in the cases of auricular flutter and complete heart-block, when the circulation is impaired, seems to suggest that diminution of the heart's output is one of the causes of its onset.

Symptoms of a reflex kind may arise from the heart itself, and, in order to appreciate how they come about, it may be useful to consider what happens to the skeletal muscles when exercised with an insufficient blood-supply. Some elderly people may be able to undertake a considerable amount of sustained effort, when it is pursued with care. If they walk on the level at a rapid rate, after a time they begin to experience a sense of weight in their feet, and by and by the lower part of the legs about the ankle-joint begins to ache. If the active walking be persisted in, the pain becomes so severe that they are compelled to abate their activities. The same inefficiency induced by exercise is noticed in individuals whose arteries are occluded from any cause. Thus I have known a man recover from a blocked femoral artery and the leg was supplied by a collateral circulation. He could walk for a considerable distance in a quiet manner; but if he hurried, after a hundred yards he was compelled to stop because of the weight and pain in the leg. The same thing happens in disease of the arteries of the leg, giving rise to what is called intermittent claudication. Here the feet in walking may become cold and the aching be so severe that the patient is compelled to stop. After standing, the feet become warm and the pain subsides.

Disease of the coronary artery may diminish the supply of blood to the heart muscle. The impaired blood-supply may be sufficient to enable the heart to act efficiently when the body is at rest; but the increased supply needed when effort is being made may not be available, and, as a consequence, we get pain and other sensations of distress. The same distress may be induced when the muscle itself becomes impaired, as from degeneration, and exhaustion is easily provoked. The mechanism by which hyperalgesia, pain, and the symptoms of distress are produced is discussed in Chapter XI. Here I point out that the first symptoms of inefficiency may arise from the heart itself.

Abnormal rhythms.—A subject of interest that needs to be worked out is the new physiology which arises when the heart takes on a new rhythm. The action of the heart in physiological and therapeutical investigations has hitherto been studied when the heart is acting in a normal manner. The clinical study of hearts with continuous abnormal rhythms, such as partial and complete heart-block, auricular fibrillation and flutter, and a combination of auricular fibrillation and complete heart-block, presents new problems which affect the manner of heart failure, the response to effort, and the reaction to drugs. Thus we are accustomed to recognize that where a heart is exposed to effort it increases its rate and output, and supplies the active organ with an increased supply of blood, while maintaining the normal supply to the other organs. I have just pointed out that in complete heart-block, there is no increase in the ventricular rate in response to effort. Under such conditions the symptoms of exhaustion become somewhat modified. Thus, in inquiry into a number of such cases, I found that with exhaustion breathlessness is not infrequent, but that they often feel as if the legs were weighted with lead, or the exertion brings on giddiness.

In abnormal rhythms, such as auricular fibrillation and flutter, we get other effects, generally associated with the great increase of the rate, so that we get symptoms arising from the excited heart action itself and from an insufficient output.

Patients are themselves distressingly conscious of the increase in the heart action, and shrink from provoking it, while the inefficient output may lead to attacks of giddiness or loss of consciousness (Fig. 141).

Objective signs of heart failure.—The objective signs of heart failure, such as dropsy and venous and hepatic engorgement, are usually spoken of as signs of back pressure ; but they are probably due to an inefficiency of the driving power. The blood passes through the capillaries at a slow rate, impairs their nutrition, and allows transudation to take place, which we call dropsy.

Under certain circumstances, this enfeebled circulation leads to great engorgement of the venous side of the circulation. Dilatation of the tricuspid and venous orifices may arise, so that we get regurgitant waves of blood sent back into the veins and the liver by contraction of the auricle and ventricle.

Under these circumstances ' back pressure ' does modify the circulation and produce definite symptoms. But these results occur in only a small proportion of cases of heart failure, and by the time they appear the heart failure has reached an advanced stage.

Principles governing the production of symptoms.—From such considerations as these we may conclude that the symptoms of heart failure are produced by an inefficient circulation in certain organs, and that the evidence of the heart failure is to be found in the functional impairment of the different organs. Moreover, such evidence is afforded in the early stages only when the heart is forced to exercise itself at the full extent of its power ; and the earliest symptom is shown by that organ which first experiences a deficiency in its blood-supply. The variableness of the symptoms of heart failure is due to the fact that different organs may be rendered inefficient in different individuals by the deficient blood-supply.

CHAPTER VII

FUNDAMENTAL FUNCTIONS OF THE HEART MUSCLE-CELLS

Myogenic doctrine.
Stimulus production.
Excitability.
Conductivity.
Contractility.
Tonicity.
Co-ordination of functions.
Characteristics of the functions of the heart muscle-fibres.

Myogenic doctrine.—While it would be somewhat beyond my province to enter into a discussion of the question whether the heart contracts in response to a nerve stimulus, or in response to a stimulus developed in the muscle-cells, it is very necessary, in order to comprehend the meaning of the signs and symptoms that arise in affections of the heart, to appreciate the phenomena which are associated with the contraction of the muscle-fibres. The conception of the meaning of the heart-beat, which we owe to Gaskell, has been supported by careful and minute analysis of the functions of the normal heart muscle-fibres; and the interpretation of the symptoms of heart affections in the light of this knowledge has revealed so clearly their true meaning as to revolutionize the study in the human subject. Even if the 'Myogenic doctrine' be ultimately proved untenable, the investigations carried out in its support have added so much of value to our knowledge of the heart's action that its conception will ever be associated with a great stride forward, not only in physiology, but also in the recognition and treatment of diseases of the heart. It is just possible that the two opposing doctrines—Neurogeny and Myogeny—may be reconciled along the lines I suggest in the following brief summary of the main points. I do not enter into much detail, but give such salient points as are necessary to appreciate the explanation of the symptoms I give in the course of this work. For fuller details the reader is referred to Gaskell's article on ' The Contraction of the Cardiac Muscle ' in Schaefer's *Text Book of Physiology*.

From the consideration of the physiology of the cell, it may be said that every function possessed by a cell in the fully developed state exists partially developed in the primitive form. However specialized the function may be, nervous, muscular, or secretory, these functions can be referred back to some property possessed by the primitive cell. The cells which constitute the primitive structure of the body all start equally endowed; and it is by a gradual process of specialization that each takes on its peculiar function, while as it acquires a high degree of specialization it gradually loses those functions it no longer exercises. The functions possessed by the primitive cells can therefore be deduced not only from the results of direct observation, but from the specialized functions of the more differentiated tissues, even if these functions be so highly developed that they bear little resemblance to those found in the primitive cell. For instance, the excitability of the cell may become so specialized as to be responsive only to certain stimuli, as heat, pain, light, sound, while all its other functions are apparently lost. If one looks at the functions of nerve- and muscle-cells in the fully developed state, it seems at first sight difficult to realize that they had originally identical functions. The primitive cells, from which the heart developed, had all the same characteristics; yet in their final evolution they present widely divergent characteristics, both in appearance and in function. That some such modification does occur must be inferred, when we witness the change in function which takes place in the evolution of the heart from the primitive cardiac tube. I therefore suggest as a working hypothesis, that in the evolution of the heart muscle-fibres certain functions of the primitive cell were retained, some of these being more developed than others according to the duties the fibres had to perform, so that while they have come to resemble muscle-fibres, they nevertheless retain, in a varying degree, some functions which are highly specialized in the nerve-cell.

The special functions which Gaskell has demonstrated are five in number, namely :

(1) The power of producing a stimulus which can excite the heart to contract—stimulus production.
(2) The power of being able to receive a stimulus—excitability.
(3) The power of conveying a stimulus from fibre to fibre—conductivity.
(4) The power of contracting when stimulated—contractility.
(5) The power to retain a certain amount of contraction even when the active movement has ceased—tonicity.

Stimulus production.—From this point of view it is assumed that the heart muscle-fibres, if supplied with appropriate nutriment, possess a power of internally secreting a material which is capable of stimulating the fibre to contract. This material is being continually secreted, and, during a pause in the heart's contraction, accumulates in the heart-cell. When sufficient has been stored to excite the heart to contract, the whole store is used up in stimulating the muscle-cell. Immediately after the contraction the store again begins to accumulate, until sufficient has been produced to excite the heart to further contraction. This function, being continuous in its action, cannot control the rhythm of the heart; but by its co-operation with the other functions a rhythmical character is given to the accumulation and destruction of this material.

Excitability.—The heart muscle depends for its contraction upon its power of receiving a stimulus—that is, upon its excitability. Immediately after the heart has been stimulated to contract, the fibres are no longer capable of further stimulation, excitability has disappeared, and the fibres are in what is called the refractory stage. The excitability begins at once to be restored, and increases very rapidly during diastole. This is demonstrated by the heart being susceptible to weaker stimuli the longer the time since the previous contraction. So long as the heart is capable of contracting, the rate of the heart depends upon the functions of stimulus production and excitability; and when the conditions are normal the equal action of both functions—the stimulus material being renewed at a uniform rate, and the restoration of the excitability taking place uniformly—a regular rhythm of the heart's action, results. Under normal circumstances, therefore, the heart's rate and rhythm are dependent upon the integrity of these two functions.

Conductivity.—In a mass of primitive cells the individual cell has a power of passing the stimulus on to neighbouring cells. This function of conductivity is possessed by the heart muscle-fibres, for the stimulus is passed on from cell to cell from the point where it originated. The possession of this function by the muscle-fibres of the heart gives them a character which is typical of certain forms of nerve-fibres; but in the heart this is not so highly developed as in the specialized nerve-fibre, the conduction of the stimulus not being so rapid in all cases, and much more easily exhausted. Like every other function of the heart, it is entirely abolished after it has been exercised; and it returns gradually. The rate at which an impulse travels also varies in different fibres of the heart. Some fibres, such as the more recently developed contractile fibres of the auricle and ventricle, conduct the stimulus with much greater rapidity than the fibres which convey the stimulus from auricle to ventricle.

Contractility.—The power of contraction is the most evident of all the functions of the heart. By the co-ordinated contraction of the fibres of the different portions of the heart, the circulation is maintained. After a contraction, this function is completely exhausted, and the power returns very gradually. Within certain limits the strength of the contraction depends upon the length of the period of rest preceding the contraction, the function gathering strength during quiescence.

Tonicity.—The functions of the heart muscle do not differ, except in degree, from those of other muscular structures; and as tone is a very characteristic property of muscular tissue, it is certain that the heart muscle will possess it, and it is shown by the fibres not relaxing to their full length during diastole. On account of the rapid action of the heart, it is not easy to demonstrate this function. Gaskell has shown that the degree of relaxation depends on the amount of tone present, and that certain drugs increase or diminish the amount of relaxation. Thus antiarin, veratrin, and digitalis prevent the relaxation of the heart muscle in the frog, so that the heart remains longer in the condition of complete contraction, the relaxation gradually becoming less and less, till finally it is almost impossible to recognize individual beats. On the other hand, solutions of lactic acid and muscarin produce the opposite effect, the heart becoming more and more relaxed, the contraction diminishing in size, till the heart stands still in diastolic relaxation. Just as certain portions of the musculature have certain functions more highly developed, it would not be unreasonable, as Gaskell says, to expect that different parts of the heart should vary in their tonicity. That this expectation is justified will be manifest when all the symptoms of heart failure are considered; and it is only by recognizing that the heart possesses this very important function that we can understand some of the most significant features of heart failure.

Co-ordination of functions.—When the complicated action of the heart is considered, it will be readily recognized that though all the fibres may be endowed with these functions, a further specialization is a necessity for the co-ordinated movement of the different parts of the heart. If all the fibres were equally endowed, then all would contract simultaneously. As it is, certain fibres at the venous end have the functions of stimulus production and excitability more highly developed than others, so that after a period of rest the contraction starts in them. The stimulus then proceeds to adjoining fibres in such a manner that the process of stimulation and contraction sweeps through the whole heart, with the result that the different chambers and the different parts of each chamber contract in that order and degree necessary to the efficient carrying on of the circulation. If any other part of the heart be rendered more excitable than the venous end, then the contraction starts there. As the stimulus then does not sweep through the heart in the normal manner, the heart's action is less efficient, and heart failure may thus arise.

Characteristics of the functions of the heart muscle-fibres.—While the heart may be said to carry on its work in consequence of its possession of these functions, there are other important features in each which have a practical bearing on the symptoms of diseases and the principles of treatment. The integrity of these functions depends on the supply of suitable nutriment, and sufficient time of inactivity to recover after their exercise. When a contraction takes place, all the functions have been exercised to the full extent of the power possessed by the fibres at the moment of stimulation. No heart-cell exhausts only a portion of its function; when stimulated, it uses all the energy which it possesses (all or nothing). For a brief period after their exercise, the functions cease to exist: recovery, however, begins at once during the period of rest, and each function in time regains its strength, so that, within certain limits, the longer the delay, the more complete is the recovery, and the more efficient is the subsequent action. It is by fully appreciating the effect of rest and proper nourishment that we gain the best conception of the principle that should underlie our treatment of heart failure. While all the functions when exercised use all the force they possess, they nevertheless manifest a quality whereby they can respond, under certain circumstances, with a greater activity. Thus the rate may be suddenly increased, and at the same time the stimulus passed from the auricle to the ventricle with increased rapidity, and the contraction be executed quicker. These changes are to a great extent under the control of the nervous system, but they imply a quality possessed by all these functions which is of vital importance to us in the study of heart failure. For, as I have already remarked, it is this power of responding to effort that gives us the clue to the real state of the heart.

When one reflects that all the fibres of the heart are not equally endowed with the same functions, and that all the functions may not always be exposed to an equal strain, it is but reasonable to conclude that conditions may arise where they are unequally affected. As a matter of fact, this is what commonly happens, and it is an interesting and important question to consider in each case of heart failure what functions are specially at fault. The significance of this question was demonstrated, when Wenckebach showed how the irregular activity of the various functions or of the various parts of the heart was made manifest by certain characteristic arrhythmias. Following up the idea of exhaustion or over-excitability of individual functions, I have sought to connect many of the symptoms of heart failure with these functions. While I do not say that my conclusions are invariably correct, they have led to some definite results of the very highest importance, and it is along these lines that advance in our knowledge will likely follow for some time.

CHAPTER VIII

DEVELOPMENT, ANATOMY, AND PHYSIOLOGY OF THE HEART

The primitive cardiac tube.
The functions of the primitive cardiac tube.
The remains of the primitive cardiac tube in the mammalian heart.
Functions of the sino-auricular node, the pacemaker of the heart.
Functions of the auriculo-ventricular node and bundle.
Functional anatomy of the heart.
The nerve supply of the heart.
    Afferent fibres.
    Cardiac ganglion cells.

WHILE I take it for granted that the reader is familiar with the ordinary text-book description of the anatomy and physiology of the heart, there are some recent investigations which have an important bearing on the clinical investigation of heart disease which need to be considered. For that reason I give here a brief *résumé* of certain points necessary for the appreciation of clinical signs.

The primitive cardiac tube.—In an early stage of the embryo's development, the heart appears as a tube. The veins from the body unite into a common cavity—the sinus venosus—at the posterior end of this tube. In the course of development this tube becomes bent upon itself, and from it, later, pouches develop which ultimately become the auricles and ventricles—the original tube still persisting and connecting them (Fig. 1). As development proceeds, the sinus venosus loses its distinctive feature as a separate structure to become incorporated in the termination of the superior and inferior vena cavæ. A small portion of tissue of a peculiar specialized kind of muscle and nerve element, in which many cardiac nerves terminate, has lately been described by Keith and Flack. The heart-beat probably originates in this structure. At the same time the original cardiac tube ceases to exist as a tube ; but it is inferred that it persists as the connecting medium between auricles and ventricles in the shape of a band of peculiar fibres—the auriculo-ventricular bundle (Fig. 2). It thus loses its function as a propelling organ, which is taken up by the auricles and ventricles.

The functions of the primitive cardiac tube.—The functions of the primitive cardiac tube and its representative in the mammalian heart need to be carefully studied, as the appreciation of the nature of its functions has the most important bearing on many cases of heart failure. Its peculiar properties have been studied most fully in the heart of the frog, also in the toad, tortoise, crocodile, etc., but, so far, only to a slight extent in the mammalian heart. In the lower vertebrates the primitive tube is still recognizable in the sinus venosus, auricular canal, and aortic bulb (Fig. 1). It has been found that the posterior end of this tube is the most excitable portion, and in consequence of this the heart's contraction starts at the sinus venosus. The remainder of the tube also possesses the faculty of starting the heart's contraction, only in a less degree than the sinus. If, how-

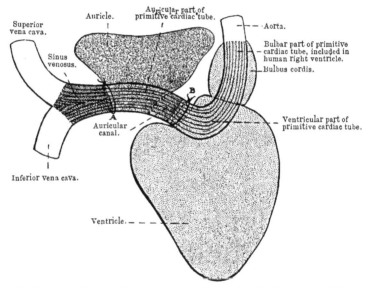

Fig. 1. Diagram of the primitive vertebrate heart, showing the development of the auricle and ventricle from the primitive cardiac tube. *A*, position of first Stannius ligature; *B*, position of second Stannius ligature. (Keith.)

ever, any part of the tube be rendered more excitable than the sinus the contraction starts from that part. The peculiarity of the primitive cardiac tube, and its relatively greater excitability than the auricular or ventricular tissue, are brought out in the following experiment by Gaskell: ' Touch the auriculo-ventricular ring of muscle (i.e. the primitive cardiac tube) with the slightest stimulus, immediately a series of rhythmical contractions occurs. It is most striking to see, after removal of the septum, how every portion of auricular and ventricular tissue can be explored up to the very edge of the ring, without obtaining more than a single contraction, while immediately the needle touches the muscular ring a series of rapid contractions results.'

The possession of the power of independent contraction by the separate portions of the heart is brought out in the Stannius experiments. When a ligature is applied or a cut made between the sinus and auricle of a frog's heart (*A*, Fig. 1), so as to sever completely the connexion, the sinus continues beating, and after a pause of varying duration the auricles and ventricles begin to beat at a rate different from, and independent of, the sinus. This rate is slower than the sinus rate, and sometimes the auricle contracts before the ventricle, sometimes the ventricle precedes the auricle, and very rarely they contract simultaneously. (Engelmann.)

If a second Stannius ligature be applied between auricle and ventricle (*B*, Fig. 1), the sinus and auricle continue beating; and after a period the ventricle takes on its own rhythm, slower than, and independent of, the other portion of the heart.

The remains of the primitive cardiac tube in the mammalian heart (*Sino-auricular node. Auriculo-ventricular node and bundle*).—The sinus venosus, which in the primitive heart normally originated the stimulus for contraction, has no representative as an independent structure in the human heart. Morphologists recognize that it has become incorporated in the great veins near the heart, and physiologists observed that the peculiar functions of the sinus venosus were found over a somewhat wide distribution. Recent observations by Lewis show that when the contraction originates from any source other than the sino-auricular node, the contraction presents abnormal features, revealed by the electrocardiograph. Until very recent times no definite remains of the sinus venosus had been found. Keith and Flack have described a small node of tissue—the sino-auricular node—at the mouth of the superior vena cava. This tissue consists of fine delicate pale fibres faintly striated, in which branches of the vagus and sympathetic nerves terminate, and is supplied with a definite artery. These observers consider that this node of tissue represents a portion of the sinus venosus, from which the heart's contraction starts. Similar tissue has so far not been found in the other veins. It is possible that some fibres may be scattered about; but, not being grouped into a definite node, they are not capable of being differentiated from the muscular fibres by which they are surrounded. The further remains of the primitive cardiac tissue are probably found lower down, arising in the right auricle and passing across the auriculo-ventricular septum to the ventricles, thus joining the auricles and ventricles. Although the presence of this bridge was inferred in the mammalian heart by Gaskell, it was not demonstrated until 1893, when first Stanley Kent, then His (junr.), described its presence and both experimentally demonstrated some of its functions. A full description of its structure and ramification was given in 1906 by Tawara, whose elaborate examination of the tissue has been of the greatest interest and importance. This bundle rises from a node of tissue—the auriculo-ventricular node—situated in the right auricular wall near the mouth of the coronary sinus. The bundle passes over the auriculo-ventricular septum below the central fibrous body and under the septal cusp of the tricuspid valve. While on the septum it divides into two, one branch passing into the left ventricle and the other into the right. In the right ventricle it continues its course as a narrow rounded bundle in the muscle-wall of the heart, till it approaches the apex, where it divides into numerous fine threads, terminating in the muscle-fibres. In the left ventricle the bundle rapidly widens out into a thin band which passes down to the apex, splitting into fine branches.

The character of the fibres constituting this bundle varies. The fibres of the auriculo-ventricular node are of the same delicate nature as those of the sino-auricular node. As this bundle passes into the ventricle the fibres change, becoming thicker, the greater part of the cell-body being undifferentiated protoplasm, only faintly striated at the circumference and containing a large nucleus. In their final distribution they are recognized as being the fibres described long ago by Purkinje. Another peculiarity of this bundle is, that it is isolated from the structures in which it is embedded by a fine sheath of connective tissue. There are numerous nerve structures in the auriculo-ventricular bundle, which have been specially studied by Gordon Wilson. He finds numerous ganglion cells, abundant nerve-fibres, an intricate plexus around the muscle-fibres of the bundle, and distinct vaso-motor nerves. Finally, it is mainly supplied by a special branch of the right coronary artery, a fact of some significance in the pathology of the heart.

Functions of the sino-auricular node, the pacemaker of the heart. —The functions of the sino-auricular node have been investigated recently in several ways. It has long been known that warming or cooling the auricular tissue near the mouth of the superior vena cava, increased or diminished the heart's rate. Excision, clamping, and freezing of the sino-auricular node have been undertaken, with no apparent effect on the heart's rate. The probable reason for this is that, while the sino-auricular node is the starting-point of the heart's contraction under normal circumstances, other portions of the auricles take on this function as soon as the node is destroyed. This explanation is rendered probable by the study of the character of the beats, as shown by the electrocardiograms. Lewis found the beats to vary according to the site at which the contractions arise. The electrocardiographic record of auricular systole which he obtained shows a characteristic form when the contraction starts at the sino-auricular node, and it is different when the contraction starts from any other portion of the auricular wall. It has also been demonstrated that when premature auricular contractions arise in the human heart, they have not the same electric character as the normal beat, and the inference is justifiable that some other portion of the

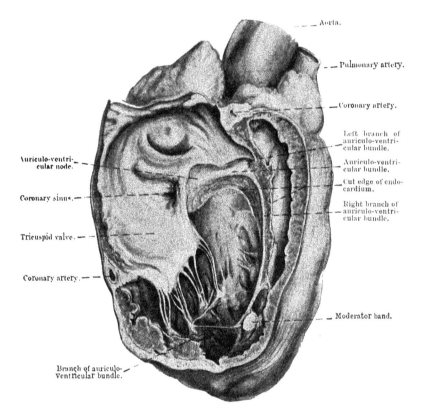

FIG. 2. Dissection showing the origin of the auriculo-ventricular bundle, and the course of the right branch in the right ventricle. The anterior and lateral walls of the right ventricle have been removed as well as a portion of the tricuspid valve. A slight dissection has been made which exposes the bundle arising in the auriculo-ventricular node, an ill-defined structure in the right auricle, near the opening of the coronary sinus. The main stem runs from the node to the auriculo-ventricular septum, where it divides into two branches, the left branch going through to the left ventricle as shown in Fig. 3, the right branch going down in the muscle of the ventricle near the endocardium as a narrow rounded band. In the specimen from which the dissection was made, it could be traced to the moderator band, which is shown cut in the drawing. Here it divided into numerous fine branches, one of which is seen passing across the cavity as a fine thread.

auricle has originated the stimulus for contraction. Moreover, in certain tachycardias the electric records demonstrate that the contractions begin at some other portion of the auricular wall than the sino-auricular node, and that, with the cessation of the tachycardia and the recurrence of

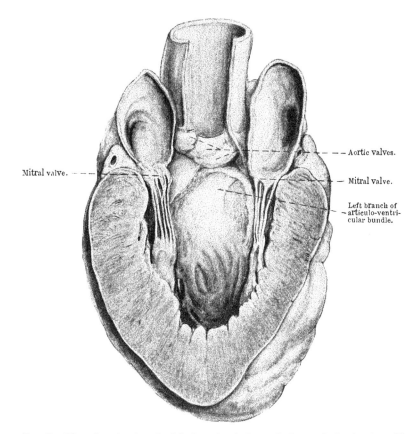

Mitral valve. ‒ ‒ ‒

‒ ‒ ‒ Aortic valves.

‒ Mitral valve.

Left branch of ‒articulo-ventri-cular bundle.

FIG. 3.   Dissection showing the left branch of the auriculo-ventricular bundle.   The posterior wall of the left ventricle has been slit open, the incision passing up through the left auricle and aorta.   The cavity of the left ventricle is exposed, and a very slight dissection made to show the left branch of the bundle entering the ventricle immediately below the septal cusp of the aortic valve.   The bundle widens out into a thin band lying immediately under the endocardium, and as it passes down the ventricle it sends branches into the muscle, until it can no longer be recognized as a separate and distinct structure.

the normal rhythm, the electric curves show a change back to that characteristic of the auricular contractions which start at the sino-auricular node.

Functions of the auriculo-ventricular node and bundle.—The functions of this bundle have been only partially·explored experimentally, though a fair inference of its functional action can be made from clinical symptoms. It has now been demonstrated that it conveys the stimulus from auricle to ventricle ; for compression of the bundle interferes with the conduction, while section stops all connexion, and the ventricle contracts at a rate quite independent of the auricular rate, as after the second Stannius ligature. An exactly similar experience is met with as a result of disease in man.

But these junctional tissues also possess the power of originating the stimulus for contraction. Proof of this conception is furnished by means of the electric curves in certain cases of abnormal rhythm. The electric curves caused by systole of the ventricle, when the stimulus for contraction enters the heart by the auriculo-ventricular bundle, have a well-defined character quite distinct from that of a beat arising in the ventricle. Thus the majority of ventricular extra-systoles show quite a different character from that of the normal beats among which they occur. In complete heart-block, the ventricular contractions yield a normal electric curve, showing that the stimulus for contraction has entered in the normal manner. As portions of the node and bundle have been destroyed, it can be assumed that the stimulus for contraction has arisen in some part of the bundle in connexion with the ventricles.

Functional anatomy of the heart.—I mention here a few of the more important features connected with the heart as a muscular organ which are of importance in this clinical study. These are based on Keith's descriptions, who has demonstrated that the heart is built of muscle bundles whose points of origin and insertion are as definite as those of skeletal muscles, and whose functions can also, to a great extent, be inferred with equal certainty. Naturally the separation of the different muscle bundles is not so complete as in skeletal muscles, there being a continuous connexion between neighbouring fibres, so that they pass gradually from one system into another.

In order to appreciate how the muscle-fibres act, and also to understand the changes that result from an increase in the size of the heart, it is necessary to comprehend how the heart is fixed in the thorax.

The pericardium is a fairly unyielding structure fixed firmly above to the cervical fascia, and below to the central tendon of the diaphragm. The aorta and the great veins, where they penetrate the pericardial sac, receive a covering from it, and these may be regarded as fixed points. The lungs also may be considered as ligaments which attach the base of the heart to the whole of the chest-wall.

The contraction of the heart starts at the mouth of the great veins. It has hitherto been assumed that regurgitation from the auricle was prevented by the contraction of the circular fibres at the mouth of the veins. Keith shows that these are too weak for the purpose, except around the coronary sinus, and that regurgitation back into the superior vena cava is prevented by the contraction of the broad band of muscle which sweeps over the roof of the auricle—the tænia terminalis. In its contraction this muscular band shuts off the vein from the auricular cavity. As the tænia is attached at the orifice of the inferior vena cava and is carried over the roof of the right auricle, it also aids in the closure of the inferior vena cava and the pulmonary veins. The pressure of the blood in the inferior vena cava, apparently renders a perfectly competent closure of the inferior caval orifice unnecessary.

Arising from the tænia are a number of other muscular bands, the pectinate fibres, which pass across the auricle to be fixed in the auriculo-ventricular septum. In their contraction, in addition to assisting the tænia in emptying the auricle, they pull up the ventricles by reason of their insertion into the auriculo-ventricular septum (A, Fig. 4).

The ventricles have themselves no real fixed point, but depend for security on the fixation of the vessels at the base of the heart. Immediately below the origin of the aorta in the heart is the central fibrous body, which is really a tendon for much of the ventricular muscle. The remainder of the ventricular muscle is inserted into the auriculo-ventricular septum. The other fixed point during contraction is the apex. It becomes a fixed point in virtue of the peculiar arrangement of the muscles here constituting the ' whorl '. A great number of fibres from different parts of the heart converge here and mutually support one another in contraction, the result being a fixed point from which the fibres can exercise traction in different directions. With the onset of the ventricular contraction, the apex of the heart rises up and presses firmly against the chest-wall. As no shortening takes place between the apex and the aorta, all the parts of the heart are drawn towards the line between apex and aorta. Hence it is that while during ventricular contraction the apex is pushed forwards, all the other portions of the cardiac surface are dragged inwards; and this explains the variation in the appearance of a cardiogram taken from different parts of the front of the chest. At the same time, as Chauveau and Keith have shown, the ventricular fibres inserted into the auriculo-ventricular septum not only diminish the size of the ventricle, but enlarge the size of the auricle by dragging down the auriculo-ventricular septum—a fact of some importance in the production of the venous pulse (B, Fig. 4).

The nerve supply of the heart.—While the heart contains within itself the power to execute its movements independently of any extrinsic nervous intervention, nevertheless nervous influences have a powerful effect in modifying the activity of the various functions of the muscle-fibres. The nerves of the heart are usually described as being of three sorts, namely, (1) inhibitory fibres passing to the heart, (2) accelerator or augmentor fibres also passing to the heart, and (3) depressor fibres passing from the heart.

The inhibitory fibres are derived from the spinal bulb by the internal branch of the spinal accessory nerve, and pass down in the vagus and reach the heart by its cardiac branches. The effects of the vagus upon the heart are varied. On division of one vagus little effect may result. If both vagi be cut the frequency of the heart is much increased. If the vagus be

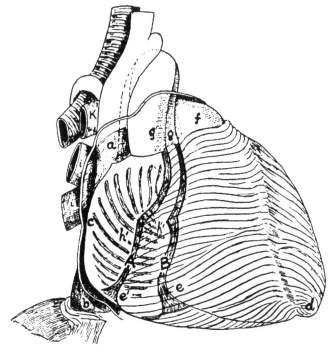

Fig. 4. Sketch of the heart to show the movements of the auriculo-ventricular groove during auricular and ventricular systole. *A*, position of groove when pulled upon by the contraction of the pectinate fibres of the auricle; *B*, position of the groove when pulled upon by the contraction of the ventricular fibres. During the diastole the groove occupies a position midway between *A* and *B*; *a*, sinus portion of superior vena cava; *b*, inferior vena cava; *c* is on the tænia terminalis; *d*, apex of the heart; *f*, pulmonary artery; *i, i*, pulmonary veins; *k*, pulmonary artery. During ventricular systole *g'* is pulled to *g* and *e'* to *e*; *h'*, musculi pectinati during auricular systole; *h"*, during ventricular systole. (Keith.)

stimulated the result is curiously varied. Its action may be said in a general way to depress the functions of the heart muscle-fibres, but it does not do so uniformly in all cases. It usually acts first on the excitability of the heart or on the stimulus production, so that the whole heart becomes slower in its action, or the whole heart may stand still for a brief period. With stronger stimulation, it may act on the conductivity of the fibres joining auricles and ventricles, and depress this function so that the ventricle fails to respond to every auricular systole. Underlying this seemingly uncertain action of the vagus is a principle which is of great importance in diagnosis and in treatment, namely, that if there be depression of one function of the heart, vagus stimulation is liable to seize upon that function and increase the depression. The fact that depressed functions are more susceptible to vagus stimulation seems to be the reason for some of the discordant results arrived at by experiments.

The accelerator fibres belong to the sympathetic system and have their origin in the spinal cord, passing out of the cord by the white rami communicantes to the upper four or five dorsal nerves. They pass upwards to the inferior cervical ganglion ; from thence they pass to join the cardiac fibres of the vagus, and so reach the heart. These fibres on stimulation increase the rate of the heart, sometimes very considerably, and, according to Roy and Adami, they increase the strength of contraction and output as well, and hence have been assumed to contain augmentor fibres.

The depressor fibre is a definite nerve which arises in the heart, and, passing upwards, joins the vagus nerve and so reaches the bulb. Stimulation of the peripheral part of the cut nerve has no effect, but stimulation of the central end causes a fall of blood-pressure through reflex action on the medulla oblongata.

Afferent fibres.—Such is a brief *résumé* of the heart nerves described in physiological text-books, but the whole matter is not included here. There is a great field of evidence which is entirely lost to the physiologist, but which is open to the clinician. The personal sensation of the animal cannot be communicated to the experimenter, nor can the changes in sensation that result from stimulation of the cardiac nerves be ascertained. In dealing with the symptoms of heart affections it will be shown that there is unquestionable evidence of a system of nerves passing from the heart to the spinal cord and the bulb. The principles involved in the production of these symptoms have not been thoroughly appreciated, and I shall enter more fully into their explanation when dealing with the reflex or protective phenomena (Chapter XI).

Cardiac ganglion cells.—The nerve-fibres of the auriculo-ventricular bundle have been referred to on p. 35. The ganglion cells in the heart have been studied by Gaskell. He says, ' What, then, are the ganglion cells in the heart ? What function do you attribute to them ? That is a question which I am ready to answer, and to answer with confidence, as follows : The ganglion cells in the heart are part of the great group of ganglion cells which are situated on the course of the small-fibred efferent nerves supplying the viscera. These cells form the outlying vagrant groups of nerve-cells which are known by the name of the sympathetic and cerebro-spinal ganglia. In the case of the heart, the ganglion cells are the cells belonging to the small-fibred efferent cardiac fibres of the vagus, just as some of the cells in the ganglion stellatum and in the inferior cervical ganglion are the cells belonging to the small-fibred efferent cardiac fibres of the augmentor nerve. There is no more reason to assign special functions to these cells than to any of the other peripheral efferent nerve-cells. They are cells connected only with the inhibitory fibres of the vagus, and as such are simply part and parcel of the mechanism of inhibition, just as the corresponding cells in the ganglion stellatum are simply part and parcel of the augmentor mechanism.'

CHAPTER IX

THE EXAMINATION OF THE PATIENT

The importance of the patient's statement.
The patient's aspect.
The patient's sensations.
The condition of other organs.
The patient's history.
The field of cardiac response.
The chief complaints.
    Breathlessness.
    The sense of exhaustion.
    Pain.
    A constriction of the chest.
    A persistent aching.
The patient's consciousness of the heart's action.
Cerebral symptoms.
    Dizziness or giddiness.
    Loss of consciousness.
    Adams-Stokes syndrome.
    Effect of a failing heart on the cerebral functions.

The importance of the patient's statement.—As a result of practical experience, the method of examination of patients has become stereotyped, and although I do not propose to depart from it, nevertheless, in view of the manner in which heart failure is presented in this book, it is incumbent on me to deal with the patient's statements with greater fullness and precision than has hitherto been the custom. The reason for this has already been given, namely, that the earliest and most valuable information regarding the efficiency of the heart is revealed by the patient's sensations in response to effort, and by the patient's consciousness of the unusual manner in which the heart may beat. From a due appreciation of the patient's sensations, the nature of the trouble will often be revealed. Moreover, in many patients the action of the heart may become abnormal at intermittent periods, so that we have to depend on the patient's description of his sensations for a knowledge of his trouble. The due appreciation of these sensations will often lead to the recognition of the nature of the complaint in many people who suffer from a cardiac affection. Some people suffer from circulatory troubles which are not directly due to the heart, and it is often very difficult to determine their origin. The recital of the patient's experiences, if made so clear that the physician can really judge of their nature, will often enable him to discriminate between sensations which are primarily cardiac in origin and those which arise from influences outside the heart.

The patient's aspect.—The appreciation of the patient's condition should begin as soon as he presents himself to us. His gait, his bearing, the colour of his face, his breathing, any peculiarity of speech or behaviour, should all be noted. If the patient is in bed, note the position he assumes and any changes in his colour or breathing in response to such effort as talking or turning over. By habit, one notices these things almost unconsciously, and their recognition guides us in the subsequent examination.

The patient's sensations.—After ascertaining the age and occupation of the patient, ask him to describe briefly the reason which led him to seek advice, so far as it appertains to his personal experiences. If it was due to a consciousness of ill health or of impaired powers, then get him to describe his sensations, briefly but concisely. Many patients become so diffuse that, unless checked and given to understand what is wanted, their description would be so confused that much time would be wasted and one would probably fail to get a clear idea of the nature of the trouble. When he refers to his sensations and their location, get him to indicate the situation by placing his hand over the region, otherwise, proud of his small anatomical knowledge, he will attribute the sensations to his viscera ; and here I may add a warning to the physician not to make a note of the sensations by attributing them to any viscus ; thus a pain should not be put down as felt in the heart, stomach, or liver, but only in the region of the body indicated by the patient, for it will probably be found on later examination that the pains are not felt in the viscus. In other words, he should make no note that might prejudge the nature of any symptom until he has before him all the evidence.

The condition of other organs.—A brief inquiry should be made regarding the other viscera, as to the state of the digestive tract, the urinary secretion, the breathing, swelling of the legs, etc. The relation of any complaint to the various activities of the other organs, as when sensations are provoked by a meal or when the stomach is empty, should be inquired into.

The patient's history.—After fully appreciating the sensations of which the patient complains, we should inquire into the past history and obtain a knowledge of the manner of life the patient has spent, particularly in relation to bodily exertion, mental worry, indulgence in food, alcohol, tobacco, and so forth. This history of other illnesses should be sought for, particularly whether there has been rheumatic fever or other febrile complaint, other forms of rheumatism, syphilis, or gout. In regard to affections occurring in families, it is not often that this affords much help in diseases of the heart ; for most diseases are the outcome of the individual's own experiences, and therefore the fact that the parent may have suffered from a heart affection, the result of some infective complaint, is of little help when the individual himself has not suffered from the same infection.

Guided by the information thus obtained, we should return again to the main complaints, and inquire when they began to appear and what induced their appearance. It is particularly necessary to appreciate the conditions and circumstances which provoke attacks of pain, breathlessness, etc., particularly in the early stages. In all cases it is necessary to find out what degree of exertion the patient can undertake with comfort. As I have pointed out, heart failure resolves itself into the question of the amount of reserve force, and consequently it is at this juncture that we begin to find out that amount ; therefore the factors which produce the first sign of discomfort need the most detailed inquiry. The sequence of the phenomena as they arise is most instructive. The patient has often only a confused notion of the order of appearance of the sensations, and the situation in which they are felt, so that it may be necessary to postpone a final opinion until a second visit, and the patient should be instructed to note, should occasion arise, the individual sensations, their location, and order of appearance. Ou a subsequent visit the account may be totally different, but often one made with great precision. It is sometimes surprising to observe that a patient, after an attack of agonizing pain, has but a very dim idea in what region it was felt. Inquiries should be made as to the presence of less obtrusive symptoms, which experience tells us to expect, but which the patient often ignores, unless his attention is drawn to them. Thus when he complains of a pain in the chest, is it associated with a sense of constriction, or, after it passes, is there a desire to micturate ? Many patients have bad dreams and even delusions, and, as Head points out, the latter are never elicited unless carefully inquired after.

The field of cardiac response.—If, up to this part of the examination, the physician has not obtained a clear conception of the manner in which the heart responds to effort, he should again carefully seek for information which will convey to him a knowledge of the heart's power to respond to effort, the amount of effort which produces evidences of heart exhaustion, and the factors which seem to favour this exhaustion. This applies chiefly to people who are able to be up and about. The manner in which young children run about conveys valuable information. In them, there is no desire to conceal their suffering, and any exertion which induces exhaustion produces such discomfort that they soon stop, and will, if properly interrogated, indicate the reason for their stopping. Hence the knowledge that children enjoy running about and playing games, and do not experience distress until they have exerted themselves as much as their healthy playfellows, will reveal to the physician the fact that, whatever abnormal sign the physical examination has brought to light, the heart's power of response to effort is not affected—a knowledge of the first importance in view of the principles underlying heart failure which have been laid down in previous chapters.

In people who can understand and appreciate their limitations, this essential knowledge is acquired by getting them to relate their experiences during some recent effort, whether playing games, walking on the flat or uphill. It is here of some use to bear in mind that some forms of bodily exercise induce exhaustion more readily than others. Thus, some folks can walk with comfort, but cycling induces exhaustion ; others, again, can cycle with more comfort than walking. One patient, a mechanic, with a badly damaged heart (Case 44) could swing his fore-hammer for many hours without fatigue, but was speedily distressed on walking uphill.

Contributory factors tending to induce exhaustion should be carefully sought for. Sleepless nights are perhaps the most potent in this respect, especially in elderly subjects. Exercise after a meal is often productive of pain and distress, while a greater amount of exercise at other times can be undertaken without discomfort. In any case where the symptoms of heart failure have come on rather rapidly, an inquiry into the amount of effort capable of being performed shortly before, may reveal the fact that the patient was able to undertake a considerable amount without distress. We may then consider that there is a fair amount of vigorous heart muscle, but that in the meantime some agency has induced exhaustion temporarily. Where there is evidence of sudden limitation of the heart's power, inquiries should be directed into the possibility of some other illness inducing the attack, such as a febrile complaint, or the sudden inception of an abnormal rhythm, as auricular fibrillation.

Many patients date the beginning of their illness from the appearance of some symptom, as angina pectoris or breathlessness. An inquiry will usually bring to light the fact that for years symptoms of distress have been gradually becoming more readily induced, until the distress has become so serious as to compel the patient to take note of his limitations.

The chief complaints.—The chief complaints from which patients with heart failure suffer are as follows : ·

Breathlessness. This first appears on the patient making some effort which was not previously attended with discomfort. The various forms of respiratory trouble are described in Chapter X.

The sense of exhaustion. Many people complain of feeling simply ' done up '. The sensation may come on after a bodily or mental effort, and particularly after some excitement. It may be a feeling of exhaustion in general, or it may be located in some definite region, as the epigastrium, or across the chest. It is a symptom common to trivial and transient conditions of heart exhaustion, and to conditions of the utmost gravity, and in the latter case usually associated with other phenomena. We should be chary of attributing the sense of exhaustion to heart conditions even in the presence of some marked abnormality, such as a murmur or irregular action, for this sensation is far more frequently vaso-motor in origin (see Chapter XVI).

Pain may appear in all degrees of intensity, and be of slight or serious import, the most severe not necessarily being the most serious, nor the slightest being of the least significance. It may come on with exertion, and at once bring the patient to a standstill. It may not appear until some hours after the exertion which induced it. It may be felt in various regions of the chest, or arms, or epigastrium, or neck. Its starting-point and radiation should always be noted, as it follows frequently very definite lines, which reveal its true origin. A pain may also be felt in other regions, as over the liver, when there is enlargement of that organ due to heart failure.

A constriction of the chest is sometimes present and often accompanies various degrees of pain.

A persistent aching in some part of the chest or arms is not infrequent in people, particularly in women, when the heart is exhausted. It is usually accompanied by *hyperalgesia or tenderness of the skin and subcutaneous tissues*. The most common site is in or under the left breast, but it may extend over a large area of the chest, particularly in the left side. (Pain and other sensory disturbances are discussed at length in Chapter XIII.)

The patient's consciousness of the heart's action.—A number of individuals may feel a peculiar action of the heart, and sometimes this consciousness alarms and depresses them, and the fear associated with it often causes them to restrict their lives. As these changes in the heart's action occur at intervals irregularly, it frequently happens that the physician has to rely on the patient's description of his sensations for recognizing the nature of his complaint. I have been able in some cases to detect the abnormal actions and have studied the sensations of the patient with the different forms of abnormal action, and from this experience I have in many cases been able to recognize the nature of the abnormalities from the patients' statements alone. Although most of these observations will be given under the different subjects, it may be convenient here to indicate some of the more frequent.

To begin with, it may be remarked that the patient is never conscious of the ' youthful type of irregularity ', so that that form need never be considered as a probable cause of the patient's sensations. The most frequent complaint is associated with extra-systoles. The sensations complained of are various, but the most frequent is the apparent pause. As it occurs frequently at night-time, some people think that the heart stands still for a brief period. The second most frequent complaint is the big beat which follows the long pause, the violent shock often causing alarm. Other sensations and their significance are described in Chapter XXVII.

The patient may be conscious of an increase in the heart's rate, lasting for periods of varying length. It may be accompanied by a sensation of fluttering in the chest or of throbbing. In the latter case it may be associated with a sudden increase of the rate, the heart's contraction arising in a normal manner. Usually some cause can be found, as excitement, or a sudden shock, and it corresponds to what is commonly taken to be palpitation. Its cessation is gradual and passes imperceptibly into the normal rate. Usually it is perfectly regular and corresponds to the condition described as palpitation on p. 174. When the increase in rate is accompanied by the fluttering sensation, it is usually due to an abnormal rhythm, giving rise to one of the forms of paroxysmal tachycardia. The patient may be conscious only of a little discomfort, or he may be so distressed that he may remain motionless until the attack passes off. If the attack persists for hours, he may be compelled to lie down and refrain from movement. Such evidences of distress are very characteristic of the attacks which arise from auricular flutter. In these cases, the rate is usually quite regular. In other cases, the rate is irregular and the patient is conscious of pauses, followed by long beats. These symptoms are usually due to auricular fibrillation. The cessation of these attacks is usually sudden, and the patient may be conscious of a few slow stray beats at the end of the attacks.

Cerebral symptoms.—There are a number of symptoms produced by the brain dependent on the inefficiency of the circulation. I exclude from consideration here the symptoms due to lesions of the blood-vessels, as rupture. The symptoms induced more directly by affections of the heart are caused by a diminished supply of blood reaching the brain, and the nature of the symptoms depends on the extent of that diminution and the period during which the diminished supply lasts.

Dizziness or giddiness.—The first stage of transient cerebral anæmia is shown by a sensation of giddiness. It is seen most characteristically in elderly people (particularly in tall people), when there is arterial degeneration. The attack usually comes on when the individual makes a sudden change in his position, as in rising from a couch. The attack may be limited to a passing sensation of giddiness, or the individual may reel and stagger and clutch at some object for support, or he may fall. In walking, a transient dizziness may come on and the individual may stagger for one or two steps. The liability to these attacks varies at different times—periods of liability varying with periods when the tendency disappears. The attacks occurring in elderly people have no special prognostic significance, as I have known persons exhibit them over a long period of years and live to over eighty years of age. Exactly similar attacks may occur where the heart fails to send sufficient blood into the brain, as in paroxysma tachycardia, where the transient increased rate is accompanied by a diminished output from the heart, or in heart-block when the ventricles stand still for a brief period.

Loss of consciousness.—Syncopal attacks or fainting, when the patient becomes limp and unconscious, occur with a diminished supply of blood to the brain. This can be brought about in a variety of ways, and is generally due to an alteration in the heart's action. I have made observations and taken tracings of several patients during syncopal attacks, and have found a variety of conditions present. The most common has been a slowing of the heart-rate, with great weakness of the pulse, so that only a slight tracing was obtained by the sphygmograph. In one case the heart was beating with great rapidity, but the pulse-beats were small and the patient lay unconscious for nearly half an hour. In another case the heart became very slow in its action with an obscure irregularity, the beats varying in strength. The more frequent forms of syncope are preceded by a preliminary sensation of extreme weakness and loss of sight. ' All became dark ' is a very frequent expression made by the patient after recovery.

There is one form of loss of consciousness which is met with in elderly people. The attacks come without warning and are of momentary duration, resembling *petit mal*. The loss of consciousness may be so transient that it may pass away before one notices a change, and the patient is only conscious of it himself, or he may seem to stare blankly for a minute, or the individual may be sitting at his desk, when his head suddenly drops on the desk, or he may be standing or walking when he suddenly falls. Consciousness at once returns and he is surprised to find himself in a strange posture. There is generally present extensive arterio-sclerosis in these cases, with an irregular heart due to extra-systoles. I am disposed to consider the attacks due to several of these extra-systoles occurring in succession, so that there is a temporary cessation or a diminution in the amount of the blood supplying the brain. Similar attacks occur in the early stages of heart-block, but tracings of the jugular pulse enable one to distinguish the condition. Another cause for the loss of consciousness has recently been recognized, namely, in the condition known as auricular flutter. Here the auricle is beating at a rate of over 300 beats per minute, and the ventricle may respond only to a few of the beats. Suddenly the ventricle may respond to every auricular beat, but the output in consequence is so small that little blood reaches the brain and unconsciousness results (see Fig. 141).

Adam-Stokes syndrome.—When the blood-supply of the brain is completely arrested, loss of consciousness results, and, if prolonged, epileptiform contractions of the muscles of the body may result. The condition of heart affection where this is seen most typically is in heart-block—when the auricle continues to beat at a normal or quickened rate, and the ventricle stands still or beats at a very slow rate. But identical cerebral phenomena may arise from other conditions when the ventricular contraction is too slow, or in the long standstill of the whole heart, probably due to vagus influence, as described by Laslett.

MACKENZIE E

The symptoms due to a diminution of the blood-supply vary according to the degree of the cerebral anæmia. Patients suffering from one of the conditions just mentioned, may show a variety of symptoms, as a feeling of dizziness, a brief loss of consciousness, or a prolonged loss of consciousness with twitchings of the muscles or even convulsions. These varying degrees depend on the frequency of the ventricular systole, the milder phenomena being shown when the ventricular standstill is prolonged, or when the contractions are at rare intervals. In heart-block the patient might have twenty or thirty brief attacks of loss of consciousness in one hour. The patient's pulse on these occasions would be found to disappear.

In one case I noted over 30 attacks of loss of consciousness in 1 hour, which occurred when the ventricle stood still for 10 seconds. When it stood still over 17 seconds convulsions followed.

How long it is possible for the pulse to disappear and recovery of con sciousness to be complete has not been determined in the human subject, nor can the observation of the pulse alone be relied upon to give information. Leonard Hill has pointed out that the merest trickle of blood may keep the brain intact, and the fact that in auricular flutter, where the unconsciousness may last for hours, the small stream of blood is sufficient to nourish the brain though not sufficient to preserve consciousness.

Effect of a failing heart on the cerebral functions.—When the heart is failing, the blood-supply of the brain is not fully maintained and certain symptoms may be detected. Thus the patient can maintain a mental effort, as in reading or in writing, though only for a short time, becoming easily fatigued. The memory for recent events becomes impaired, and what the patient may read is imperfectly retained. In more severe cases *hallucinations* may appear and may take various forms. The patient may imagine that some one is hiding behind a door, and though in conversation admitting the unlikelihood of such a circumstance, yet when left alone the hallucination returns with a sensation of terror. Or the patient may wake up and imagine he sees objects, as an arm projecting from the ceiling, or the sound of some one on the stair, or of soldiers marching past in the street. Head has dealt very fully with this matter, and points out that the patient usually conceals these hallucinations until he is directly questioned concerning them.

Delusion may arise in patients with heart disease, who are taking full doses of digitalis, but it is the digitalis intoxication which causes this mental disturbance.

CHAPTER X

RESPIRATORY SYMPTOMS

Breathlessness, or air hunger.
The sense of suffocation.
Inability to stop breathing.
Quiet, rapid breathing, free from distress.
Continuous laboured breathing.
Laboured breathing brought on by exertion.
Attacks of breathlessness (cardiac asthma).
Cheyne-Stokes respiration.
Slow respiration.
Pulmonary hæmorrhage.
Acute suffocative œdema of the lungs.

THE respiratory symptoms arising in the course of heart affections are so numerous, and the conditions causing them so multifarious, that it is impossible to deal exhaustively with this subject. The factors concerned in the production of any one of the forms of respiratory trouble are often difficult to recognize, and I shall not attempt any strict analysis of these factors, but limit myself to the more apparent clinical forms that accompany heart affections.

Breathlessness, or air hunger.—There is normally a 'desire to breathe', and under certain circumstances this may be intensified so that there is a ' hunger ' for air. The sense of air hunger compels laboured breathing, so that the term ' breathlessness ' includes the subjective sensation and the objective symptom. The centre for respiration in the medulla is influenced by its blood-supply and its nervous connexion with the periphery. A free blood-supply is necessary to supply oxygen and remove the carbonic acid ; and an insufficient interchange of these gases is betrayed by an increased activity of the centre, thus giving rise to breathlessness. The respiratory centre is also receptive to peripheral stimulation, as from sensory nerves of the skin and from cardiac and pulmonary nerves.

An absence of the sense to respire may occur for a short period, as in the apnœic stage of Cheyne-Stokes respiration. John Hunter gives a curious account of an attack from which he suffered, when he lay pulseless but conscious ; observing he did not breathe, and had no desire to do so, he thought he must die if he did not breathe, and by an effort of will continued to breathe until his pulse returned and the automatic respiration was established.

The sense of suffocation.—This is difficult to describe, and is referred usually to the upper part of the chest and throat. The mechanism is obscure. It is a frequent accompaniment of heart affections, from temporary weakness of the heart to the gravest forms of heart disease, and its significance may be slight, or in serious heart trouble it may be a very grave sign. This sense of suffocation may appear in healthy people after violent and prolonged exertion, such as racing or rowing.

Inability to stop breathing.—I have been struck by the fact, while taking tracings of the jugular and other pulses, that many patients are unable to stop breathing. When asked to hold their breath, they will shut their mouths, but are unable to stop breathing through the nose. If the nose be pinched, they then complain of distress (air hunger). This condition only arises in extreme heart failure, and as the heart regains strength we may recognize the fact by the ability to hold the breath.

Quiet, rapid breathing, free from distress.—In many cases of heart failure, when the patient is lying quiet, no definite symptom can be found save that of a respiration more rapid than normal. There is no distress, and the symptom is apt to be overlooked. Sometimes I have failed to recognize it, until I have come to analyse tracings where the respiratory movements had been taken. Where, as sometimes happens, a patient describes certain feelings (as angina pectoris) which we are bound to recognize as cardiac in origin, but where physical examination reveals no sign of mischief, the recognition of more rapid respiration may prevent us from viewing too lightly the condition of the patient. This symptom is of the greatest importance in patients suffering from affections of the heart, particularly in mitral stenosis, in exhausting diseases like typhoid fever, and in all conditions that compel the weakly, and particularly the elderly, to lie on their backs, as e. g. when suffering from a broken leg. In such cases the lying in bed, while favouring the work of the left ventricle, embarrasses the work of the right by restricting the respiratory movement. As a result of this restraint of the ribs, the breathing becomes shallow. The effect is to retard the flow of blood through the less mobile part of the lungs, and in consequence stasis at the base of the lungs results.

Continuous laboured breathing.—This occurs only when the heart failure is so extreme that the reserve force is exhausted. The patient cannot lie down, but sits up, breathing in short quick gasps. The slightest exertion, such as is entailed by changing to a more comfortable position, immediately aggravates the distress. This form of breathing is best seen in cases of dilatation of the heart with the rapid irregular pulse due to auricular fibrillation, and, in fact, the whole respiratory distress is often the outcome of the embarrassment due to this condition of fibrillation (Chapter XXX). With slowing of the heart's action and other evidences of cardiac improvement, the respiratory distress gradually disappears, but is liable to be brought on by exertion.

Laboured breathing brought on by exertion.—This is a symptom common to a great many affections besides heart troubles, but its association with an inefficient heart is so common that it should at all times lead to an inquiry as to the condition of the heart. It may occur with every form of heart affection. It is of very great use in estimating the strength of the heart, as its appearance indicates in a rough way the degree of exhaustion ; the slighter the exertion provoking it, the less is the reserve power of the heart. On the other hand, improvement may be indicated by the gradual return of the ability of the patient to undertake with comfort greater exertion. The forms of exertion that induce it are very puzzling. Some patients can lift great weights, and pursue the hard work associated with their calling, yet cannot walk up a slight hill without complaining of being short-winded ; or they suffer in the same way on going into the cold air. Some can cycle in comfort, while others cannot cycle, but can walk with comfort on the level. I cannot explain these and other peculiarities, but note them as clinical facts.

Attacks of breathlessness (cardiac asthma).—A form of respiratory distress which comes on usually in the night, sometimes suddenly arousing the patient from sleep, has received the name of ' Cardiac Asthma '. An attack of this sort is sometimes the first serious sign of heart trouble, though, on inquiry, an account can usually be obtained of a period prior to the attack when there was a distinct limitation of the field of cardiac response. The patient may have gone to bed in his usual health and according to his usual custom, and after three or four hours' sleep he is awakened with a feeling of suffocation, and an intense desire to breathe deeply. He sits up in bed, and breathes in deep and laboured fashion. A sense of great prostration may add to his suffering. Wheezing sounds may appear in the chest, and he may cough up some frothy phlegm. The attack may last for half an hour or longer ; then the breathing becomes quieter, and he is able to lie down, though he keeps starting up, and finally assumes a position with his head and shoulders raised, passing the remainder of the night in uneasy slumber. Once these attacks begin they are apt to continue, and the nights of the patient often become periods of great distress. The fear of the attack may keep the patient awake, and should he drop off to sleep, he awakes with a start at the first sign of embarrassed breathing.

The class of case which shows this condition most characteristically is the elderly, and those who suffer from arterial and cardiac sclerosis. They frequently have a high blood-pressure, and the heart is usually regular except for the presence of occasional or frequent extra-systoles. In these cases we sometimes find the best examples of the pulsus alternans. The cause of this form of asthma is not quite clear. I have found the greatest distress induced by this condition in many cases insusceptible to treatment ; but I have given massive doses of oxygen in a few cases with very gratifying success. In most cases this symptom is a very grave sign, and usually indicates an exhaustion of the heart so extreme that only a very slight improvement can be hoped for, especially when associated with the pulsus alternans and other signs of heart exhaustion. Similar attacks of breathlessness occur at the end of the apnœic stage of Cheyne-Stokes respiration, and I am not at all sure, from recent observations I have been making, that all cases of cardiac asthma may not arise from this apnœic stage. The matter needs further investigation.

Cheyne-Stokes respiration.—In all cases of serious heart failure, associated with breathlessness, quiet observation should be made when the patient is perfectly still, and nothing attracting his attention. Under such circumstances, the patient's breathing may occasionally be found to take on a peculiar rhythmical character. Instruction should also be given for the attendants to note the character of respiration during sleep. The character of the breathing is a rhythmical variation in the size of the respiratory movements—a gradual passage from a state of complete or almost complete cessation to a condition of breathing where the respiratory movements are deep and laboured. When the breathing gradually slows and ultimately stops, the patient's mental condition frequently becomes a blank, and is accompanied usually by twitching of some muscles, especially to be noticed in those of the hand and arm. With the resumption of the breathing, he wakes, and may resume a conversation that he had been pursuing before the slowing of the breathing set in.

Usually no material change can be detected in the action of the heart during the diverse phases of respiration. Sometimes, however, certain changes may appear in the pulse coincident with the respiratory phases, as the appearance of the pulsus alternans during the respiratory phase, or its intensification, if already present. The blood-pressure may fall 5 or 10 mm. Hg. during the apnœic stage.

Usually the patient is unaware of the occurrence of this periodic respiration, and it causes him no distress. On the other hand, it may occasion acute distress : the patient may drop off to sleep, and this form of respiration gradually appears, and during the apnœic stage the patient awakes with a most distressful sensation of suffocation. So terrible is this that patients, though extremely exhausted, may spring suddenly out of bed in an extremity of terror.

The great majority of cases of Cheyne-Stokes respiration are brought on by, or associated with, degenerative changes in the myocardium, arterial disease, and high blood-pressure. It disappears with the sudden fall of blood-pressure due to dilatation of the heart. It may be made temporarily to disappear by massive doses of oxygen ; or on the inhalation of small quantities of CO_2 (Pembery). Haldane and Poulton have produced the condition by forced breathing, and conclude that the periodic breathing is due to the ' disappearance of the (indirect) excitatory effects of want of oxygen in the respiratory centre '. G. A. Sutherland has shown me tracings from a child where marked Cheyne-Stokes breathing occurred, the rate during the respiratory stage reaching 160 respirations per minute.

In the great majority of cases of arterio-sclerosis and Bright's disease, the appearance of Cheyne-Stokes respiration is usually the beginning of the end, the patient dying within a few months or weeks, or even a few days of its onset. It may be present in cases of extreme heart failure, associated with auricular fibrillation and auricular flutter. In these conditions it is not of serious significance, inasmuch as it disappears when the ventricular rate slows under digitalis, and the patient may live a useful life for years afterwards.

Cheyne-Stokes respiration must be kept distinct from certain other forms of periodic respiration. Hibernating animals show a form of periodic respiration, also some children during sleep. It appears also in some cases of tubercular meningitis.

Loss of consciousness does not always ensue during the apnœic stage of Cheyne-Stokes respiration, as shown by the following instance. I saw in consultation a clergyman, aged fifty, who had a paralytic seizure two years previously, resulting in an ordinary hemiplegia. When I saw him he was lying in bed quite conscious, extremely prostrate, with a pulse rate of 180 per minute, with typical periodic respiration. During the apnœic stage he was quite conscious, and could talk intelligently ; his voice was faint and reedy in quality, diminishing in loudness towards the end of his remarks. His medical attendant told me he had suffered off and on from this condition for three years. This case corresponds to a description given by John Hunter, who says, ' A gentleman had a singular asthmatic affection, and his breathing gradually stopped and again gradually recurred, but became violent, and thus constantly and alternately held two or three minutes, and when the breathing ceased yet he spoke although but faintly.'

Slow respiration.—There are a number of individuals in whom the respirations during rest are much slower than normal, 7 to 10 per minute. The slow respiration induces an irregular action of the heart, due to stimulation of the sino-auricular node. The condition is probably due to vagus stimulation, and I have seen it occur from the administration of digitalis.

Pulmonary hæmorrhage.—Bleeding from the lungs is not an infrequent complication in heart failure. It is most commonly seen in the terminal stages of arterio-sclerosis, with the fall of blood-pressure that indicates dilatation of the heart and stasis of blood in the lungs. In these cases the expectoration is either blood-stained, or it is almost entirely composed of lumps of dark clotted blood. In the post-mortem examination there are usually found several hard patches of ecchymosed blood at the base of the lungs. In the young with mitral stenosis, profuse hæmoptysis may occur, and is generally a sign of extreme gravity.

In other forms of heart affection, especially in the later stages of auricular fibrillation, hæmorrhage more or less free may occur, and give the patient considerable relief, and be followed by no serious consequence. In fact, if we find the patient on the whole with a fair amount of reserve force, whatever the nature of the heart lesion, there need be no immediate alarm from a free hæmoptysis when due to cardiac trouble.

A serious form of hæmoptysis arises from a pulmonary infarct, or a pulmonary apoplexy; in these cases the symptoms are extremely varied in severity. Thus I have seen patients with phlebitis of the veins of the leg, or after confinement, die in a few minutes with symptoms of great respiratory distress. In some cases I have seen the most intense dyspnœa with gradual loss of consciousness go on for four or five hours, and then suddenly the dyspnœa ceases and the consciousness returns. After twelve hours the patient has expectorated large quantities of pink-stained jelly-like mucus. I have also seen cases of pulmonary infarct, as after a fracture of the tibia, where the only evidence was the expectoration, for three or four days, of dark-coloured blood, in small quantities at a time, followed by complete recovery. Presumably the difference in the symptoms in these cases depended on the size of the infarct or the extent of the apoplexy.

Acute suffocative œdema of the lungs.—A peculiar form of œdema, of which I have only seen a few cases, is that in which the patient is suddenly seized with breathlessness, usually during the night, followed speedily by the welling out of the mouth and nose of large quantities of froth. Sometimes the patient succumbs within an hour of the commencement of the attack, at other times after a few days. The conditions giving rise to it are obscure, and it occurs in a great variety of cases, and mitral stenosis seems slightly to predispose to its occurrence.

CHAPTER XI

REFLEX OR PROTECTIVE PHENOMENA

Classification of symptoms in visceral disease.
Insensitiveness of the viscera to ordinary stimuli.
The mechanism by which pain and other reflex phenomena are produced in visceral disease
    (the viscero-sensory reflex).
The purpose of visceral reflexes.
Why pain is referred to regions remote from the organ.

Classification of symptoms in visceral disease.—When the symptoms of visceral disease are carefully analysed there appears a great similarity in the nature and origin of certain of them, which permits of their division into three groups : first, symptoms due to changes in the organ itself—in the case of the circulatory system, changes in the movements of the heart and blood-vessels ; second, symptoms observed in remote organs and tissues which suffer indirectly from the primary lesion—for instance, jaundiced skin in liver affections, uræmic convulsions in renal disease and dropsy, œdema or albuminuria in heart failure ; third, reflex or protective phenomena, which form the subject of this chapter.

While the character of the symptoms in the first two divisions depends on the size and specific function of each organ, the reflex phenomena produced by all organs have a great resemblance. This is particularly the case with all the hollow muscular organs. They have similar origins and their reflexes are similar in character, and are only modified by the special development of each. In spite of the seeming dissimilarity in the form and function of the digestive tube, uterus, ureter, and heart, they are fundamentally the same, and the reflexes associated with them are of a like nature. Hence the nature of obscure symptoms in affections of the heart may be revealed by an inquiry into the meaning of similar phenomena presented by these organs, which have at first sight so little affinity with it.

Insensitiveness of the viscera to ordinary stimuli.—In order to appreciate the reflex symptoms in visceral disease, we must keep in mind the functions of the nerves that supply them.

The nerve-supply of the body is included in the two great systems, the autonomic and the cerebro-spinal. The autonomic includes the whole of the sympathetic nerves, and certain cerebral nerves, of which the vagus is the only one that concerns us here.

The tissues and organs supplied by the nerves from the autonomic system, are not endowed with sensation in the sense in which the term is used in regard to tissues supplied by the cerebro-spinal nerves. The skin, muscle, and other tissues of the external body-wall are readily sensitive to all forms of stimuli that produce such sensations as touch, pain, heat, and cold, whereas the viscera supplied only by the autonomic system are totally irresponsive to such stimuli. Thus such organs as the heart, stomach, bowels, liver, kidney, can be cut, torn, burnt, and no sensation elicited. Yet, as we know, pain of a most excruciating character can arise from visceral affections. Harvey describes how he touched the exposed heart of the son of Viscount Montgomery and found it without sensation. Surgeons in pre-chloroform days incidentally refer to the insensitiveness of the viscera. Thus Richerand describes how, in operating in the neighbourhood of the heart, he found the pericardium insensitive, and I have repeatedly verified this observation in cases where the ribs have been resected.

The following experience illustrates the insensitiveness of the viscera, and at the same time affords an insight into the manner in which visceral pain arises. I had occasion to resect the bowel in a conscious subject under the following circumstances. He had an umbilical hernia, and had worn for years a pad tightly pressed over it, until the skin had ulcerated. The ulceration had finally penetrated into the bowel, and his food was discharged through the fistula. It was resolved to resect the bowel, but the patient would not be anæsthetized. Observing that the skin was already ulcerated, and that the tissues forming the external wall were not very sensitive, so that the abdominal cavity could be opened with little pain, I reasoned that the after-operation could be performed painlessly. It turned out as I had expected, and I was able to break down numerous old and recent peritoneal adhesions, to detach them from the liver and bowel, to resect a piece of bowel and mesentery, and to stitch these structures without the patient experiencing the slightest sensation. But I found that he occasionally groaned with pain when I was not touching him, and watching to see the cause I found that the upper part of the resected bowel, which was laid on one side in a warm aseptic cloth, occasionally passed into peristalsis, contracting from a wide tube to a thick fleshy rod ; when this happened the patient groaned with pain. I asked him where he felt the pain, and he passed his hand invariably over the umbilical region. I started the peristalsis several times by slightly pinching the bowel, and each time the patient felt the pain. Here before my eyes was the cause of the pain, and the seat of origin of the pain was at least twelve inches away from the part in which the pain was felt.

From this experience the following deductions can be made : first, that the stimuli that produce pain and other sensations in the external body-wall are not adequate to produce these sensations when applied to the viscera ; second, that violent contraction of non-striped muscular fibres can produce pain, but the region in which the pain is felt is different from that in which the contracting muscle lies.

This isolated experience has been confirmed by many other observations I have made, and also by the observations of Lennander, and in part confirms the experiments made by Haller more than 150 years ago upon animals, when he showed that they were indifferent to severe mutilation of their viscera, so long as the external body-wall was not interfered with.

These experiences compel one to look for an explanation of the production of visceral pain other than that which suffices to explain its production from the stimulation of the external body-wall ; and the following explanation seems satisfactorily to account for the matter, and to explain the peculiar nature of the sensory phenomena that arise in visceral disease.

The mechanism by which pain and other reflex phenomena are produced in visceral disease (the viscero-sensory reflex).—When a nerve that terminates in a sense organ is stimulated in any part of its course from the periphery to the brain, a stimulus is conveyed to the brain of a kind similar to that induced when the peripheral end-organ is stimulated. Thus the stimulation of any part of the optic nerve or auditory nerve gives rise to the sensation of light or of sound. In the same manner, if a sensory nerve be stimulated in any part of its course through the brain, spinal cord, or trunk of the nerve, the resultant sensation is referred to the peripheral distribution of the nerve in the external body-wall.

Fig. 5 is a diagram representing the brain and spinal cord (S.C.) with a sensory nerve (S.N.) passing from the skin (Sk) through the spinal cord to the brain. A stimulus applied to the skin, or to the sensory nerve between the skin and the cord, or to the sensory nerve in the cord, gives rise to a sensation referred by the brain to the portion of skin innervated by the nerve, though the stimulus may have affected the nerve after it had left the skin. In the diagram, a viscus (H) is represented, and its nerve (Sy. N.) is seen passing to the spinal cord. In the normal processes of life, a stream of energy from the viscera is continually passing by the afferent nerves to the spinal cord, and continuously playing upon the efferent nerves that run to muscles, blood-vessels, and so forth. These processes are conducted so that they give rise to no appreciable sensation. If, however, a morbid process in a viscus gives rise to an increased stimulation of the nerves passing from the viscus to the spinal cord, this increased stimulation affects neighbouring centres. If it excites the sensory nerve represented in the diagram as passing from the skin to the brain, the resulting sensation will be referred by the brain, not to the viscus, but to the peripheral distribution of the sensory nerve. Thus it was that when, in the course of the operation which I have described, the bowel contracted, the resulting pain was referred not to the bowel, but to the peripheral distribution of the sensory nerves in the region of the umbilicus; thus the pain in visceral disease is seen to be of a reflex character—*a viscero-sensory reflex.*

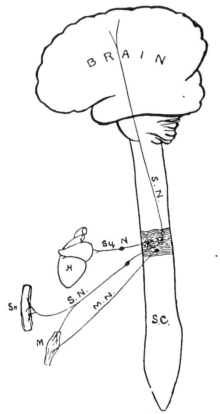

Fig. 5. Diagram showing the mechanism producing visceral pain. From the viscus *H*, an abnormal stimulus is conveyed by the sympathetic nerve (*Sy. N.*) to the spinal cord *S.C.* On reaching the cord, the abnormal stimulus spreads beyond the sympathetic centre, and affects nerve-cells in its immediate neighbourhood. The cells so stimulated react according to their function, the sensory causing a sensation which the brain recognizes as pain, and refers to the peripheral distribution of the sensory nerve (*S.N.*) in the skin (*Sk*) or muscle (*M*), the motor (*M.N.*) producing contraction of the muscle (*M*). The abnormal stimulation may leave a portion of the cord abnormally irritable (shaded portion), so that the tissues supplied by nerves from that portion of the cord are hyperalgesic, and attacks of pain, as of angina pectoris, are more easily provoked.

In the diagram there is shown a motor nerve (*M.N.*) arising in the cord and passing to a muscle (*M*). The stimulus from the viscus (*H*), passing into the spinal cord, may excite the cells of origin of the motor nerves, with the result that the muscle is stimulated to contract ; hence we get the *viscero-motor reflex*. This reflex is best seen in affections of the abdominal viscera when the abdominal wall becomes hard, due to tonic contraction of the muscles.

When a portion of the spinal cord becomes violently stimulated by reason of a visceral affection, that portion of the cord may remain for a lengthened period in an over-excitable state, so that all the nerves that arise from this portion of the cord may be much more easily stimulated. This can be demonstrated in many cases of visceral disease by the hyperalgesic state of portions of the external body-wall, and by the exaggerated motor reflexes. In such instances, stimulation of the skin or muscles, as by light pinching between finger and thumb of such weak force that normally it would only result in the sensation of touch, is felt by the patient as pain. Light stroking of the skin with a pin-head may be felt as pain, and produces very readily a strong reflex contraction of the muscles whose nerves arise from the same portion of the cord. A further result of this *irritable focus* in the cord is that the visceral stimulation more readily induces pain, and not only may the original attacks of pain (as in angina pectoris, renal and biliary colic) be more easily induced, but stimuli from other sources may induce the attack of pain. Thus in cases of gall-stones with hyperalgesia of the external body-wall over the region of the liver, the ingestion of the food into the stomach may give rise to much pain in the hyperalgesic tissues.

The purpose of visceral reflexes.—Reflexes have been studied with the greatest minuteness, and the work of Sherrington demonstrates the extraordinary variety and complexity of the spinal reflexes, but their purpose has been to a great extent overlooked. The main purpose of many reflexes has been either to remove the body from the reach of injurious influences, or to interpose a firmly contracted muscle between the agent threatening the injury and the organ. It may even be true, as Herbert Spencer suggests, that the evolution of muscles and the segmentation of the body was due to the necessity of protection when the external body-wall changed from an insensitive hard carapace to a sensitive mobile covering. The way that the protective mechanism comes into play, is by exalting the sensitiveness of reflexes. Thus if an organ suffer injury, as by inflammation, the surrounding portion of the external body-wall immediately has its protective functions exalted. This is usually accomplished by increased sensitiveness of the skin and underlying structures, so that touch arouses at once a strong and vigorous contraction of the protective muscles. These muscles themselves become much more sensitive to pain, and, as painful stimuli are the most provocative causes of reflexes, acutely tender muscles may remain permanently contracted.

To illustrate the meaning and purpose of visceral pain and allied phenomena, a case of gastric ulcer may be taken. The ulcer may be situated on the posterior wall and at the cardiac orifice of the stomach, while the sensation of pain is referred to the epigastrium. Here the skin and muscles may be found exceedingly tender to touch and light pressure. The reflex contraction of the underlying recti muscles is extremely lively and powerful. If you try gently to palpate the stomach, these muscles at once become so strongly contracted that it is utterly impossible to feel what is underneath. What is Nature doing ? Manifestly it is interposing a most efficient barrier between the intruding hand and the diseased organ—the whole being a protective mechanism. Had the stomach only been sensitive, the hand would have reached the stomach, but by the reflex mechanism the external body-wall is made sensitive, and the powerful reflex contraction of the muscles effectively guards the stomach from injury. The same protective mechanism is involved in joint-disease. Thus the shoulder-joint may be found immobile. Put the patient under chloroform and all the muscles relax, and a grating may be detected on moving the joint. It is evident that here the injured joint required protection, and the muscles responded to their first and primitive duty.

Pain itself, Hilton pointed out, has the same purpose, that is to say, protection. It commands at once cessation of any action that induces it; and this protective function is seen nowhere more clearly than in heart affections.

Why pain is referred to regions remote from the organ.—In a great many instances the pain is referred to situations remote from the organ giving rise to it. Thus the pain of biliary colic may be felt in the epigastrium, the pain of renal colic in the testicle, the pain of heart affections in the arm.

The reason for this is that in the course of development, the tissues that in a low scale of life immediately covered the organ, have been displaced. Thus the pain felt in the testicle in renal calculus is due to the fact that in its journey down to the scrotum, the coverings of the testicle receive a twig from the first lumbar nerve, from which the kidney is also innervated, and when the centre of this nerve in the spinal cord is stimulated, as in renal calculus, the pain is felt in the testicle, and exquisite pain may be elicited on pressing the testicle. On the other hand, one never finds the skin of the scrotum hyperalgesic in these cases, but only the deep covering of the testicle, because the scrotum is supplied by the sacral nerves.

CHAPTER XII

The Relation of the Heart to Cerebro-spinal Nerves

The relationship of the heart to sensory nerves.
Cutaneous distribution of the cervical and upper dorsal nerves.
Herpes zoster and sensory disorders.
Areas in which pain and hyperalgesia are felt in affections of the heart.
Hyperalgesia in acute dilatation of the heart and liver.
Symptoms in the head and neck (vagal reflexes).
The pain of angina pectoris as a viscero-sensory reflex.
The viscero-motor reflex.

In the last chapter the principles and purpose underlying the production of pain and other sensory disturbances in affection of the viscera were discussed ; in this and the two following chapters the application of these principles to the study of the heart will be dealt with.

The relationship of the heart to sensory nerves.—In order to appreciate the mechanism of the pain felt in affections of the heart, the manner in which the upper dorsal nerves are distributed should be borne in mind. Ross has pointed out that in the primitive vertebrates before the development of the limbs, each spinal nerve is distributed segmentally round one half of the body (Fig. 6). The upper dorsal nerves are, therefore, entirely distributed over the body-wall and to the tissues covering the heart. The upper limbs, as they bud out from the trunk in their development, drag with them away from the trunk portions of the cervical and upper dorsal nerves, so that parts of the first and second dorsal nerves are distributed to the ulnar border of the forearm and inner surface of the upper arm. Thus, a stimulus originating in the heart and affecting the cord area of the first and second dorsal nerves, would be felt in the lower vertebrate as pain over the heart, whereas in man it would be felt in the upper arm or in the forearm (Fig. 7). This peculiar distribution of the sensory nerves to the chest and arms resulting from the development of the limbs, provides a unique field for observing the mechanism of sensory disturbance in affections of the heart.

Cutaneous distribution of the cervical and upper dorsal nerves.—In order to appreciate more fully the regions in which pain is felt, and the hyperæsthetic fields in heart failure, it will be advisable to bear in mind the distribution to the skin of the nerves implicated. The cervical nerves, from the second to the fourth, supply the skin of the back of the head, the neck, and the shoulders. The fourth cervical also descends to the front of the chest at least as low as the third rib, where they overlap with the second dorsal supply. The fifth and sixth cervical nerves are distributed in the arm, in an area roughly described as the outer half of the upper arm, the radial half of the forearm, and part of the thumb. The seventh cervical is distributed to the hands and fingers, the eighth also to the ring and little fingers, to the ulnar border of the hand, and with the first dorsal supply the ulnar half of the forearm. The second and third dorsal are distributed on the inner half of the upper arm, axilla, and chest, meeting and overlapping with the fourth cervical, as already stated (Fig. 7). The fourth and fifth dorsal are distributed to the chest, the latter descending as low as the upper part of the epigastrium. It must be borne in mind that each spinal nerve practically divides into three parts after the junction of the posterior and anterior nerve roots, viz. a posterior, a lateral, and a ventral. It is the lateral and ventral divisions that are involved in the

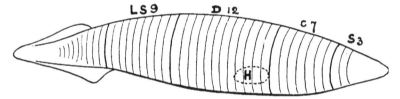

Fig. 6.   Diagrammatic representation of a primitive vertebrate animal to show the distribution of the sensory nerves.   For clearness of comparison the number of segments is represented to be the same as in man, and the heart occupies the same position.   Each nerve is shown as limited in its distribution to one segment (after Ross).

supply to the arm, the posterior divisions being distributed to the skin of the back. Thus, then, with the exception of the posterior divisions, the nerves from the fourth cervical to the second dorsal are distributed to the arms. The second dorsal nerve (occasionally also the first) does send branches to the front of the chest. There is thus an interesting test provided in considering the distribution of any sensory abnormality—pain or hyperæsthesia—that arises in the chest. If it affects a series of nerve centres in succession, it will not pass up the chest and over the clavicle, but will descend on the inner aspect of the arm to the ulnar border of the hand (Fig. 7). In like manner pain arising in the neck, and produced by stimulation of a descending series of the cervical nerve roots, will proceed down the chest for only a short distance, and then be deflected down the outer portion of the upper arm to the radial border of the hand.

Herpes zoster and sensory disorders.—Many years ago, while studying these sensory phenomena, I was struck by the resemblance of the situation occupied by the eruption in herpes zoster to the situation of the pain and hyperæsthesia in certain cases of visceral disease. Up to this time the eruption in herpes zoster had been described only in relation to the peripheral nerves ; but inasmuch as these nerves are usually composed of fibres from more than one nerve root, no very satisfactory information had resulted. I recognized the fact that herpes zoster was probably due to the affection of the root of the nerve (probably the ganglion on the posterior root), as Head and Campbell have since demonstrated ; with this knowledge, the area in which the eruption and hyperalgesia occur becomes intelligible and instructive. Frequently there is evidence that more roots than one are affected, but these are generally neighbouring roots. It is difficult to say when one nerve root only is affected. There are other symptoms present besides the herpes zoster that help to complete the picture, and to indicate the direction in which neighbouring nerve roots are distributed to the skin. The most important of these other symptoms are pain and hyperalgesia of skin and subcutaneous tissues, and when the eruption is scanty or absent it is difficult to decide whether these phenomena are not due to some visceral disease.

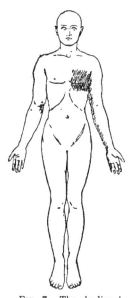

Fig. 7. The shading in the left chest and arm and inner side of the right elbow shows the distribution of the hyperalgesia after several attacks of angina Pectoris. The pain was felt in these regions during an attack. (Case 54.)

Areas in which pain and hyperalgesia are felt in affections of the heart.—In the great majority of cases the pain complained of in heart affections is referred to some part of the chest-wall, most frequently under the left breast, and across the middle of the chest at different levels. In many cases it may at first be limited to a small area in the chest (Fig. 8) and later radiate from the starting-point in different directions, chiefly towards the axilla and down the left arm (Fig. 7). It is curious how difficult it is to get an exact account of the region where it is very severe, unless the patient is asked carefully to observe while the pain is felt. The most common region into which the pain radiates is shown in the shaded area of Fig. 7, and it is interesting to compare the area with the distribution of the eruption in a case of herpes zoster (Fig. 9). In some cases the presence of hyperalgesia permits the areas to be mapped out. When the radiation of the pain follows some seemingly erratic course, it is possible that it is due to an abnormal nerve distribution. Thus in Case 29, the attacks of pain extended into the left arm and affected with great severity the ball of the thumb ; and Fig. 10 is a sketch I made during one of the many examinations, and its accuracy was confirmed by the patient, who was an educated and intelligent

man. Shortly after 1 made these observations, 1 saw a case of herpes
zoster, where the eruption in the arm and hand occupied the same peculiar
distribution as in Fig. 11, which is taken from a photograph.

Although, in the great majority of cases, the pain arises in the chest and
radiates into the arm, in some cases the pain arises in the hand or arm
and radiates to the chest, and in a few cases the pain may be restricted to
the arm (Cases 22 and 31). I witnessed in two patients attacks of this sort,
and during the attack they nursed their arms across the chest and rocked

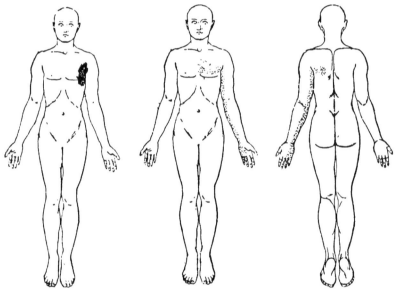

FIG. 8. The shading in   FIG. 9. The dotted region shows the distribution of the
the left chest shows the area   eruption in a case of herpes zoster. It has the same distri-
of hyperalgesia after the first bution on the left side as the hyperalgesia in Fig. 8.
attack of angina pectoris.
(Case 54.)

themselves backwards and forwards in an agony of pain. The pain is
sometimes referred to the insides of one or both elbow-joints; thus, one
man complained of pain striking with great severity across the middle of
the chest and on the inside of the left elbow. He could not tell where
the pain came first, nor which was the most severe. In this connexion it
is interesting to note an experience related by Sherrington. Ou applying
a mustard plaster to the upper part of his chest, after a few minutes he became
conscious of a disagreeable smarting pain in the inner side of the left elbow.
This can only arise from the stimulus passing from the skin of the chest
to the central nervous system, and then stimulating the centre of the sensory

nerves which supply the skin of the elbow. In Fig. 7 there is a shaded area in the inner side of the right elbow, which represents an area of acute hyperalgesia, which I detected in this patient (Case 54). The pain may extend to the same region on the right side, but as a rule it is less severe, and in some instances it is entirely limited to the right side and may be of great severity.

An experience of another kind showed the relation of the distribution of pain to the sensory nerves. While investigating the goose-skin (pilo-

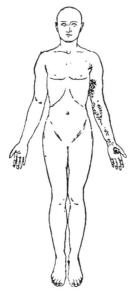 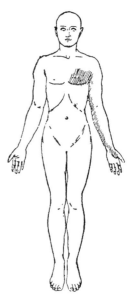

FIG. 10. The shading shows the region in which pain was felt during an attack of angina pectoris. (Case 29.)

FIG. 11. The dotted line shows the distribution of the eruption in a case of herpes zoster. Compare this area with that in Fig. 10.

motor reflex), I was wont to rub lightly and briskly the skin under the left breast. As a result a local goose-skin eruption would appear, and occasionally this would spread up the chest and down the inside of the left arm. The eruption would be accompanied by a chilly sensation spreading to the same region and reaching down as far as the little finger. I tried this experiment on one patient (Case 22), who also suffered from angina pectoris, and he said he felt the chilly sensation. I asked him to describe the region in which the sensation was felt, and with a look of surprise he remarked, 'It is just where I feel the pain,' and he indicated the inner sides of the upper arm and forearm.

We may get the pain, in rare instances, extending down the arm in the region of distribution of the fifth and sixth cervical nerves. Thus in one patient who suffered from extreme attacks of heart failure, and who had mitral stenosis and auricular fibrillation, the pain struck with great severity in the left side of the neck and extended down the outer side of the shoulder and arm to the elbow. After the pain subsided the skin of the neck became very tender.

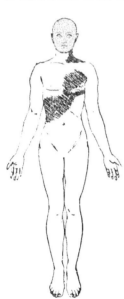

Hyperalgesia in acute dilatation of the heart and liver.—In a few cases of paroxysmal tachycardia, especially that due to auricular fibrillation, I have noticed marked sensory disturbances follow the dilatation of the heart and liver, which occurs in consequence of the abnormal rhythm. The shaded areas in Fig. 12 show the region where the skin was found tender in one patient (Case 51). There was a diffuse ill-defined patch over the liver which merged into the cardiac area. There was also tenderness of the left neck, the sterno-mastoid being very sensitive to pressure. Within a few hours of the cessation of the attack of tachycardia all the symptoms had disappeared, and the heart and liver had diminished markedly in size. Such phenomena are not infrequently present in more chronic attacks of heart failure, with dilatation of the heart and liver.

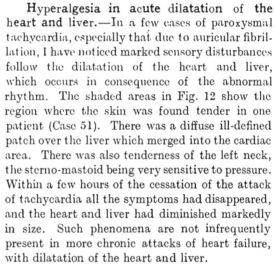

FIG. 12. The shaded area in the abdomen, chest, and neck shows the distribution of the continuous hyperalgesia in a case with rapid dilatation of the heart and liver in a case of paroxysmal tachycardia (auricular fibrillation). (Case 51.)

Symptoms in the head and neck (vagal reflexes).—So far the symptoms that have been referred to are those in association with the sympathetic nerve supply. In carefully examining the patients I became aware of distinct sensory abnormalities in other fields. The most conspicuous of these was tenderness on lightly pinching the sterno-mastoid and trapezius muscles. That the muscles themselves are tender admits of no doubt. The skin and subcutaneous tissues may be pinched without evincing any abnormal tenderness; but, when the muscle substance is pinched, tenderness, sometimes exquisite, is evoked. Finding the sterno-mastoid and the trapezius so frequently tender, and having regard to the nerve supply, the spinal accessory, with its known association at its origin with the vagus, I considered that the transmission of the irritation to the spinal accessory was from the heart by the vagus. While the abnormal sensitiveness of the sterno-mastoid muscle and of the trapezius are the most constant phenomena, there are frequently sensory disorders in other places. Thus, pain may be felt in the neck, in the head, back and front, and along the lower jaw (Cases 27 and 42). Hyperalgesia may also be present in these areas, and the patient may complain of pain in swallowing after an attack of pain felt in the jaw and throat. These areas demonstrate the connexion of the nerves so affected at their centres with the vagus. As a rule the sensory phenomena occurring in the head and neck, are associated with those occurring in the upper dorsal and lower cervical nerves. As a matter of routine, in many cases it is my custom to press over the second left rib in the nipple line, over the upper dorsal vertebræ, pinch the left sterno-mastoid muscle and the trapezius immediately above the spine of the scapula. If sensory phenomena are present, they are usually manifested in one, if not in all, of these areas. In some cases all are extraordinarily sensitive, and, excepting some obscure pains, no other sensory disorder may be present. Other reflexes of vagal origin are sometimes met with during or after an attack of angina pectoris, as an abundant flow of saliva (Case 28), or the secretion of a large quantity of pale urine of low specific gravity (Case 23).

The pain of angina pectoris as a viscero-sensory reflex.—The usual description given of the pain in angina pectoris, is that it is felt in the heart and shoots into the arm, or that there are two pains, a local pain in the heart, and a referred pain in the arm. If, however, a careful analysis be made of all the symptoms present, facts will be found that practically demonstrate that in angina pectoris there is but one kind of pain, and that its production is in accordance with the law I have attempted to establish, namely, that it is a viscero-sensory reflex. It is not in every case that one is able to demonstrate the truth of this hypothesis, but the conclusions drawn from observations made in suitable cases may legitimately be applied to others. Shortly, these observations are, that the pain in the very gravest cases may be felt in regions distant from the heart, as in the left arm ; that this pain is identical in character with that felt over the heart ; that the pain may originally start in parts distant from the heart and gradually approach and persist over the heart ; and lastly, that the tissues of the external body-wall over the heart may be found extremely hyperalgesic after the pain has passed away. From this last fact it is inferred that, inasmuch as the seat of pain corresponds to the region of hyperalgesia, therefore the pain was felt by the hyperalgesic nerves. To assume otherwise is to ignore a principle that explains satisfactorily the sensation of pain wherever arising.

The viscero-motor reflex.—So far I have dealt mainly with the viscero-sensory reflex, but no less striking evidence can be found of the viscero-motor reflex among the group of symptoms included in the term ' angina pectoris '. Some would limit the term ' angina pectoris ' to that class of cases where, in addition to the pain, there is a sense of constriction in the chest, amounting to the sensation at times as if the chest were gripped in a vice, or as if the breast-bone would break. I am convinced that these sensations of constriction arise from spasm of the intercostal muscles, and correspond to the hard contraction of the flat abdominal muscles, in affections of the abdominal viscera. If one watches a case of what is called ' muscular rheumatism ', where the intercostal muscles are affected, and where these muscles are stimulated by the slightest movement to violent cramp-like contractions, one cannot but be struck by the resemblance to the description, given by the gripping sensation experienced by patients suffering from certain affections of the heart. I have watched the attacks in such cases, and could find no difference between them and those where the sense of contraction was the chief symptom in heart disease. Moreover, I have seen in consultation a few cases where angina pectoris had been diagnosed in mistake for this muscular contraction. The viscero-motor reflex may be present alone, or, as is more commonly the case, it may be associated with the pain, and the symptoms may arise at different times owing to an attack (Case 8). The sense of constriction due to this viscero-motor reflex is seen best in the elderly, where it may be considered a symptom of one form of the terminal affections of the heart due to senile changes. I have found it a precursor of steadily advancing cardiac weakness, and although, for a time, considerable relief may be afforded, the changes in the heart are so advanced that in the nature of things only one end can be looked for. In such cases pain may be absent.

CHAPTER XIII

SENSORY DISORDERS AS A RESULT OF HEART AFFECTION

Conditions in which angina pectoris is induced.
Conditions giving rise to attacks of angina pectoris.
Conditions predisposing to an attack.
Association of angina pectoris with exhaustion of the muscle of the heart.
Cardiac exhaustion and the susceptibility to nerve stimulation.
The sensory phenomena produced by over-exertion in healthy hearts.
Sensory disturbances in weakened hearts.
The significance of sensory disturbances.

Conditions in which angina pectoris is induced.—If a large number of cases be studied, symptoms of angina pectoris will be found to arise in patients with the most diverse forms of lesion, and even in patients without any evidence of cardiac disease. In the appendix I quote a number of cases from which it will be seen that angina pectoris can arise in cases of overstrain, aortic aneurism, aortic valvular disease, atheroma of the coronary arteries, myocardial degeneration or enfeeblement of the heart muscle from poor nourishment, increased arterial pressure, sudden changes in the rate and rhythm of the heart, temporary conditions of an obscure origin, and ' senile ' changes.

It would seem that identical symptoms produced from conditions so diverse cannot be directly due to the organic lesion, to the aortic aneurism, to the disease of the coronary artery, to the increased peripheral resistance, or to the variations in rate and rhythm. We must therefore look for a cause common to all these conditions.

Conditions giving rise to attacks of angina pectoris.—In order to find out what this common cause may be, consideration of the conditions giving rise to an attack of angina pectoris will help materially. In the first place it is to be noted that angina pectoris, in many of the conditions cited, appears usually as a late symptom, after the heart has been struggling a long time against the obstacles opposed to its efficient action, or after the nutrition of the muscle has been impaired by gross pathological changes in the coronary artery, or when the muscle fibres have become impaired through slowly advancing degeneration of the fibres. We find, further, that many patients when at rest do not suffer from pain, but that any cause inducing increased work on the heart provokes an attack. Bodily exertion in any form, excitement, increased peripheral resistance (as in exposure to cold air), or when the heart is suddenly embarrassed by a new rhythm, may bring on directly an attack of angina pectoris. That is to say, in predisposed individuals all circumstances which throw more work on the left ventricle induce an attack of angina pectoris.

Conditions predisposing to an attack.—That a muscle should evoke disagreeable symptoms when over-fatigued is a principle applicable to all muscular structures of the body. In looking at the coronary arteries in certain typical cases of angina pectoris, one can reasonably infer one way in which the attacks are brought about. In some cases the coronary arteries are so narrowed as scarce to permit the entrance of a pin. During life the stream of blood must have been greatly reduced, and if it were sufficient to supply the muscle during rest, it was demonstrably insufficient while the heart was in a state of activity. In this respect there seems to be a distinct affinity between the origin of the pain in these cases, and in those cases of what is called 'intermittent claudication', as described on p. 25.

Pain is the chief characteristic of extreme exhaustion. The exhaustion of the heart muscle may be caused by a diminished supply of blood, as in coronary obstruction by deficient nutriment in the blood, or by a diminution of active muscular tissue due to fatty and fibrous degeneration of the heart muscle. There are, indeed, many cases where it is difficult to explain the rationale of the process by which exhaustion is produced, but in studying large number of cases, it affords a reasonable guide for the appreciation of the patient's condition ; and this aspect will be brought out in the discussion of prognosis and treatment. The one thing that is necessary to insist on here is that angina pectoris is not a disease ; but that it is merely a group of symptoms which afford no clue as to the real nature of the heart's complaint, so that inquiry must be made for other evidences which will elucidate this problem.

Association of angina pectoris with exhaustion of the muscle of the heart.—Such considerations lead to the conclusion that angina pectoris arises from certain conditions of the muscular substance of the heart, when the contraction meets with a resistance greater than it can efficiently overcome, whether a fairly strong muscle struggles against an increased resistance (as when there is great peripheral resistance or a narrowed aortic orifice), or whether a weak or degenerated muscle has opposed to its contraction a normal or even a lowered pressure, but a pressure greater than the weakened muscle can readily overcome, or where a heart has for a long period been exposed to effort with insufficient time for rest and recuperation. The view that angina pectoris is an outcome of exhaustion of the heart muscle, is supported by the fact that it is frequently associated with other evidences, connected with or due to such exhaustion as dyspnœa, cardiac asthma, the pulsus alternans, Cheyne-Stokes respiration.

Cardiac exhaustion and the susceptibility to nerve stimulation.— It is a well-recognized fact that seemingly identical lesions of the heart give rise to different phenomena in different people. This difference is seen especially in the reaction of different individuals to pain-producing stimuli. It is probably because of this individual peculiarity that we find angina pectoris the expression of a trivial lesion in some, and the expression of a grave lesion in others, while in many pain is absent in even the most advanced cases of disease and heart failure. Experience has taught me to look upon angina pectoris from a twofold aspect, an expression of cardiac exhaustion and also an expression of a susceptible nervous system. The possibility of the latter condition will be recognized, when it is remembered that, in many cases, there is undoubtedly present an irritable focus of the spinal cord in the region from which cardiac and cerebro-spinal nerves arise. It is necessary in every case to understand the sensibility of the individual to peripheral stimuli, for it is because of this that we get such typical attacks of angina in highly neurotic individuals.

The sensory phenomena produced by over-exertion in healthy hearts. —It has already been pointed out that when a heart is forced to do work beyond its normal capacity, or, in other words, after the reserve force has been exhausted, sensations of distress arise. The sensations may vary, at first a slight breathlessness, a sense of suffocation, referred to the throat, or a tightness across the upper part of the chest. These are the signs usually experienced by healthy people whose hearts have for the time being been subjected to a severe strain, as in running or rowing in a race. In addition to these sensations, pain may be induced, and be followed by other sensory disturbances, as hyperalgesia of the skin and subcutaneous tissues of the left chest-wall. Such phenomena always appear in some portion of the field shaded in Fig. 7. Thus a healthy youth of 16 years went for a cycling holiday in a hilly country. On the first day he rode a great distance and was much spent. On the second day he covered about 100 miles on a hilly road, and collapsed at the end of the day with a sense of suffocation and pain in his left chest. Next day a short ride brought on the pain, and he returned home, and I examined him the third day after the onset of the pain. I could detect nothing wrong with him from a physical examination. There was an ill-defined area of tenderness around the left breast. I advised him to go about quietly, avoiding all exertion which induced the pain. This he did, and from time to time he tested his running powers, only to find that as soon as he had run a few hundred yards the pain returned. After a few months it was less readily induced, and by the end of the year he was as fit as ever, and now, six years later, he is in good health. A healthy medical man, aged 32, went shooting one hot day in the summer. His life had been somewhat sedentary. He climbed a steep hill, carrying his gun and ammunition. At the top, he was seized with a stabbing pain, which lasted

for a few moments. Next day he discovered an area of tenderness around
the left nipple, and consulted me. I could detect no abnormality in the
heart. This was eight years ago, and he is still actively and energetically
engaged in his work, with no signs of heart weakness. I could quote
a number of similar instances (as Case 2); but these suffice to show the
intimate relation between the cardiac and sensory nerves, and the production of sensory disturbances by healthy hearts. The same mechanism
is at work, only the disturbance is more easily induced.

Sensory disturbances in weakened hearts.—If a systematic examination be made of all patients who complain of weakness, breathlessness on
exertion, and palpitation, a considerable number of them will be found
to have some area of tenderness on the left side of the chest, particularly
under the left breast. The area is sometimes quite small, but in many cases
it is of considerable extent. Some of these folks complain of a dull aching
pain at times in this region, and others have sudden stabbing pain, while
in some the pain comes on with great severity, and is accompanied by
other phenomena, so that it is indistinguishable from an attack of angina
pectoris, or rather it is an attack of angina pectoris.

The majority of these cases are highly-strung nervous people, and
especially women. They have frequently been exposed to some strain,
mental or physical, and their cardiac symptoms may be but a part of the
manifestation of ill health. We find such symptoms frequently at the
menopause, or when the patient is subject to some other complaint, as
intestinal stasis or poisoning from some microbic infection. I have watched
such individuals for over twenty years; some of these have suffered from
typical attacks of angina pectoris; so that the presence of these sensory
phenomena was not indicative of a grave heart lesion, but was due to an
exhaustion of the heart in individuals with a very sensitive nervous system
(Cases 6 and 7).

These areas of hyperalgesia are extremely common with actual disease
of the heart, as in auricular fibrillation, and in other conditions where
heart failure is present. So acute may the hyperalgesia be, that I have
seen cases where the tenderness of the skin in the left chest was so great
that the diagnosis had been made of a neuritis.

The significance of sensory disturbances.—If we leave aside for the
moment the question of angina pectoris, associated with heart affections, which
will be dealt with in the next chapter, the presence of these sensory disturbances is of very great value to the clinician. In many cases of actual heart
disease, recognizable by other means, the sensory disturbances may be
ignored; and an approximate idea of the heart's efficiency may be obtained
without taking them into consideration. On the other hand, there are
a large number of people who really suffer from cardiac weakness in whom
the hyperalgesic area is the only phenomenon, apart from the patient's

statements, which the physician can detect—the physical examination revealing no abnormality. I have for a long while been accustomed to search for the presence of these hyperalgesic areas, by lightly pressing the skin of the chest and lightly pinching the pectoralis major muscle, where it forms the anterior wall of the axilla, and the sterno-mastoid and trapezius muscles. The sensitiveness of these structures will be found to vary ; and it will always be found that the patient's statements of great exhaustion will correspond to periods of greater sensitiveness of these structures. Moreover, in many cases where the complaints are obscure or unsatisfactory, the presence of the hyperalgesia will reveal to us the fact that, notwithstanding the absence of physical signs, there is in this symptom demonstrable evidence of the exhaustion of the heart muscle. With this recognition we can search for the circumstances which may have induced the exhaustion.

CHAPTER XIV

ANGINA PECTORIS

Mechanism by which the symptoms of angina pectoris are provoked.
Conditions inducing an attack.
Character and duration of an attack.
The symptoms present during an attack of angina pectoris.
  Pain.
  Constriction of the chest.
  Feeling of impending dissolution.
The state of the heart and arteries.
Symptoms of an attack.
Establishment of a tendency to recurrence of the attacks.
Prognosis.
Treatment.
  Improvement of the condition of the heart.
  Treatment during an attack.

Mechanism by which the symptoms of angina pectoris are provoked. —In the three preceding chapters I gave the reasons for assuming that the symptom complex, called angina pectoris, belongs to the class of reflex protective phenomena, where the symptoms are evoked by a viscus reflexly stimulating certain areas in the central nervous system. The stimulus from the heart to the spinal cord irritates the nerve-cells in close proximity to the nerve conveying the stimulus from the heart. The nerves thus irritated, respond and exhibit the evidence of their peculiar function, that is, sensory nerves, by pain felt in their peripheral distribution, and motor nerves, by contraction of the muscles. In this way we get the peculiar distribution of pain in affections of the heart, and the sense of constriction of the chest-wall. This violent stimulation of the spinal cord may leave, after its subsidence, an irritable focus in the cord, rendering that portion of the cord more susceptible to stimulation, so that it becomes easier for future attacks of angina pectoris to be provoked. This irritable focus can be demonstrated to exist in some patients by the hyperalgesic state of the skin and muscles, and other subcutaneous tissues in the region where the pain was felt. So sensitive may this irritable focus become, that an attack of angina pectoris may be provoked by a stimulation reaching the focus from regions other than the heart. I have further suggested in the foregoing chapters that these phenomena are not the outcome of the gross lesion found in cases of angina pectoris, but are due to the exhaustion of the heart muscle. If this view be kept in mind, the examination of patients is greatly facilitated, and the grounds for a rational diagnosis, prognosis, and treatment are laid.

Conditions inducing an attack.—Angina pectoris is rarely the outcome of an acute affection, though it may in rare instances arise in the course of an acute or subacute infection (Cases 5 and 86); it is usually led up to by a period of gradual exhaustion, except when some event suddenly embarrasses the heart in its work, as in coronary embolism, or the onset of an abnormal rhythm (Case 79). The onset is, in the majority of cases, induced by some extra effort on the part of the heart. This need not be an effort of unusual severity; it occurs more frequently when the individual is using his powers in a way which formerly required no very marked strain. The cause may be of the nature of bodily exertion, mental excitement, exposure to cold air, or anything that calls for more work on the part of the heart. In most cases the attack does not come on at once, unless the effort is persisted in, as in walking up a hill; and the first warnings of heart exhaustion are ignored. The attack of pain may not come on for some minutes or even hours after the causal exertion has ceased, indeed it may arise after the patient has been resting in bed. In some severe cases, the attack of pain may come on at intervals, when the patient has been exposed to no exertion, particularly in cases where the attacks have been frequent, and a tendency to them has been established. One of the most common provocative cases of angina pectoris is a full stomach. Many patients feel the attacks only when they begin to walk after a meal. They may be pulled up two of three times after walking 50 or 100 yards. In some, the pain leaves them after a time and they can walk miles without distress. In many severe cases, the attacks may be provoked with great ease, and from sources that call for no extra effort on the part of the heart. Thus I have seen attacks arise from the mere stimulation of the skin under the left nipple, and from slight movements of the left arm, while the right could be used freely and forcibly without giving rise to an attack (Case 22). In these cases, there is probably an extremely irritable focus in the cord (p. 61).

Character and duration of an attack.—The attacks may be so slight at first as to pass almost unnoticed; and it is only after they become more frequent and severe that the patient's attention is called to the fact that he had previously experienced some discomfort. In the more simple cases, the pain may not be very severe, and, appearing after some violent exertion, may never again show itself. Instead of pain, it may be but a slight sensation of constriction across the chest, that calls for a deep inspiration to relieve the tension. The more severe attacks imperatively command a cessation of all efforts, and here all degrees of suffering may be experienced. During the attack the patient may stand still in a position of rigid immobility,

afraid to move or to speak, scarcely daring to breathe; or he may kneel
down and rest his head on a chair, or roll on the floor in an extremity of
agony; or the patient may become unconscious, and, in rare cases, may die.
If the pain is located in the arm, he may nurse it across his chest, rocking
backwards and forwards. The face may become pale or flushed, and beads
of perspiration may roll down the forehead. The attack may terminate
with the expulsion of air from the stomach, unconsciously sucked into it
during the attack.

In most cases the attack lasts for a few seconds; but it may continue
with great severity for several hours, yielding only to chloroform or large
doses of opium. Such severe cases may die during the suffering.

The symptoms present during an attack of angina pectoris.—The chief
symptom is pain; there may be also a sense of constriction across the chest,
a sense of suffocation, and a sense of impending death. Occasionally other
reflexes may be present, such as a flow of saliva from the mouth, and an
increased secretion of urine. These symptoms are not all present in every
attack, nor are they always present in the same degree. There may be
a slight pain, or a slight sense of constriction across the chest. Or the pain
may be of the utmost severity, with constriction of the chest so violent that
the patient feels as if his breast-bone was about to break.

Pain.—Pain is usually referred to some portion of the distribution of
the upper four left dorsal nerves in the chest and arm. Sometimes the pain
may be felt as low as the distribution of the sixth dorsal nerves in the epigastrium, and as high as the eighth and seventh cervical in the ulnar border
of the forearm and hand. It is rarely felt in similar areas on the right side,
and sometimes it is felt in the neck and back of the head, in the upper cervical
nerves, whose roots are in close association with the vagus. The pain is
usually felt across the chest, and may remain stationary there; or it may
radiate in a very definite manner into the axilla, and down the arm to the
ulnar border of the forearm and hand. When it does this, it may stop for
a brief period in the upper arm or forearm, and be felt there most violently.
On the other hand, the pain may start in the arm and radiate to the chest,
where it remains with great severity for a time. These regions have already
been described (Chapter XII).

Constriction of the Chest.—Arising along with the pain, or following it, or
quite independent of the sensation of pain, is a sense of constriction, which
I have reasoned is due to the reflex stimulation of the intercostal muscles
(p. 61). It may be so slight as to be felt only as a mere tightness across
the chest following exertion; or it may grip the chest so firmly that the
patient has to stand still and take a great deep inspiration to relieve the
spasm of the muscles. In its most violent form, it adds greatly to the
suffering of the patient, when pain is also present. Thus a man, aged 48
(Case 8), who had violently exerted himself, felt a pain in his chest come

on gradually some minutes after the exertion. As the pain increased, he called on me, and I asked him if he felt his chest constricted. He said, ' No.' A few hours later, the pain increased in severity ; then suddenly he felt his chest gripped with a violence so great that it added, he said, indescribably to the terror of his suffering. It was only relieved by large doses of opium. Next day he felt for a short time, when in bed, as though that ' awful gripping were coming on ', and he lay for ten minutes with perspiration pouring off him, in the dread of its return.

Feeling of impending dissolution.—This, I presume, is the result of violent stimulation of the nervous system, comparable to what happens when any other viscus is violently stimulated, as after a blow in the epigastrium, or on the testicle. On rare occasions the patient faints during an attack, and may die during the faint.

The state of the heart and arteries.—During an attack of angina pectoris some marked changes occur in the heart and blood-vessels, and it is impossible to say whether these changes are the cause or consequence of the attack of pain. The heart may show a sudden increase in rate, an abnormal rhythm ; and I have obtained records of a number of cases where irregularities occur, such as extra-systoles, but the real nature of some of the irregularities I do not understand. I give in the appendix a record of some of these cases. Some patients are conscious of a fluttering of the heart when the attack is on, and in one case of aortic disease, while I was testing the sensitiveness of the skin of the left breast, the heart suddenly became increased in rate from 90 to 130, accompanied by a severe attack of angina pectoris. Most cases suffer so severely that it is not possible to obtain reliable records. The blood-vessels are also profoundly affected in many cases. A rise in the blood-pressure, with a constriction of the blood-vessels, is sometimes well marked, particularly in cases of aortic valvular disease (see Cases 38 and 42), but this is far from being a common occurrence ; for I have frequently felt the pulse become soft and scarcely perceptible during an attack, while in one case it disappeared, and the individual became unconscious for a brief period, finally dying while I was watching him. My experience, therefore, is that though no perceptible change may occur in the heart's action in many cases, there are certain cases where the attacks are accompanied by profound change in the heart's action, whose nature I am unable to explain.

Symptoms after an attack.—The patient feels greatly exhausted after the attack has passed off. Sometimes the pain does not completely disappear, and an uneasy painful sensation may last. The end of an attack may coincide with the expulsion of air from the stomach, and as this is usually accompanied by a sense of relief, the attacks are often supposed to be of gastric origin. I have watched these patients, and have no doubt that the air has been sucked into the stomach during the attack. This air suction is seen most characteristically in nervous people, especially women, and is referred to more fully on p. 91. Some patients have a desire to micturate, and the urine secreted is always abundant, pale, and of low specific gravity. In some patients, areas of hyperalgesia of the skin appear in some portion of the field in which the pain had been felt. In the first attacks it may be limited to a small patch, as in Fig. 11, but with recurring attacks the area may spread wherever the pain is felt, as in Fig. 12. This subsequent exhaustion is not always present. The patient may appear sprightly and active as soon as the pain subsides. This was such a marked feature in one patient that his family would not admit the gravity of his condition, and were greatly shocked when he died during an attack.

Establishment of a tendency to recurrence of the attacks.—I have already described how an irritable focus may be produced in the cord after a violent stimulation from a visceral lesion (shaded area in Fig. 5, p. 60). This may be manifested by an area of hyperalgesia in some part of the body, and in those that exhibit this hyperalgesia, attacks of angina pectoris come on with very little provocation. Even when there is no distinct evidence of hyperalgesia, the stimulation of the skin or the movements of the muscles of the arm may induce an attack. I have on several occasions inadvertently brought on an attack while testing the sensibility of the skin and deeper tissues over the præcordium. Visiting a patient one day, who suffered from violent attacks, I found him feeding himself entirely with his right hand. When I asked him why he did not use his left, he said he was afraid to do so, as sometimes the movement of the left arm induced an attack. He died a few hours after, during an attack (Case 22).

Prognosis.—The tragic circumstances surrounding certain cases of angina pectoris, have so oppressed the profession and the laity that an altogether exaggerated opinion has been formed of the gravity of this complaint. If it be realized that angina pectoris is but the expression of an exhausted muscle, and that the exhaustion may arise from any cause that overtaxes the heart, a truer appreciation of the meaning of the symptoms will be obtained. The estimation of the gravity of the cases does not depend upon the violence of the symptoms. A severe attack is not necessarily serious, nor is the mildest free from danger. The importance of the symptoms must be estimated by an examination of the conditions that have induced the muscular exhaustion. This is, as a rule, not a matter of much difficulty, if one carefully searches for a predisposing cause. The age of the patient, the conditions of his or her life, work, worry, nourishment, over-indulgence in tobacco, and, in the case of women, the number of children she has borne, her menstrual functions, all lead to the recognition of the nature of the muscular exhaustion. If the probabilities point to the absence of progressive arterial degeneration and degeneration of the heart muscle, the patient may on the whole be assumed to have a favourable future. If one has reason to suspect that the symptoms have appeared in the early days of advancing senile changes, when the patient, ignoring the limitation of his powers, follows the manner of his life pursued in vigorous manhood, then the probabilities are that, with rest and care, the heart will recover from its exhaustion, and be able to carry on its work at a lower level for many years in comfort. The prognosis is most serious when it occurs with marked evidence of general degeneration, arterial and cardiac, where there is little response to treatment, and where the attacks are induced with slight provocation. The presence of other phenomena, such as cardiac asthma, the pulsus alternans, Cheyne-Stokes breathing, is an additional evidence of such advanced exhaustion that the outlook becomes very grave. In all cases it is well to suspend judgement until a period of treatment has been tried ; the treatment to include the suspension of all forms of effort which induce or predispose to the attacks. This is especially important where there is evidence of a progressive lesion in the heart, as in the cases of syphilis affecting the aorta and its valves. If, in spite of treatment, the attacks keep on recurring, and with little provocation, then the outlook is very serious. Nevertheless, there are cases so severe that for months a patient may scarcely be able to walk across the floor without inducing an attack, when rest for a long period may restore the heart and induce a cessation of the symptoms.

It is important to bear in mind that angina pectoris is the outcome of disturbance in two systems, the circulatory and the nervous. From the fact that apparently similar lesions may be present with and without angina, we are led to surmise that the lesion is not the sole factor. Moreover, the susceptibility of the nervous system varies so much in different people, that the aspect which the disease presents is influenced greatly by the difference in the individual. In discussing the production of sensory disturbances, it was shown that repeated attacks broke down the resistance of the nervous system, and even injured the central nervous system, so that an irritable focus in the spinal column was produced, and as a consequence, stimuli reaching that focus from other sources might produce attacks of angina pectoris (Case 22). Any form of mental excitement may cause the heart to beat rapidly and violently, and, in the predisposed, give rise to attacks of angina. When, therefore, we estimate the factors, the state of the nervous system must be inquired into ; and if we find evidences that it is in an irritable state, we must take this fact into consideration. Many cases of so-called ' pseudo-angina ' are nothing more than a peculiarly sensitive nervous system, with some temporary cardiac enfeeblement, as in neurotic young women or women about the menopause, and in many women with valve lesions. In elderly subjects, we may get evidence of a highly sensitive nervous system, shown by the patches of flushing which may appear suddenly in the cheeks, neck, or chest.

The difficulty arises where there is undoubted advanced cardiac disease in people with a neurotic constitution ; for the nervousness of manner may be in a great measure the outcome of the cardiac disease and suffering. A painstaking inquiry into all the circumstances, especially if it be found that at times the individual can undertake a good deal of effort, will generally give a good guide. When we find that a moderate amount of effort invariably induces the pain, even if the amount of nervousness in the individual, man or woman, is striking, judgement should be reserved until a period of treatment has been tried.

The following is the method I employ to estimate the condition of a patient suffering from attacks of angina pectoris. I get from the patient a description of his sensations when pain is present, and the position in which it arises and in what region it may spread, and where it holds him with the greatest severity. Then I inquire into the duration of the different attacks, their manner of onset and offset, and find out if there is any accompanying phenomena, as a gripping sensation, the sensation of collapse or exhaustion, which may accompany or follow the attack, whether saliva pours from the mouth, or whether there is a call to micturate after an attack. With a thorough comprehension of the nature of the attack, I next inquire into the very first time any sensation of a disagreeable kind appeared and the circumstances under which it appeared. Frequently one gets a history of slight unnoticed attacks of pain or other signs of limitation, it may be years before, while in other cases the attacks may come on without any previous history of exhaustion being present. Then I find out the circumstances which induce an attack, whether they arise in response to effort and especially after meals, or excitement, or if they come on when at rest in bed. Inquiry is then directed into the history of the individual, seeking for evidence of a possible infection of the heart by rheumatism, syphilis, etc. Then the life which has been led, in regard to work, worry, food, drink, and tobacco, should be considered.

Then a thorough knowledge of the patient's response to effort must be acquired by finding out how he reacts to varying amounts of bodily effort under different circumstances, and the greatest amount of effort he can do under favourable circumstances. A physical examination should next be made ; the aspect of the individual and the manner of telling his tale will already have given an idea of the type of individual. The radial artery is noted in regard to the thickness of its wall. The character of the pulse and the blood-pressure are noted. Any irregularity is differentiated. If the symptoms indicate rather an advanced condition of exhaustion, then a tracing of the radial pulse should be taken to see if there is a tendency to the pulsus alternans. It may be necessary to take a long tracing to catch an extra-systole, as it is after the extra-systole that the pulsus alternans tends to appear. Then the state of the heart, the myocardium, and the valves should be noted.

Following on this inquiry, the condition of other organs, as the lungs, should be observed, whether there is any tendency to cardiac asthma, Cheyne-Stokes breathing ; the kidneys, and the digestive tract, should also be considered.

In estimating the condition of individual cases, I go on the following lines. If I find that the attacks have been induced by severe bodily exertion, in a man who had previously been in fair health, then I gather that the severe exertion had profoundly exhausted the heart, especially if the subject is under 50 years of age, and if rest be possible, a good prognosis may be given, though it may be many months before the tendency to the pain disappears (Case 2). The same opinion is given where we find a woman who has had for years insufficient rest, and in whom attacks of angina are readily provoked (Case 7). In advancing years, about 50 and over, attacks may be induced under peculiar circumstances, as after a meal. In these a favourable prognosis can be given when we find that at other times the individual can take a considerable amount of exertion, as walking briskly five or ten miles. We can gather from this that there is present a store of good functioning muscle, but that it is embarrassed by some mechanism induced by the meal (Case 9).

We may find that the attacks have arisen in a man getting on in years, who has been leading a vigorous life at a greater pace than he had twenty years before, or he may have undertaken some effort which he was wont to do with ease, but had not attempted for a long time. In such the prognosis is good, for with a period of rest and a life at a lower level he may go on for an indefinite number of years, with a tendency to recurrence when he does not respect his advancing years (Cases 8, 9, and 13). Attacks may arise from some passing affection of the heart, and the nature of the affection is usually so obscure that it is impossible to recognize it (Case 12), while in other cases we can detect evidence, such as a change in the rhythm (Case 79), or the presence of a temporary affection (Case 86). We may suspect some such condition, when an otherwise healthy person is suddenly seized with an attack.

The presence of an active lesion can sometimes be detected, particularly when it appears in the aortic valves ; and the progress depends on one's power to check the advance of the disease, so that a prognosis should be reserved till a course of treatment has been given. This especially applies to syphilitic lesions (Cases 37, 38, and 40). Angina is frequently associated with aortic lesions, and the attacks are easily provoked and often most intractable (Case 42). These patients may live for many years, suffering greatly at times (Case 39). In the more grave cases, the pain is always induced by effort ; and there are times when they are unable to undertake any effort without distress. This indicates such profound exhaustion of the heart muscle that judgement should be suspended till a period of rest has been tried. This may be followed by a respite (Cases 14, 18, and 19), while in some cases the respite is only slight (Cases 24, 25, and 27), and in others no improvement takes place and death follows (Cases 22 and 28). When the attacks of pain are associated with cardiac asthma, or Cheyne-Stokes breathing, or the pulsus alternans, a very grave condition is present (Cases 24 and 27).

Treatment.—Treatment naturally divides itself into two heads, namely, the improvement of the condition of the heart, and the giving of relief during an attack.

Improvement of the condition of the heart.—For the first of these it must be borne in mind that the attack is the expression of an exhausted muscle, and the treatment requires a careful inquiry into the conditions inducing that exhaustion. First and foremost, a stop must be put to that form of exertion which has induced the attack, and any other conditions that predispose to it must be avoided, such as work, worry, sleeplessness, over-indulgence in food and alcohol, tobacco, and so forth. The next step is to place the heart in such a position that it will regain its reserve force, that is, the heart must be given less to do. This does not necessarily mean that the patient should rest in bed, but he should restrict his movements as much as possible. Here the habits and condition of the patient will have to be considered, and each individual separately treated. To stop an individual altogether from his work and engagements may seriously affect his business affairs and aggravate his condition by mental worry. It is best, as a rule, to permit him to follow some particular kind of work that does not put a strain upon his heart. When feasible, a complete change of habits and life, as free from over-exertion as possible, is most beneficial, such as a good holiday spent in the manner that affords the maximum of enjoyment and requires the minimum of effort. In the cases that do not yield to such limited restriction, and when the attacks are demonstrably the outcome of an advanced exhaustion of the heart, then absolute rest in bed is necessary. In other conditions the treatment should follow the lines that I have laid down in the chapters upon treatment. Of remedies and methods supposed to cure, the name is legion. Happily in their prescription the above suggestions are also included, and the benefit so accruing is too often attributed to the remedy or method. I have in several individual patients tried various so-called remedies, and I find on the whole, that if the patient is not worried, has plenty of sleep, and leads a fairly restful life, he does as well without any special drug treatment as he did with it. In certain cases, especially in neurotic subjects and those with aortic disease, there is a great tendency for the attacks to be provoked by a slight stimulus, as exertion or emotion. Even with rest in bed this tendency may not cease. For such patients I have been accustomed to prescribe bromide of ammonium, and to push it until the patient becomes drowsy and apathetic. In most cases the susceptibility to attacks is greatly diminished when this stage is reached. The patient should be kept under the influence of the drug for a week, when the quantity should be gradually reduced. When this drug has failed I have had to resort to chloral. In administering the drug, the dose depends upon the effects, and the drug should be carefully pushed until undoubted effects are induced—that is, until the patient becomes drowsy and apathetic.

In those cases of angina pectoris, where the attacks come on while walking after a meal, the food should be taken in small quantities, and so dry in quality as to necessitate thorough mastication. The food should be taken at regular and frequent intervals, so as to avoid any sense of exhaustion, and the patient should rest after each meal for half an hour.

As many patients of a neurotic type suffer from angina pectoris, the mental factor should always be considered. The term angina pectoris conveys to their minds such fearful associations, that they readily become depressed and miserable. A careful study of each case will show that, in the majority, the attack is the outcome of a temporarily exhausted muscle, and the patient can have his mind relieved by the assurance that the prognosis is a good one. In the after-treatment of such cases, careful management is needed, in order that they should not always be reminded of their complaint. Hence systems of dieting, where the patient at each meal has to reflect if the ingredients are injurious to his heart, should be rigidly avoided. Most dietetic systems are the outcome of a fad, and based on an imperfect knowledge of digestive and metabolic processes, as in the exclusion of common salt and lime salts from the meals. For the same reason, ' health resorts,' where people congregate and discuss their ailments, should be avoided.

Treatment during an attack.—The slighter attacks require no treatment. When they become more severe, rapidly acting vaso-dilators should be administered, such as hot drinks, hot water with whisky or brandy, the nitrites, of which the best and most speedy is amylnitrite, by inhalation. This drug is not successful in all cases, but in many its action is rapid, and the relief is generally complete. When it is successful, it has been inferred that the patient had previously constricted arterioles, or increased arterial pressure, and that the pressure was reduced, and so the heart was eased. This is not the full explanation. A patient with cardio-sclerosis had an attack of angina pectoris in my consulting-room. I took his blood-pressure, and found it 190 mm. Hg., and then administered to him nitrite of amyl : it acted instantaneously, and gave him perfect relief. After fifteen minutes I again took his blood-pressure and found that it had risen to 200 mm. Hg. Though the pressure was higher, he had no pain. I inferred that the action was similar to that of a man who puts on a hat that is too tight ; at first there is no pain, but gradually, by the summation of stimuli, discomfort comes on and increases in intensity ; he removes the hat from his head, and obtains relief. He replaces the hat in the same position, and, although it is as tight as before, the pain has permanently disappeared : so that the temporary removal of the summating stimuli seems to be the reason for the relief afforded in the particular case mentioned.

In place of nitrite of amyl, trinitrin in tablets of $\frac{1}{100}$ and $\frac{1}{50}$ of a grain may be used, or nitro-glycerine. When the nitrites fail to relieve the patient, we are forced to use chloral or morphia in doses sufficient to give relief. I have found occasionally that chloral acts beneficially, not only in relieving the somewhat long attacks, but in preventing the attacks recurring, when given in repeated small doses of 3–5 grains and also when given at night to induce sound sleep.

In advanced cases where the suffering comes on mainly at night, it is occasionally very difficult to give the patient relief, except by the hypo-dermic injection of morphia or an inhalation of chloroform. Massive doses of oxygen have in some cases, as in cardiac asthma, been followed by marked benefit, and should be tried.

CHAPTER XV

HEART AFFECTIONS AND A HYPER-SENSITIVE NERVOUS SYSTEM

Reaction of visceral disease on the central nervous system.
Pseudo-angina pectoris, a useless and misleading term.
Exaggerated sensory phenomena with and without valvular disease.
Exaggerated sensory phenomena, with pathological changes in the heart.
Characteristics of the sensory phenomena.
Air suction.
Prognosis in cases with exaggerated sensory symptoms.
Treatment.

IT not infrequently happens that the most common forms of disease are the most difficult to describe. I attempt here the analysis and explanation of the symptoms present in certain cases which are frequently met in actual practice. As the symptoms show great variety in number and intensity, numerous attempts have been made to divide them into groups; and we find them under various guises, as neurotic hearts, cardiac neuroses, cardiac neurasthenia, pseudo-angina pectoris. I have endeavoured to find the underlying principles which provoke these manifold symptoms, as their due appreciation is of prime importance in the management of these cases.

Reaction of visceral disease on the central nervous system.—In describing the symptoms of angina pectoris, I have endeavoured to show that the symptoms arise from a reflex stimulation of the central nervous system. But the heart and the nervous system can react upon one another in other ways than by reflex stimulation. In heart affections, as in affections of all other viscera, there is a tendency for the central nervous system to become hyper-sensitive (I use this word for want of a better), whereby symptoms of nervous origin are readily evoked. This applies more particularly to the production of sensory phenomena, where a comparatively small visceral lesion gives rise to an irritable focus in the spinal cord, and to severe suffering and widespread areas of hyperalgesia, or to certain mental states where the patients sometimes become 'nervous' and apprehensive. The result of the association of heart affections with these latter, may be summed up in the expression that the cardiopath tends to become a neuropath.

This mental state is seen very characteristically in both men and women. If they have been told that they have a murmur, or an irregular heart, or if they are conscious of an extra-systole, or suffer actual distress of a cardiac origin, they become extremely apprehensive. The hyperalgesia, so common in the breasts of women suffering from some slight heart trouble, is a constant source of worry, and some are continually imagining that the abnormal soreness is an indication of serious disease. This apprehension is unfortunately too often aggravated by the warnings of the physician, who estimates the significance of the symptoms too seriously, or will neither admit nor deny the gravity of the condition.

The combination of cardiac and nervous exhaustion may be brought about in another way. People with a tendency to 'nervous debility', or who have acquired it from some other cause, may develop some cardiac trouble, functional or organic. In such people, the reflex symptoms are greatly exaggerated. Thus one of my patients with aortic and mitral disease, experienced no sensory phenomena until she developed a gastric ulcer. This gave rise to great pain, and to a widespread area of hyperalgesia of the skin and muscles in the left side of the abdomen. Soon after this she began to suffer from pain from the heart affection, and the hyperalgesia finally embraced nearly the whole of the left chest. The patient lived for many years after the appearance of these symptoms; and a pyloric ulcer and aortic and mitral valve disease were found on post-mortem examination.

In all these cases, we must exercise a great deal of judgement. It frequently happens that in patients with a demonstrable cardiac lesion the symptoms are estimated too seriously, and the case looked upon with greater gravity than need be. On the other hand, if there be no murmur or irregularity, the case is liable to be treated lightly as one of 'pseudo-angina pectoris' or neurasthenia.

Pseudo-angina pectoris, a useless and misleading term.—It is time the term 'pseudo-angina pectoris' was dropped out of medical literature. While it may be convenient to group under indefinite terms many conditions of whose nature we are ignorant, it should be borne in mind that this grouping is but provisional, and a confession of our ignorance of the real nature of the complaint. With advance in our knowledge, first one complaint and then another should be placed in a group whose cause is definite and known. In this way many cardiac terms, such as tachycardia, embryocardia, bradycardia, have been employed loosely, and now should never be employed unless a definition be given of what is meant.

The term 'angina pectoris' is employed to designate a group of symptoms evoked by the heart, of which pain is the most distinctive. As angina pectoris is sometimes associated with grave organic lesions, we find such cases referred to as 'angina pectoris vera'. The term 'pseudo-angina pectoris ' is applied to cases in which the pain resembles that of angina pectoris vera, but is due to some other cause than heart disease, or in which the pain arises from the heart with no organic lesion. In regard to the former class, if the pain is due to some other viscus, e.g. the stomach, as sometimes happens, why call it ' pseudo-angina pectoris ' ? If it is due to the stomach, why not say so ? In regard to the latter class, the employment of this term is due to a total misconception of the nature and mechanism of visceral pain. The fundamental cause of the pain is the same in the case of the heart as in that of any other viscus, and the pain is as readily induced in the heart as in the stomach. As we would never dream of calling a stomach pain a ' pseudo-gastralgia ', so we need not call a heart pain ' pseudo-angina '.

I deal with the matter at length, as the employment of a fine-sounding term has too often sufficed for a diagnosis, so that no inquiry into the real nature of these symptoms has been undertaken. In the great majority of cases, when a patient complains of a pain in his chest which radiates into his arm, in the area shaded in Fig. 7, the pain is of cardiac origin. The only other conditions in which I have found pain to occupy this characteristic site, was in herpes zoster affecting the upper dorsal nerves, certain rare forms of gastric affection, pleurisy, and pleurodynia. In one case, I thought I had to deal with a case of angina pectoris until the herpetic eruption revealed the true nature of the complaint. In pleurisy and pleurodynia occurring in the left chest, the pain is always aggravated by the movements of respiration. It is quite conceivable that other conditions may give rise to pain having this distribution, but that is no reason for calling them pseudo-angina pectoris.

The characteristic distribution of the pain and other sensory phenomena at once excludes hysteria, for in the latter the symptoms do not follow the anatomical distribution of nerves. When an hysterical patient feels a pain in this region, it may be assumed that there is probably some cardiac trouble in addition to the hysteria.

Exaggerated sensory phenomena with and without valvular disease. —A great many people with a demonstrable cardiac lesion, as of the mitral valves, develop sensory phenomena in an exaggerated form. This is particularly seen in some women in whom the reserve force is exhausted. Such folks may struggle on for a long time, working hard and ignoring their earlier symptoms of a limitation of the field of cardiac response, determined not to give in. Finally the nervous system shares in the exhaustion, and the breakdown is brought about with an extreme development of the sensory phenomena ; thus attacks of pain, sometimes of great severity, may be felt across the chest and extending into the left arm, or more often the complaint may be of a dull aching pain of varying severity, but distinctly worse at the end of a day's work. The hyperalgesia may spread over a very extensive area, and sometimes is extremely acute.

On account of the manifest lesion in the heart, these cases are not un-frequently diagnosed as cases of angina pectoris of a severe and dangerous form ; and I have known patients lead a life of great restriction for many years under this mistaken notion. The attacks are indeed those of angina pectoris, but are not dangerous, and are an evidence of exhausted heart muscle, and disappear with the restoration of the reserve force.

On the other hand, we have mothers of families with no heart murmurs, who for many years have worked hard from morning till night, whose sleep has been disturbed by ailing or fretful children, and who finally break down with exhausted heart and nervous system (Cases 6 and 7). Some of my most typical cases have been in young women, whose sleep has been disturbed frequently every night for many years to attend to an ailing parent. This constant strain night and day exhausts the strength. These patients suffer from heart pain, sometimes with the classical symptoms of angina pectoris.

With suitable management they eventually recover, though recovery is usually very protracted, the patients sometimes having to lead very quiet lives for months, or even years. Similar symptoms may arise in others who have been exposed to worry and anxiety, or who have suffered from sleeplessness, while others may suffer when there is no apparent reason for the exhaustion.

Exaggerated sensory phenomena, with pathological changes in the heart.—The possibility that in all these cases there may be slowly pro-gressive lesions affecting the heart muscle and valves, should be kept in mind, especially in cases over 40 years of age. There is nothing to tell whether it is so or not, for the superficial arteries may be quite normal in appearance, and the blood-pressure give no sure information. This needs to be specially insisted on when these exaggerated phenomena appear in women between 50 and 60. I have seen a number of patients develop all the sensory phenomena in an extremely exaggerated form, becoming weaker until they were unable to leave their beds ; some have become unconscious, and died ; others regained consciousness, and after a time sufficient strength to go about for years. After their recovery, I have been surprised to find an aortic systolic murmur, which had not been present prior to the break-down. Some of these have remained liable to attacks of angina ; one dropped down dead, and in another, who died from subsequent heart failure, there was marked sclerosis of the heart muscle, coronary arteries, aortic valves, and aorta. In syphilitic affections of the heart, particularly where the aortic valves are involved, the first sign to draw the attention of the patient is the occurrence of pain of unusual severity. This may happen even before any aortic lesion is detected by physical examination (Case 40).

Characteristics of the sensory phenomena.—There are some special points in these cases that distinguish them from those who do not have the same susceptible nervous system. The suffering may not be as severe as in the more grave forms of angina pectoris, but it is more lasting and comes on after periods of continuous exertion. Sometimes it is limited to the left arm, if that arm has been much employed in work, as in washing or baking. It is frequently associated with extreme tenderness on pressure of the tissues of the left chest and neck, especially the left breast, the pectoralis major and sterno-mastoid muscles. After testing the tender skin and muscles by slightly pinching the skin and muscles between the fingers and thumb, the tissues thus stimulated become extremely sore, and the aching lasts for hours afterwards. When the patient is suffering from severe pain, the mouth may become dry and parched, and large quantities of pale urine may be passed, as happens in cases where the angina pectoris is of very grave significance.

Air suction.—Another symptom is extremely common in these cases— the belching of air. One searches text-books in vain for any hint as to the nature of this symptom, and though it is extremely common in all neurotic people, its significance is almost invariably misunderstood. A detailed and satisfactory account is given by Wyllie, and it is to this article I owe enlightenment as to the meaning of this symptom.

The chief feature is the noisy expulsion of air from the stomach. Patients complain of attacks of flatulence, and in these attacks seemingly expel large quantities of air ; but, if closely watched, they will be seen first to suck air into their stomachs. Before expelling the air, they unconsciously close the glottis, fix the muscles of the abdominal wall, then expand the chest. As no air goes into the lungs, and the diaphragm is raised, the pressure in the stomach becomes negative. By this process they suck air into the stomach. After sucking in a quantity, they expel it with considerable force, and often with a good deal of noise. Many people can do this at will, others only in certain states of excitement. Some have ' attacks of flatulence ' in the middle of the night, and such attacks are due to air swallowing, or more correctly air suction. As Wyllie points out, these attacks can be stopped by making the patient open his mouth widely, and keeping the jaw propped open by a large cork between the teeth, a procedure which prevents the air suction.

I have watched several patients during an attack of angina pectoris, and when they stand seemingly immobile, they unconsciously suck air into the stomach. Immediately the pain subsides the air is expelled, and the patient is apt to attribute the relief he has experienced to the coincident and demonstrable act. This very obvious phenomenon has led many observers to imagine that the attack was gastric in origin, and hence the group of gastric ' pseudo-anginas '.

This association of air suction with attacks of angina pectoris, which is sometimes found in men, is extremely common in women. As air suction is frequent in women, it is sometimes mistaken for an hysterical symptom, and its relationship to a real heart attack is apt to be overlooked. As a matter of fact, attacks of air suction are apt to arise from any exciting cause, and attacks of angina pectoris readily induce them. In some it occurs so readily that it may come on before the real suffering. Thus, one lady who suffered from extreme arterial degeneration had severe attacks of angina pectoris, which disappeared after a long period of rest in bed. When she got about again she could walk on the level with comfort, but the slightest hill brought on discomfort, which if not heeded resulted in great pain in the chest. As a rule, however, before the pain became severe she began to suck in and to expel air. She would rest a minute and start again, but soon had to stop, and expel ' more wind ', as she put it.

Prognosis in cases with exaggerated sensory symptoms.—If care be taken to differentiate between the patients who exhibit exaggerated nervous phenomena due to progressive organic lesions, especially when there is a history of syphilis, and those due to exhaustion apart from a progressive lesion, the prognosis can be made with fair certainty. Recovery almost invariably results in the latter class, though it may be delayed for a long time. Naturally, the complication producing the nerve exhaustion must be taken into account ; and if due to other visceral affections, the prognosis depends also upon their nature.

When there is an organic lesion, as myocardial degeneration, or valvular disease, on the whole the exaggerated nervous phenomena do not add to the gravity, but, it has even seemed to me, act favourably in many cases, for the early exhaustion is attended by such an amount of suffering that the heart is protected from more extensive exhaustion of its reserve force.

Treatment.—It is of the first importance that we should appreciate the nature of the trouble in these cases, and bear in mind the part played by the nervous system. In cases where we are satisfied there is no progressive lesion, the nervous element is the chief consideration, and the sufferings of many of these patients are aggravated by the consciousness or dread of some serious affection of the heart. Having satisfied ourselves as to the real nature of the trouble, we should first of all reassure the patient. In a great many cases success in treatment depends on this, and we can often see patients at once made well, or greatly improved, when they become fully reassured. This is more particularly the case, when the patient has previously been alarmed by being told that the condition was serious. The peculiar mental factor that makes this class of patient the stay and support of many forms of empirical or semi-empirical treatment, should be kept in mind. As suggestion plays an important part in the numerous special methods of cure, it should be used intelligently by medical men, and in a legitimate manner ; that is to say, the patient should be reassured from the standpoint of a full knowledge of his condition.

There is a great tendency for the physician to attach too high an importance to a case with exaggerated nervous symptoms, where there is an organic lesion of the valves. I have seen many patients lead lives of great restriction, with a certain amount of fear, on account of the supposed seriousness of heart trouble. Women have had attacks of angina pectoris, and have been forbidden to undertake their household duties. Great numbers have gone to health resorts at great expense and inconvenience, year after year, to perform the 'cure', because in their days of suffering they had experienced benefit. When there is a valvular murmur, we must carefully inquire into the conditions that have induced the heart exhaustion and the attendant suffering, and consideration of the whole of the facts will enable us with certainty to recognize the real nature of the phenomena. We can often with certainty reassure the patient that with suitable treatment the suffering will, to a great extent, disappear, and that, though the organic trouble may persist, with intelligent management there is good ground for hope of a fair restoration to health. In many cases one is able to do more, to point out that the suffering is a safeguard, its first appearance being an evidence that the patient is exhausting the reserve force of the heart, and that such restrictions are necessary to guard against further exhaustion.

This intelligent appreciation of symptoms is of service in other ways. Thus, when patients become conscious of an extra-systole, they are often subjected to long courses of treatment, usually inefficient, by their medical attendant, or by some special method. The mere reassurance of the harmlessness of the symptoms would have done more good than all the treatment. As an illustration, I cite the following experience. A professional football-player consulted me because his heart 'stopped' at times. He had been seen by two doctors, who forbade him to play, and put him on digitalis and strychnine. This cessation of work was a serious matter to him, because if he could not complete his engagement for the season, he lost the chance of a benefit match, which he looked upon as a reward at the end of his services as a footballer. Except that he was frightened and nervous, I found him in all respects a healthy man, save for a somewhat frequent extra-systole. I told him he could start playing at once, and that when he was conscious of his heart stopping he was to pay no attention to it. He at once resumed his engagements, and completed his term with no discomfort. He told me that at the beginning of one match he was painfully conscious of his heart's irregularity, and felt he must retire, but reflected upon what I had told him, dashed into the game, and in a few minutes forgot all about his trouble, and said he never played better in his life.

I use this illustration to emphasize the fact that neither the exaggerated sensory and mental sensations, nor the symptoms giving rise to them, should be the guide, but what effort the heart can undertake without discomfort.

Besides reassuring the patient, steps should be made to remove him or her from any conditions that conduce to the exhaustion, such as over-work, worry, nursing a sick relative. Discretion must be used, and the patient's circumstances considered. When the patients are well-to-do, a complete change in the mode of life is often very efficacious, and they may be sent away, the choice of the place depending on the patient's tastes. If they can undergo some physical effort, a holiday may be recommended that includes some exertion, such as hill-climbing, cycling, golfing, or ' sight-seeing '—town or country—provided the occupation interests the patient. They may be sent to some watering-place, and may indulge in the special treatment adopted there—for the sake of doing something, and getting what benefit hydrotherapy may convey. My patients have gone to all sorts of places, and those who went to the seaside and indulged in sea-bathing got more benefit than those who frequented the more vaunted inland spas, home or continental. The life there is more bracing, and there is less opportunity to meet all sorts of neurotics ; and the baneful habit of comparing experiences is thus not so easy to indulge in.

The vast majority of patients cannot go away and leave their posts, and these form the class with which the general practitioner has often a great deal of trouble. With patience and perseverance, however, much can be done for them ; and in many instances the doctor can give great help to some of the most deserving patients he has to treat. The mother of a family has to keep going, the tired daughter has to nurse the ailing parent. In all these cases there will be found, almost invariably, insufficient sleep, or sleep frequently disturbed ; and this is often the real cause of the trouble, and in addition renders the patient peevish and irritable. Much can be done by suggesting different devices to promote the patient's rest. In many cases we have to resort to drugs ; and happily the most efficacious hypnotics in these cases are also the safest, namely, bromides (particularly bromide of ammonium), which should be given until the patient sleeps soundly. Often they produce drowsiness and languor during the day, and the patient may complain of being weaker than ever. This is no contra-indication, but rather the contrary, for the languor induces idleness and restfulness ; for less work is done and patients are not so irritable, and the heart is not so easily excited. After a few weeks, if the dose be gradually diminished, it will often be found that in the meantime the patient's condition has wonderfully im-proved. The necessity of duties being fulfilled prevents the possibility of any immediate recovery, but by the judicious administration of the bromides, patients can be tided over trying periods for months or years.

' Heart tonics ' in these cases are of little use. Even if they had the action they are supposed to possess, it is doubtful if their administration would be wise. It is not a whip which an overworked horse needs, but rest.

The nourishment of the patient often leaves much to be desired. In the case of women, the household duties and the cooking take away the appetite, and they content themselves with stuff easily swallowed and stimulating—hot fluids, tea, coffee, and spirits. The food should be taken in small quantities and often, and should be fairly dry to ensure slow mastication. It is sometimes a good plan to suggest a dietary of a very simple nature. Find out what food the patient prefers, and, if it is rational, so arrange the diet that every few hours may bring a change, even if it be but an egg at one time, and a dry biscuit and a few tablespoonfuls of milk at another. In all cases stimulants should be forbidden. The great exhaustion brought about by the long weary hours of work and suffering is often speedily temporarily relieved by spirits ; but these are just the people who ultimately find solace in increasing quantities, until the habit becomes all too powerful.

CHAPTER XVI

VASO-MOTOR SYMPTOMS

The vaso-motor nerves. Origin and distribution.
Function of the vaso-motor nerves.
Agents influencing the vaso-motor nervous system.
The sense of exhaustion and syncope.
Vaso-motor angina pectoris.
The circulatory symptoms in the X disease.
The cause of the X complaint.
Treatment.

The vaso-motor nerves. Origin and distribution.—There is a system of nerves distributed to the blood-vessels, over which they exercise a marked control. These nerves belong to the vaso-motor system, and are intimately associated with the peculiar functions of the organs and tissues to which they are distributed. The chief vaso-motor centre is on the floor of the fourth ventricle. There are other centres at various levels in the central nervous system ; and the nerves from these centres, in their distribution, form a part of the sympathetic nervous system, and many reach their peripheral destination along with the spinal nerves.

Function of the vaso-motor nerves.—Their chief function is to regulate the supply of blood to the different organs and tissues. As in the processes of life, the various organs are called into activity, now one organ, then another being especially active, and as the supply of blood to the organ varies with activity and inactivity, these vaso-motor nerves regulate the supply by varying the lumen of the small vessels (arteries, capillaries, and veins). In carrying out this work they are stimulated in the proper manner by an intricate series of reflexes. While the harmonious activity of the different organs is characteristic of what we call health, and the individual is barely conscious of the action of his various organs, except by the vague sensation of well-being, the inharmonious action of the vaso-motor nerves may lead to a disturbance of this sense of well-being and produce discomfort or distress.

The evidence of the presence of these vaso-motor nerves can be demonstrated in the human subject in innumerable ways, both from central stimulation and peripheral : as, for instance, the flushing and paling of the face by emotion, and the various reactions which follow the scratching of the skin by a pin-head, or the application of heat and cold.

An undue sensitiveness to vaso-motor stimulation may be inherited or acquired, and in consequence we get a series of phenomena which often cause such distress that the advice of the physician is frequently sought. The most extreme form of over-action is seen in such instances of vaso-contraction as result in fingers becoming cold and numb, often causing considerable distress, and in some instances leading to the death of some portion of the tissues. An extreme instance of the vaso-motor effect is noted in Raynaud's disease, where a localised constriction of the arterioles cuts off the blood-supply to the tissues. A persistent over-dilatation of the blood-vessels of the skin is sometimes met with in certain toxic conditions, as in exophthalmic goitre, where the dilatation of the arterioles gives rise to a persistent sensation of warmth. Not infrequently in middle-aged or elderly people of a neurotic habit, patches of the skin in the cheeks, neck, or chest, may suddenly become deeply suffused of a bright red colour. As these people not infrequently complain of cardiac distress and even angina pectoris, the presence of these symptoms may be taken to indicate a neurotic tendency, and so enable us to recognize that the symptoms of distress may be due partly to a hypersensitive nervous system. Apart from such well-recognized instances, there are a great number of people who suffer from a variety of distressing sensations, of obscure origin, but in whom the vaso-motor system plays an important part. As these sensations are frequently imagined to be associated with cardiac conditions, it is necessary to give them some consideration.

Agents influencing the vaso-motor nervous system.—The vaso-constrictor nerve-fibres are distributed to the muscle-fibre in the middle coat of the arterioles. Their termination here can be influenced by certain substances introduced into the circulation. Thus suprarenal extract injected into the jugular veins causes a rise of blood-pressure, which, however, lasts for a very short time. Extracts of the pituitary body have a like effect.

It is probable that the high blood-pressure, in such diseases as Bright's disease, is produced by some substance being retained in the blood which stimulates the vaso-constrictor nerves.

Certain substances have an opposite effect. Commercial peptone, injected into the veins of an animal, causes dilatation of the peripheral arterioles, with a fall of blood-pressure. The nitrites act in a similar way, only their action is very transient.

The sense of exhaustion and syncope.—Many individuals complain at times of a sense of fatigue easily provoked under certain circumstances. If there should happen to be some unusual cardiac phenomenon present, as a murmur or an irregularity, it is usually assumed that the exhaustion is the outcome of the cardiac condition. I have already pointed out that the evidence of heart exhaustion is fairly characteristic, and that the sensation of exhaustion is rarely primarily cardiac in origin. As a rule it is really due to vaso-dilatation in certain regions, with a depletion of blood in other organs, as the heart or the brain. Thus some people walking on a close damp day with heavy clothing, speedily experience a sensation of great exhaustion. If they sit down or lie down, it speedily passes off. Pembrey has pointed out that the reason soldiers faint on the march on a hot day is that the warmth produced by their heavy clothing and the exertion has induced such dilatation of the vessels of the skin, that anæmia of the brain results and the soldiers faint. It is for this reason that lads faint when kept standing, and women faint when being fitted for a dress. In such cases, the syncope arises from temporary dilatation of the great abdominal veins. If a hutch rabbit is suspended by its ears, the blood drains into the abdominal veins, and the animal becomes unconscious and dies. In some people there is a tendency for the blood to accumulate in the big abdominal veins. I have been able to demonstrate this by the following

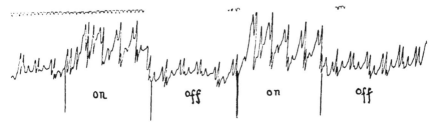

on   off   on   off

FIG. 13. Tracing of the jugular pulse while pressure was applied to the abdomen (*on*). The jugular vein increased in size, while on removal of pressure (*off*) the vein became less distended.

method. If a suitable case be laid down and gentle firm pressure applied with the open hand over the abdomen, the veins of the neck will be seen to swell up. The tracing (Fig. 13) was taken during this procedure. The receiver was placed over the internal jugular vein in the neck, and pressure applied to the abdomen, and during the pressure the change in the jugular vein was graphically recorded—the great rise in the tracing being due to the distended jugular vein. I have seen such patients greatly benefited by wearing a tight abdominal belt. Thus a tall lady in cycling on a hot day had frequently to get off her bicycle, and lie down by the roadside to recover from an impending attack of syncope. At my suggestion she wore a tight abdominal belt, and the tendency to syncope disappeared, but returned when she tried to do without the belt. The best instance I have had of this accumulation of blood in the great abdominal veins, was in a man who complained of inability to work or to walk about because of a sensation of great exhaustion and giddiness. When lying down nothing could be detected amiss, but as soon as he stood up he became gradually more and more giddy till he was compelled to sit down. It was found that, on standing, his heart became very rapid in its action. A tight abdominal belt was applied, and he was at once able to walk about and follow his occupation. On several occasions records were taken of his pulse while standing, at first with his belt on, when the pulse was quiet and regular ; then a few minutes after the belt was removed, when the heart's action became rapid and irregular. The nature of the abnormal action was examined by means of the electrocardiograph and polygraph by Lewis and Marris, who found that during the rapid action of the heart, contraction originated in a region near the node (probably a true nodal rhythm).

Some people who suffer from attacks of angina pectoris have the attacks readily produced if they walk after a meal. It is possible that dilatation of the splanchnic vessels during digestion, combined with the dilatation of the blood-vessels of the muscles exercised in walking, causes a depletion of the supply of the blood to the heart itself, and so induces the speedy exhaustion of the reserve force, which provokes the pain. As these attacks are more readily provoked in the morning after breakfast, it may be that the response of the coronary artery after a night's rest is not sufficient to supply the heart muscle with enough blood to meet the calls made upon the heart, but that later the heart becomes more abundantly supplied.

Vaso-motor angina pectoris.—Nothnagel called attention to a series of cases, where the attacks of angina pectoris were associated with evidence of vaso-constriction. The idea that vaso-constriction is a common cause of angina pectoris has gained ground, but, as a matter of fact, it is of rare occurrence, and certainly not the cause in the majority of cases. Some cases of angina pectoris experience an attack when they go into the cold air. In them there are some organic changes in the heart ; and the increased peripheral resistance caused by the cold embarrasses and exhausts the heart. But there are rare cases in which the cold may induce such vaso-constriction, that angina pectoris may occur in hearts not previously the seat of disease. Thus a patient, aged 30, whom I had under observation for a number of years, complained of the miserable sensation of exhaustion and chilliness which she experienced during cold weather. On a few occasions, she suffered from attacks of pain in the chest, of which the following is an example. On a raw November Sunday morning, she went to teach in a Sunday school. The room was cold, and she felt chilly. Still feeling chilly, she went to church—a cold damp building. The sensation of cold got worse, and towards the end of the service she began to feel a pain in her left chest. She gradually got worse ; and on reaching home it became of great severity and extended from her left chest and down her left arm. She was put to bed with hot bottles and given hot drinks, and when she became warm the pain subsided. In rare instances attacks of angina are provoked only in cold weather—during the summer or while living in a warm climate the individuals may be quite free from them and able to undertake considerable effort. In such cases, it is very difficult to say what are the data on which a trustworthy opinion should be based. I have watched quite a number who restricted themselves during cold weather, or avoided it by going abroad, and who lived useful lives for many years. On the other hand, I have seen one individual who died suddenly three years after the first sign. He was 42 when he died, and, save for a history of ptomaine poisoning six years before he died, there was no evident cause for his suffering. The attacks of pain were so persistent during the cold weather, while he was quite free from them in the summer, that he went to Australia during two winters, and while returning to this country from his last visit he died on board ship. There was nothing to be detected in a physical examination, during the last two years of his life, when I had him under observation. The heart was normal in size, its sounds clear, and blood-pressure 130 mm. Hg., and in warm weather he was able to undertake a considerable amount of effort, such as walking 10 to 15 miles without distress.

In diseases of the aortic valves, especially where there is marked regurgitation, the vaso-motor system becomes unusually sensitive. I am not at all clear of the mechanism by which it is brought about, but it can be demonstrated in several ways, as, for instance, the difference in the arterial pressure in the legs and arms (see p. 138). In certain of these cases, there is a tendency to attacks of angina pectoris, and associated with or causing the attacks, there is marked constriction of the blood-vessels. Several cases have been recorded where the constricted arteries have been noted ; and the violent beating of the heart has caused the bed on which the patient was lying to shake. Case 42 illustrates the peculiar sensitiveness of the vaso-motor system to mental stimulation, with the tendency to attacks of angina pectoris.

The circulatory symptoms in the X disease.[1]—There is another class of cases of somewhat indefinite character, that needs to be recognized in order to appreciate other forms of heart trouble. The class I allude to will be recognized by every practitioner, as they form a considerable portion of the community. The individual is spare and thin ; the face is often drawn and lined, sometimes even in the young. It is usually pale, though

[1] I employ the term ' X disease' for the reason that I do not know the nature of this complaint. Many physicians call members of this class ' neurasthenics ', and are content to leave the matter there. This is simply to give a complaint a name, which is so satisfying that the fact is often lost sight of that the name sheds no light upon the complaint and is nothing but a cloak for ignorance. If the term ' X disease' be employed, it will be a glaring acknowledgement of our ignorance, and will lead to a constant endeavour to clear up the mystery surrounding these cases.

in some the face is ruddy, and the nose is red in cold weather. The hands are usually cold; and they tell you their circulation is feeble. They are always worse on raw cold days, and feel chilly and ill after a cold bath.

Cold hands are sometimes associated with a peculiar roughness and thickness of the skin. The fingers may become white and numb; 'dead' is the term often applied. Exposure on a very cold day may cause the condition to be so extreme that pain in the finger ends is very severe; and in one case I have seen a slight gangrene follow. The nose is often red, and the association between dyspepsia and the red nose is extremely common in these individuals. There is very often dilatation of the stomach, associated with accumulation of blood in the abdominal veins. This latter can be demonstrated in the manner described on p. 98 (Fig. 13). In some cases the increased swelling and pulsation of the jugular vein can be seen to occur during quiet respiration, the swelling of the vein occurring during inspiration. The cause of the swelling in this condition is that pressure on the abdomen empties the abdominal veins into the right heart, so that there is less accommodation for the blood returning by the superior vena cava; hence the jugular vein distends. Inspiration causing a descent of the diaphragm compresses the abdominal contents, including the large veins, against the unyielding wall, and brings about the same result.

The heart itself in these cases is sometimes slightly dilated; and there may be mitral and tricuspid systolic murmurs. They are very evanescent, present at one minute and gone the next. Sometimes we can detect them at the beginning of an examination, and in a few minutes they have disappeared. The rate and rhythm of the heart often vary. Sometimes it is rather slow, and sometimes it is irregular, the irregularity usually being respiratory, though occasionally extra-systoles are present; and then the patient if conscious of them is often greatly frightened, particularly if the doctor does not convincingly reassure him. Hesitation or doubt on the part of the doctor hangs like a cloud over the patient. On account of the presence of some of these symptoms, these cases are often mistaken for cases of heart disease, and many individuals in consequence are subjected to prolonged treatment, which, being ineffective, depresses the patient, interferes with his business affairs, and may send him all over the world in search of a 'cure'. I have never seen heart failure occur in any of these cases; and this assurance is often more effective than any special form of treatment.

I have been particularly struck with the slow respiration in a number of these cases. It may fall as low as seven per minute, and the patient be free from any distress, and quite unconscious of any trouble. It is then that the heart rhythm is most affected, and the swelling of the vein during inspiration and from pressure on the abdomen occurs most characteristically. The nature of this irregularity is fully described in Chapter XXVI.

A healthy individual can sometimes produce this irregularity by simply breathing slowly and deeply, at the rate of seven or eight per minute.

The complaints are extremely varied, and many have a fixed idea that certain organs are at fault ; and it is true that some trouble, usually slight, may be found in some organ. Thus we find gastric and bowel complaints extremely common, though other viscera may also be at fault and complained of. The patient's mental condition is curious and interesting. Some of them are sane, level-headed, and extremely intelligent. To these the bodily suffering is nothing more than a grievous and troublesome affliction. In others it leads to irritability and peevishness in temper. Some become introspective, and are deeply concerned about their bodily or spiritual affairs. It alters their views of material things ; cranks and faddists, political religious, and dietetic, are common among them, often exhibiting strenuous enthusiasm for their particular ideas. Another astonishing feature in these cases is the remarkable way in which a temporary recovery may take place. For weeks some of these individuals may go about miserable and ill, taking little food, finding that little too much for the digestion, and searching for some kind that will suit them—when suddenly they feel better. Their recovery may last for weeks or even months, but they generally relapse.

Now this peculiarity leads to another characteristic of this complaint—unbounded and unreasoning belief in what they take to be the cause of their recovery, diet, drug, methods of exercise, operation. It is because of this tendency to recover that there are so many cures. If one reads between the lines of the testimonials in favour of certain remedies, empiric or recognized by authority, we can see that it is this class of case that is being treated. It is especially among them that faith-cures abound ; and these are the people who swell the ranks of Christian Scientists. Emotional excitement, whether of love or religion, always relieves this kind of person ; and so when religion comes into play we get the various forms of faith-healing. Many women feel extremely well when pregnant.

The diagnoses of medical men are as numerous and varied as the complaints of the patient. The gynæcologist diagnoses some pelvic disorder ; the surgeon sees the source of all the trouble in an appendix, a dilated stomach, or a wandering kidney ; while the physician recognizes the disease according to the bent of his studies—a heart affection, visceral stasis, gastroptosis, neurasthenia, atonic dyspepsia, and so forth. So minute indeed are some of the diagnoses, that we find them classified further as cardiac, gastric, mental, or renal neurasthenias.

The cause of the X complaint.—Although I have sought long and earnestly for an explanation of this complaint, I must confess that I have but an imperfect conception of its origin. As I say, it never leads to heart failure or to death, so that its cause can only be one of speculation. Seeing it is so often associated with digestive troubles, it at once occurs to the mind that it may be due to absorption of a toxic substance from the intestines. In support of this view is the fact, that it is so often associated with constipation and dilatation of the stomach. It is seen very typically in cases of gastric ulcer, especially occurring at the pyloric orifice, with pyloric stenosis and dilatation of the stomach. So frequent is this association that I always examine my patients carefully for gastric ulcer. I have seen several cases greatly improved after a gastro-enterostomy has been performed; and treatment directed to the digestive tract is the one which I have found most beneficial on the whole. Nevertheless, there are cases in which we can detect no digestive trouble, and in some we get other visceral affections. Thus I have seen the condition acquired in people who have had much suffering for years from other complaints, as renal calculus. There is no doubt that several different complaints are included in this description, but so far it is not easy to see on what grounds we should separate them.

Treatment.—When, after an examination, we find there is no trouble, as a gastric ulcer, the confident reassurance of the patient may do a great deal, especially if he has been told that he has a heart complaint and has been treated for it. Then any digestive troubles, such as constipation, should be corrected; and the patient encouraged to lead a life interested in his affairs and duties, and to take as much exercise in the open air as his circumstances will permit. During periods of depression, sleeplessness, and worry, a course of ammonium bromide for a week or ten days will often tide over the troublesome time.

CHAPTER XVII

INSTRUMENTAL METHODS OF EXAMINATION

The sphygmograph.
The polygraph.
The clinical polygraph.
The ink polygraph.
The electrocardiograph.

IN the examination of the vast majority of patients, the diagnosis can be made independently of instrumental methods. It must not be inferred from this that graphic records can be dispensed with, for the power to diagnose the great majority of cases comes through the information obtained by this means. Though it is not necessary for a physician himself to take records, he must be familiar with their interpretation in order that he may appreciate and apply the results.

There have been many methods devised to record the movements of the circulation, but here I will only deal with those which in my hands have yielded very satisfactory results. The essence of a method should be simplicity, for the more complicated the processes the more unsuitable it becomes for practical clinical purposes. In hospitals with large staffs of assistants, the more elaborate methods may be usefully employed, but for the practitioner who studies his own patients, the simpler the method the better.

The sphygmograph.—It is scarcely necessary to enter into a full account of the construction of the various sphygmographs. They have been so frequently described in text-books that their construction is familiar to all medical men. They are all practically constructed on the same principle. A steel spring is laid upon the radial artery at the wrist in such a manner that, while it compresses the artery, it does not obliterate it. Attached directly to the spring is a long lever, or a series of small levers, that magnify the movements of the spring. The free extremity of the lever presses lightly against a strip of paper, whose surface has been blackened by the smoke of burning camphor or turpentine, the strip of paper passing at a uniform speed by means of a clockwork arrangement. Although I have worked with several instruments, I find the Dudgeon to be the handiest and most useful. Into all sphygmographic records, certain errors, due to defects of the instruments, creep. Some of the more elaborate instruments may be freer from defect than the Dudgeon; but so long as one is cautious not to read into the tracings movements evidently due to instrumental errors, the Dudgeon sphygmograph is quite serviceable for a great many practical purposes, and more particularly for giving a true and accurate record of the occurrence of pulse-beats.

The polygraph.—There are many perceptible movements due to the circulation that the sphygmograph fails to register ; and when it is required to record these movements other instruments have to be employed. The method most commonly adopted has been by conveying, by means of a tube containing air, the movements to be registered to a tambour on which there rests a lever. The excursion of the lever is recorded on a revolving drum covered by smoked paper. Two or more tambours being used with their levers placed one above the other, the simultaneous record of different movements can be readily effected.

The elaborate and bulky apparatus required has restricted the employment of this method to such narrow limits, that numerous points of interest in clinical medicine have been either overlooked or misunderstood. In my investigations into the nature of the venous pulse, I had at first to use this unwieldy instrument ; but its cumbersomeness compelled me to devise a much simpler and more effective apparatus.

The clinical polygraph. In my early days when investigating the action of the heart, I attached a tambour to the upright stem of a Dudgeon sphygmograph in such a manner that I was able to obtain, at the same time as the radial pulse was being recorded, some other movement, as the jugular pulse, apex beat, or carotid. As, however, there was a good deal of inconvenience in the blackening and varnishing the papers, and as it was not possible to get a long tracing upon the heart's rhythm, I discarded this for the ink polygraph.

The ink polygraph (Fig. 14). The essential parts of the instrument are a small cup (*E*, Fig. 14) for receiving the impressions of the pulsations, a tube for transmitting the impressions to a tambour (*B*, Fig. 14) and lever, with pen (*F*, Fig. 14).

The small cup for receiving the impressions (which will be referred to hereafter as the ' receiver ') is simply a small shallow vessel, circular in shape, one and a half inches in diameter and half an inch in depth. The open mouth is applied over the pulsating part so that its edges are closely adapted to the skin ; and all communication with the outer air is excluded. From the roof of the receiver rises a narrow pipe, half an inch in length. To this pipe is fitted an india-rubber tube three to four feet in length, the other end of which is connected with the tambour. A modification of this receiver is required when tracings of the liver pulse are taken. The ' liver receiver ' (*B*, Fig. 15) is larger, being five inches in length, two inches in breadth, and one inch in depth, its open edges slightly curved on their long axis. A small air-hole is made at one end near the roof. In employing the ' liver receiver ', the position of the lower margin of the liver having been ascertained, the receiver, held in the right hand, is laid lengthwise across the abdomen, its lower edge being two inches below the liver margin, and the end with the air-hole towards the middle line. Steady continuous pressure is applied to the lower margin of the receiver till it presses deeply into the abdomen; and then the upper margin is adapted closely to the skin. In this manner, a considerable portion of the lower liver edge is embraced by the receiver. If the forefinger of the right hand is now applied over the air-hole, the

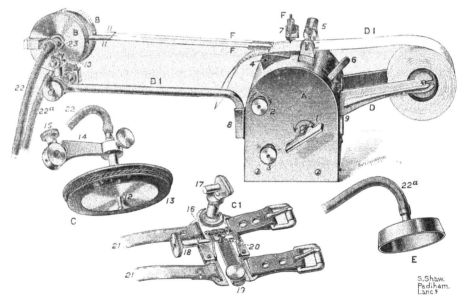

FIG. 14.   The Ink Polygraph.

movements of respiration and liver pulse will be communicated to the lever. If the patient stops breathing, the liver movements are alone transmitted.

The case A (Fig. 14) contains the clockwork for the roller which unwinds the roll of paper D, and also the separate clockwork which moves the time-marking pen F. B B are the two tambours, and F F their levers. The writing pens in Fig. 14 are narrow-grooved wires, one end fixed to the bottom of a small cistern at the free extremity of the lever. The other end of the grooved wire is adjusted to barely touch the paper. The ink is put into the tiny cistern, and it flows along the groove to the pen point by capillary attraction. Recently, these pens have been greatly improved by making a shallow groove in the lever act in place of the cistern. If the pens are kept clean, and the ink is free from dust, they serve their purpose most admirably, and are ever ready for use. Red ink is better than the black inks, as it does not corrode the pens. As the radial pulse is the most service-able of standards, a special method is employed to record it. A splint (C 1) is fastened to the wrist in such a manner, that the pad of the steel spring falls on the radial artery, and is pressed down by an eccentric wheel (18), until a suitable movement is transmitted to the spring by the artery ; then the broad tambour (C) is fitted on to the splint so that the knob (12) falls on the moving spring. This wrist tambour is connected to the tambour B by india-rubber tubing (22, 22), and the movements of the radial pulse are recorded by the lever F. The shallow cup (receiver) E is placed on the pulsation which it is desired to record ; and the movement is conveyed to the lever F of the other tambour. In this way, simultaneous with the radial pulse, a record can be obtained of the apex beat, carotid, jugular, or other pulses.

To record the respiratory movements, a bag can be substituted for the receiver E.

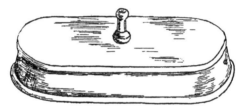

FIG. 15. The Liver Receiver (half size).

By turning the screw (3) the rate at which the paper passes can be quickened or slowed at will. This is of the greatest use ; for it often happens that in quickly succeeding events a wider interval may be required, whereas in recording respiratory movements a slow rate is best. As the time-marker registers one-fifth of a second, and is driven by a separate clockwork, the rate of the recorded movements can always be ascertained with absolute accuracy.

It has been suggested that another tambour should be added to record a third movement ; and I have tried this, but have practically discarded it, as, though it might be of use occasionally, it would complicate the apparatus unnecessarily. When one is making observations single-handed, the two tambours are quite sufficient to occupy the attention. With a little practice, this apparatus can be used with the greatest facility. In the course of a few minutes the different movements can be recorded, with the patient sitting up, or in the recumbent position.

When the tambour is strapped to the wrist to take the radial pulse, one hand is always free to start the machine, and to replenish the ink or regulate the rate, the other hand holding the receiver over the movement to be recorded.

The electrocardiograph.—It has long been known that the contraction of muscle gives rise to electrical changes. Waller pointed out that if the legs or arms were used as leads and connected with a galvanometer, the electrical reactions which occur with the contraction of the heart, would affect the magnet.

Einthoven invented the string galvanometer, by means of which the movements of the heart can readily be registered. In this instrument a thread of platinum or other suitable material is placed between the poles of a magnet. As it lies in this magnetic field, the thread becomes very sensitive to the

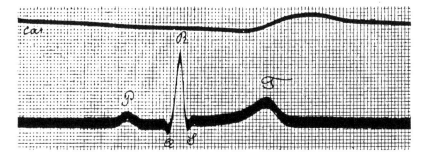

FIG. 16, for which we are indebted to Professor Einthoven, shows a portion of a carotid curve and a single beat of an electric curve. The abscissæ are divided at intervals of 0·01 sec. ; the ordinates are divided at intervals of 10^{-4} volt. The lead, as in all figures shown, was from right arm and left leg. In this, as in all figures also, corresponding points of time are directly vertical to each other. P represents the auricular and Q, R, S, and T the ventricular contraction.

slightest electric change. The right arm and left leg or right arm and left arm are immersed in a suitable basin containing salt and water, in which there is a sheet of copper. This sheet of copper is connected by wires with the thread lying between the poles of the magnet. The electric disturbances caused by the movements of the heart chambers are conveyed to the thread and cause it to execute a very slight movement. A series of lenses is so arranged that by means of an arc light, the shadow of the thread is thrown upon a movable photographic plate, in such a manner that the movement of the thread, when influenced by the electrical changes of the heart, is photographed.

The electrocardiogram obtained from a normal acting heart, shows a series of movements due to the contraction of the auricles and ventricles (Fig. 16 and 17). In a cardiac revolution, the first wave P is due to the contraction of the auricle ; this is followed by a series of waves, the result of the ventricular contraction. The first of this series is a steep sharp wave R, which falls equally rapidly, and is followed by a negative wave S. This is again followed by a slower rising wave T, of less height than R.

While the waves shown in Fig. 16 are present in all normal acting hearts, they may show slight variations. These variations become marked in certain diseased conditions. Thus, hypertrophy of one ventricle more than

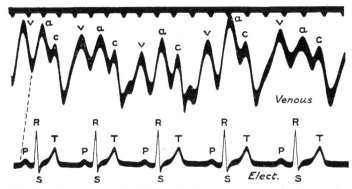

FIG. 17. Simultaneous records of time, in $\frac{1}{5}$ sec., venous and electrocardiographic curves. The delay in the venous curve is due to the air transmission employed, to the delay in transmission from auricle to neck, and to the fact that the electric change slightly precedes the contraction. From a patient in whom the P–R and a–c intervals show slight prolongation, but in whom the curve is otherwise normal.

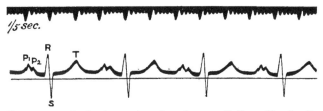

FIG. 18. From a case of mitral stenosis and aortic regurgitation. Showing the prolongation of P–R interval, a splitting of P, and an increase in S.

another gives rise to peculiarities in the ventricular complex; so also hypertrophy of the left auricle induces a modification of the P waves (Fig. 18).

It is, however, in the bringing to light of abnormal rhythms, that the galvanometer is of the greatest service. We know that the heart's contraction may start in any portion of the heart muscle, if that portion is independent of the normal pacemaker, or is more excitable than the pacemaker. When this occurs, a modification of the character of the electric curves gives a clue to the source of the contraction. Lewis has demonstrated experimentally the peculiar character of the electrocardiograms, when the auricular contractions start from places other than the normal; and he has been able to recognize, in the clinical electrocardiogram, abnormal rhythms arising from different regions in the auricle. When the ventricular contractions arise in a normal fashion, the waves R, S, and T follow one another with characteristic shape and sequence, and it has been suggested that these characteristics are due to the stimulus for contraction entering

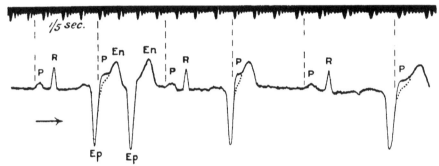

FIG. 19. The curve shows three beats in which the normal P–R sequence is observed, and four extra-systoles of the ventricle. The P waves which are regular are superimposed upon the extra-systolic curves in three places (dotted lines).

FIG. 20. From a case of auricular fibrillation, showing the absence of the normal wave P, and the presence of irregular waves having fixed relationship to other events.

the heart by a definite path (the auriculo-ventricular bundle), stimulating first the base, passing to the apex, and returning to the base. When a stimulus arises in the ventricle itself, as in cases of ventricular extra-systole, then an anomalous curve is obtained, quite different from that of the normal (Fig. 19), suggesting that the contraction has arisen from some part of the ventricle itself, a suggestion confirmed by experiment, where identical curves can be obtained by the artificial production of a ventricular extra-systole.

The recognition of this fact is of importance, as it shows that in such conditions as auricular fibrillation, the auricle is thrown out of gear and

acts in a very abnormal fashion, giving rise to a peculiar and characteristic electrocardiogram ; yet it is still the source of the ventricular
stimulation, inasmuch as the characteristic normal ventricular complex is
maintained, indicating that the stimulus for contraction has entered the
ventricle by the normal path (Fig. 20). This is also a point of some interest
in complete heart-block. Here the separation of auricle from ventricle is
complete, so that the ventricle contracts quite independently of the auricular
stimulus, yet the ventricular electrocardiograms show a perfectly normal

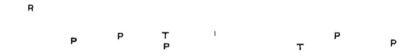

FIG. 21. From a case of complete heart-block, showing the dissociation of auricle and
ventricle.

outline, indicating that the stimulus has entered the ventricle by the normal
route, that is, by the auriculo-ventricular bundle (Fig. 21). As the nodal
portion of the bundle is destroyed in these cases, we must infer that the
remaining portions of the bundle are capable of originating and transmitting
the stimulus for ventricular contraction.

Certain of the peculiarities induced by abnormal rhythms and disease
of the heart muscle will be referred to in the text. I do not deal with them
at great length, but would refer the reader to Dr. Lewis's writings for a full
exposition of the subject. It is to him I am indebted for taking the records
and interpreting the curves in the great majority of my cases.

CHAPTER XVIII

The Position and Movements of the Heart

The position of the heart.
The standards for recognizing the events in a cardiac revolution.
Conditions of the chest-wall permitting the recognition of certain movements of the heart.
The nature of the movements graphically recorded.
The apex beat.
Interpretation of a tracing of an apex beat due to the systole of the left ventricle.
The auricular wave.
Retraction of yielding structures in the neighbourhood of the heart during ventricular systole.
Liver movement due to cardiac aspiration.
Epigastric pulsation.
The apex beat due to the right ventricle.
Significance of the inverted cardiogram.
Alteration of the apex beat due to retraction of the lung.
The shock due to the ventricular systole.

The position of the heart.—Professor Waterston has lately been reinvestigating the position of the organs in the human body; and he has furnished me with the following result of his observations on the heart:

' Both the position and the form of the heart present considerable variation in different individuals of the same age and sex, hence it is impossible to lay down a rigid statement of what is normal in the position or form, except within fairly wide limits.

' It may be stated, first of all, that in the female, the heart is slightly smaller than it is in the male, and that in old age there is a diminution of the size of the heart which may be considered to be normal. In the child, the heart lies at a somewhat higher level than in the adult—this difference being possibly associated with the large size of the liver in the child.

' Apart from these variations associated with age and sex, the individual variations are probably to be associated with the different shapes of the chest, and with the varying height of the diaphragm, which are found in different individuals.

' I have recently made a number of observations upon the position of the heart as a whole, and of its chambers in relation to the chest-wall, by a method of projecting orthogonally the outline of the ribs, the sternum, and heart on to a flat surface.

' Fig. 22 shows an average result obtained in this way, from an adult male. It will be seen, from the figure, that the anterior surface of the heart is of a quadrilateral shape. The whole of the right border is formed by the right auricle, and the same chamber constitutes the whole of the heart which lies on the right side of the sternum. The right ventricle con-

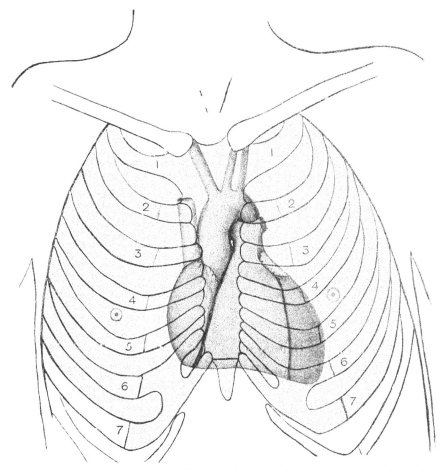

Fig. 22. An accurate delineation of the relation of the heart to the anterior chest-wall obtained by orthogonal projection (Waterston).

stitutes the greatest part of the anterior surface and lies behind the sternum and to its left, while the left margin and the apex of the heart are formed by the left ventricle. Only a very small portion of the left auricular appendix appears on the anterior surface, at the root of the pulmonary artery, and it is quite insignificant.

MACKENZIE

' It is quite usual to find the apex of the heart behind the sixth costal cartilage, and the lower margin of the heart is frequently found at a lower level than is usually given, namely the lower border of the body of the sternum; and it descends behind the ensiform cartilage.

' The greatest vertical and transverse measurements of the projected outline of the heart measure four and a half to five inches in the adult male. Frequently, however, one of these dimensions is increased, usually the vertical, while the transverse diameter is somewhat diminished. This shape of the heart is associated usually with a long narrow chest.

' These observations have been made on the cadaver in the horizontal attitude, and may be taken to indicate accurately the position and shape of the heart in that condition.

' If these outlines are compared with the outlines taken during life in the vertical position, by the orthodiagraph (Fig. 23), it is found that there is a difference in the results obtained, indicating that the position of the heart is different. In the vertical attitude, during life, the heart lies at a lower level, and the lower border of the heart descends behind the ensiform cartilage to a varying degree, and the right ventricle comes to lie behind the upper part of the abdominal wall in the infracostal angle. This descent is associated with the descent of the diaphragm which occurs in the change from the horizontal to the vertical position.

' It is further found that the movements of respiration affect the position of the heart very considerably, and especially the level of the lower border, which rises in expiration and sinks in inspiration. The upper border, on the other hand, is not so much altered, but the right and especially the left borders are influenced especially at their lower ends. The left margin, as is shown by Fig. 23, was found in expiration to move to the left side to a distance of as much as one inch.'

The standards for recognizing the events in a cardiac revolution.— Owing to their easy recognition and determined place in the cardiac cycle, the carotid and radial pulses form the most certain standards for finding out the place of other movements in a cardiac revolution. In describing the tracings frequent references will have to be made to these standards, and more particularly to that period during which the semilunar valves are open, which is indicated in some tracings by the space E. When it appears in the radial tracing, it corresponds to the effects of the ventricular systole upon the radial pulse—that is to say, to the actual pulse-wave—and not to the true time of the occurrence of the ventricular systole, for the pulse-wave having a longer distance to travel, the period E will be later in the radial than in the apex or carotid tracings.

Conditions of the chest-wall permitting the recognition of certain movements of the heart.—The movements of the heart in a healthy person are often so obscured by the lungs, that only very little change is

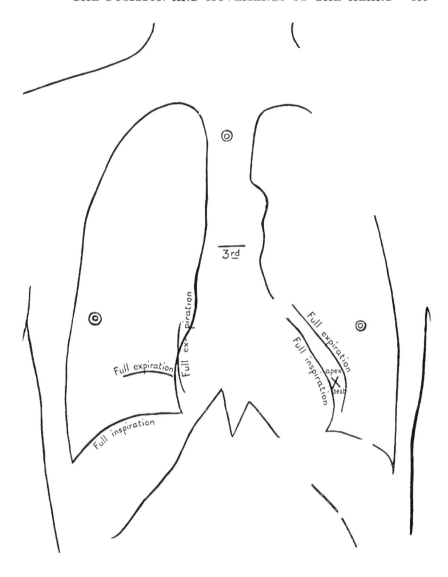

FIG. 23. The position of the heart and blood-vessels in the chest obtained by the orthodiagraph
(Ritchie).

discernible in the external chest-wall. In many cases the lungs are so voluminous, or the chest-wall so fat and thick, that no movement can be detected.
But when a large surface of the heart is directly exposed to a thin chest-wall,
the heart being normal or increased in size, and the lung displaced, a series
of movements of the chest-wall, due to the contraction and expansion of
the heart, can be recognized. The movements thus discernible are not the
same in all cases, but depend on which part of the heart's surface comes in
contact with the chest-wall and other yielding structures. These movements take place so rapidly, that it is difficult to interpret their significance
by the unaided senses. Many writers on this subject have drawn elaborate,
but nevertheless erroneous, conclusions from such unaided observations ;
and it seems to me that accurate observations by the graphic method alone
can furnish a clear and definite explanation.

The nature of the movements graphically recorded.—The movements of the heart that are most readily recognized, are those connected
with the systole and diastole of the ventricles. Movements directly due
to the auricles are so obscured by the larger and more vigorous movements
of the ventricle, that it is doubtful if they are ever capable of recognition.
The movements most readily recognized are : first, the apex beat ; second,
the filling of the ventricles ; third, the emptying of the ventricles ; and
fourth, the shock communicated by the sudden hardening of the ventricular
walls as they pass into systole.

The apex beat.—The chief movement, and the one which is usually
most apparent, is that caused by the forcible outward projection of the
apex of the heart during the ventricular systole—the apex beat. This is
generally described as ' the lowest and outermost point of the heart which
strikes against the chest-wall '. In healthy adults, it is usually felt in the
fifth left intercostal space, immediately inside the nipple line. It may,
however, be situated in the fourth interspace, and outside the nipple line
in children and in some adults. In disease of the heart, it alters its situation
with the increasing size of the heart. This forward thrust occurs, when the
left ventricle is in contact with the chest. As will be shown later, a movement of another description occurs, when the right ventricle constitutes the
so-called apex beat. That the apex beat due to the left ventricle is a distinct
displacement of the heart forward, can be recognized by the senses of touch
and sight.

During the whole time occupied by the systole of the ventricle, the apex
is usually kept projecting into the interspace, so that the palpating hand
recognizes the forward thrust, and in such a tracing as Fig. 24, the lever
taking the tracing is kept raised during the whole time of the outflow
from the ventricle (space E'). If the left ventricle is much hypertrophied,
the same movement can sometimes be detected in two or three interspaces.
If the interspaces be fairly open and the chest-wall thin, and the tip of the

finger be thrust into the third or fourth interspace near the sternum, the right ventricle can be felt hardening, and remaining thus hardened in contact with the finger during the whole period of the ventricular systole. It cannot, however, be averred that in this case there is a forward thrust. The heart here is always in contact with the chest-wall, and the finger pushed into the interspace during the diastole, in all likelihood, impinges against the lax ventricular wall. As soon as the ventricle hardens, the finger recognizes

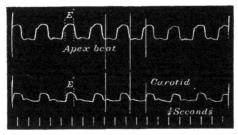

FIG. 24.   Simultaneous tracings of the apex beat and the carotid pulse, showing the 'systolic plateau' in the cardiogram during the outflow from the ventricle (E').

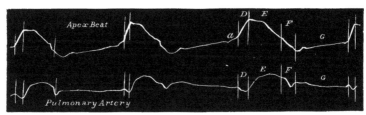

FIG. 25.   Simultaneous tracings of the apex beat and of the pulsation in the pulmonary artery. *a* represents the small wave due to the auricular systole. The time during which the ventricle is passing into systole is represented by the space (D) emptying (E), relaxing (F), filling (G). While this tracing was being taken the cylinder was rapidly rotated. The letters D, E, F have reference to the same periods in the cardiac revolution as in Fig. 47.

this hardening as something pushing against it. This sensation of a thrust is sometimes actually synchronous with an indrawing of the soft structures filling up the interspace (Fig. 30).

Interpretation of a tracing of an apex beat due to the systole of the left ventricle.—A tracing of the apex beat or cardiogram is a diagrammatic representation of (*a*) the forward movement of the apex of the heart, while the ventricular muscle is beginning to contract (space *D*, Fig. 25); (*b*) the retention of the apex beat against the chest-wall while the ventricles are emptying (space *E*, Fig. 25); (*c*) the backward movement of the apex of the heart, while the ventricular muscle is relaxing (space *F*, Fig. 25); (*d*) and the gradual swelling of the ventricle during diastole (space *G*, Fig. 25).

(a) *The period of commencing contraction of the ventricular muscle—the presphygmic interval* (space *D*, Fig. 25).—During this period the pressure within the ventricle is rapidly rising. The auriculo-ventricular valves close as soon as the pressure within the ventricle rises above that in the auricle, and the semilunar valves open as soon as the pressure in the ventricle rises above that in the aorta. This last occurs at the end of the period *D*, Fig. 25, and is usually indicated by the abrupt termination of the upstroke.

In Fig. 25 simultaneous tracings were taken of the pulsation in the pulmonary artery and of the apex beat. As the beginning of the pulse in the pulmonary artery indicates the opening of the semilunar valves, so it is

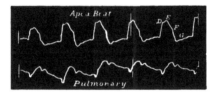

FIG. 26. Simultaneous tracings of the apex beat and of the pulsation in the pulmonary artery. The letters have the same significance as those in Fig. 25.

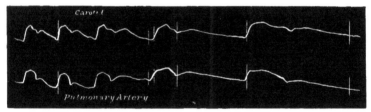

FIG. 27. Simultaneous tracings of the pulses of the carotid and pulmonary arteries. After the third beat the cylinder was rotated rapidly.

found that the end of the period *D* corresponds exactly with the beginning of the pulsation of the pulmonary artery. When this figure was taken, the cylinder was rotated rapidly, in order to separate the events as widely as possible. When the cylinder rotates at a slower rate, this period is represented by an almost perpendicular line (Fig. 26).

It will be noted that the termination of the upstroke corresponds exactly with the beginning of the outflow of the ventricle into the artery. These tracings were taken from a lad, suffering from phthisis of the left lung, which had retracted from the heart, and through the thin chest-walls the various movements could easily be observed. In the second left interspace there was a marked pulsation, and tracings of this, taken at the same time as the carotid pulse, left no doubt as to its being caused by the pulmonary artery (Fig. 27). It will be noticed that the carotid pulse appears just a very little

later than the pulmonary.   Here also, after a few beats, the cylinder was
rapidly rotated, with the hand, to separate more widely the different events.

(b) *The period of ventricular outflow* (space *E*, Fig. 25).—When the
pressure in the ventricles exceeds that in the aorta and pulmonary artery
the semilunar valves open, and the blood flows out from the ventricles.
During this period the apex is usually kept stationary, pressing against the
chest-wall, and in many tracings (as in Fig. 28) it is shown by a fairly level
line—the ' systolic plateau '.   In place of a flattened top representing the
period of ventricular outflow, the tracing may continue to rise (as in Fig. 24),
indicating that the ventricle is still slightly shifting.   On the other hand,
the tracing sometimes rapidly descends (Fig. 25 and 26).   I cannot but
think that this is due to the ventricle shrinking away from the interspace
during its systole, the receiver perhaps not being exactly over the apex.
I shall show later on, that this shrinking can be demonstrated in various
places, and I have found evidence of it immediately under a diffuse apex

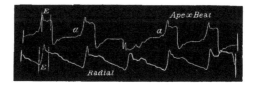

Fɪɢ. 28. Simultaneous tracings of the apex beat and of the radial pulse,
showing the ' systolic plateau ' and the small wave (*a*) due to the auricular
systole.   The third beat in the apex tracing is obliterated by the movement of
inspiration.

beat.   The movement producing the apex beat is really a displacement
of the heart forward, and while the heart is thus displaced, the ventricles
shrink as they empty themselves.   The termination of the ventricular
outflow is occasioned by the pressure in the aorta becoming higher
than that in the ventricle.   The semilunar valves close in consequence,
and the ventricular muscle then relaxes ; the termination of the systolic
period is indicated in the cardiogram by a sudden descent.

(c) *The period of relaxation of the ventricular muscle* (space *F*, Fig. 25).
—With the relaxation of the ventricular muscle the apex retreats from
the chest-wall, as is indicated by the slanting downstroke in the tracing, or
where the tracing is already falling during the ventricular outflow by a more
rapid descent (Fig. 25 and 26).   During this period, the ventricular pressure
rapidly falls until the stage of complete relaxation, when the pressure inside
the ventricles becomes lower than that inside the auricles.   When this
occurs, the auriculo-ventricular valves open.   The apex then has reached
its greatest distance from the chest-wall, and in the tracing the lowest
point is reached.

The time of the opening of the auriculo-ventricular valves is usually
a very definite landmark in apex and jugular tracings, and, in consequence,
is a useful standard for measuring the sequence of events in tracings of
irregular heart action. It is recognized as the lowest point reached in tracings
of the apex of the left ventricle, and it is just before the fall of the wave *v*,
in tracings of the jugular pulse. Its time corresponds nearly with the bottom
of the aortic notch in tracings of the radial pulse. It is represented by the
perpendicular line 6 in many of the tracings given later.

(*d*) *The period of filling of the ventricles* (space *G*, Fig. 25).—Upon the
opening of the auriculo-ventricular valves, the blood flows from the auricles
into the ventricles ; and as the ventricles distend the heart pushes against
the intercostal space, and slightly raises the lever. This period is marked
in the tracing by a gradual ascent. Frequently, however, the heart fails
to affect the tissues in the interspace during this period, so that no indication
of the filling of the ventricles is obtained ; in such a tracing as Fig. 24,
for example, and in many others given in the text, the whole of this period
is a blank, so far as information regarding events in the cardiac cycle are
concerned.

The auricular wave.—In some tracings from the apex there is occasionally found an abrupt, though slight, rise immediately preceding the
beginning of the ventricular systole (*a*, Fig. 28 and 29). This is due to
a sudden increase in the contents of the ventricle, caused by the contraction
of the auricle, and may be termed the auricular wave.

The auricular wave is not always perceptible in apex tracings, but when
present it often gives valuable information. Normally, it precedes the beginning of the wave due to the ventricular systole by about one-tenth of a second
(space between 1 and 2, Fig. 29). Sometimes this interval is increased ;
and then it may indicate a delay in the passage of the stimulus from
auricle to ventricle. In cases of heart-block, it may be recognized during
the ventricular pauses. Its absence may be of no significance, but it is
to be noted that it is never seen in cases with auricular fibrillation, even
when immediately before the starting of this abnormal rhythm, it had been
a conspicuous feature.

Retraction of yielding structures in the neighbourhood of the heart
during ventricular systole.—When the ventricles expel their contents,
they must of necessity shrink. This shrinkage occurs abruptly, and
with considerable force. The yielding tissues in the neighbourhood of the
heart are dragged upon, and evidence of this dragging can be obtained
from a variety of sources. John Hunter originated the idea that the systole
of the ventricles would have a tendency to produce a vacuum, and thus
expedite the flow of the venous blood into the chest. Evidence of this
'cardiac aspiration' affecting the lungs, has been obtained by a number
of observers. The tracings of Mosso and Delépine of the movements of

the column of air in the respiratory passages, due to the cardiac aspiration, correspond exactly with those obtained from the præcordium (Fig. 30), from under the liver (Fig. 31 and 32), and from the epigastrium (Fig. 33 and 34).

In Fig. 30 this drawing-in of tissues in the intercostal spaces over the heart is demonstrated. It was obtained from a boy aged 14. The apex beat was well marked in the fourth interspace outside the nipple. At the same time that the apex was thrust outwards, the skin and subcutaneous

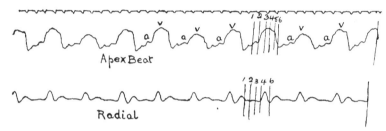

FIG. 29. The apex tracing shows a slight wave, a, due to the contraction of the auricles distending the ventricles and beginning one-tenth of a second before the ventricular systole. For explanation of the numbered perpendicular lines see Fig. 50.

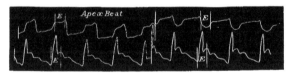

FIG. 30. Simultaneous tracings of the heart movements (upper tracing) and of the radial pulse. The first part of the upper tracing was taken from the apex beat in the fourth interspace immediately outside the nipple, while the latter part was taken in the same interspace near the left border of the sternum. In the first part the cardiogram shows a 'systolic plateau' during the ventricular outflow (E); in the other part the cardiogram is inverted, i. e. there is a depression during this period (E).

tissues over the same interspace inside the nipple were drawn in. In Fig. 30 the tracings of the apex beat were taken simultaneously with the radial pulse for four beats. The clockwork was then stopped, and the receiver, which had been applied over the apex, was placed over the præcordium inside the nipple, and the 'inverted cardiogram' of the last portion was obtained. The space E represents the duration of the outflow from the ventricle ; and this period, which in the apex tracing shows a flattened elevation, shows a great depression in that obtained from the front of the heart. The ascending limb of the apex tracing corresponds to the period, during which the ventricle is contracting (space D, Fig. 25). This period in the inverted cardiogram is represented by a slight rise, due to the shock of the contracting ventricle. No blood as yet has escaped from the ventricle. As soon as the semilunar valves open, the blood rushes out of the ventricle, the ventricles diminish in size, and the yielding tissues of the interspace sink in and cause the great fall, as represented in the inverted cardiogram (space *E*, in the latter half of Fig. 30).

Liver movements due to cardiac aspiration.—Not only can this aspiration be demonstrated as affecting the pliable tissues immediately in contact with the heart, but in suitable cases it can be shown to produce a distinct excursion of the liver. All writers referring to this movement

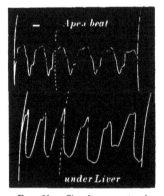

FIG. 31. Simultaneous tracings of the apex beat and of the movement of the liver. When the ventricle empties, the liver is drawn up, and this causes the fall in the tracing.

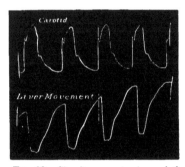

FIG. 32. Simultaneous tracings of the carotid pulse and liver movement. With the appearance of the carotid pulse there is a sudden fall of the lower tracing, due to the liver being drawn upwards by the emptying ventricles.

of the liver, speak of it as a downward thrust during the ventricular systole. Careful tracings demonstrate that this movement is quite of the opposite nature—it is a drawing-up of the liver during the ventricular systole. In Fig. 31 the apex beat is taken at the same time as the movement of the liver.

The receiver, taking the liver movement, being applied to the under surface of the organ, a retraction of the liver upwards corresponds with a fall in the tracing, and vice versa. It will be seen that the movement of the liver upwards takes place during the ventricular systole, while the downward movement is due to the diastolic filling of the ventricle. In Fig. 32 the movement of the liver is recorded at the same time as the carotid pulse. It is seen that as soon as the carotid pulse appears, the liver is drawn up, and remains there until the end of the ventricular systole, after which the liver gradually falls down.   I do not mean that the excursion of the liver is one of considerable extent, but the movement is so great as to be obvious to the palpating hand.   It is distinct from a pulsation of the liver, which is a periodic swelling of the liver, while this is a displacement of the liver *en masse*.

Epigastric pulsation.—The causes which may produce a pulsation in the epigastrium are : (*a*) a dilated right heart ; (*b*) a hypertrophied left ventricle ; (*c*) the abdominal aorta ; and (*d*) an aneurysm of the abdominal aorta.

In the later stages of typhoid fever and other exhausting diseases, epigastric pulsation is an ominous sign of cardiac enfeeblement.   The movement consists of an alternate swelling and retraction of the epigastrium. It is invariably assumed that this swelling or pulsation is due to the right ventricular systole, and that it is of the same nature as the outward protrusion constituting the apex beat.   If this form of epigastric pulsation is carefully

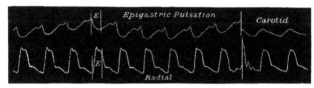

FIG. 33.   Simultaneous tracing of the epigastric pulse, due to a dilated right heart, and of the radial pulse.   The epigastric pulse shows a retraction during the ventricular systole (*E*), and a protrusion during the filling of the ventricle.

timed with the carotid pulse, it will be found that the epigastric pulse, protrusion, or swelling, precedes the carotid pulse, and that the retraction of the epigastrium corresponds in time to the carotid pulsation.   The apex beat is rarely available in these cases, on account of the right heart pushing the left ventricle backwards.   In the tracings of the epigastric pulse (Fig. 33), the radial pulse is taken as the standard of time.   The time occupied by the pulse travelling from the heart to the wrist being allowed for, it will be found that the great fall in the epigastric pulse corresponds exactly with the ventricular systole (*E*).

The patient from whom this tracing was taken was dying from pernicious anæmia.   At the post-mortem examination, a needle pushed through the epigastrium, at the place where the tracing was obtained, was found to have penetrated the right ventricle.

In Fig. 34 a similar tracing is given, except that there is a slight interruption at *c*, on the line of descent.   This will be found to correspond exactly to the time of the abdominal aorta, taken from the middle of the abdomen, a few beats of which are also given.   This small wave (*c*) is due to the impulse imparted to the tissues by the pulse of the underlying aorta.   Epigastric pulsation, due to hypertrophied left ventricle, has the same character as an apex beat (Fig. 35). Epigastric pulsation, due to the abdominal aorta, presents quite a different character from that due to a dilated right ventricle, as shown in Fig. 36, where the pulse corresponds in character and time with the radial pulse. An epigastric pulsation, due to an aneurysm of the abdominal aorta, would assume the time and character of the abdominal aortic pulse (Fig. 36).

FIG. 34. Shows the same features as Fig. 33, with the exception of the small wave (c) occasioned by the shock communicated to the episgastrium by the abdominal aortic pulse. A few beats of the abdominal aorta are also given.

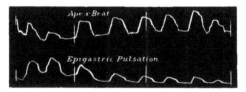

FIG. 35. Simultaneous tracings of the apex beat and of the epigastric pulsation, due to a hypertrophied left ventricle.

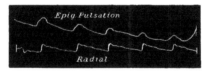

FIG. 36. Simultaneous tracings of the epigastric pulse, due to the abdominal aorta, and of the radial pulse.

The apex beat due to the right ventricle.—Accepting the usual clinical definition of the apex beat ' being the lowest and outermost part of the heart's impulse ', a totally different form of beat is found when the right ventricle causes this movement. In certain cases of dilatation of the right heart, nearly the whole anterior aspect of the heart is composed of the right auricle and ventricle, the left ventricle forming but a mere strip of the border (see Fig. 177 and 178). This portion of the left ventricle is situated so far back that it is covered by the lungs, and does not reach the chest-wall. Hence it is that ' the lowest and outermost part of the heart ' in contact with the chest-wall, is the right ventricle. The character of the apex beat now corresponds exactly with that of the liver movements, of the epigastric pulse, due to enlarged right heart, and of the inverted cardiogram in Fig. 30. In place of the outward thrust during the systole, as in the apex beat due to the left ventricle, there is an indrawing of the tissues.

Fig. 37 was taken from a youth, aged 18, with simple dilatation of the heart, and free from valvular disease. There was marked pulsation of the jugular veins, a few beats of which are given. The apex tracing shows a great depression during the period of ventricular outflow (*E*). This period is immediately preceded by an abrupt rise, due to the shock communicated to the chest by the sudden hardening of the ventricular wall. Although corresponding with the period *D* (in Fig. 25) in the left ventricular apex

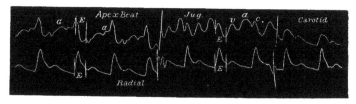

Fig. 37. Tracings of the apex beat, jugular pulse, and carotid pulse (upper tracing), taken at the same time as the radial. The apex tracing is due to the right ventricle, and shows a depression (*E*) during the ventricular outflow. The sharp elevation preceding *E* is caused by the shock of the contracting ventricles. This is preceded by a small wave (*a*), which is due to the contracting auricle distending the ventricle, and corresponds in time exactly with the wave *a* in the jugular pulse, which is due to the contracting auricle sending a wave of blood back into the veins.

tracings, I am inclined to think that the rise here is an instrumental fault, due to the violent shock communicated by the sudden and forcible ventricular contraction. This period is preceded by a small wave (*a*) in the tracing, identical with the similar rise, in Fig. 28 and 29, of the left ventricular apex beat. It is due in this case, as in those, to the distension of the ventricle by the auricular systole. It occupies exactly the same period in the cardiac revolution as the wave *a* in the venous pulse, which is produced by the systole of the right auricle. The space *E*, in all the tracings, represents the period of ventricular outflow as it affects the different pulses. One can, therefore, readily and with certainty refer the different events to their causes. Thus we know that the wave of contraction arising in the auricle passes on to the ventricle, that between the auricular outflow and the ventricular outflow a period, the presphygmic interval (*D*, Fig. 25), exists during which the ventricle is contracting and raising its pressure until it opens the semilunar valves. Thus the presphygmic period in the apex tracing exactly corresponds to the period between the summit of the wave *a* in the venous pulse, due to the auricular systole, and that of the wave c, due to the carotid pulse. A few beats of the carotid are given, which can be taken as a standard of time to verify all these points. The period G is due to the filling of the ventricle.

Significance of the inverted cardiogram.—It is asserted in text-books that an indrawing of the apex, during systole, of the ventricles is a diagnostic sign of adherent pericardium. I have had several cases where I have got at one time tracings of the apex beat due to the left ventricle, and at other times tracings due to the right ventricle, with indrawing during systole ; and at the post-mortem examination, there has never been found any signs of adherent pericardium.

The fact that ' the lowest and outermost point of the heart which strikes against the chest-wall ', may be due to the right ventricle should be borne in mind. Whenever that occurs, the cardiogram is an inverted one—that is to say, there is a shrinking of the heart from the chest-wall during the

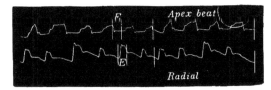

FIG. 38. Simultaneous tracings of the apex beat, and of the radial pulse. The rise in the apex tracing resembles the usual characters present in a tracing of the apex beat due to the left ventricle. On analysis, it is found that the elevation is during the diastole, and the fall (E) during the systole, of the ventricle.

systole, and a protrusion during the diastole of the ventricles. This is not always recognizable at first sight. Being somewhat familiar with the form of various apex-beat curves, I generally have no difficulty in recognizing cardiograms due to the left ventricle. But when from a patient I took Fig. 38, I certainly was misled in the first instance. The abrupt rise and fall bear a close resemblance to an apex-beat curve, due to the left ventricle. Careful measurements of the radial and apex tracings show that the elevation in Fig. 38 was not at the period of ventricular systole, but occurred during ventricular diastole, while the systolic period (E) corresponded with the fall in the tracing. It is necessary to insist upon this view, because inferences drawn from the apex beat alone are liable to lead one into error. Even so careful an observer as Keyt has mistaken the nature of such an apex-beat tracing, and imagined in consequence that he detected an extreme delay in the appearance of the arterial pulse. I have observed similar errors of interpretation in the tracings of other writers. It follows, then, that for a guide to any event occurring during a cardiac revolution, the arterial pulse is the only safe and reliable one. When the apex beat is taken as a standard, careful inquiries should be directed to ascertain its true nature. While it is true in the majority of instances that the cardiogram from the right ventricle is ' inverted ', I have taken tracings with a systolic plateau from the third and fourth interspaces near the sternum ; but, as I have had no post-mortem examination in these cases, I am not sure of the part of the heart producing these curves. The whole subject of cardiography is in great need of thorough and painstaking investigation.

Alteration of the apex beat due to retraction of the lung.—If one watches the progress of a case of advancing heart failure over a period of years, marked changes will sometimes be detected, not only in the character, but in the position of the apex beat. In the earlier stages of heart failure, due to mitral disease, for instance, the left ventricle may be pushed back by the distended right ventricle, so that it is entirely covered by the lung, and the apex beat may then be due to the right ventricle. In course of time, from pressure of the enlarged heart, the lung is compressed and recedes, leaving a large surface of the heart bare to the chest-wall. In such cases, the apex beat may be found in the posterior axillary line, and in the eighth interspace. The tracing obtained then is one due to the left ventricle.

The shock due to the ventricular systole.—I am of opinion that a good deal of confusion, in regard to the correct interpretation of the heart movements, has arisen from associating the shock conveyed to the chest-wall, when the ventricles pass into systole, with the apex beat. The apex beat and this impulse have become so connected that it is assumed that they are one and the same thing. The apex beat due to the left ventricle is a movement which lasts during the whole of the ventricular systole ; the shock caused by the ventricular contraction endures but a short space of time, and occurs while the ventricular muscle suddenly hardens, and corresponds with the upstroke only of the apex beat (D, Fig. 25 and 26). It is this shock which sends the lever so high in Fig. 28 and 37, at the beginning of the ventricular contraction. In the tracings of the epigastric pulse (Fig. 33 and 34), and of the movement from the front of the heart (Fig. 30), this shock causes the sharp elevation just before the fall (E) due to the emptying of the ventricle. Thus, in noting the time of the shock and watching the epigastric pulse, for instance, as in Fig. 33 and 34, one could see that the retraction of the epigastrium followed it. If one associated the shock with the apex beat, it would therefore be assumed that the protrusion corresponded with the systole, and the retraction with the diastole. It frequently happens that this shock is the only movement of the heart, discernible on examining the chest. It is often markedly present in dilatation of the heart, when the heart's surface in contact with the chest-wall is entirely made up of the right ventricle and auricle. In such cases, it must not be assumed that the shock is the evidence of the contraction of the right ventricle only. It is impossible to distinguish the shock, due to the right ventricle, from the shock due to the left. The reason I insist upon this is because the perception of this shock has been assumed to be an evidence of the right heart contracting, when the absence of a beat in the radial pulse was supposed to indicate the absence of a contraction in the left ventricle. As will be shown later, this sort of evidence is not only unreliable but actually misleading.

CHAPTER XIX

Superiority of the digital examination.
What is the pulse ?
Inspection of the arteries.
Digital examination of the arteries.
    The condition of the walls.
    The size of the artery.
    Character of the pulse.
    The pulse-rate.
    The size of the pulse-wave.
    The impact of the pulse-wave on the finger.
    The rhythm of the pulse.
    The two radial pulses compared.
The value of a sphygmogram.
Definition of a sphygmogram.
Events occurring during a cardiac revolution revealed by the sphygmogram.
Features of the sphygmogram due to instrumental defect.

Superiority of the digital examination.—In the examination of the arterial pulse, several methods may be employed, as exploration by the finger, by graphic records, and by instrumental measurement of the arterial pressure. By far the most important of these methods is the first. There is a tendency to exalt the others at the expense of the digital, but no apparatus can ever replace the trained finger. No doubt the other methods can give very definite information of a limited kind, but in diagnosing the patient's condition, they should only supplement the digital examination.

The mechanical methods can be of use, however, in enabling us to appreciate the meaning of the sensations felt by the finger; and the attempt should always be made to correlate these sensations with the results obtained by the more elaborate means.

Warning must be given against estimating the patient's condition by the study of the pulse alone; any definite result obtained, must only be employed as one of a group of symptoms on which the ultimate opinion is based.

What is the pulse ?—In order fully to appreciate the study of the arterial pulse, it is essential to have a proper conception of the true nature of what it is we perceive when we examine the pulse with the finger. Broadbent very properly calls attention to a universal misconception of what the pulse is, and points out that it is not an expansion of the artery due to the blood discharged into the aorta. Marey says that the expansion is so slight that many physiologists have denied its existence, and he states that Poiseuille has demonstrated, that in the larger arteries a slight expansion with each systole does take place. No doubt the aorta and its primary branches are somewhat dilated by the injected blood; but whatever the expansion may be in them, in the carotid and radial it must be very minute. To feel the pulse or to take a tracing, it is necessary that the artery should be flattened against the bone. Lister states that it is for this reason that surgeons, operating in close proximity to a large artery, may be utterly unconscious of its neighbourhood, unless they inadvertently wound it, or recognize its pulsation by having compressed it against some resistant structure. The visible movements of the artery are extremely deceptive. They often give the appearance of contracting and expanding; but if the movement be critically examined, it will be found to be, in reality, a displacement of the artery. A straight artery, like the carotid, resembles somewhat a cord

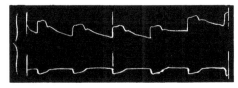

Fig. 39. The upper tracing was taken with the receiver over the carotid artery, at the same time as the lower one was taken with the receiver placed by the side of the carotid artery. The lower tracing is the inverse of the upper.

that is periodically tightened and slightly relaxed. During the systole of the ventricle, the carotid is straightened and tightened, and it becomes slightly relaxed during the ventricular diastole. In persons with thin necks, this movement can be studied. If we place one receiver over the carotid and one alongside it, and have the movements properly registered, the one tracing will be found to be the exact reverse of the other (Fig. 39). If the artery expanded during the ventricular systole, it would naturally thrust out all the tissues surrounding it, and the tracing from the side would then be an exact duplicate of the one taken from the front of the artery. The movement, then, of the beating carotid is one of displacement of the whole vessel, not a dilatation and contraction of the vessel.

A similar confusion arises in studying an artery when it is tortuous. In looking at the radial when it is tortuous, one can readily imagine that the rising and falling of the artery is really a distension and contraction of the artery. But if a suitable case be taken, where, in the course of the tortuous artery, there is a short lateral bend, the movement can be demonstrated to be due to the displacement of the artery, and not due to expansion and contraction of the artery. If the pad of the sphygmograph spring be placed close to the artery on the concave side of the bend, and a tracing taken, it will be found that during the ventricular systole, the bend is exaggerated, the artery being pushed farther away from the straight course, and during ventricular diastole the bend diminishes. If tracings be taken of the pulse in such a radial artery at the same time as the carotid pulse (Fig. 40), it will be found that the radial gives an inverted tracing, comparable to that in the preceding figure. If the visible movement were due to the expansion and contraction of the artery, the lever would, on the contrary, rise during systole and fall during diastole, as in an ordinary sphygmogram.

What we recognize, then, as the pulse is the sudden increase of pressure within the artery pressing against our finger, when we compress the artery. With the cessation of the ventricular systole, the resistance to our finger steadily diminishes, until the next ventricular systole suddenly rises. Broadbent uses the following apposite illustration : ' Such a pulsation can

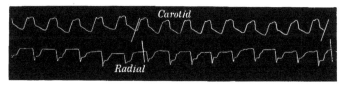

FIG. 40. Simultaneous tracings of the carotid and radial pulses. The radial tracing was taken by placing the pad of the sphygmograph by the concave side of a bend of the tortuous radial artery. During systole, the artery receded from the sphygmograph, and returned during diastole, and hence the tracing obtained is an ' inverted sphygmogram '.

be felt on a large scale by placing the foot on the inelastic leather hose of a fire-engine in action, in which there can be no expansion.'

To speak of the pulse as being the expansion and contraction of the arterial walls, or ' the swinging backwards and forwards of the arterial wall ', is not only to use language of exaggeration, but to convey a totally erroneous conception of what the pulse really is.

Inspection of the arteries.—Inspection of the arteries reveals in health but little movement. Conditions giving rise to forcible action of the left ventricle, may render the pulse visible in some of the superficial arteries. Exertion, excitement, or the febrile state may induce visible beating of the carotids, while this is a marked feature when the arteries are tortuous and atheromatous, and in such a disease as exophthalmic goitre. In free aortic regurgitation, not only is there marked pulsation of the carotids, but pulsation is visible in numerous superficial arteries in various situations. The tortuous character of superficial arteries is visible in arterial degeneration.

Digital examination of the arteries.—It is usual, in the routine examination of the pulse, to place two or three finger-tips on the radial artery near the wrist. The fingers are laid on the artery, and moved upwards and downwards and across the artery, at first gently, and then with more pressure. By this procedure, a knowledge of the size of the artery and the conditions of its walls is acquired. Steady pressure being applied in order to obliterate the pulse, the force required to attain this gives an idea of the arterial pressure, and of the character of each individual pulse-wave. It is a good thing to practise the digital examination of the pulse with sphygmographic tracings, taken at the same time. By this means, the character of the pulse will be better appreciated by the finger.

The condition of the walls.—We recognize the yielding nature of the arterial coats in healthy arteries. In degeneration of the coats the arterial walls may be universally thickened, or contain bead-like patches of indura- tion, as in atheroma, or the artery may have become a rigid tube, as in calcareous degeneration.

The size of the artery.—The variations in size depend entirely upon the degree of relaxation of the muscular coat of the artery. A large artery is not necessarily significant of a strong pulse, nor a small artery of a weak pulse. An increase in the size of the artery frequently implies diminished opposition to the work of the heart. The size of the artery can sometimes be readily appreciated by lightly rolling it under the fingers. At other times it can only be detected, when the pulse is elicited by firm pres- sure at the place where we expect to find it. This difficulty may occur where there is a good-sized artery embedded in a fat, well-padded wrist, or where the artery is small and contracted. On the subsidence of a fever, a notable diminution in the size of the artery can often be readily recognized.

Character of the pulse.—The trained finger is as yet the best guide we have, in judging the character of the blood-stream within an artery. The knowledge necessary to determine what is normal, and what is abnormal, can only be acquired by the constant study of the pulse. The finger-tips become so educated in course of time that we readily appreciate the sensation, conveyed in compressing an artery.

The pulse-rate.—The reckoning of the pulse-rate should be made at a late stage in the examination. When abnormally rapid, it should be again counted when the patient has regained his composure. It is best enumerated in two separate half-minutes, to ascertain if the heart is acting quite steadily. In children, unless asleep, abnormal frequency is often very unreliable as a guide, as the presence of the doctor often keeps up a continued excitation of the heart. While the rate of the pulse normally indicates the number of the contractions of the left ventricle, it sometimes happens that these are so weak that some of the pulse-waves are not per- ceptible to the fingers. In such cases, the pulse is usually slow or irregular in rhythm. To appreciate the significance of the pulse-rate, due regard should be paid to the age and idiosyncrasies of the patient, and to the ailment from which he suffers.

The size of the pulse-wave.—The trained finger can recognize a great variety in the apparent volume of the wave itself. Some waves seem to roll up under the finger, passing gradually away, while others pass quickly, giving a mere flick to the finger.

The impact of the pulse-wave on the finger.—This may be quick and abrupt, and the pulse-wave quickly disappear (pulsus celer), or the impact may approach the finger gradually and gradually subside (pulsus tardus). Although the pulse-wave occupies such a short space of time, yet the sensitive finger readily recognizes these different features.

The rhythm of the pulse.—The beats usually follow one another at regular intervals, and should be of equal strength. The divergences from the normal rhythm are numerous, and the usual terms employed to distinguish them are, in my opinion, both unsatisfactory and misleading; but this subject is fully entered into later. In estimating the rhythm of the pulse, one's whole attention should be concentrated upon the observation. If one does not exclude other thoughts from the mind, a variation in the pulse-rate and strength may apparently be felt. This is due to a failure to appreciate the pulse, during a remission of the attention. I have not only been conscious of this myself, but in cases where it was important to note the fact, as in pneumonia, I have found my colleagues describing irregularity as being present, when careful examination revealed a perfectly regular pulse.

The two radial pulses compared.—Finally, the two radial pulses should be compared, and any difference in the character of the beats noted. A difference in the strength of the two pulses may be due either to an abnormal distribution of the arteries on one side, or to an interference with the lumen of a vessel on one side. A difference in the character of the pulse usually occurs only in the latter case. The two most frequent conditions altering the character of the pulse on one side, are the presence of an aneurysm or of an atheromatous plate, diminishing the lumen of the vessel, on the proximal side of the place where the pulse is examined.

The value of a sphygmogram.—Although the sphymogram represents the variations in arterial pressure, and although it can give information in this respect, yet there are so many sources of error, that it cannot be trusted implicitly. Its greatest service is in giving an accurate record of the movements of the left ventricle. However eloquent may be the words of a writer, he cannot in a page convey as clear an idea of the rhythm of a heart as a simple pulse-tracing; and if writers had given us more pulse-tracings, their works would have been greatly enhanced in value. It is because it gives us a permanent and accurate record, that a tracing of the arterial pulse is of such great value. When we seek to find the nature of any movement of the circulation by recording it graphically, the arterial pulse is the best and most useful standard, by which we can find its position in the cardiac cycle, as will be shown later.

Definition of a sphygmogram.—When the spring of a sphygmograph is so accurately adjusted on an artery that it does not obliterate the artery, when the arterial pressure is at the lowest, and still slightly compresses the artery, when the arterial pressure is at the highest, the spring will oscillate with each variation of pressure within the vessel. This oscillation being communicated to the lever and recorded on the tracing-paper gives us a series of wavy lines, which represent the variations of the pressure within the artery. A sphygmogram may, therefore, be defined as a diagrammatic representation of the variations of pressure within an artery. If we knew exactly the amount of pressure exercised by the spring, we should be able to obtain the value of each movement. But the possibilities of error are so numerous, that it is useless to draw conclusions from the amount of pressure supposed to be exercised. From the examination of a tracing we obtain information on three different points : first, concerning the rate and rhythm of the heart's action ; second, concerning the sequence of certain events occurring in a cardiac revolution ; third, concerning the character of the blood-pressure within the artery.

Events occurring during a cardiac revolution, revealed by the sphygmogram (see diagrams, Fig. 47 and 50). (a) *The systolic period.*—If we take a sphygmogram, we can divide the cardiac cycle into two periods : one (E, Fig. 41) during which the aortic valves are open, and the ventricle pours its contents into the aorta, and another (G, Fig. 41) during which the aortic valves are closed, and the ventricle is in diastole. For the sake of convenience in describing sphygmograms, these two periods will be referred to as the systolic and diastolic periods, although in the space G the presphygmic and postsphygmic periods of the ventricular systole are included (Fig. 47). The character of the systolic portion varies very much in different individuals. These variations depend mainly on the amount of resistance offered by the arteries to the ventricular systole. In such a tracing as Fig. 41, there is first an abrupt rise (p), then a fall followed by a continuation of the wave s at about the same level. This period is usually described as being divided into two, the abrupt rise being spoken of as the primary or percussion wave, and the latter portion as the tidal or predicrotic wave (the papillary wave and outflow remainder wave of Roy and Adami). This division has led to the idea that these represent two different events in the pulse itself. As a matter of fact, the abrupt rise p above the level of the wave s, is due to instrumental defect, and the whole period E is occupied by the ventricular pressure forcing blood into the arterial system, and corresponds with the period E in Fig. 47. In cases where the arterial pressure is low relatively to the strength of the ventricular systole, these two waves are so blended together that so-called percussion and tidal waves can no longer be differentiated (Fig. 42). The whole of this period E in the tracing will hereafter be referred to as the systolic period, and the wave s as the systolic wave, as it represents the period of ventricular systole, when the ventricle and arterial system are in free communication.

(b) *The diastolic period.*—With the closure of the aortic valves, the arterial pressure falls rapidly to the bottom of the aortic notch (n, Figs. 41 and 42). In the tracings, this is seen to be at the beginning of the diastolic period. This fall is interrupted by a distinct rise in the pressure represented by the dicrotic wave d. There has been a good deal of discussion concerning

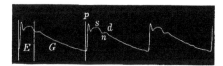

Fig. 41. Sphygmogram of the radial pulse. The space E is the period of ventricular systole when the aortic valves are open ; the space G the period of ventricular diastole ; s is the pulse-wave due to the ventricular systole ; n the aortic notch ; d the dicrotic wave ; and p a wave due to instrumental defect.

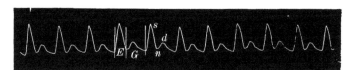

Fig. 42. The letters have the same significance as in Fig. 41.

the cause of the dicrotic wave. The following explanation seems to me the most probable. The semilunar valves are so delicately constructed, that they readily respond when the pressure on one side rises above that on the other. As soon as the aortic pressure rises above the ventricular the valves close. At the moment this happens, the valves are supported by the hard, contracted ventricular walls. The withdrawal of the support, by the sudden relaxation of these walls, will tend to produce a negative pressure wave in the arterial system. But this negative wave is stopped by the sudden stretching of the aortic valves, which, on losing their firm support, have now themselves to bear the resistance of the arterial pressure. This sudden checking of the negative wave starts a second positive wave, which is propagated through the arterial system as the dicrotic wave. After the dicrotic wave, the arterial pressure-curve gradually falls. Occasionally there are slight waves in the fall, but these are of doubtful import.

Features of the sphygmogram due to instrumental defect.—In the study of sphygmographic tracings, one has always to bear in mind that certain features may be due to the instrument itself. Speaking generally, these instrumental features occur where there are sudden and forcible

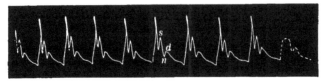

FIG. 43. A strong-beating ventricle has jerked the lever high above the true systolic wave, and the falling lever has made an artificial notch on the systolic wave *s*. The true pulse-curve is probably represented in the dotted tracing.

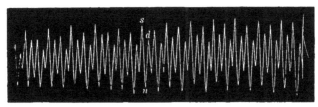

FIG. 44. The forcible changes in pressure have exaggerated the height and depth of all the waves.

changes in the arterial pressure. The most frequent of these is the jerking up of the spring by the systolic wave itself. Then the next most frequent is the formation of a notch on the tracing of the systolic wave, due to the sudden fall of the spring after being jerked high up, as in Fig. 43. Occasionally one finds the aortic notch artificially deepened by the sudden lowering of the pressure, as in Fig. 44.

CHAPTER XX

ARTERIAL PRESSURE

The cause of arterial pressure.
Methods of measuring the blood-pressure.
Increased blood-pressure.
Hyperpiesis.
Effect on the heart of increased peripheral resistance.
Increased arterial pressure and heart failure.
Prognosis of high blood-pressure.
Treatment of high arterial pressure.

The cause of arterial pressure.—When the left ventricle contracts it drives the blood into the arterial system. The escape through the arterioles and capillaries is retarded, so that the blood continues to flow after the ventricle has ceased to contract. As a consequence of this, the arteries are slightly distended during ventricular systole, and their elastic coats compress the column of blood within them after the ventricular systole is over, and thus maintain a degree of arterial pressure during the period in which the ventricle is not acting. The ventricular force is thus stored up by the distension of the elastic coats of the arteries, and liberated during the ventricular diastole.

The chief factors, therefore, concerned in the maintenance of arterial pressure are the ventricular systole, the peripheral resistance, and the elastic recoil of the arteries. The viscosity of the blood is also a factor in the raising of the arterial pressure.

Methods of measuring the blood-pressure.[1]—Of late years many instruments have been devised to measure the arterial pressure. The majority are constructed on the principle of compressing the brachial artery with an air-bag embracing the upper arm. Air is pumped into the bag, and its pressure is measured by a mercury manometer in connexion with it. When the pressure is raised sufficiently to obliterate the radial pulse, we obtain the only really trustworthy standard, and it is this I refer to hereafter as ' arterial or blood pressure '. Attempts have been made to estimate the systolic, mean, and diastolic pressures by observing or recording the

---

[1] There is no use trying to get an accurate record of the blood-pressure in cases of continuous irregular action of the heart, such as auricular fibrillation. The size of the beats are always varying, and any attempt to gain even an approximate figure to represent the blood-pressure is little more than guesswork, so that observations based on such results are not only unreliable but absolutely misleading.

movements, communicated to the column of mercury by the compressed artery. It is found that, during the gradual compression of the artery, oscillations due to the pulse-beat occur in the mercury. These oscillations begin, gradually reach a maximum, and gradually decrease as the pressure is raised or lowered. Far-reaching deductions have been drawn from the changes in these oscillations. As the cause of these oscillations is not understood, the attempts to estimate the mean or diastolic pressure from them is little better than guesswork, and in practice it will more likely tend to mislead than to give reliable information (see diagram, Fig. 45).

The force required to obliterate the pulsation in the radial artery is fairly easily ascertained, and from it certain limited inferences may be drawn. It is doubtful if it represents the actual arterial pressure within the artery,

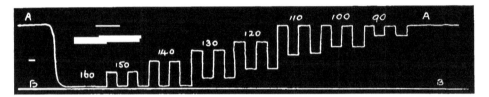

FIG. 45. Diagram to show the nature of the oscillations of the mercurial column in estimating the blood-pressure. A and B represent the walls of the brachial artery. At 160 the lumen of the artery is obliterated by the pressure of an air-bag embracing the upper arm. As the pressure is gradually lowered in the bag, each beat of the artery produces a movement of the mercury in the manometer, the movement being represented by the elevations in the diagram. With diminution of pressure there is at first a gradual increase in the extent of the movement, followed by a gradual decrease until the pressure in the air-bag ceases to compress the artery. From this it is shown that there is no definite period which can be said to correspond to the systolic, diastolic, or mean blood-pressure.

for an escape can take place imperceptible to the finger, and certain external conditions may affect the pressure. It is usually assumed, for instance, that the arterial wall and its coverings offer such a slight resistance as to be negligible. Russell, on the other hand, asserts that the thickening or contraction of the artery may have a very considerable effect, and that thick, sclerosed, and contracted arteries may offer such resistance that a considerable proportion of the pressure may be spent in overcoming it. Oliver has shown that the pressure obtained by instruments may vary in different arteries in the same individual. Hill, Rowlands, and others have shown that in aortic regurgitation the pressure in the femoral artery may be much higher than in the brachial, as much as 100 mm. Hg. By immersing the trunk in hot water, these differences disappear. This remarkable difference is probably due to some modification in the arterial wall, but its nature I do not understand.

There are a great many different instruments devised to take the arterial pressure. Most of them are somewhat cumbrous, and some patients resent the disagreeable sensation produced by compressing the upper arm. Hence these methods are not likely to receive that general application, which the need for ascertaining the blood-pressure requires. L. Hill has recently invented an extremely simple and practical method. In place of a cuff surrounding the upper arm, he uses a small bag, which is compressed over the radial artery, until the pulse disappears below the place of compression. The bag is connected with a very simple manometer, which can be carried in the waistcoat pocket.

Erlanger and Gibson have invented methods for graphically recording the blood-pressure. The tracings from Gibson's apparatus seem very instructive; but I have no experience in the use of his apparatus.

A great deal has been written about blood-pressure and its estimation in practical medicine; but it must be confessed that much of it has been of little practical value, and much careful observation, extending over many years, on individual patients, will be necessary before any sure and certain result is obtained. The remarks I make on the subject are based on the examination of numerous patients, in the endeavour to ascertain some sure foundation, on which to base the application of the method in the clinical examination of heart affection.

Increased blood-pressure.—In many cases, one can corroborate by instrumental observation the knowledge previously acquired by the finger, that the pressure in the arteries increases in certain diseased conditions, as Bright's disease, and with advancing years. As the increased pressure of advancing years is associated with arterial changes, the question of cause and effect is a very difficult one to solve. On the one hand, the changes in the blood-vessels undoubtedly tend to raise the blood-pressure, while it is contended that these are induced by the blood itself, containing ingredients that provoke a contraction of the arterioles, in consequence of which the muscular coat hypertrophies. A rise in pressure seems to induce atheromatous degeneration, and this in turn causes a rise in pressure. The fact is undoubted, that arterial changes and high blood-pressure are very frequent phenomena in advanced life. The changes are so insidious, that they rarely come under consideration until they are well established. One may infer, indeed, that such changes are occurring in middle life, when one notices a tortuous radial artery, but it is rare that the condition gives any cause for anxiety until it is well established.

It is a mistake, and one made not infrequently, to consider the high blood-pressure as if it were a disease. Happily the efforts employed to reduce the blood-pressure, are usually of little effect. In order to appreciate the meaning of high blood-pressure, it is well to consider the condition associated with its production, for I think it has a significance beyond that of being a manifestation of disease.

I have already pointed out that the arterial pressure is maintained chiefly by the force of the left ventricle, the peripheral resistance, and the elastic recoil of the arteries. The necessity for the pressure is the regular and equable supply of blood to the organs and tissues. Between the heart and tissues there is an intimate association, whereby the supply to the tissues and organs is moderated by their requirements—the heart beating more forcibly and more rapidly, and the peripheral resistance diminishing, when there is an urgent need, by the exercise of the functions of the organs. With advancing age, three great changes occur in the blood-vessels. The elasticity of the arteries diminishes. The result of this is, that there is no longer the same equable maintenance of the pressure during diastole. The arteries approximate the condition of rigid tubes, where the force exerted by the left ventricle is not sufficiently stored up in the elastic coats, to be liberated during diastole. The loss of this assistance necessitates increased force of the ventricular contraction, and, therefore, an increase of the pressure during ventricular systole. In the arterioles there may be an increase of the muscular tissue, and this implies an increase in functional activity with an increase of the peripheral resistance. These are the two factors that are generally assumed to be the cause of increased blood-pressure; but there is a third which has not received that consideration to which it is entitled, namely, the diminution of the capillary field. This can be recognized in various ways, as, for instance, the thinning and wasting of the skin and subcutaneous tissues, and by the absence of oozing in surgical operations. The manner in which it raises the blood-pressure is simply by narrowing the passage of outflow.

Hyperpiesis.—In the routine examination of patients, we meet occasionally with some, usually middle-aged, sometimes young, who show considerable fluctuations in blood-pressure. Periods of high arterial pressure (hyperpiesis of Clifford Allbutt) may be associated with some discomfort, as mental dullness, headache, &c. These periods can be cut short by a smart purge, bodily exercise, &c., or they disappear from no ascertainable cause. It is possible that such periods of high arterial pressure are due to faulty metabolism; but they will be found to recur in spite of the greatest care in diet. It is said by some that these periods of high blood-pressure are the cause of arterial degeneration, but, with an imperfect knowledge of all the factors, we are not in a position to decide.

Effect on the heart of increased peripheral resistance.—I have mentioned that the connexion between the heart and the tissues is so intimate, that the demand from the tissues is responded to by stronger contraction of the heart. When, therefore, one or all of these causes increasing the peripheral resistance are in action, the heart, in order to supply the tissues with blood, has to exert more force in its contraction. It accommodates itself to its ever-increasing burden by calling upon its reserve, and the only evidence that it has more to do, is in the limitation of its field of response. One can almost say, when an individual realizes the fact that a hill is not climbed with the ease and comfort with which it used to be done, that already the heart is meeting an increased peripheral resistance, and there is already a slight exhaustion of its reserve force. This, as we know, is a very gradual and long-continued process, beginning insidiously in the fourth decade of life, and coinciding with the time at which athletes abandon the exercises that call for long and severe exertion.

As the changes that increase the peripheral resistance tend slowly but surely to advance, the work of the heart becomes ever greater, the field of response becomes more limited, till finally the patient's attention is called by some disagreeable sensation to the fact of the great limitation, and so we get the evidence of heart failure.

But this is not all. The changes that have taken place in the arterial walls in the periphery have, at the same time, been affecting the arteries of the heart, with the result that the muscle-fibres are imperfectly nourished and degenerate. It is in these cases of long-standing high blood-pressure that we find the most striking evidence of degenerative changes in the heart muscle, associated with arterial degeneration, and it is wonderful how long a heart extensively degenerated can maintain a high blood-pressure.

Such cases of degenerated arteries and long-continued high blood-pressure end by a degenerated artery giving way and causing cerebral apoplexy, or by failure of the heart. The latter may come about in various ways : by a sudden change in the inception of the heart's contraction—for it is in these cases we frequently find the extra-systole and auricular fibrillation—by gradual exhaustion of the heart's strength, often with angina pectoris, and on rare occasions by rupture of the heart. There may occur a somewhat sudden fall in the arterial pressure from dilatation of the heart. When this occurs, there is a sudden change in the character of the symptoms, which I have given in some detail in the chapter on dilatation of the heart (Chapter XXXVIII).

Increased arterial pressure and heart failure.—From such considerations, it will be realized that we may have heart failure without fall of blood-pressure ; and this consideration brings clearly into view the fact that heart failure in these cases is primarily a matter of exhaustion of reserve force. In cases of valvular disease, there may be marked failure of the heart with little or no fall in blood-pressure, and recovery may ensue with little or no rise in blood-pressure.

Prognosis of high blood-pressure.—There has been so much nonsense talked and written about high blood-pressure, that I am constrained to draw attention to our extreme ignorance of the cause and consequence of raised blood-pressure. That we are totally ignorant of the cause, does not prevent many people adopting heroic measures for reducing it, without even considering the wisdom or necessity for so doing. That it may be a physiological process for the benefit of the organism is seldom considered. It would not be exaggerating to say that the present state of our knowledge of this subject is so wanting in trustworthy data as to warrant neither a sound prognosis nor a rational therapy. In some cases it is associated with manifest disease of the arteries or the kidneys, and here a grave prognosis can safely be ventured; but the high blood-pressure forms but one datum, and the older physicians could have given as sound a prognosis before the invention of the instrument for estimating the blood-pressure.

It must be borne in mind that it is only within recent years that observations approaching accuracy have been in use, and that no one has watched individuals for a long enough time to acquire the knowledge of the variations of pressure which accompany a healthy life. When what has been considered an increase has been detected in an individual, he has been subjected to treatment, and if he has continued living as a normal man, this has been attributed to the measures prescribed for his raised blood-pressure. We constantly see individuals proceeding to some spa for treatment for high blood-pressure, and the spa physician puts an individual through some rigid régime, and, finding the pressure fall, imagines that his treatment has saved the patient from arterio-sclerosis. I have repeatedly seen such cases, and have taken the blood-pressure before and after their visit to the spa, and have detected no difference, notwithstanding that they have brought back a letter from the spa physician telling of the wonderful way the blood-pressure has been reduced. One constantly meets with individuals who have been under continued treatment for years, because they have had a blood-pressure supposed to be high. The inefficiency of treatment to reduce the pressure, has produced in them a state of depression at times approaching panic.

I give here the grounds I have employed for a prognosis in these cases ; grounds which are no doubt slight and inefficient, but, so far as I have tested them, of quite a distinct value.

Although I had been studying blood-pressure for years, and used various instruments, it was only in 1905 that I obtained an instrument of some reliability, namely, the Martin modification of the Riva-Rocci. I used only the method by which the disappearance of the radial pulse is detected, when the pressure in the armlet obliterates the pulse—what is called the systolic pressure—though I am not sure that it actually represents the systolic pressure—nevertheless it is a safe standard from which to measure variations. I took records of a good many people whom I could keep under observation. In some I found the pressure vary remarkably. At some examinations, it would be 180 mm., a few days later it would be 120. I could find no cause for such variations. In some liable to attacks of angina pectoris, the liability was as great when the blood-pressure was low as when it was high. Some with high blood-pressure got heart failure, or apoplexy, and died; others lived and pursued their occupations with no limitation for the years I have been able to watch them. When I came to inquire into the difference between these various types, I found that the former were always associated with evidences of disease of the heart, kidneys, or blood-vessels, of such an extreme degree that a sure prognosis could have been given apart from the blood-pressure. On the other hand, those who pursued a normal life presented no changes in other organs, beyond what one would consider compatible with their time of life. In giving a prognosis, therefore, I am accustomed to review critically the condition of the kidneys, the state of the arteries (inquiring if there has been any hæmorrhage), and the condition of the heart, with particular reference to its size and functional efficiency. It is on the result of such a review, with the knowledge of the blood-pressure, that I base a prognosis: that is to say, if the size of the heart is within normal limits and the heart's power not restricted, then the prognosis is favourable; and the less favourable prognosis is based on the limitation of the heart's power—which is usually associated with an increase in the heart's size.

Treatment of high arterial pressure.—In a long series of observations on the effects of drugs and diet which my colleagues and I have carried on at the London and Mount Vernon Hospitals, we have been struck with the futility of the methods and drugs usually recommended to lower blood-pressure. Such drugs as the nitrites have only a transient effect, when they do affect the blood-pressure. Many of the observations with the nitrites have been made on the young with healthy arteries, and the conclusions drawn from them have been applied in the treatment of the senile with degenerated arteries. As a matter of fact, we found that in the elderly the blood-pressure was often quite unaffected by fairly large doses of the nitrites.

When there is heart failure aggravated by high pressure, the best line of treatment is to ease the load and give the heart rest, to regain some store of reserve force. There is no use in trying to reduce the blood-pressure by administering drugs of the vaso-dilator class. Luckily, the administration of these drugs is of little effect, and little or no permanent lowering can be obtained by their use. It is manifest that with changed arteries, and a diminished capillary outflow through obliteration of the capillary vessels, a high blood-pressure is necessary to supply the organism with blood. If it were possible to reduce the blood-pressure permanently, in a man who for years had a blood-pressure of 180–200 mm., the result would be impaired nutrition of the organism. If the final breakdown of these patients be watched, it will not infrequently be found that the blood-pressure does fall to 150 or 140 mm. Hg., and the result is at once the appearance of the signs of extreme heart failure—dropsy, enlarged liver, œdema of the lungs, &c.

(see Case 35). So serious is the significance of a fall of blood-pressure in patients with degenerated heart muscle, even with attacks of angina pectoris, that the persistent fall of pressure is an evidence of the final exhaustion of the heart, though the anginal attacks may cease.

The principle I pursue with most success, is to place the patient under conditions that give the heart less work to do, carefully avoiding ' cardiac tonics ' and ' vaso-dilators ', restricting the diet, evacuating the bowels, and permitting such exercise as the patient can undertake without distress, according to the lines laid down in the chapter on treatment (Chapter XLVI).

CHAPTER XXI

The Venous Pulse

What the venous pulse shows.
Inspection of the jugular pulse.
Methods of recording the jugular pulse.
The recognition of the events in a jugular pulse.
Description of the events in a cardiac cycle.
The causes of the variation of pressure in the auricle and in the jugular vein.
Standards for interpreting a jugular tracing.
The carotid wave.
The notch on the ventricular wave.
The diastolic wave.
Changes due to variation in the rate of the heart.
Method of analysing a tracing.
The ventricular form of the venous pulse.
Anomalous forms of the venous pulse.
Conditions giving rise to a venous pulse.

What the venous pulse shows.—The consideration of the circulation has so far been mainly concerned with the effects of the contraction of the left ventricle. When the apex beat is studied, or the characters of the arterial pulse analysed, our purview is limited almost entirely to the doings of the left ventricle. The arterial pulse, indeed, gives us a direct knowledge of the left ventricle's action during but a portion of the cardiac cycle, namely, during the period when the aortic valves are open. When they are closed, we are no longer directly cognizant of what is happening in the left ventricle. We come now to the study of a subject, which gives far more information of what is actually going on within the chambers of the heart. In the venous pulse, we have often the direct means of observing the effects of the systole and diastole of the right auricle, and of the systole and diastole of the right ventricle. The venous pulse, therefore, presents a greater variety of features, and may manifest variations due to disease which the study of the arterial pulse fails to reveal.

Inspection of the jugular pulse.—In examining a patient for pulsation in the jugular vein, it is generally best that he should lie down, though in some rare cases, where the veins are greatly distended, the pulsation can only be recognized when the patient sits up. The pulsation is most commonly limited to the internal jugular veins, and these veins, lying alongside the carotid arteries, are never visible, being covered at the root of the neck, not only by the skin and sterno-mastoid muscle, but by a variable quantity of adipose tissue ; one, therefore, recognizes the venous pulse only by the character of the movements communicated to the structures covering the vein. In that form of the venous pulse in which the principal wave is due to the auricular systole, the sudden collapse of the tissues covering the vein is more striking than the protrusion. If one further carefully times this collapse, it will be found to be synchronous with the arterial pulse. The pulse in the internal jugular vein is, in diseased conditions, sometimes mistaken, even by experienced observers, for ' beating of the carotids '. But the carotid pulse is always abrupt and sudden in its protrusion of the covering tissues, and gradual in the shrinking. Furthermore, when one finds a small radial pulse and a large pulsation in the neck, one may safely conclude that the neck pulsation cannot be carotid, unless under very exceptional circumstances (as aneurysm). When the pulsation is in the more superficial veins, as the external jugular, facial, or superficial thoracic veins, the collapse of the vein synchronous with the carotid pulse is usually easy of recognition. In another form of venous pulse, where the pulsation is due to the ventricular systole, the engorgement of the veins is usually so great, the arterial pulse so small, and the cardiac mischief so evident, that the recognition of the venous pulse is comparatively easy.

Methods of recording the jugular pulse.—Usually, the movements of the vein are best recorded with the patient lying down, the shoulders slightly raised, the head comfortably supported by a pillow, and turned slightly to the right in order to relax the right sterno-mastoid muscle. The receiver (E, Fig. 14) is placed over the jugular bulb immediately above the inner end of the right clavicle, with just sufficient pressure to shut off the interior of the receiver from the outer air. One may have to shift the receiver about to get the best movement. The relation of the jugular bulb to the surrounding structures is shown in Fig. 46, where the circle above the clavicle indicates the position of the receiver.

Sometimes better tracings are got higher up in the neck, or from the left side. In great engorgement of the veins, it may be possible only to get a tracing when the patient is sitting up. The continued action of the sterno-mastoid in laboured breathing, may prevent a tracing of the jugular pulse being obtained.

The recognition of the events in a jugular pulse.—There is still much that is obscure about some of the details of the venous pulse, and several of these are still the subject of controversy. In the following interpretation I deal with the salient points, which have thrown most light upon the obscure features of the heart's action. The movements of the venous pulse are usually more numerous than those of the arterial, and in the tracings a number of waves are present. As each of these indicates a rise of pressure in the veins, the tracing can only be properly interpreted when the force producing each rise of pressure is known ; and for this purpose the time of appearance of each wave in the cardiac cycle must be established. This is done by taking tracings of the venous pulse, at the same time as some movement whose position in the cardiac cycle is definite, and the arterial pulse, carotid or radial, is the most reliable. The apex

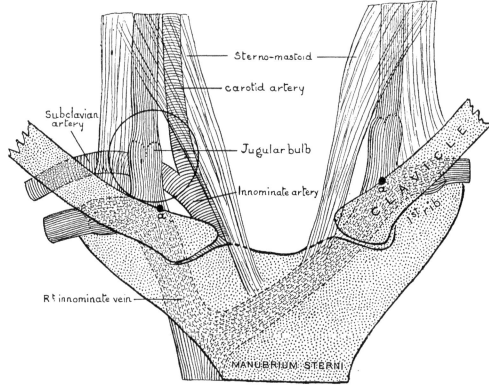

FIG. 46. Shows the relation of the internal jugular vein to the carotid and subclavian arteries, and to the sterno-mastoid muscle. The circle represents the position of the receiver in taking a tracing, and is seen to cover not only the jugular vein but also portions of the carotid and subclavian arteries. The spot at *a* is one inch from the internal end of the clavicle. (Keith.)

beat is often useful and convenient, but care is necessary in the employment of the apex beat, as has already been pointed out (p. 124).

Description of the events in a cardiac cycle.—In the diagram (Fig. 47) there is represented a series of movements, due to various forces that occur during one cardiac cycle. If a wave be found in the vein, and if its time of occurrence be ascertained by referring to the place it would occupy in this diagram, we can usually find its cause by noting what force

is operative at that period. It must be added that while this diagram repre-
sets with fair accuracy the chief events in a cardiac revolution, it is not
asserted that it is correct in every detail. Authorities are not quite agreed
on several small points, but it is sufficient for the purpose I have in
view.

What we have here presented are, the curves representing the variations
of (1) the pressure within the auricle ; (2) the pressure within the ventricle ;

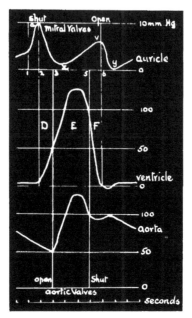

Fig. 47. Semi-diagrammatic representation of the auricular, ventricular,
and aortic pressures during one cardiac revolution. *D*, the presphygmic period of
the ventricular systole ; *E*, the sphygmic or pulse period ; *F*, the postsphygmic
period. The figures 1, 2, 3, 5, and 6 have the same significance as those in Fig. 50.
The divisions on the bottom line represent tenths of a second. (After Frey.)

(3) the pressure within the aorta. The spaces embraced by the perpendicular
lines represent, respectively, the time during which the semilunar valves are
open (*E*) and the auriculo-ventricular valves are shut (*D*, *E*, *F*). I would
direct attention to the presphygmic period *D*, when the ventricular pressure
is rising, but has not yet opened the aortic valves ; and to the postsphygmic
period *F*, where the ventricular pressure is falling after the closure of the
aortic valves. The curves indicating the pressures are approximately
correct, but are utilized here to show the periods when variations take place
in the pressure. Though the events in the diagram represent what happens

in the left side of the heart, there can be no doubt that the changes on the right side are of the same character.

The causes of the variation of pressure in the auricle and in the jugular vein.—The auricular pressure in Fig. 47 shows a series of rises and falls, and these correspond to those in a venous pulse (Fig. 48). The forces operative in producing the variations in the auricular pressure, are also acting in producing the jugular pulse. (The curves of auricular pressure by different physiologists are very perplexing, some getting a rise of varying duration during ventricular systole. I select Frey's as the simplest and probably the truest.)

The auricular wave (a) and fall (x).—The rise *a* in the jugular pulse, Fig. 48, corresponds with the first abrupt rise *a* in the auricular pressure-curve, Fig. 47, and both are due to the systole of the auricle. Neglecting the wave *c*

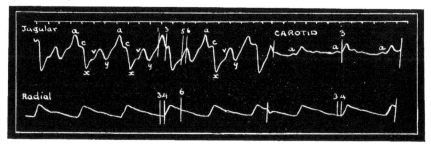

Fig. 48. Simultaneous tracings of the jugular and radial pulses and of the carotid and radial. The elevations *a* and *v*, and falls *x* and *y*, in the jugular tracing correspond to those in the auricular pressure-curve in Fig. 47.

for discussion later, the fall *x* in the jugular pulse corresponds to the fall *x* in the auricular pressure-curve, and occurs at the time the ventricle is in systole. The fall is due to three factors : (1) the relaxation of the auricle after its systole ; (2) the dragging down of the auriculo-ventricular septum by the ventricular muscle, enlarging the auricular cavity as described on p. 39, and Fig. 4 ; (3) the diminished intrathoracic pressure in consequence of the expulsion from the chest of the contents of the left ventricle. When there is a delay in the ventricular contraction, the factors may be separated as in Fig. 153, p. 263, where *x* is due to the first factor, and *x'* to the second and third factors.

The ventricular wave (v).—The rise *v*, after the fall *x* (Fig. 48), is due to the storing of blood in the auricle during the time of the ventricular systole, and corresponds with the second rise (*v*) in the auricular pressure-curve in Fig. 47. The termination of this rise in both figures is sudden, and due to the opening of the auriculo-ventricular valves. *While the beginning of this rise is very variable, its termination is one of the most certain periods in the cardiac cycle, indicating as it does the time of the opening of the tricuspid valves.* The variableness in its beginning is due to the fact that it owes its origin to the quantity of blood stored in the auricle during ventricular systole; and this varies in individual cases, and also in the same individual, with exertion and respiration. The blood comes mainly from the periphery, pouring into the auricles through the veins. When the auricle becomes filled, the surplus distends the superior vena cava and jugular veins, and hence appears in the tracing as a wave. Another source is sometimes regurgitation through the tricuspid orifice. It is necessary to bear this in mind, as the failure to recognize how tricuspid regurgitation would be manifested in the venous tracing has led to a total misconception of the meaning and nature of the ventricular form of the venous pulse. It has been assumed that, in tricuspid regurgitation, the blood sent back into the veins would appear in

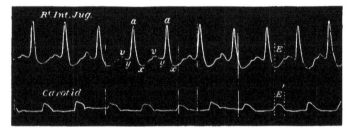

Fig. 49. Simultaneous tracings of the jugular and carotid pulses, showing that the waves in the jugular correspond in time with the waves of increased auricular pressure in Fig. 47. In this patient the tricuspid valves were partially destroyed and the orifice therefore markedly incompetent, so that there was free tricuspid regurgitation. The wave *v* is therefore partly due to blood regurgitating from the right ventricle.

the jugular at the same time as in the carotid. In this assumption, the effects of a dilating auricle between the ventricle and veins has been overlooked; as a matter of fact, what happens is merely an increase in the amount of blood accumulating in the auricle during the ventricular systole, and this causes the appearance of the wave *v* to be somewhat premature. Thus, for instance, Fig. 49 is from a case where there was a damaged tricuspid valve so that regurgitation took place, and the wave *v* is seen to be of small size, beginning early in the time of the ventricular systole (period *E*).

I call this wave *v* the ventricular wave, because of its association with the systole of the right ventricle. Thus the termination of the wave is due to the relaxation of the right ventricle and opening of the tricuspid valves; it is often made up of blood sent back through the incompetent tricuspid orifice by the systole of the right ventricle; though this wave may be small and of brief duration in the auricular form of the venous pulse, it becomes increased in size, and the main or only wave in the ventricular form of the venous pulse.

The fall (*y*), in Fig. 47 and 48, is due to the blood, that has been stored in the auricle during ventricular systole, flowing into the ventricle after the opening of the tricuspid valves. Then, as the ventricle becomes filled, stasis in the auricle and veins takes place, causing the rise between *y* and *a*, Fig. 47 and 48, till the auricle again contracts.

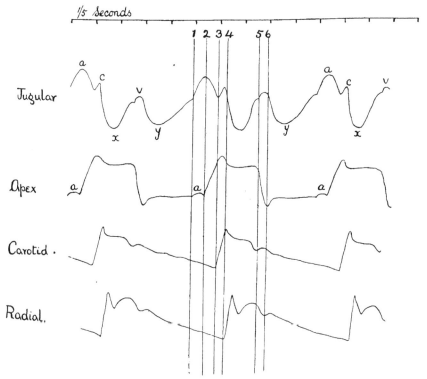

FIG. 50. Tracings of the jugular pulse, apex beat, carotid and radial pulses. The perpendicular lines represent the time of the following events: 1, the beginning of the auricular systole; 2, the beginning of the ventricular systole; 3, the appearance of the pulse in the carotid; 4, the appearance of the pulse in the radial; 5, the closing of the semilunar valves; 6, the opening of the tricuspid valves (compare with Fig. 47).

Standards for interpreting a jugular pulse.—Such are briefly the main factors concerned in the production of the auricular form of the venous pulse. It is at times difficult to interpret the tracings, so that it is necessary to have definite standards to help in deciphering certain obscure features.

In Fig. 50 I have placed, below the jugular pulse, tracings representing the apex beat and the carotid and radial pulses, to show the relation in time of certain events in these various movements. The numbered perpendicular lines indicate the simultaneous events in the jugular pulse, the apex beat, the carotid, and the radial pulse. The perpendicular lines facilitate the comparison of the tracings at definite points in the cycle, and have the same significance in the later tracings : 1, the beginning of the auricular systole ; 2, the beginning of the ventricular systole ; 3, the opening of the semilunar valves and the appearance of the carotid pulse ; 4, the beginning of the radial pulse ; 5, the closing of the semilunar valves ; and 6, the opening of the tricuspid valves. The time is recorded in fifths of seconds in this and other tracings.

Although the carotid pulse and the apex beat can sometimes be usefully employed as a standard, it will be found that the radial pulse is, on the whole,

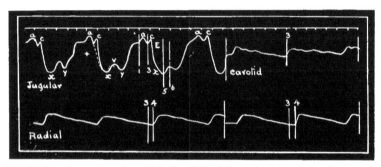

Fig. 51. Simultaneous tracings of the jugular and the radial pulses in the first part of the tracing and of the carotid and the radial in the latter part. The jugular pulse is of the auricular type. a, auricular wave ; c, the carotid wave ; v, the ventricular wave ; x, the auricular depression ; y, the ventricular depression. These letters have the same significance in all the other tracings, and the numbered perpendicular lines have the same significance as those in Fig. 50.

the most convenient in practice. A certain loss of time takes place in the transmission of the wave to the radial pulse, and this can be estimated by taking simultaneously with the radial a few beats of the carotid, as in Fig. 48 and 51, in which the space between 3 and 4 shows the loss of time between the appearance of the carotid and the radial pulse. This loss being allowed for, one can always find a definite period in a jugular tracing which corresponds to any event occurring in the neck due to the ventricular systole. I also employ a very useful period, namely, that portion of the ventricular systole during which the semilunar valves are open (period marked E in some tracings). Its duration can be found in the radial tracing, extending from the beginning of the upstroke to near the bottom of the dicrotic notch. It corresponds to the time between the perpendiculars 3 and 5 in all the carotid, jugular, and apex tracings given here. In the neck the period E begins with the carotid pulse. There is a slight delay between the opening of the aortic valves and the carotid pulse, but it is so short (one-fiftieth of a second) that it may be ignored. The space E in the radial tracing begins about one-tenth of a second behind the same period in the neck.

Another important standard is that of the opening of the tricuspid valves (perpendicular line 6 in all the tracings), which in jugular tracings is always indicated by the beginning of the fall of the wave v. In the apex tracing this event occurs at the bottom of the fall, after the systolic plateau, as in Fig. 29 and 50, and in the radial, at the bottom of the dicrotic notch.

The carotid wave.—In the tracing in Fig. 50, 51, and 52, in addition to the waves a and v, which have already been described, there is another wave marked c. In Fig. 46 it will be seen that the subclavian and carotid arteries lie in such close proximity to the jugular vein that the receiver covers a portion of these arteries. In consequence of this, the stroke of the arterial pulse affects the tracing from the jugular, and produces the wave

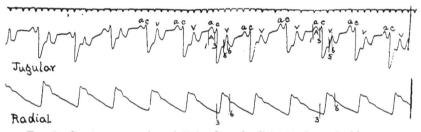

Jugular

Radial

FIG. 52. Simultaneous tracings of the jugular and radial pulses from a healthy man. The letters and numbers have the same significance as in Fig. 50.

c, which I have called the carotid wave. A considerable amount of discussion has taken place in regard to the cause of c; but if an observer will carefully take tracings higher and higher up in the neck, he can easily satisfy himself of its nature, for it gradually assumes the character of a tracing from the carotid artery. The recognition of c as due to the carotid (or carotid and subclavian) helps much in the analysis of tracings from the neck, particularly when there is a delay between the auricular and ventricular systole, the duration of the a–c interval being the best measure of the delay. (Experimental observations show that faint waves may occur in the veins about the time of the carotid wave, produced in some obscure way by the systole of the ventricle, but the carotid and subclavian impact is the main, and for practical purposes the only one, that need be considered.)

The true venous curve would follow the dotted line in Fig. 50.

The notch on the ventricular wave.—In a great many cases, the wave v has a notch, followed sometimes by a considerable rise, on it just before its termination (perpendicular line 5 in Fig. 50). It corresponds in time to the closure of the semilunar valves, and the following rise in v occurs between the closure of the semilunar valves and the opening of the tricuspid valves (postsphygmic interval, F, Fig. 47). The exact cause of this notch is still a matter of dispute—no satisfactory explanation being yet forthcoming. I have often employed it as a useful guide in measuring the period when the semilunar valves close, and it is represented by the perpendicular line 5 in all the tracings.

The diastolic wave.—Occasionally a wave may be detected in slow-acting hearts, shortly after the opening of the tricuspid valves (h, Fig. 53).

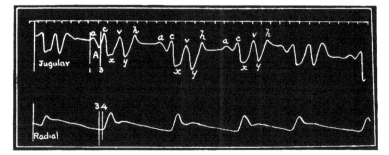

Fig. 53. Shows a diastolic wave h in the jugular tracing. Rate 48.

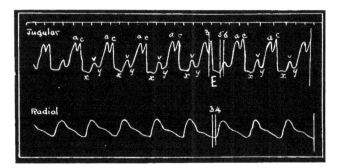

Fig. 54. In increase of the heart's rate the period between y and a becomes shortened, so that the auricular wave, a, follows immediately after v (compare with Fig. 52 and 53).

A. G. Gibson and Hirschfelder describe this as due to the inrush of blood into the ventricle, floating up the cusps, and causing a transient closure of the tricuspid valves. Thayer and Gibson also describe a sound heard occasionally at this time.

Changes due to variation in the rate of the heart.—When the heart's rate increases the shortening of the cycle takes place mainly at the expense of the diastolic period. In the venous tracing, the first effect is shown by the disappearance of the period of stasis, the wave a following immediately on the ventricular wave v (Fig. 54); with still greater increase in the rate, v and a become blended (Fig. 55). In Fig. 56, the variation in the jugular pulse due to variation in rate is seen. Here there is an irregular rhythm with periods of slow rate and periods of increased rate. It will be seen that the fall y disappears during the rapid period, while the waves a and v become blended.

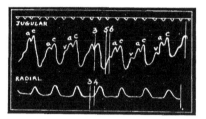

FIG. 55. With great increase in the rate the waves v and a become blended.

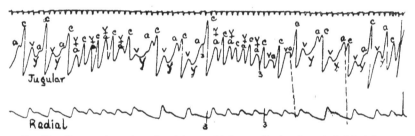

FIG. 56. Shows an irregular pulse of the youthful type. During the period of the infrequent rate, the a waves in the jugular pulse are separated. During the more rapid rate, the shortening of the diastolic periods causes the a and v waves to fall together.

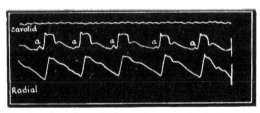

FIG. 57. In tracings from the neck the small wave, a, due to the auricular systole may be the only evidence of the jugular pulse.

Method of analysing a tracing.—In the tracings given so far, the waves have been distinct and well marked. It often happens that the jugular pulse is extremely small, so that we only get a slight movement due to the auricle, the main portion of the tracing being due to the carotid, as in Fig. 57. At other times the movements of the neck seem mere dancing vibrations, and the record obtainable shows a series of small undulations.

But with the radial pulse as a standard, one can definitely assign each undulation to the force producing it. Thus in Fig. 58, we can analyse the tracing by the following procedure : Make a downstroke (4) parallel with the perpendicular line at the beginning of the radial tracing, at the beginning of a radial pulse-beat. As the carotid pulse occurs nearly one-tenth of a second before the radial, draw the perpendicular line 3 one-tenth of a second in front of 4. Measure the distance from the perpendicular line at the beginning of the tracing to 3. Draw a downstroke in the jugular tracing, at the same distance from the one at the beginning. This will be found to fall at the beginning of a small wave, which, therefore, must have been due to the carotid, and so mark it c. The auricular wave occurs one-fifth of a second in front of c, and so the wave a can only be due to the auricular systole. In Fig. 50, p. 151, it was shown that the opening of the tricuspid valves (per-

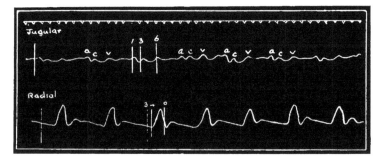

Fig. 58. The movements in the neck seemed dancing vibrations, but an analysis of a tracing refers each movement to a definite cause.

pendicular line 6) often coincides with the bottom of the dicrotic notch in the radial tracing. If now a perpendicular line (6) be drawn at this period in the jugular tracing, it will be found to fall at the end of a wave, v, which must therefore be the ventricular wave.

By strictly following such a method as the foregoing, little difficulty will be experienced in analysing the great majority of tracings.

The ventricular form of the venous pulse.—In Fig. 59 and 60 are tracings of the jugular pulse. At a glance these are recognized to be totally different from the form of the venous pulse just described. The waves, v, in Fig. 59 and 60 are due to the blood being forced back through the tricuspid orifice into the veins by the contraction of the right ventricle. In a sense its origin is identical with the wave v in the auricular venous pulse, as in Fig. 48 and 49, but appears earlier in the cardiac cycle (synchronous with the carotid pulse) because *there is not now a dilating auricle interposed between the vein and ventricle.* When we come to analyse tracings of the ventricular venous pulse with a standard movement, as in Fig. 59, we discover there is no evidence of an auricular wave, nor of a fall corresponding to the fall x in the auricular venous pulse—in other words, there is one great wave (v) synchronous with the ventricular systole, and one great fall (y) synchronous with the ventricular diastole. Another point to be noticed is that the

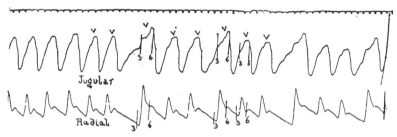

FIG. 59. Simultaneous tracings of the jugular and carotid pulses, showing one large wave v, synchronous with and due to the ventricular systole, and one large fall, y, synchronous with and due to the ventricular diastole. There is no sign of an auricular wave, and the jugular pulse is therefore of the ventricular type, and the rhythm of the heart is continuously irregular.

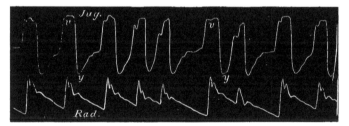

FIG. 60. Simultaneous tracings of the jugular and radial pulses, showing the ventricular jugular pulse, i.e. one large wave, v, synchronous with and due to the ventricular systole, and one large fall, y, synchronous with and due to the ventricular diastole. The rhythm of the heart is continuously irregular. When there are long pauses the tracing of the jugular gradually rises before the next large wave, on account of stasis in the veins. When the pause is short there is no sign of stasis, or only a slight wave, as on the second beat, where it might simulate a wave due to the auricle, but the real cause is seen to be stasis in the veins when the pause is longer.

rhythm frequently is irregular, and that when there is a long diastolic period there is a rise in the tracing due to the vein filling, as after the long pauses in Fig. 60.

There are three conditions which produce the ventricular form of the venous pulse :—

(1) The onset of auricular fibrillation. This is by far the most frequent cause of the change in the venous pulse from the auricular to the ventricular

type. In the great majority of cases, it is accompanied by the complete and disorderly irregularity of the heart's action, as shown in Fig. 59 and 60. The appearance of the ventricular form of venous pulse in auricular fibrillation is always accompanied by a series of other manifestations, which will be fully described in the chapter on auricular fibrillation (Chapter XXX). Occasionally the rhythm is quite regular, but the rate is always slow, as in Fig. 61.

(2) Great distension of the right auricle. Here there is great engorgement of the right heart, so that the auricle becomes embarrassed in its action, and the *a* wave in the jugular pulse diminishes in size and disappears,

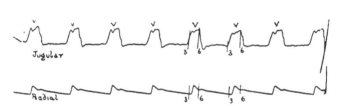

FIG. 61.   Jugular and radial tracings from a case of auricular fibrillation. The jugular
pulse is of the ventricular form, and the rhythm is quite regular.

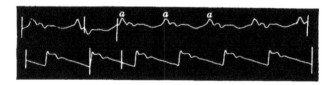

FIG. 62.   Tracings of a slight movement in the jugular vein taken at the same time as the
radial pulse. The wave *a* is due to the systole of the right auricle (Case 11).

while the *v* wave increases in size and occupies the whole period of ventricular systole. With recovery and diminution of the engorgement, the auricular wave reappears. It is to be noted that the rhythm in these cases is always regular. This manner of production of the ventricular venous pulse is, however, very infrequent, far less common than my earlier observations led me to suppose, for the vast majority of cases of the ventricular venous pulse are due to auricular fibrillation.

(3) In certain forms of regular tachycardia, where the heart's contraction starts in an abnormal focus. In these cases, the engorgement of the heart is so great, that each ventricular systole sends back through the auricle into the veins large waves of blood. So forcible may these waves be, that they are mistaken sometimes for beating of the carotid (compare Fig. 62 and 63).

Anomalous forms of the venous pulse.—It is not always easy to appreciate the various events in the jugular pulse, during abnormal action of the heart. In certain cases of auricular fibrillation, this difficulty is not infrequently met with. The tracing from the neck in such instances as in Fig. 64 shows marked variation in the character of the waves. These variations are due sometimes to the differences in the fullness of the veins, produced by variation in the rate and the phases of respiration. Another class often causes so much difficulty that I failed to interpret the waves. In auricular flutter and paroxysmal tachycardia the varying relationships of

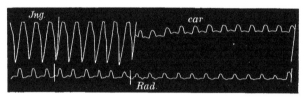

Fig. 63. Simultaneous tracings of the pulsation in the jugular bulb and in the radial, and of the carotid and radial pulses, during an attack of paroxysmal tachycardia, taken eighteen hours from the beginning of the attack (Case 11).

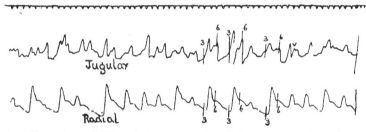

Fig. 64. Shows the variability of the jugular pulse of the ventricular form due to the respiration and variation in rate. Taken from a patient with auricular fibrillation.

the action of the auricles and ventricles produce such a medley of waves that frequently I have failed to interpret satisfactorily the tracings obtained from the neck (see Chapter XXXI).

Conditions giving rise to a venous pulse.—To a great extent we are even at this day quite at a loss to explain all the conditions, that give rise to a venous pulse. Most people in good health show it, while in cases of marked heart failure it may be entirely absent. Some people when in robust health show no signs of it, but if they become slightly debilitated the venous pulse may appear in the neck. It is frequently absent in the aged, though they are otherwise well. In some cases of pernicious anæmia, the venous pulse may be a very prominent symptom; in others it may never appear. Some women during pregnancy develop a large venous pulse, others only develop it during the puerperium, while others never show the slightest sign of it. In irregular action of the heart, it may assume in certain cases enormous proportions ; in other cases there is not the slightest sign. A man may show it during one attack of heart failure, and during another and more grievous attack it may be absent.

I have endeavoured to find out the reason for this variability, but though in some cases I have been able to connect its appearance and disappearance with definite changes in the heart, yet on the whole the matter is one which still puzzles me.

CHAPTER XXII

ENLARGEMENT AND PULSATION OF THE LIVER

Reflex or protective symptoms.
Signs of enlargement of the liver.
Pulsation of the liver.
Conditions producing enlargement and pulsation of the liver.
Jaundice.
Different forms of the liver movement.
Differential diagnosis of liver enlargement.
Prognosis.
Treatment.

THE symptoms arising from enlargement of the liver due to heart failure, receive little consideration from clinicians, and are very frequently overlooked or misunderstood. To a certain extent, this is due to the fact that this enlargement may appear at such an advanced stage of cardiac failure, that the diagnosis and treatment can be determined without paying particular attention to the liver symptoms. Graham Steell includes the enlargement of the liver as one of the cardinal symptoms of heart failure, and Salaman has given a very suggestive analysis of the pathological changes and the conditions inducing them ; but clinicians generally have dealt with the subject in a most perfunctory manner. While it is true that the conditions producing these liver troubles imply an advanced stage of heart failure, yet the recognition of the symptoms have an important bearing on diagnosis and treatment in many cases. The symptoms, due to changes in this organ, are not always easy to understand, but that is no reason for ignoring them.

Reflex or protective symptoms.—Usually in the early stages of liver enlargement, we find evidences of the intervention of the protective mechanism (see Chapter XI, p. 62). While the liver may be only one or two inches below the ribs, the muscle wall of the upper part of the right half of the abdomen becomes hard and tender. This tenderness is invariably put down to the liver itself, and the manner in which this 'tenderness' is usually demonstrated, is by eliciting pain on pressing the finger into the patient's abdomen. But if the extent of the hyperalgesia and the size of the liver be mapped out, it will be found that the former is far more extensive than the latter, and sometimes extends round to and affects the erector spinæ muscles. In some cases, the skin and subcutaneous tissue also become tender, but they rarely become so sensitive as the muscles. Sometimes there seems an increased tenderness where the liver is reached, but this will be found to be due to the more effective compression of the muscle between the finger and the liver. There are many other ways, by which the resourceful observer can demonstrate the tissue in which the tenderness is present.

The consequence of this muscular hyperalgesia is manifested in various ways. If the patient is going about, he may suffer severe pain across the upper part of the abdomen or in the back, this probably being due either to increased engorgement of the liver, or to the increase of the pain in consequence of the exercise of the hyperalgesic muscles. This tenderness and rigidity of the abdominal muscles interferes with the respiration of the patient. He cannot breathe deeply, and attempts to do so are painful, hence there results rapid and shallow breathing, with further embarrassment of the right heart and a tendency to pulmonary stasis.

With long-continued persistence of the enlargement, all the sensory phenomena disappear, the abdominal wall becomes lax, and sometimes the edge of the liver can be grasped.

Signs of enlargement of the liver.—It is not always easy to make out the enlargement of this organ. The contracted muscles often prevent the palpation, and even percussion helps but little. Ascitic and gaseous distension add further to the difficulty. But with care and gentleness in palpation, one may overcome the resisting muscles. Even when the edge of the liver cannot be made out, the peculiar sense of resistance conveyed to the exploring hand may reveal the enlarged liver. Other methods may be adopted, such as pushing the liver forward with one hand while the other explores the front. When the muscles relax and the hyperalgesia disappears, there is no difficulty in finding out the enlarged liver, except when there is great distension of the abdomen.

Pulsation of the liver.—When the liver is enlarged from heart failure, it not infrequently pulsates. If the abdominal muscles are lax, there is no difficulty in recognizing this. If one hand presses on the liver behind, and the other is laid on it in front, the latter is heaved up and down with the pulse. Even where there is a considerable amount of muscular contraction, exploring the edge of the liver with the liver receiver will often reveal the pulsation (pp. 105 and 106).

There are two forms of liver pulse, corresponding to the two forms of venous pulse—an auricular (Fig. 65), and a ventricular (Fig. 66). When a liver pulse and a jugular pulse are both present in the same individual, they are always of the same form. In Fig. 67, a tracing of an auricular jugular pulse is taken simultaneously with a tracing of the auricular liver pulse. In Fig. 68, the tracing of the ventricular jugular pulse is seen to be identical with the liver pulse in Fig. 66, both tracings being from the same patient.

Conditions producing enlargement and pulsation of the liver.—
I have already remarked on the variety of conditions producing the jugular pulse; and there is a like difficulty in understanding the conditions which

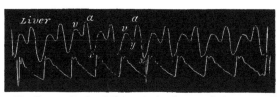

FIG. 65.   The liver pulse is of the auricular form and shows a well-marked auricular wave, *a*.

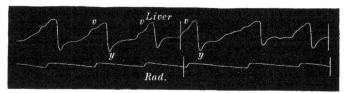

FIG. 66.   The liver pulse is of the ventricular form, showing no auricular wave.

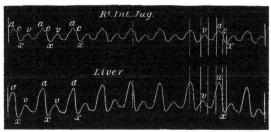

FIG. 67.   Simultaneous tracings of the jugular and liver pulses, showing the correspondence between the waves *a* and *v*, and the absence of the carotid wave *c* from the liver pulse.

give rise to liver enlargement. Cases otherwise identical in their symptoms, and suffering from heart failure due to the same cause, may differ in this particular, some showing enlargement of the liver, and others failing to do so. Similarly, it is not always quite clear why some pulsate while others do not. To a certain extent, I think this is due to the condition of the right auricle. It takes some force to distend the liver, and normally the right auricle has not sufficient strength, so that as long as the right auricle contracts and dilates in its normal place in the cardiac cycle, it prevents the ventricle exercising its force on the liver. When, however, the auricle is not contracting in a normal manner, the ventricle drives the blood through the incompetent tricuspid orifice with such force that the liver pulsates. It is in the cases of auricular fibrillation, that we most frequently find the liver pulsating. When the auricular fibrillation or certain forms of tachycardia are transient, the liver may quickly enlarge and pulsate, and with cessation of the attack as quickly subside and cease to beat—the liver pulse being of the ventricular form (Fig. 69).

Reasoning that it requires some force greater than the normal strength of the right auricle to produce pulsation of the liver, I at first drew the conclusion that an auricular liver pulse indicates hypertrophy of the right

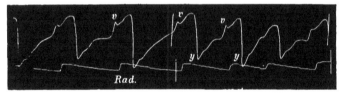

FIG. 68. Simultaneous tracings of the jugular and radial pulses. The jugular pulse is of the ventricular form and is identical with the liver pulse in Fig. 66, both being taken from the same patient.

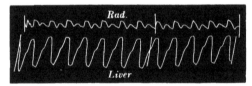

FIG. 69. Simultaneous tracings of the radial and liver pulses during an attack of paroxsymal tachycardia towards the end of life (Case 72).

auricle, and as this occurs most characteristically in cases of tricuspid stenosis, I regarded the auricular liver pulse as diagnostic of tricuspid stenosis. All the cases that had shown this auricular liver pulse during life, whose hearts I examined post-mortem, showed tricuspid stenosis. But I have now had a number of cases showing this form of liver pulse, in which I doubt if I am justified in assuming tricuspid stenosis. Turnbull and Wiel have recorded a case from my clinic in which there was an auricular liver pulse and no tricuspid stenosis.

Jaundice.—Jaundice is a frequent accompaniment of enlargement of the liver ; though of itself of little importance, it should be kept in mind that a slight jaundice may be misleading. Many patients with advanced heart failure and with auricular fibrillation get rapidly thinner. In these, the liver is sometimes greatly enlarged, so that the wasting of the patient, the enlargement of the liver, and the jaundiced tint, present the features of malignant disease of the liver; and I have seen cases presenting these symptoms thus wrongly diagnosed.

Different forms of the liver movement.—Many writers refer to an 'arterial pulsation' of the liver, and I have often wondered what they mean, particularly as no details are ever given. I have never found any condition that could come under this heading, and I suspect that some observers have mistaken the movement of the liver, when it is pulled up and down with the systole and diastole of the ventricle, for a pulsation, particularly as it is sometimes mentioned in connexion with aortic regurgitation. Wherever there is much cardiac enlargement, movement of the liver is produced. Even in patients with normal hearts but with lax abdominal wall, this up-and-down movement can be recognized. It has already been referred to on p. 122. Here I need only point out, that the conditions in which it occurs are generally very different from that of the heart failure in which the true liver pulsation occurs. A tracing of this movement

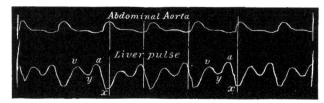

Fɪɢ. 70.   Tracings from the abdominal aorta and the liver. The liver pulse is of the auricular type.

sets the matter at rest, as the fall due to the ventricular systole does not begin until the opening of the aortic valves and the expulsion of blood from the chest, which is practically synchronous with the carotid pulse. In the ventricular form of liver pulse, on the other hand, there is a rise during ventricular systole. A tracing of the liver movement can be distinguished from the auricular liver pulse, in that the fall in the latter case precedes the carotid pulse.

There is generally little difficulty in distinguishing the pulsation of the abdominal aorta from that of the liver pulse. In cases where the ventricular liver pulse is present, it is very rarely that the abdominal aorta can be felt, and the characters of the tracings are not likely to be confused. The auricular form of liver pulse is still more distinct in character from that of the abdominal aorta, as shown in Fig. 70.

Differential diagnoses of liver enlargement. — There are cases occasionally met with where there is dropsy, ascites, enlargement of the liver, which resemble heart failure so much that they are not infrequently mistaken for it. In a few cases which I have seen, my suspicion has been aroused by the absence of any signs of dilatation of the heart and absence of cardiac dyspnœa. Careful inquiry into the habits of the individual may reveal a history of long-continued indulgence in alcohol. With such a history, one can conclude that the case is one of hypertrophic cirrhosis of the liver. Moreover, these livers never pulsate. The enlarged liver in auricular fibrillation with jaundice, simulating carcinoma of the liver, is referred to on p. 308.

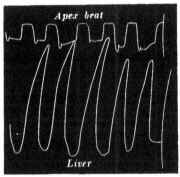

FIG. 71. Simultaneous tracings of the apex beat and of the liver pulse. The liver edge was below the level of the umbilicus, and the pulsation of great size.

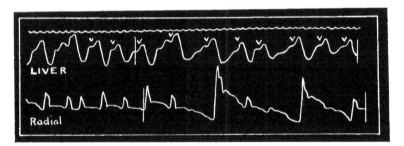

FIG. 72. Tracings of the liver and radial pulses during a period of extreme heart failure (auricular fibrillation).

Prognosis.—Liver enlargement and pulsation from cardiac disease indicate a very advanced stage of heart failure. In cases where the heart failure is secondary to a rheumatic affection of the heart with mitral disease, it may only appear during the attacks of heart failure to which the patients are liable. The enlargement subsides with improvement; and if the heart's restoration be good, the patient may have no signs of the liver enlargement for many years. Some patients with auricular fibrillation secondary to rheumatic affection of the heart may, for years, have a big pulsating liver (Fig. 71); in others the enlargement appears during temporary heart failure.

In some of these the exhibition of digitalis may cause the subsidence of the liver in a couple of days. Fig. 72 was taken from the liver of a man which was pulsating as low as his umbilicus. In a couple of days, all signs of the liver below the ribs had gone. The enlarged liver coming on in paroxysmal tachycardia is a serious symptom, as it indicates a tendency to dilatation and inefficiency of the heart. Also in the heart failure due to cardio-sclerosis with the permanent auricular fibrillation, it is a very grave symptom, especially when the heart failure is due to extensive degeneration of the cardiac muscle, and does not respond to the influence of rest and digitalis. Enlargement of the liver in muscle failure, due to chronic alcoholism, is a bad sign.

Treatment.—Though no treatment is directed specially to the liver enlargement, the effect of the rigid tender muscles in embarrassing the respiration should be borne in mind, and suitable attempts made to put the patient in a comfortable position, so that he can breathe more easily ; and the pain due to the enlarged liver should call for the cessation of all exertion that induces it. A smart mercurial purge may sometimes afford considerable relief.

CHAPTER XXIII

INCREASED FREQUENCY OF THE HEART'S ACTION

The normal rate.
Classification of cases of increased frequency.
Those cases in which the heart is suddenly stimulated to increased rate by mental excitement.
Cases which respond to a call upon the heart's energy by increased frequency.
Cases in which the heart's rate is continuously increased.
Cases in which the increased frequency of the heart occurs in irregular paroxysmal attacks.
The cause of increased frequency of the heart's action.
Prognosis.

The normal rate.—The rate of the heart varies very considerably according to age, sex, and individual peculiarities. At birth, the rate is usually from 130 to 140 per minute. With advancing years the heart slows down gradually : between 9 and 10 the average is about 90 ; at 20, about 74 ; at 30, from 66 to 76 ; it remains at about this latter rate until over 50, when it gradually begins to increase in frequency. At all ages very considerable variations may be met with, and the table which follows, compiled by W. A. Guy in Todd's *Cyclopædia*, gives a fair idea of these variations.

'The following table presents the number of the pulse at each quinquennial period throughout the whole life. The averages for the first eight periods were each founded on 50 observations, of which half were made on males and half on females. The average for the period from 76 to 80 is deduced from the same number of facts similarly divided. For most of the other periods the averages are derived from 40 observations, 20 on males and 20 on females. Where the number of observations is less than this, it is stated in a note.'

Age.	Max.	Min.	Mean.	Range.
2–5	128	80	105	48
5–10	124	72	93	52
10–15	120	68	88	52
15–20	108	56	77	52
20–25	124	56	78	68
25–30	100	53	74	47
30–35	94	58	73	36

Age.	Max.	Min.	Mean.	Range.
35–40	100	56	73	44
40–45	104	50	75	54
45–50	100	49	71	51
50–55*	88	55	74	33
55–60	108	48	74	60
60–65	100	48	74	60
65–70	96	52	75	44
70–75	104	54	74	50
75–80	94	50	72	44
80 and upwards†	98	63	79	35

The heart's rate is greatly increased by exertion, even in those who are in good training. Deane found the pulse-rate over 200 per minute in a professional dancer, at the end of a dance. It quickly subsided to the normal rate. According to Pembrey and Todd, the increase in rate is somewhat greater in the trained than in the untrained; but the decrease in the rate to normal is more rapid in the trained man, though there are so many exceptions to this rule, as to make it of very little use in estimating the heart's strength.

Classification of cases of increased frequency.—In considering the conditions that give rise to increased frequency of the heart's action, we are confronted with such a great number that it is impossible to deal with them all. What I propose to deal with here is the abnormal increase of pulse-rate, and certain conditions other than febrile which induce the rapidity of the pulse. These may fittingly be discussed in four groups : (1) those cases where the heart is suddenly stimulated to increased rate by mental excitement ; (2) those cases in which the heart responds to a call upon its energy by increased frequency; (3) those cases in which the heart's rate is continuously increased; (4) those cases in which the periods of increased rapidity take place in irregular paroxysmal attacks.

Those cases in which the heart is suddenly stimulated to increased rate by mental excitement.—The susceptibility of the heart to mental excitement varies greatly ; and in many cases it is so persistent that it is impossible for the physician to get a correct idea of the rate during an examination, as the presence of the physician acts as the exciting cause. This often creates a difficulty where there is reason to suspect some lesion of the heart. The rapid action may bring out a murmur or an irregularity, and this may be taken as evidence of disease. It is in such cases that hearts to all intents and purposes healthy may show these signs : therefore the opinion should rather be based on the knowledge of what the heart can do when exposed to effort. In the majority of cases who present themselves for life insurance or for entrance into the services, this knowledge can be acquired by getting a history of how they have undergone some effort entailing hard bodily

* Twenty-two observations.   † Twenty-nine observations.

effort. In the young, I have sometimes been able to induce brief periods of slowing, by making them breathe slowly and deeply, and I look upon this as a sign that the heart is probably sound according to the views expressed on p. 187.

Cases which respond to a call upon the heart's energy by increased frequency.—The cases in the first of these groups, those in which the heart responds to an increased call upon its energy by increased frequency, show in reality but an exaggerated form of the normal condition. When we find that a patient is seized with palpitation or rapid heart action after mounting a few steps, we recognize as abnormal that which would have been regarded as normal, in an individual who had run half a mile at the top of his speed. In other words, this increased rate is an evidence that the field of the heart's response to effort is greatly reduced. A further deduction can be made from observing these patients, viz. that exhaustion of the reserve force heightens the excitability of the whole heart, for not only is the rate increased, but the contraction sweeps through the heart with greater rapidity and the systoles of the chambers are of shorter duration. The increased frequency should always lead one to seek the cause from which it arises. The conditions underlying it are too numerous to mention, but they all in the end point to enfeeblement or irritability of the muscle of the heart. In all exhausting diseases, and after convalescence from such a wasting sickness as typhoid fever, the heart's rate can be greatly increased by even very moderate exertion. In the various anæmias (chlorosis, pernicious anæmia, malignant cachexia), and in poisoning of the heart chiefly, the rapid heart action is very often the symptom to which the patient's attention is first called. In organic affections of the heart, as in the various forms of myocarditis, in fatty degeneration of the myocardium, and in valvular disease when there is only a small amount of reserve force in the muscle, increased frequency of the pulse on exertion is extremely common. Many of the patients whose ailments are included in the foregoing groups, when at rest, have a pulse beating about or not much above the normal rate. The heart then seems to be capable of sustaining the demands of the circulation, but seems to be working near the exhaustion of its reserve energy. On exertion, this reserve energy is speedily exhausted; and in order to make up for its inability to respond to the demand of the tissues for more blood by giving stronger ventricular contractions, it responds by giving a greater number of feebler and less complete contractions.

In addition to the increased rate, there is usually hurried and laboured respiration, and this too occurs whether a strong heart is overstrained by a great effort, or a weak heart by a slight effort. Not infrequently in elderly people, before the interference with respiration can arise, the patient in making an effort is stopped by a feeling of weight or oppression within the chest, or even by pain striking across the chest, sometimes severe, sometimes slight, but in all cases imperiously demanding a cessation of the effort.

It is as impossible to indicate, with any approach to accuracy, when a pulse-rate is abnormal on moderate exertion, as it is to indicate what the pulse-rate should be in health under similar circumstances. The increase is often so marked that its recognition is beyond dispute. Thus, in making a patient sit up or turn over in bed, a rise of five to ten beats a minute may not be worthy of much attention; but if the increase is fifteen to thirty beats, then there is distinct evidence that we have to do with some condition that has exhausted the heart's reserve power. This increase of the pulse-rate beyond the normal on moderate exertion, does not give any clue to the nature of the condition that has reduced the heart's reserve power. As already indicated, these conditions are so numerous that an examination for other symptoms must be undertaken to discover them.

As moderate exercise often occasions a remarkable increase in rate in healthy hearts (up to 120–140 in rapid walking) it is not advisable to consider the increase in rate as an evidence of impairment. It will be found that where the increase is due to cardiac enfeeblement, it is accentuated by exertion, and there is always accompanying it a sensation of distress or discomfort, and these are better guides to the estimation of the heart's condition.

Cases in which the heart's rate is continuously increased. (a) *Valvular disease.*—The second division, in which the heart maintains a frequency beyond what we recognize as within the limits of health, also includes a great variety of heart conditions. We have among these the series of valvular diseases of the heart, with the muscle exhausted, it may be from struggling against the obstruction caused by the valve lesion, or with the muscle itself suffering from an associated degeneration. Not only do such hearts respond to effort with marked increase in frequency, but even during rest the heart may beat with abnormal rapidity, regularly or irregularly. This forms a very important factor in arriving at an estimate of the strength and condition of the organ, especially in aortic valvular disease. The other symptoms of heart failure present will help in indicating the stage at which the patient has arrived.

(b) *Affections of the myocardium.*—Apart from patients with manifest valvular disease of the heart, there are many whose pulse is rapid, and in whom no disease of the heart can be detected by physical signs. The chest-wall may be thick and fat, or the lungs so voluminous that the actual size of the organ cannot be satisfactorily defined. The sounds, though free from murmur, may be so slightly modified that no certain inferences can be drawn from them. Yet that serious mischief is present, is but too often demonstrated by watching the after-history of these cases. If we exclude, for the present, the consideration of neurotic and poisoned hearts, the cause of the rapid action in all cases is really associated with a want of strength in the muscular wall. In valvular disease this is usually spoken of as failure of compensation, the notion being that the heart muscle is embarrassed by the back pressure. In degeneration of the wall, fatty or fibrous, the weakening of the wall is directly due to this degeneration. In impaired hearts overstrained from excessive exertion, the weakness of the wall is the principal cause of the whole train of symptoms associated with the failure of the heart, and invariably there is present some damage to the muscle, which renders the heart unable to undertake the work which causes the strain. In arriving, therefore, at an estimate of the value of the pulse quickening, a consideration of the other symptoms present will be necessary to recognize what is the cause of the increased pulse-rate in each special case. The circumstances, age, and condition of the patient, will help much in recognizing the rapid pulse due to actual degeneration of the heart-wall. But there is a series of cases in which it is difficult to account for the rapid pulse, especially when it occurs in the apparently strong, in the prime of life. In these cases there is generally a history of hard work, or periods of excessive muscular exertion or poisoning. Sometimes the condition receives a special name, as ' the soldier's heart '. Medical men whose practice lies amongst workpeople subjected to such muscular exertion, are familiar with a similar condition. The heart overstrain is most evident amongst those with a tendency to obesity and who indulge rather freely in alcohol. The symptoms are mainly a rapid pulse, and shortness of breath on exertion. The recent advances made in the recognition of abnormal heart action, have shown that a good many recorded instances of ' overstrain ' are due to the sudden inception of auricular fibrillation, or other abnormal action. As probably these abnormal rhythms are always the outcome of disease processes in the walls of the auricle, the particular effort which was supposed to cause the ' overstrain ', was really the factor in starting an abnormal rhythm in a diseased heart.

(c) *Pregnancy.*—It may be noted that an increased pulse rate is often present in pregnant women, but there the cause is but temporary, and a certain amount of recovery follows delivery. But, in my experience, there is often left a certain amount of cardiac weakness, shown by a distinct limitation of the field of cardiac response.

(d) *Toxic conditions.*—There are a great many agents which invade the heart, and, among other changes, increase its rate, such as alcohol, arsenic, the products of bacterial infection, &c., and these are dealt with in the chapter on poisoning of the heart (Chapter XXXVI).

(e) *Neurotic cases.*—There is a group of people who exhibit a rapid pulse in whom no heart lesion can be detected, and whose future history demonstrates that no serious cardiac lesion existed. These people exhibit other symptoms more prominently associated with the nervous system, and are described in Chapter XV.

(*f*) *Exhausting diseases.*—It is always well to bear in mind that a persistent quick pulse may be the earliest symptom of some exhausting condition (as pernicious anæmia), or of the onset of malignant disease (as cancer).

(*g*) *Exophthalmic goitre.*—The essential features arising from the circulation in many cases of exophthalmic goitre, it seems to me, are the abnormal and persistent dilatation of the arterioles, and a heart acting with a force relatively great to the resistance opposed. These are indicated by the rapid and forcible pulse-wave felt by the finger, and the visible pulsation of the superficial arteries and the carotid. The corresponding sphygmographic features are a high upstroke and rapid fall, so that the dicrotic notch is near the base line (Figs. 73 and 74). The rate of the pulse may be greatly increased, up to 140–160 per minute. The same factors, the unusually forcible injection of the blood into the arteries of low blood-pressure, are

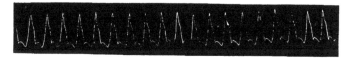

FIG. 73. From a female aged 40, suffering from exophthalmic goitre. Rate 120.

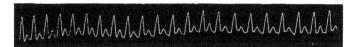

FIG. 74. From a female aged 22, suffering from exophthalmic goitre. Rate 120.

present in aortic regurgitation. Though the beating of the carotid is due to similar causes in the two cases, the low arterial pressure at the end of diastole is different. In exophthalmic goitre, the dilatation of the arterioles and capillaries is the sole cause, whereas in aortic regurgitation there is in addition the backward flow into the ventricle through the incompetent valves. The condition of the circulation in exophthalmic goitre is also comparable to that in some forms of sthenic fever, where the heart beats forcibly and the arteries are relaxed.

Another evidence of the relaxation of the arterioles is to be found in the subjective sensation of warmth, felt by some sufferers from exophthalmic goitre. They rarely complain of cold in winter, however lightly clad they are ; and this is not infrequently the cause of matrimonial disputes, for while the ailing wife feels warm in bed during winter with few blankets, the healthy husband feels the cold keenly. This feeling of warmth has supplied me with the indications for the only treatment of this class of case, that I have found both grateful and beneficial to the patient, namely, the periodic stimulation of the vaso-motor nerves by cold baths. Whenever the feeling of warmth

has been present, I have found these baths do good; and when there is
nervousness and muscular tremor the administration of the bromide of
ammonium has been of great service.

Cases in which the increased frequency of the heart occurs in
irregular paroxysmal attacks.—This class includes cases of 'palpitation'
and 'paroxysmal tachycardia'. There are quite a number of different
conditions included under these terms, and no clear idea is usually given
of what is meant. A very useful and practical division may be based on
the manner, in which the heart's contraction starts. In the vast majority of
cases of transient rapid heart-action, the heart's action is perfectly normal;
the rapid action of this class will be spoken of here as 'attacks of palpitation'.
In another class of patient, the heart's contraction does not start at the
normal place; to this latter class, the term 'paroxysmal tachycardia' is
limited; and the cases are described in the chapters on auricular fibrillation
(p. 231), auricular flutter (p. 237), and paroxysmal tachycardia (p. 251).

The rate in the first class rarely exceeds 170 beats per minute, and the
rhythm is regular except for the presence of an occasional extra-systole; in
the latter class the rate may reach 300 beats per minute, and the rhythm
is frequently irregular. The manner in which attacks of palpitation and
paroxysmal tachycardia stop is, as a rule, distinctive. In the former case
the rapid action subsides gradually, while in paroxysmal tachycardia,
the ending is abrupt and often accompanied by one or more slow strong
beats.

Another difference of considerable practical importance has been brought
out by Lewis, who has shown that in tachycardia arising from the normal
starting-place, the rate varies with effort and rest, while in the tachycardias
arising from an abnormal focus, with a regular rhythm, this variation does
not occur.

In the following paragraph I describe, under 'palpitation', the more
common forms of temporary rapid action of the heart.

Palpitation.—This may occur in people suffering from a great variety
of complaints. The patient is usually conscious of the change in the heart's
action, feeling the rapid beats and sometimes describing them as gentle,
sometimes as hard and hammering. These latter sensations may occur
with little or no increase in frequency. In cases of valvular disease with
limited reserve force, slight physical effort or mental excitement may
readily induce an attack. Even in the healthy, certain mental states may
induce an attack, while when the system is weakened from disease the
liability to attack is much increased. It is in certain neurotic subjects,
particularly females, that one sees the complaint attain its most distinctive
features. There may be no organic affection of the heart, and though
frequent attacks may ultimately induce exhaustion of the reserve force,
yet, as a rule, they do not appreciably shorten life. Anything that startles

the patient, whether a sudden noise or mental perturbation when awake, or uncomfortable dreams when asleep, readily induces an attack. But it may supervene from more obscure causes, evidently caused by reflexes from organs more or less remote (stomach, uterus), or from undiscernible sources. When a severe attack comes on, the patient may become painfully aware of the violent action of the heart. She prefers to sit upright, draws deep inspirations, and moves uneasily from side to side, with the hand pressed over the heart. It is accompanied by sensations of a distressing nature, such as a sense of suffocation, and a fear of impending dissolution. When it subsides it leaves the patient exhausted.

During the attack the pulse is usually increased in frequency. The artery may be of fair size ; sometimes, however, it is very small. The impact of the pulse-wave on the finger is sudden, and sharp, and of extremely brief

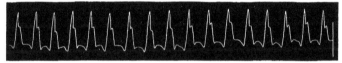

FIG. 75. During an attack of palpitation. Rate 105.

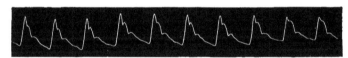

FIG. 76. Tracing of the normal pulse of the patient from which Fig. 75 was obtained.
Rate 64.

duration. The tracing, Fig. 75, taken during an attack of palpitation, shows a high upstroke with a great fall, so that the arterial pressure at the bottom of the dicrotic notch is nearly as low as at the end of the diastolic period—an evidence that, in addition to the excited heart, there is great relaxation of the arterial wall. Fig. 76 is from the same patient, when the heart was acting quietly.

We occasionally meet with patients in whom the pulse is extremely rapid for a period, sometimes for a few minutes, sometimes for a few hours, with no other sensation than that of exhaustion, the attack quietly subsiding (Fig. 77). The causes are so obscure that it would be mere guesswork, in the majority of cases, to attribute it to any one cause.

The cause of increased frequency of the heart's action.—Apart from cases due to nerve excitation, and the abnormal rhythms, it is extremely difficult to account properly for this abnormal increase in rate. All the parts of the heart participate in the excitability. It is not due merely to a dilatation of the heart ; for we may have hearts greatly dilated that show no marked rapidity of action ; and there may be hearts of normal size which may for a long time beat with great rapidity. Apart from the neurotic cases, it might be assumed that an intoxication of the heart, or a deficiency in some nutriment, is the fundamental cause that renders the tissues more irritable. That the whole tissue is involved, and not merely the cardio-motor centre, is demonstrated in many cases by the quicker contraction of the chambers, and the accelerated conduction of the stimulus from auricle to ventricle. Thus in Fig. 77 the tracing shows a very minute a–c interval, while, notwithstanding the abnormal rapidity of the heart's action, the excitability of

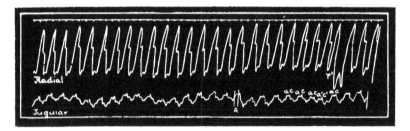

Fig. 77. Simultaneous tracings of the radial and jugular pulses. The rhythm is normal, the rate 164 per minute. There is an auricular extra-systole (a' and c' in the jugular tracing and r' in the radial).

the auricular muscle was so great that a premature auricular systole actually appeared.

Prognosis.—A number of people whose hearts beat too frequently, show no sign of heart trouble. We then can gauge their condition by their reserve force. Apart from cases with a previous rheumatic history, or of serious heart mischief, I have found that people with continuous rapid hearts gradually recover so far as the heart's condition is concerned, and even cases of exophthalmic goitre may gradually recover with the heart slowing down. If an alcoholic will but mend his ways before he has induced organic changes in his other organs, the heart shows a wonderful power of recovery. Manifestly, in the other ailments, as tubercular and malignant diseases, the future progress of the case is to a certain extent independent of the heart affection. I do not like the continued rapidity (over 90) in cases with valvular lesions, especially of the aortic valve, as it is usually associated with a serious impairment of the myocardium ; and if they do not respond to treatment they generally speed on to a fatal issue.

CHAPTER XXIV

Definition of the term ' bradycardia '.
Normal bradycardia.

Definition of the term ' bradycardia '.—The term 'bradycardia' has been used when the arterial pulse was slow ; and from this it has been inferred that the whole heart was slow in its action. The result of this usage has been to employ the term in many cases quite inappropriately. Thus it is most commonly used in association with the condition known as ' heart-block ', a condition, as will be shown later, where the ventricle alone beats slowly, the auricle pursuing a normal or even accelerated rate.

In order to differentiate between the different forms of slow pulse-rate, it is necessary to make observation of the movements of the various chambers of the heart. If this is done, it will be found that the cases of diminished frequency of the *pulse* can be divided into four classes : (1) Those where all the chambers of the heart participate in the slow action (normal brady-cardia) ; (2) where the slow pulse-rate is due to a missed beat, the ventricle having contracted, the resulting pulse-wave being too feeble to reach the wrist (Figs. 93 and 94) ; (3) certain cases of auricular fibrillation ; (4) where the stimulus is blocked between auricle and ventricle so that the auricle beats at its normal rhythm (Chapter XXXIV), or where there is auricular flutter and the ventricle does not respond to all the auricular systoles (Chapter XXXI) ; (5) where the vagus slows the heart, producing stand-still of the whole heart for irregular periods (Chapter XXVI).

Normal bradycardia.—This only occurs when all the chambers of the heart participate in the slow action. The demonstration of the character of the slowing is best shown by tracings of the jugular pulse with the radial (Fig. 78) or apex beat (Fig. 79), where the auricle is seen to beat at the same rate as the ventricle. There are a number of people in the enjoyment of perfect health, whose pulse beats regularly about fifty per minute. Those of whom I have kept a record were mostly tall men. In a great many people of spare habit, who suffer also from the X disease (p. 100), the heart-rate may fall under fifty beats per minute. In some of these, a rise of temperature of one or two degrees may actually make the pulse beat slower.

There are other conditions which may induce a slowing of the heart's pulse, such as increased arterial pressure in Bright's disease, in gout, and in certain cases of arterial degeneration. In pregnancy the pulse may also be occasionally slow. Jaundice is said to have a considerable power in slowing the pulse, but I myself have never found it.

Occasionally we find patients losing their memory, and the pulse will be found to be very slow—between forty and fifty beats per minute. Further, certain phases of respiration may slow the pulse, and also the exposure of

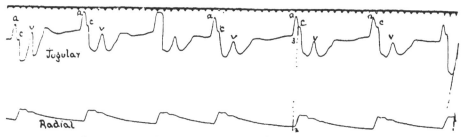

FIG. 78. Infrequent pulse from a healthy acrobat. Rate 26–30 per minute. The jugular pulse shows that all the chambers of the heart participate in the infrequent action.

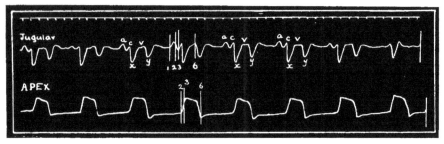

FIG. 79. Simultaneous tracings of the jugular pulse and apex beat, showing the participation of auricle and ventricles in true bradycardia. Rate 50 per minute.

the body to the cold air or to cold baths. So far as I have observed, I have never found any serious result from such slowing of the heart, and I have watched patients whose pulse may frequently be found about fifty per minute, for fifteen and twenty years.

I have recently seen two cases with pulse-rates, in one, 36 per minute, in the other, sometimes lower than 30 per minute. The latter was an acrobat, 40 years of age, and he was himself aware of the slow heart-rate for twenty years. It would usually fall to its lowest during the night, and he would sometimes wonder if it would not stop altogether, the pauses lasting so long. During the day the slow periods varied with periods of increased but usually irregular action, as in Fig. 81.   Colonel Deane made a careful study of this man during his work and at rest, and reports that immediately after violent exertion the rate would be 140, falling in two minutes to 64 on stopping the exertion.   Tracings of the jugular pulse (Fig. 78) and electro-cardiograms showed that all the chambers of the heart participated equally in the slow action.   The other case was a clergyman, 54 years of age, who only complained of feeling tired after a hard day's work.

CHAPTER XXV

THE IRREGULAR ACTION OF THE HEART

Significance of irregular action of the heart.
Places where the heart's contraction may start.
Classification of irregularities.
    Irregularities arising in the sino-auricular node (sinus irregularities).
    Extra-systoles.
    The irregularity due to auricular fibrillation.
    Irregularities due to auricular flutter.
    Irregularities due to failure of the conducting power of the auriculo-ventricular bundle.
    The pulsus alternans.

Significance of **irregular action of the heart.**—Irregular action of the heart is of importance in indicating the mechanism of many of the heart's actions, and a knowledge of this mechanism is essential to the proper diagnosis of pathological changes. As it is a subject of some complexity, I give in this chapter a brief review of the more important points bearing upon irregular rhythm, and a classification of the more common forms.

Irregularities are of such great frequency, and their presence so readily recognized by both patient and physician, that it is necessary clearly to differentiate the different forms and to recognize their meaning and significance. Until a few years ago, their nature was shrouded in obscurity, and in consequence the mystery regarding them in a great measure oppressed both patient and physician. The fact that, in some instances, irregularity was associated with grave conditions of the heart, led to the supposition that all irregularities were signs of some grave mischief. In consequence of this, many patients are subjected to unnecessary fears, made to carry out elaborate methods of treatment, and have imposed upon them burdensome and unnecessary restrictions.

The advance that has been made in the knowledge of this subject within recent years, positively constitutes a revolution. By the combined efforts of clinicians and experimental physiologists, what was recently a complete mystery is now one of the best understood matters in the whole science of medicine. Not only has the scientific aspect been followed out so that we now recognize the different kinds of irregularities, but by watching individual cases for years and noticing the changes that have taken place with advancing years, and observing how people with irregular hearts have borne the stress of life, I have endeavoured to obtain a clearer conception of the bearing of the different irregularities upon the future history of the patient.

Places where the heart's contraction may start.—The normal starting-place of the heart's contraction is in the node of tissue, described by Keith and Flack, at the mouth of the superior vena cava. In describing the functions of the heart muscle, it was pointed out that any part of the muscle was capable of starting the contraction, and that it was because the venous end was the more excitable that the normal rhythm started there. When another part of the heart muscle becomes, from any cause, more excitable than the sino-auricular node, then the contraction starts at that more excitable part, and an abnormal rhythm results. If a break should occur in the bundle joining the auricle and ventricle, the two divisions of the heart will beat separately and independently, as is shown in the Stannius ligature. In what is called ' heart-block ', such a separation occurs, and auricle and ventricle beat at independent rhythms.

Classification of irregularities.

(1) *Irregularities arising in the sino-auricular node (sinus irregularities).*— The heart's contraction arising normally in the sino-auricular node is set to a regular rhythm. This sinus tissue may be excited or depressed as by nerve influence, and irregularities may then occur. This form of irregularity is characterized by a varying length of the cardiac cycle, mainly of the diastolic portion, the pulse-beats being always of equal size or nearly equal size, and presenting no ' imperfect systoles ' or ' missed beats '. The variation usually corresponds with certain phases of respiration. It is most frequent in the young, but is occasionally present in adult life (see Chapter XXVI).

(2) *Extra-systoles.*—Here an auricular or ventricular systole, or both together, may start prematurely and independently of the rhythm of the sino-auricular node. They occur occasionally in an otherwise regular heart ; a premature beat of the radial pulse is felt, followed by a long pause, or there may simply be a long pause (intermittent pulse). Sometimes these extra-systoles may occur with greater frequency, every second beat being of this nature (pulsus bigeminus), or a few may follow one another in rapid succession (multiple extra-systoles). When they are so small as to be imperceptible to the finger, it might seem as if the heart were beating extremely slowly. On auscultation, synchronous with the premature beat, two short, sharp sounds are heard—the first and second sound of the premature or extra-systolic contraction. These sounds are very characteristic of this condition (Chapter XXVII).

(3) *The irregularity due to auricular fibrillation.*—In this irregularity, beats of varying size follow one another at varying intervals ; sometimes

the irregularity is extreme, sometimes scarcely perceptible, but careful analysis will usually show variations in the length of the cardiac cycle. This irregularity is usually associated with marked diminution of the heart's power, sometimes extreme, at other times only indicated by a limitation of the field of cardiac response when the patient makes an effort. It may occur at all ages after the first few years of life. The heart's rate is, as a rule, more frequent than normal, and it may be extremely rapid temporarily (paroxysmal tachycardia) or continuously ; when continuously rapid, it may slow down and beat about 70 to 90 per minute. In some cases, it is less frequent than normal (see Chapter XXX).

(4) *Irregularities due to auricular flutter.*—Under certain circumstances, the auricle may beat at a great rate, 250–300 beats per minute, and the ventricle may not respond to all the auricular contractions, so that an irregularity in its action results. Irregularities of this sort are of extraordinary variety; sometimes the ventricle is rapid and regular, and then the pulsus alternans may appear (Chapter XXXI).

(5) *Irregularities due to failure of the conducting power of the auriculo-ventricular bundle.*—This is due to the ventricular systole dropping out, in consequence of the stimulus for contraction not reaching the ventricle. This condition is rare, but may occasionally occur in influenza and other infectious complaints, and in old and recent rheumatic hearts, especially after digitalis, and in hearts with degenerate heart muscle. A more extreme form of the condition is known as heart-block. This condition may be suspected, when there is a complete pause in the radial pulse with absence of heart sounds (Chapter XXXIV).

(6) *The pulsus alternans.*—The irregularity in this form is due to the varying strength of the beats, a big beat alternating with a small one, the rhythm usually being regular or very slightly altered (Chapter XXXIII).

(7) There are forms of irregularity which we meet on rare occasions; but so far a sufficient number of these forms have not been obtained to warrant a full description. Some of them are referred to in Chapter XXVIII.

CHAPTER XXVI

SINUS IRREGULARITIES (THE YOUTHFUL TYPE OF IRREGULARITY)

Character of the irregularity.
Etiology.
Symptoms.
Associated symptoms.
Diagnostic significance of the youthful type of irregularity.
Treatment.

Character of the irregularity.—As the sino-auricular node, situated at the mouth of the superior vena cava, possesses in a degree higher than any other part the power of rhythmically producing the stimulus for contraction, the rhythm of the whole heart follows normally the time set by this portion of the primitive tissue. While, normally, this rhythm is a fairly regular one, as a matter of observation we find a great many people who show a variation, sometimes slight, sometimes marked, in the duration of the cardiac cycle. There is a much greater constancy in the duration of the systolic period of the cardiac cycle than of the diastolic. With the increase of the pulse-rate, the shortening of the period of the cardiac cycle takes place almost entirely at the expense of the diastolic portion. In sinus irregularities, it is the variation in the length of the diastolic period that is the chief characteristic. In the rapid pulse, we find the duration of the diastolic period reduced, so that with increase of rate this irregularity disappears. On the other hand, when the heart gradually slows in its action, this form of irregularity is prone to occur, so that we find it best in the young and in some adults after a febrile attack or during slow respiration. Typical instances of sinus irregularity are given in Figs. 80 and 81. In Fig. 80, the irregularity is seen to be due to variations in the length of the diastole of the heart (period G), the systolic period (E) remaining constant. The jugular tracings show that the right auricle (a), and ventricle (v), participate in the same irregularity as the radial pulse.

Etiology.—It is generally agreed that this irregularity is of vagus origin. Normally, there is a certain degree of inhibition maintained by this nerve, but its centre may become unusually susceptible to impulses from other parts, and these are transmitted reflexly to the heart. This is well seen in some cases where the vagus is more excitable. In certain cases, the reflex stimulation of the vagus will produce an alteration of the heart's rate, by the respiration. A more striking illustration of the reflex effect by swallowing is found in Figs. 258 and 259, where it not only slowed the sinus rhythm, but depressed the conductivity of the auriculo-ventricular fibres, so that the stimulus from auricle to ventricle was occasionally blocked. In these tracings, it is further to be noted that the vagus effect is not

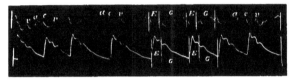

FIG. 80. Simultaneous tracings of the jugular and radial pulses, showing the agreement in rhythm of the right auricle and ventricle (waves *a* and *v*) with the radial pulse, in the sinus form of irregularity. The irregularity is seen to be due to variations in the length of the diastolic period (spaces *G*).

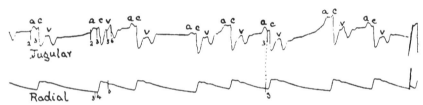

FIG. 81. Simultaneous tracings of the jugular and radial pulses, showing that the auricle participates in the irregularity, and that there is no premature contraction during the long pauses (sinus irregularity).

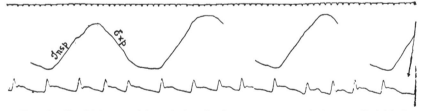

FIG. 82. Youthful type of irregularity showing respiratory variations—a diminished frequency during expiration and an increased during inspiration.

immediately produced and does not at once pass off, but lasts some little time. Thus, in Fig. 259, there is shown a secondary slowing some seconds after the swallowing. The reason I dwell upon this, is because this sinus arrhythmia is often distinctly respiratory in origin, though the pulse variations do not always correspond with identical phases of the respiration (Fig. 82).

In the dog, this irregularity is very common, and disappears on section of the vagus. An irregularity identical with Fig. 84, due to vagus stimulation, is shown in Fig. 83.

Symptoms.—This irregularity is easily recognized. To the finger the pulse-rate is continually changing, usually with respiration, and the beats are equal in strength. On auscultation, the sounds are heard clear and distinct, and the interval between the first and second sounds is constant. By the ear, the varying difference in the diastolic period can be made out

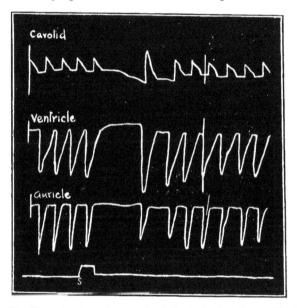

Fig. 83. Shows the effect of vagus stimulation in the dog's heart. The downward movements in the tracing of auricle and ventricle are due to the systole. The vagus was stimulated at *s*, and produced a standstill of the whole heart. (Cushny.)

more easily than by the pulse. In some instances, the slowing may occur frequently (Fig. 81) or at rare intervals, and affect only one or two beats, as in Fig. 84, and there may be at first some difficulty in recognizing the nature of the irregularity ; but when the condition of the patient in other respects is taken into account, the nature of the irregularity can be inferred with certainty. Such an irregularity from any other cause would show evidence of severe heart trouble (as heart-block or the auricular fibrillation), whereas in such cases there is no evidence of heart trouble, or but the very slightest. Tracings of the jugular pulse at once determine the nature of the irregularity by showing that the auricle is also subject to the same influence.

Associated symptoms.—These are merely incidental, the irregularity itself causing no subjective symptom. When some incidental phenomenon such as syncope appears, an undue importance may be attached by the physician to the irregularity. Many young folks have syncopal attacks, and this irregularity, being the only abnormal feature found by the physician, is often the ground on which unnecessary alarm and unnecessary treatment are based.

Although in the vast majority of cases the slowing of the heart, presumably due to vagus action, gives rise to no symptoms, particularly in the young and when of respiratory origin, yet the period of standstill may be at times so long as to produce an effect on the brain. The patient from whom Fig. 84 was taken, had attacks of giddiness at times, and the pauses in the heart's action were often longer than those figured here.

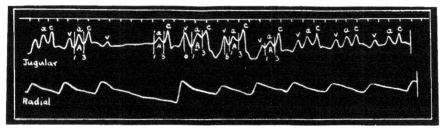

FIG. 84. Occasional slowing of the whole heart due to inhibitory nerve influences on the sinus. The a–c interval (space A) is not affected by the variations in rate. (Compare with Fig. 83.)

Diagnostic significance of the youthful type of irregularity.—By means of the electrocardiograph, Lewis has detected this irregularity at birth. Nicholson has demonstrated its presence in infants, Watson Williams in healthy schoolboys, and Deane in athletic soldiers, and I have found it in a great number of healthy individuals, so that one can safely look upon it as a normal circumstance.

Seeing that the youthful type of irregularity is present in perfectly healthy hearts, it occurred to me to consider the question : Was its presence an evidence of a healthy muscle ? The importance of this question has been forced upon me by the fact, that I have repeatedly seen in consultation young people confined to bed and drastically treated because of its presence. When it appears after a febrile attack, and especially after an attack of rheumatic fever, it has frequently been looked upon as undoubted evidence of some affection of the heart, particularly if associated with a systolic murmur. It is well understood that for a long time after an invasion of the heart by an acute infection, such as occurs in rheumatic fever, a long period of rest is needed, so that the inflamed heart may not be exposed to fatigue. In the confused symptomatology hitherto prevailing, irregularities, especially combined with murmurs, have been considered evidence of an inflamed heart. Contrary to this view, I have come to look upon the presence of this irregularity as an evidence that the heart has escaped infection, when the rate has fallen below 70 beats per minute. The reason for this suggestion arose from the consideration of the conditions in which this irregularity is present, namely, when the heart is free from any excitation. It is at these periods that the vagal effect which produces the irregularity, is capable of acting. When the heart is stimulated, whether as a result of exertion, excitement, bodily effort, fever, or infection, then this vagal action disappears. Hence, when, after the subsidence of the fever, the heart slows down and this irregularity appears, it is an evidence that all exciting causes (including infection) have gone, and therefore we can be justified in assuming that the heart has escaped damage, and that there is no need for the precautionary treatment which is called for where there is a suspicion of persisting infection. Even the presence of a systolic murmur need not render this view improbable, as will be seen in the discussion of the significance of murmurs (Chapter XL). This view I have put in practice for ten years, and so far it has proved trustworthy in every case, although with extended observation it may have to be modified. I have had a few cases where, from the character of the murmurs and the size of the heart, it is evident there had undoubtedly been infection of the heart during an attack of rheumatic fever, and, some months after, this irregularity was present. In them, the rate was over 80 per minute, and subsequent observations two or three years after showed that the heart had made a very good recovery. Where the heart has been affected, it is possible that the appearance of this irregularity may show that the active stage of the infection has ceased. At all events, I have never seen the presence of this irregularity in an acute infection or with a progressive lesion of the heart muscle. But, as I have said, this is a matter for further observation ; and I would suggest that it is a very good subject to follow up for those who see many cases of rheumatic fever. It will require, however, long and patient observation, and individual cases will need watching for many years.

Treatment.—I have repeatedly seen cases subjected to a great many different forms of treatment for this irregularity. From what I have just said, it will be realized that it calls for no special treatment, as its presence indicates that the heart is healthy.

CHAPTER XXVII

THE EXTRA-SYSTOLE

Definition of the term ' extra-systole '.
The character of the irregularity.
Recognition of the extra-systole.
The different forms of extra-systole.
The ventricular extra-systole.
The interpolated extra-systole.
Simultaneous occurrence of the normal auricular systole and of the ventricular extra-
    systole.
The auricular extra-systole.
The extra-systoles arising in the auriculo-ventricular node (nodal extra-systole).
Conditions inducing extra-systoles.
Sensations produced by extra-systoles.
Prognosis in cases with extra-systoles.
Treatment.

Definition of the term ' extra-systole '.—There are so many conditions that simulate extra-systoles, that a good deal of confusion exists
in regard to what really constitutes an extra-systole, and it is therefore
necessary to define the term. As the stimulus for contraction arises normally
in the sino-auricular node, and as the stimulus passes from this place to
the auricle, then to the ventricle, so that there is a sequence of stimulation
and contraction of auricle and ventricle, I would suggest that the term
' extra-systole ' should be limited to those premature contractions of
auricle or ventricle in response to a stimulus from some abnormal point
of the heart, but where, otherwise, the fundamental or sinus rhythm of
the heart is maintained. Where a continuous dominant rhythm arises from
other sources, as in heart-block and auricular fibrillation, premature contractions may arise in the ventricle, and these also may be included under
the definition of extra-systole.

The character of the irregularity.—The extra-systole in cases with
the normal or sinus rhythm is usually recognized by the occurrence of
a premature beat in the radial pulse, followed by an abnormally long pause,
as is shown in Fig. 85, where the two small beats are extra-systoles. It
may appear only at rare intervals, or it may occur at frequent irregular
intervals, or regularly after every 1, 2, 3, 4, or more, normal beats, as
in Figs. 86, 87, 88, 89. Sometimes periods may occur at fairly regular
intervals, during which several extra-systoles may appear. Fig. 90 shows
such a period, during which there are three radial beats followed by long

pauses, but the jugular tracing shows that, during these pauses, an extra-systole occurred which failed to affect the radial pulse. In this case, these

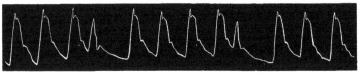

FIG. 85. The small beats are due to extra-systoles.

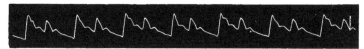

FIG. 86. Pulsus bigeminus due to an extra-systole occurring after each normal beat.

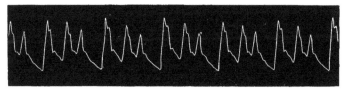

FIG. 87. Extra-systole occurring after every two normal beats.

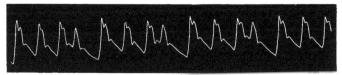

FIG. 88. Extra-systoles occurring after every three normal beats.

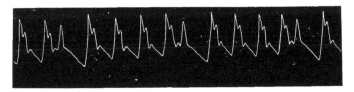

FIG. 89. Extra-systoles occurring after every four normal beats.

periods appeared after every four or five normal beats throughout the examination.

The ventricular contraction causing the extra-systole may be so weak that no wave is perceptible to the finger in the radial, though it may be detected in the sphygmogram, as in Figs. 91 and 92. In some cases, it may even not appear in the sphygmogram; but the heart's sounds, or a tracing of the jugular pulse or apex beat at the same time, show that during the long pause in the radial pulse the ventricle contracted, but not with sufficient strength to send a wave into the radial artery (Figs. 90, 93, 94).

In these cases, the pulse is described as 'intermittent', or, if the extra-systoles occur regularly after each normal beat, the pulse at the wrist

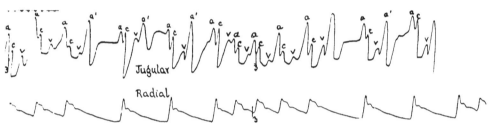

FIG. 90. Shows periods of normal heart action varying with periods in which the extra-systoles occur. There are two periods of irregular pulse-beats (three pulse-beats in each period). The jugular pulse shows that, after each of the pulse-beats, there is a large wave a', due to a premature contraction of the auricle. On account of the size of the wave, it can be inferred that the ventricle was also in contraction, so that the auricular contents could not go forward into the ventricle, but were sent back into the veins.

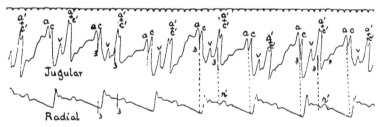

FIG. 91. The radial tracing shows a premature beat or extra-systole after each normal beat (pulsus bigeminus). The jugular tracing shows a large wave $a'+c'$ occurring at the same time as the extra-systole; showing that the auricles and ventricles contracted at the same time.

appears extremely slow, and the case may be put down as 'bradycardia', or heart-block. It may be differentiated by the observation of the jugular pulse or apex beat, or by auscultation.

Recognition of the extra-systole.—I find in practice that many people have a difficulty in distinguishing an extra-systole from other forms of irregular heart action; and I wish to insist on the ease of its recognition in the great majority of cases by means of auscultation. The regular sequence of sounds is interrupted by two short, sharp sounds, followed by a long pause, as is represented in the diagrams, Figs. 95 and 96. Sometimes the extra-systole is so weak that only one feeble sound can be detected. It may be confidently accepted that when such sound or sounds are heard, during an ' intermission ' of the pulse, the irregularity is due to the occurrence of an extra-systole. The only exception is partial heart-block with mitral stenosis, where, in very rare instances, a sound due to the auricle may be perceived during the pause. This usually happens only after digitalis administration, and there is always a presystolic murmur present.

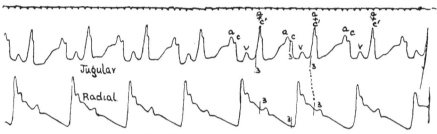

FIG. 92. Shows the same features as Fig. 91.

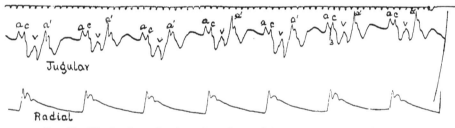

FIG. 93. The jugular pulse shows large beats a' during the long pause in the radial, indicating that the auricles and ventricles contracted, but that the ventricular contractions were too weak to produce a wave in the radial pulse sufficiently large to affect the sphygmograph.

In many cases, if the hand be placed over the heart, the short premature contractions of the extra-systole can be perceived. This extra-systolic contraction may be of considerable force, and some writers have erroneously imagined that when this happened it was due to the right ventricle contracting while the left stood still.

The different forms of extra-systole.—It has already been said that, if any portion of the heart becomes more excitable than the sino-auricular node, then the heart's contraction will proceed from this place. If such a place be continuously excitable, then we get a continuous abnormal rhythm. If it is only transiently excitable, then we get simple premature contractions, their frequency varying and depending on the degree of excitability. In the human subject, we can sometimes recognize whether these premature contractions arise in the auricle, or ventricle, or in the auriculo-ventricular node or bundle.

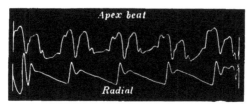

FIG. 94. Simultaneous tracings of the apex beat and of the radial pulse. There are two beats of the apex to one radial pulse.

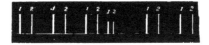

FIG. 95. Diagram representing the sounds of the heart with occasional extra-systoles.

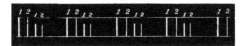

FIG. 96. Diagrammatic representation of the sounds of the heart in a case of such rhythmical irregularity as is represented in Figs. 91–94.

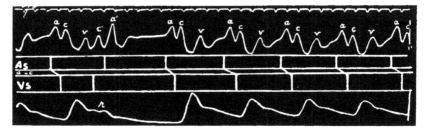

FIG. 97. Represents a common form of ventricular extra-systole. There is a long pause after the extra-systole (r). In the jugular tracing and in the diagram this is seen to be due to the failure of the stimulus from the auricle (a′) to provoke a ventricular contraction.

The ventricular extra-systole.—The simplest form of extra-systole is where a premature beat of the ventricle occurs, followed by a long pause. This is shown in Fig. 97, where the small beat in the tracing is seen to occur soon after the preceding beat. It is followed by a long pause. The explanation is afforded by a study of the jugular pulse (upper tracing).

The waves a are due to the auricle and are seen to occur with perfect
regularity. They are all followed by a wave c, due to the carotid pulse,
except in the case of the wave a', which is preceded by a wave from the
carotid, c'. This carotid wave c' corresponds to the small premature wave
r in the radial pulse, and means that the carotid pulse in this case has
preceded the auricular wave in the jugular pulse—in other words, the ventricle has contracted before the auricle. This will be readily understood,
if the diagram inserted between the jugular and radial tracings be studied.
The downstroke in the upper compartment represents the systole of the
auricle, and corresponds with the auricular waves a in the jugular tracing.
They are seen to occur with perfect regularity. The downstrokes in the
lowest compartment represent the ventricular systoles, and correspond with

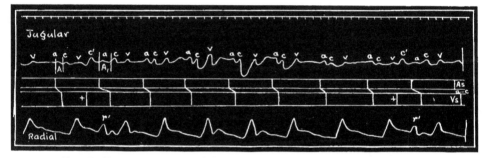

FIG. 98. Simultaneous tracing of the jugular and radial pulses, showing the interpolation
of ventricular extra-systoles (c', c' and r', r') represented in the diagram by the downstrokes
+ +. The downstrokes in the space As represent the auricular waves (a) in the jugular,
and the downstrokes in the space Vs represent the carotid waves c, and the slanting lines
connecting them represent the a–c interval.

the waves c and c' in the jugular and with the radial beats. The slanting
lines in the mid-space represent the passage of the stimulus from auricle
to ventricle. It will be seen that the contraction of the ventricle is dependent
on the auricular contraction, except in the case of the premature contraction c', when the ventricle precedes and is independent of the auricular
systole. The long pause which follows the premature beat, is seen to be
due to the fact that the ventricle stands still, until the next auricular beat
stimulates it to further contraction.

The interpolated extra-systole.—Such is the usual way in which an
extra-systole of the ventricle is produced. But in rare instances the ventricle
not only gives rise to a premature contraction, but responds to the subsequent auricular systole as well, in which case we get a ventricular beat (Fig.
98) in the radial pulse without a corresponding auricular beat in the jugular.
The interpolated diagram shows the manner in which these beats arise.

In Fig. 97 and 98, the premature or ventricular extra-systole preceded the auricular contraction, as shown by the wave c' preceding the wave a'. In Fig. 99, the extra-systole c' follows at a short distance the auricular wave.

Simultaneous occurrence of the normal auricular systole and of the ventricular extra-systole.—In the illustrations I have given of the ventricular extra-systole (as in Fig. 97 and 98), in the jugular tracing the carotid wave c' was seen to precede the auricular wave a'. In these

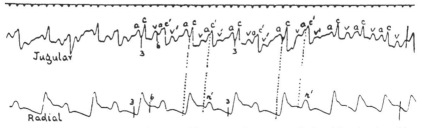

Fig. 99. Every second radial beat r' is small and premature (pulsus bigeminus), and is due to an extra-systole. In the jugular tracing, it will be seen that the wave c' occurs after the wave a, but at a shorter distance than the normal a–c interval.

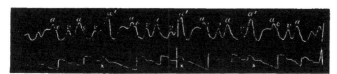

Fig. 100. Simultaneous tracings of the jugular and radial pulses. The small beats × × × are extra-systoles. The auricle preserves its rhythm during the irregular periods in the radial pulse. The wave a' is the auricular wave during the premature contraction of the left ventricle. The absence of the ventricular wave v, after the wave a', indicates that the right ventricle had contracted early, evidently synchronous with the premature contraction of the left ventricle, the large wave following a' being due to stasis.

instances, the normal rate was rather slow. In most instances, however, they fall together—the auricular contraction occurring during the ventricular contraction. In consequence of this, the auricle cannot empty its contents into the ventricle, and hence a big wave is sometimes sent into the jugular. In patients with a well-marked jugular pulse, this is readily recognized by the eye. In other cases, the jugular pulsation is only to be seen when this big wave is sent back.

In Fig. 100, the waves a and a' are due to the auricular systole, and occur at regular intervals. The waves a' are, however, much larger than the waves a, and the reason for the increase in size is found in the fact that at that time the ventricle was also in systole, causing the extra-systole.

In Fig. 101, a simultaneous record of the apex beat and jugular pulse shows the premature contraction of the ventricle *o*, at the same time as the large auricular wave *a'*, so that here also we have evidence of the simultaneous contraction of auricle and ventricle during a ventricular extra-systole. When there is a large jugular pulse, the increased size of the auricular wave occurring during the extra-systole of the ventricle may not be so marked. We can frequently recognize that an extra-systole of the ventricle has taken place when there is no radial beat, by the increased size of the auricular beat in the jugular pulse.

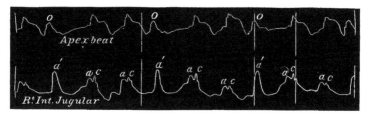

FIG. 101. Simultaneous tracings of the apex beat and of the jugular pulse, showing the rhythmical appearance of the auricular wave during the irregular periods in the apex tracing. The small beats *o o o* are extra-systoles of the ventricle.

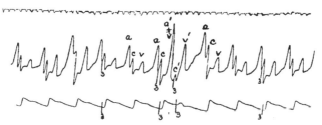

FIG. 102.   Shows an auricular extra-systole—the premature wave *a'* falling on the wave *v* of the previous ventricular systole.

The auricular extra-systole.—When an extra-systole arises in the auricle, the sounds of the heart and the radial tracing present exactly the same features as when a ventricular extra-systole occurs; and it is only by a simultaneous record of the jugular pulse that the one can be differentiated from the other.   In Fig. 102 and 103, the radial pulse shows premature beats (*r'*), which can be readily identified as extra-systoles.

In the jugular tracings the carotid wave *c'* is preceded by an auricular wave *a'*, and the only inference that can be drawn is that *a'* is due to an extra-systole of the auricle, which is followed by an extra-systole of the ventricle, producing the carotid and radial beats *c'* and *r'*.   In Fig. 102, the wave *a'* falls on the *v* wave of the preceding ventricular systole, and is, therefore, of great size.

o 2

In such instances as these, the auricle is supposed to contract in reply
to a stimulus from some source other than the sinus, and the long pause
after the extra-systole is due to the fact, that the stimulus from the sinus
arising at its normal time fails to provoke the refractory auricle to contraction. This is brought out in the intercalated diagram in Fig. 103, in
which, above the upper space, are arrows representing the sinus stimulation.
In the diagram, it will be seen that there is no response to the sinus stimula-

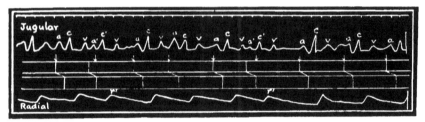

Fig. 103. Shows auricular extra-systoles (a') followed by ventricular contractions (c', r')
The arrows in the diagram represent the sinus stimulation, and the long pauses after the extra-
systoles are seen to be due to the fact that the auricle did not respond to the sinus stimulation.

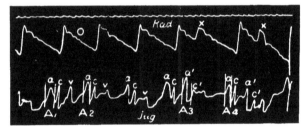

Fig. 104. Shows two premature or extra-systoles of auricular origin ($\times$). The waves c' in
the jugular tracing occur at the same time as the small premature beats ($\times$) in the radial
tracing, and are therefore due to the carotid. These are preceded by premature waves a' due
to the auricle. The interval a'–c' (space A_3) is greater than the average a–c interval (A_2), and
is much greater than the following a–c interval (A_4).

tion after the extra-systole, but that auricle and ventricle remain quiescent
till the following sinus stimulation excites them to a contraction. In these
two illustrations, the irregular period is equal to two cardiac cycles, the
explanation being obvious from the study of the diagram in Fig. 103. In
most cases of auricular extra-systole, the irregular period is less than two
cycles, as is shown in Fig. 104 and 105. The reason given by Cushny and
Wenckebach, and usually accepted, is that the stimulus arising in the
auricle passes back to the sinus, and stimulates the sinus, so that its stored
energy is exhausted, and it begins to build up anew the stimulus material.
As soon as it has again reached the excitable stage, it starts off the contrac-

tion. Thus in the diagram (Fig. 106), representing the events in Fig. 105, the stimulus is represented coming down from the sinus to the auricle, but at the extra-systole (+) the stimulus is represented by an arrow passing back to the sinus, so that the sinus responds to the retrograde stimulation. After this premature stimulation, the sinus rests for a normal period, and starts off again at the normal rhythm. This irregular period, due to the auricular extra-systole, is so frequently shorter than two normal beats, that this is usually assumed to be the manner in which it is brought about. While it offers a plausible explanation, it cannot be said in any sense to have been proved, and there are other possibilities which need consideration

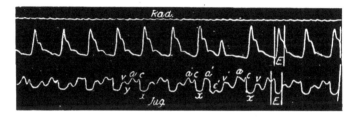

FIG. 105. Shows an extra-systole of auricular origin at a'. This tracing is interpreted in the diagram, Fig. 106.

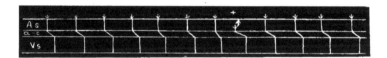

FIG. 106. Diagram representing the events in Fig. 105. The extra-stimulation at + is represented arising in the auricle, passing back and disturbing the sinus rhythm. Note the lengthened a–c interval after the auricular extra-systole.

before it can be finally accepted. As, however, they are still speculative, it would not be convenient to discuss them here.

The extra-systoles arising in the auricular-ventricular node (nodal extra-systole).—So far the recognition of extra-systoles as ventricular or auricular has been comparatively easy. There is a third class which has hitherto not been sufficiently considered, and which, in my opinion, has been wrongly interpreted. The characteristic feature of these extra-systoles is that auricle and ventricle contract prematurely and together. Thus in Fig. 107 the auricular wave a' in the jugular appears prematurely, and obscures the appearance of the carotid waves,—the time when the latter were due can be ascertained by measuring the time between the extra-systole in the radial pulse, and the preceding beat. That the auricle did not contract at its normal time is evident by the absence of any wave at

why not interpret 'auricular extra-systoles' were being premature discharges from sinus.

the time of the arrow in the intercalated diagram during the irregular period, which is the time when it was due. Here, then, we have evidence that both auricle and ventricle contracted prematurely and simultaneously. In the ventricular and auricular forms, no difficulty is found in recognizing that the extra-stimulation must have affected either one chamber or the other, but in this form we have to consider where a stimulation could arise that would at once affect both chambers. If all the possibilities be con‑ sidered, we are driven by a process of exclusion to attribute the source of this stimulation to the tissue that joins auricle and ventricle, and almost to a certainty to that portion described as the auriculo-ventricular node. Probably the extra-systoles shown to occur in the jugular tracing of Fig. 93 are also nodal in origin.

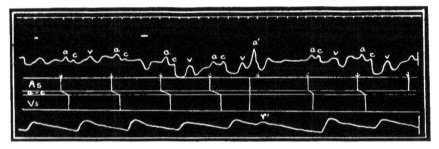

Fig. 107. Shows a nodal extra-systole (a′ and r′); the auricular and ventricular systoles as shown in the diagram are premature and simultaneous.

Conditions inducing extra-systoles.—In the careful examination of young and old, it is surprising to find how frequently the extra-systole is detected in healthy and robust subjects. This was first impressed upon me, while pursuing an investigation into the circulatory changes in pregnant women. I used to take tracings as a routine in women before, during, and after pregnancy, and detected it so frequently that I came to look on it as an ordinary event. Nor was their occurrence limited to, or connected with the pregnant state. Extending my observations to all cases, I collected tracings from several thousands of individuals who showed extra-systoles, and found that these extra-systoles could be detected in healthy people at all ages after infancy. They are rare before 20 years of age, increasing in frequency up to 40 years, and are very frequent between 40 and 50 years of age, and I was led to expect them in every one over 60 years of age. The vast majority of people are quite unconscious of their presence.

The slight changes which take place in the muscle of the heart, as years advance, are the probable cause for their greater frequency in the elderly.

In rheumatic affections of the heart, after the acute stage has passed, where the muscle is affected, there is a great tendency to the occurrence of the extra-systole.

There are many agents which may provoke extra-systoles in the predisposed. Not infrequently we may detect extra-systoles at the beginning of an examination, when the individual is somewhat excited. At other times they occur when the individual is in bed, when it would seem that the slow-acting heart gives the opportunity for some excitable part of the heart to start the contraction.

Indiscretions in food and drink may readily induce these extra-systoles, so much so that some folks only complain of them when they have eaten large meals, and especially with alcohol. Occasionally they occur only after some particular article of diet, such as tea.

Tobacco readily induces them in some cases. One of my colleagues, who is now 59 years of age, has been conscious of them, after smoking, since he was 18 years old. He was warned of the danger of tobacco in producing them, but he has smoked heavily, and is to-day a healthy vigorous man.

Digitalis readily produces them in some people, particularly when it slows the heart in auricular fibrillation.

Sensations produced by extra-systoles.—The majority of people are unconscious of their presence, but some are conscious of a quiet transient fluttering in the chest when an extra-systole occurs ; others are aware of the long pause ' as if their heart had stopped ' ; while others are conscious of the big beat that frequently follows the long pause. So violent is the effect of this after-beat, that in neurotic persons it may cause a shock, followed by a sense of great exhaustion ; some have a suffocating sensation rising in the throat, which may cause them to cough. Most patients are unconscious of the irregularity due to the extra-systole, until their attention is called to it by the medical attendant. Both being ignorant of its origin, and it being characteristic of human nature to associate the unknown with evil, patient and doctor are too often unnecessarily alarmed. When a series of extra-systoles follow one another, it is possible that the output from the heart is so small that giddiness and syncope may result.

Prognosis in cases with extra-systoles.—Extra-systoles or intermittent heart, as they are sometimes called, occur so frequently, and are viewed by the profession so seriously, that it is necessary to indicate their bearing on the individual's future. Hitherto their cause has been unknown, and individuals showing them have been considered unfit for admission into the services, military, naval, and civil, and have been considered unsuitable for life insurance or have been penalized with increased premiums ; and they have been made miserable for life by the vague prognostications of danger, and have been subjected to prolonged and quite unnecessary treatment.

The fact that the occurrence of an extra-systole is due to some part of the heart's structure being temporarily more excitable than the normal starting-place, has led to the idea that it may be an evidence of some disease process. A certain amount of confirmatory evidence for this supposition is found in the fact, that people with undoubted disease of the heart do show extra-systoles, and that extra-systoles have sometimes been found to precede the appearance of grave disturbances of the heart's action, as auricular fibrillation (Case 51). For these reasons, there has been a tendency to view extra-systoles as signs of some gravity. If, however, the subject be studied from a wider and more practical outlook, it will be found that extra-systoles in themselves are not signs of any specific injury to the heart, nor should a prognosis of any gravity be based on their appearance alone. I have watched individuals for over twenty-five years who have presented extra-systoles, sometimes with greater frequency than at other times; and these people have led laborious lives, and have never shown the slightest symptoms of heart failure, or any other evidence of heart impairment. I have had similar experiences with people who have shown all forms of extra-systole, auricular, ventricular, and nodal. I have watched young people grow into manhood and lead vigorous lives. I have watched elderly people live beyond 80 years of age, in whom I had detected extra-systoles at the age of 60, and when they did die the cause of death was not primarily cardiac failure. A short time ago, I was consulted by a man aged 69 years, and whom I found in a fair state of health. He presented auricular extra-systoles at frequent intervals; and when I remarked upon this, he told me that they had been present for over fifty years. When he was 18 years old, he should have gone to India to take up an appointment for which he had been specially educated, but was prevented because on a medical examination these extra-systoles were detected, and the doctors said he was unfit. He tried for other appointments, but the presence of this irregularity stood in his way. He had ultimately to seek a livelihood by other means, which had entailed great bodily strain for many years. Time and again he had submitted to prolonged treatment, without avail, for the purpose of curing this irregularity. He had oftentimes been made miserable and depressed by the grave prognostications of his medical advisers, and had, up to the time when I saw him, been under the apprehension that he had some obscure heart affection which might prove fatal at any moment.

From such facts as these, that healthy men and women may present this form of irregularity, it can be gathered that extra-systoles in themselves are signs of no significance so far as the efficiency of the heart is concerned. Where there is heart failure, it will invariably be found that other evidences are present; and the prognosis is to be based upon these evidences, and not upon the presence of the extra-systole. Even in cases where it is reasonable to assume that some lesion causes the frequent occurrence of the extra-systole, or where a series may follow one another so that the circulation is interfered with, there are always other signs present which, if duly appreciated, will guide to a prognosis.

It may therefore be stated that when the extra-systole is the only abnormal sign, the prognosis is a favourable one, and where it is associated with other signs, the prognosis is to be based upon these other signs.

Treatment.—The patient is usually unconscious of the presence of these extra-systoles, and may be alarmed by his doctor telling him that he has an intermittent or irregular heart. The patient may be conscious of the pause and may feel frightened lest the heart should stand still, and he is painfully aware of the big after-beat. As these extra-systoles frequently occur in the night, when the heart is otherwise acting slowly, patients, particularly neurotic individuals, are greatly distressed. As the presence of extra-systoles and the patient's consciousness of them cause great mental distress, it is always necessary in treatment to take the whole mental state into consideration. The alarm is often aggravated by the inability of the doctor to recognize the significance of the irregularity, and by his subjecting the individual to a long course of treatment, or sending him to some health resort which advertises itself as a cure for heart affections. As all attempts at cure are often unavailing, many individuals go through life, obsessed with the idea that they have a serious affection of the heart. The first duty of the physician is clearly to recognize the nature of the trouble, and to relieve the patient's mind so far as this irregularity is concerned. There is absolutely no cause for alarm. I frequently see members of our profession greatly distressed, because they themselves have detected this irregularity. They have sought in text-books for an explanation of their trouble, and, finding nothing but vague statements, they have become oppressed by the mystery of their trouble. The intelligent explanation of the nature of the irregularity has at once dispelled this fear. So it is necessary that we should, with confidence based on knowledge, reassure the patient in the first instance as to the innocent nature of the complaint. When some digestive disturbance, or such articles as tobacco, tea, or coffee, predispose to extra-systoles, the alteration of the diet and the omission of the offending article are quite sufficient to stop their occurrence.

In neurotic people, when their occurrence causes distress, especially during the night, ammonium bromide (20 grains two or three times a day) usually gives relief after a few days. In the vast majority of cases drugs are of no use in stopping them. Many drugs have a reputation for stopping them, even digitalis, which as a matter of fact readily provokes them in certain cases ; but it will be found that there are periods during which the extra-systoles are of frequent occurrence, and long intervals during which they are absent, and the cessation of the extra-systoles is, in these cases, quite independent of the drug. When they persist for months and years, no form of treatment appears to be of use in stopping them. I have carefully pushed many drugs in these persistent cases ; and I have seen individuals who have been subjected to all sorts of treatment ; but I have been unable to find any drug or method which was effectual in stopping them. Many people are entirely free from them, while they take plenty of healthy exercise in the open air, but have them when leading a somewhat sedentary life, so I sometimes prescribe more exercise in the fresh air.

CHAPTER XXVIII

SOME RARE FORMS OF CARDIAC IRREGULARITY

Sino-auricular block.
Blocked auricular extra-systoles.
Escaped ventricular beats and nodal beats.
Multiple extra-systoles of auricular origin.
Multiple extra-systoles of ventricular origin.
Causes of multiple extra-systoles.
Prognosis.

IN addition to the more common forms of cardiac irregularity described in Chapter XXV, there are a few rare forms which call for a passing attention.

Sino-auricular block.—We occasionally meet with cases which show a pause in the contraction of both auricle and ventricle, of such a character that it is assumed that the stimulus has arisen in the sino-auricular node, but has failed to reach the auricle. This is shown by the sudden dropping out of a cardiac cycle, as revealed by polygraphic and electrocardiographic methods. This condition is not of much significance so far as the heart efficiency is concerned.

Blocked auricular extra-systoles.—As a rule the ventricle responds to auricular extra-systoles. Sometimes the stimulus from the auricle fails to reach the ventricle, when there is an auricular extra-systole. ' In these cases, there may be found a delay between the auricular and ventricular systoles, as in Fig. 108, when the $a'-c'$ interval (space A') after the auricular extra-systole is much longer than the normal $a-c$ interval (space A). In other instances, the stimulus fails to reach the ventricle and we get a pause in the radial pulse. When the extra-systole occurs after each normal beat, the blocking of the stimulus may result in an infrequent ventricular rate, which accounts for the slow pulse seen in Fig. 109. This is a different mechanism from that which happens in partial heart-block, where two normal auricular beats occur to each ventricular beat, as in Fig. 163. In the latter case, the auriculo-ventricular bundle is damaged, so that every second normal auricular systole fails to get through. With the blocked auricular extra-systole, there is no reason for assuming that the bundle is damaged, but possibly that the disturbance induced by the extra-systole has caused a depression of conductivity. The occurrence of auricular extra-systoles, in which the ventricle responds to some and not to others, may give rise to a very irregular rhythm, as in Fig. 108, 109, and 110. The tracings,

Fig. 108–10. were taken from an apparently healthy youth with no cardiac infirmity.

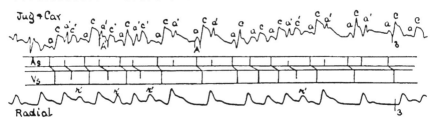

FIG. 108. Tracings from the jugular and radial pulses showing the frequent occurrence of auricular extra-systoles (a', c', and r'). The interval between the extra-systolic auricular and ventricular contractions (space A') is much greater than the normal a–c interval (space A). Some of the extra-systolic auricular contractions fail to produce ventricular contractions, causing the long pause in the radial tracing. In the interpolated diagram the shortened downstrokes represent extra-systoles and show diagramatically the delayed response or block.

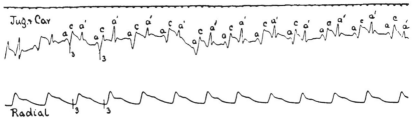

FIG. 109. Shows an infrequent radial pulse (60 per minute). The jugular tracing shows that after each normal beat there is an auricular extra-systole (a') which is blocked, so that the ventricle does not respond.

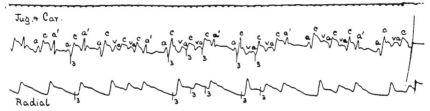

FIG. 110. Shows an irregular radial pulse due to the occasional occurrence of blocked auricular extra-systoles (a').

Escaped ventricular beats and nodal beats.—In a few cases, I have met with peculiar rhythms due to the beats rising somewhere near the node. This is best seen in cases of partial block, where what is called ' escaped ventricular beats ' occur. Here, when the pauses between the ventricular

beats are somewhat prolonged, the ventricle tends to go off on independent
beats.   This is seen in Fig. 111, where there is a partial heart-block, and a
pulse-beat appears at the same time as the auricular wave in the jugular.   In
Fig. 261, there is a standstill of the whole heart, and the ventricular escaped

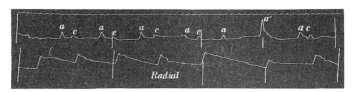

Fig. 111.   Tracing from a case of partial heart-block, due to influenza. The large wave
in the jugular tracing is due to the auricle contracting at its normal period at the same time
that the ventricle contracts from another source (escaped ventricular beat).

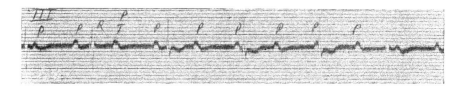

Fig. 112.   Electrocardiogram from a case of partial heart-block, due to digitalis. The
auricular contraction causes the elevation P, and the ventricular contraction, the high sharp
summit R. The last three or four ventricular contractions are independent of the auricular
contractions.

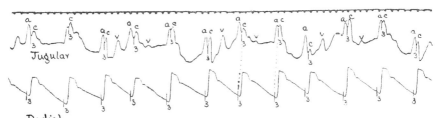

Fig. 113.   An irregular pulse due to escaped ventricular contractions, shown by the
shortened a–c interval.

beat occurs at the same time as the auricular beats. Fig. 112 is an electrocardiogram of a case of partial block, and there is an escaped ventricular
beat which occurs during auricular systole. The character of the ventricular
beat is the same as the other normal beats of the heart, so that we can
infer that stimulation for contraction must have entered the heart by the
normal path, and the stimulus must have arisen in the auriculo-ventricular
node or bundle.

On a few occasions, I have met with a curious irregularity during which the auricular rhythm was irregular, and then nodal beats occurred. Fig. 113 is a tracing of such an instance ; it shows some beats where the distance between the auricle and ventricle is so slight as to prove that the ventricular contraction was independent of the auricular stimulus. Fig. 114 is an electrocardiogram of a similar case ; and it shows that occasionally the ventricle contracted independently of the auricle, and, as the ventricular contraction gives a normal electrocardiogram, we can conclude that the stimulus for contraction arose here in the auriculo-ventricular node or bundle.

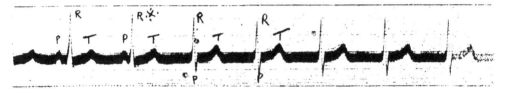

Fig. 114. Electrocardiogram showing an altered action of the heart after the first two beats. The summit P is due to the auricular contraction, and the summits R and T are due to the ventricle. The third ventricular beat is independent of the auricular contraction. After this, auricle and ventricle contract together (probably a true nodal rhythm).

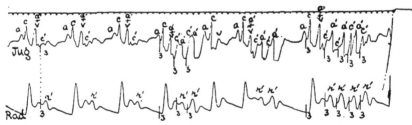

Fig. 115. Multiple auricular extra-systoles (r'). One auricular extra-systole occurs after each normal beat in the first part of the tracing, and several in the latter part of the tracing.

Multiple extra-systoles of auricular origin.—In certain cases, we may meet with a somewhat confused irregularity or short periods of tachycardia, which are due to a series of extra-systoles. In Fig. 115 there is in the first part of the tracing a bigeminal pulse which the jugular tracing shows to be due to an auricular extra-systole, alternating with a normal beat. This part of the tracing was taken while the patient held his breath. When breathing freely, in place of one extra-systole, two, three, or five would follow one another before a normal beat occurred as shown in the latter part of the tracing. A somewhat similar condition is seen in Fig. 116, where an auricular extra-systole (a') occurs after two normal beats. These extra-systoles are ' blocked ', having no ventricular response. These are followed by a series of auricular extra-systoles (a'), and the ventricle responds to the abnormal auricular beats, and the end of the tracing shows that the normal rhythm is resumed. In this patient, paroxysms of tachycardia would frequently occur, lasting for several minutes, and the radial pulse would then show the pulsus alternans. Fig. 117 shows the end of such a paroxysm.

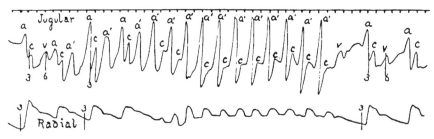

FIG. 116. Simultaneous tracings of the jugular and radial pulses during one attack of paroxysmal tachycardia. The first cardiac cycle in the jugular tracing shows the normal events (a, c, v). The second cycle shows the normal waves a and c, but the wave following, marked a', occurs earlier than the wave v in the previous cycle, and is due to a premature or auricular extra-systole, but is not followed by a c wave or by a radial pulse-beat. The next two normal a, c waves are each followed by an auricular extra-systole (a') with no ventricular response, as shown by the absence of the c wave and the radial pulse-beat. These are all 'interpolated auricular extra-systoles'. After these there follows a series of auricular premature beats (a'), to which the ventricle responds as shown by the c waves and the small radial pulse-beats.

The onset of the paroxysm always coincides with great distension of the jugular veins, which is shown in the tracing by the greater amplitude of the auricular waves a'.

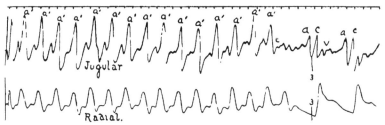

FIG. 117. From the same patient as Fig. 116, taken at the end of a long paroxysm. It shows the same features as Fig. 116, but here there is a well-marked alternation of the radial pulse-beats during the paroxysm.

Multiple extra-systoles of ventricular origin.—As a rule, only a few beats of this kind occur, as in Fig. 118, where it will be seen that the auricular wave a pursues a regular undisturbed course, while two radial beats occur prematurely. In one case (Case 80) with auricular fibrillation and heart-block, ventricular extra-systoles were of frequent occurrence. This patient was always conscious of their presence, and sometimes recognized that a few would follow each other. Towards the end of his life, he had periods when the extra-systoles would persist for a short time, so that the ventricular rate would suddenly rise from 30 beats per minute to 70. When these ceased, the ventricle would stand still for short periods, during which the patient would lose consciousness and become convulsed. He knew when a paroxysm was on, and could tell us when an attack of loss of consciousness was impending.

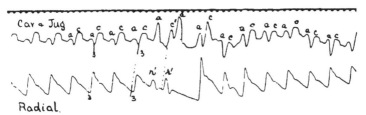

FIG. 118. Two ventricular extra-systoles (r') are seen to occur together in this tracing.

Causes of multiple extra-systoles.—So far it is only possible to surmise the cause of these multiple extra-systoles. It is just possible that there is some irritable focus in the muscle of auricle or ventricle, giving rise to them. So far as the ventricular cases are concerned, in all the cases which I have seen there has been distinct evidence of myocardial disease.

Prognosis.—In the few cases of short attacks of tachycardia of auricular origin which I have seen, the individuals did not seem much embarrassed by the peculiarity ; and I have not followed them for long enough periods or in sufficient numbers to express an opinion. I am disposed to look on the ventricular form as distinct evidence of advanced myocardial degeneration. Each case, however, must be judged on its merits, and on the broad principles which I have laid down for the estimation of the value of obscure signs (Chapter V).

CHAPTER XXIX

ABNORMAL RHYTHMS

The cause of abnormal rhythms.
Result of onset or offset of an abnormal rhythm.
The bearing of abnormal rhythms on the efficiency of the heart and their reaction to stimuli and drugs.

The cause of abnormal rhythms.—So far we have considered the irregularities which occur, when the normal action of the heart is maintained, or interrupted at intervals by a few beats arising in an abnormal place. As has been stated, different parts of the heart muscle or of structures contained in the heart muscle are capable of originating a contraction or a series of contractions. The reason that they do not exercise this function in health, is because the rapidity of forming the stimulus material is greater at the sino-auricular node than at any other part of the heart. As with each contraction of the heart the whole material is for the time being destroyed, each part has to form another supply, and in health the sino-auricular node does this most rapidly and is therefore the most excitable part. If from any cause some other part of the heart becomes more excitable, in such a manner that it can produce this stimulus for contraction more rapidly than the sino-auricular node, then the contractions will start there, and produce occasional beats or a continuous series of beats, as in extra-systoles or paroxysmal tachycardia ; or if the sino-auricular node itself becomes too slow in its stimulus production, then some other part of the heart may start off before it (as in extra-systole or escaped ventricular beats); or if the stimulus for contraction fails to reach all portions of the heart, then such portions may themselves start to beat independently of the sino-auricular node, as in complete heart-block.

As we have seen, in the study of extra-systoles, that abnormal beats may arise independently of the sino-auricular node, producing extra-systoles of auricular, ventricular, and nodal origin, so we get continuous rhythms of a similar origin. Up to recent times it was impossible to recognize the nature of a great many forms of abnormal action of the heart. With newer methods and a fuller knowledge of the physiology of the heart, we are able to recognize a considerable number of these abnormal actions, although there still remain many kinds which we cannot yet appreciate.

Result of onset or offset of an abnormal rhythm.—Before entering on the description of some of the more common of the abnormal continuous rhythms, it may be convenient to draw attention to some of their features, which have very important and practical bearing on their clinical aspect.

When one rhythm of the heart takes precedence of another, if the succeeding rhythm is a slower one, there is a pause of varying duration before the new rhythm starts. If, for instance, a tracing of an attack of paroxysmal tachycardia be taken at the time the attack ceases, one or two normal beats will be slower than the normal rhythm which goes on (Fig. 116 and 117). In affections of the auriculo-ventricular bundle, at one period there is merely a delay in the passage of stimulus from auricle to ventricle; at a further stage, the ventricle may occasionally not respond to the auricular contractions, and at a later stage the ventricle may respond only to every two, four, or eight auricular contractions. Usually there comes a stage when the auricular stimulus fails to reach the ventricle, and the ventricle takes on its own infrequent rhythm. Immediately the auricular stimulus fails to reach the ventricle, it stands still, and ceases to contract for periods of varying lengths. It is at this stage that attacks of loss of consciousness and epileptiform convulsions are particularly apt to occur (see Fig. 168).

When an abnormal rhythm arises in the ventricle in complete heart-block, the cessation of the abnormal rhythm is also followed by a pause before the idio-ventricular rhythm is again taken up (see Case 80).

The bearing of abnormal rhythms on the efficiency of the heart and their reaction to stimuli and drugs.—Although abnormal rhythms are here dealt with as separate conditions, it must be borne in mind that they are always the outcome of a myocardial lesion, and that the future of the patient depends on the nature and extent of the lesion, and whether the heart can carry on an efficient circulation hampered by the abnormal rhythm. Moreover, this abnormal rhythm reacts to stimuli different from the reaction of a normal heart. Thus excitation, which calls for a greater activity, may be met in a different manner according to the nature of the abnormal rhythm, so that we get varied results in people with auricular fibrillation, auricular flutter, and heart-block. Not only may the heart affected by an abnormal rhythm respond in a different manner from the normal-acting heart, but so varied are the individual peculiarities that we get a great many peculiar responses. The effect of remedies on a heart affected with abnormal rhythms, is different from that on the normal-acting heart, as seen in the action of digitalis in auricular fibrillation, which again differs from the action of digitalis in auricular flutter, while the insensibility of the ventricle in heart-block to all forms of cardiac stimulation is a peculiar and marked feature.

CHAPTER XXX

AURICULAR FIBRILLATION

The importance of recognizing auricular fibrillation.

Type of case showing auricular fibrillation.

Personal experiences in the recognition of auricular fibrillation.

What is auricular fibrillation ?

Conditions inducing auricular fibrillation.

Duration of auricular fibrillation.

Effect on the ventricles.

    Rate.

    Rhythm.

The size of the heart.

The jugular pulse in auricular fibrillation.

Fibrillation waves.

The electrocardiogram in auricular fibrillation.

Changes in the heart's murmurs.

Auricular fibrillation and digitalis.

Effect on the heart's efficiency.

Causes of heart failure in auricular fibrillation.

Clinical characteristics.

    The patient's history.

    The patient's sensations.

    Character of the pulse.

Symptoms of heart failure.

Auricular fibrillation and angina pectoris.

Prognosis.

Treatment.

    General.

    The use of digitalis.

    Method of administration.

    Danger in the administration of digitalis.

The importance of recognizing auricular fibrillation.—The most important of the continuous abnormal rhythms is that which is due to fibrillation of the auricles. The recognition of this condition and the symptoms associated with its presence, is the most important discovery yet made in the domain of the functional pathology of the heart; and few physicians are aware of its significance. The symptoms directly due to auricular fibrillation, and the symptoms of heart failure induced by this condition, are so clear and definite, that we have little difficulty in recognizing this condition as a distinct clinical entity. Its recognition is not of mere academical importance, but is of the greatest practical value; for when we recognize the

P 2

various symptoms, they afford us grounds for a sure diagnosis, a safe prognosis, and for a rational line of therapy in a large proportion of cases of serious
heart failure. The great frequency of its occurrence renders it imperative
that all practitioners should become familiar with its symptomatology; for
60 or 70 per cent. of all cases of serious heart failure met with in practice
owe the failure directly to this condition, or have the failure aggravated
by its presence. Some of the symptoms have been overlooked in the past,
while the significance of others has not been appreciated. Moreover, the
response of hearts affected with auricular fibrillation to remedies differs so
much from the response of all other forms of heart action, normal and
abnormal, that the recognition of its characteristics materially alters the
views universally held as to the action of drugs upon the heart.

Type of case showing auricular fibrillation.—Before setting out in
detail the features characteristic of auricular fibrillation, it might be convenient to appreciate the kind of case which shows this condition. The most
common evidence is an irregular action of the heart of a very disorderly
kind. It is that form of irregularity so frequently met with in the elderly,
and in patients with hearts damaged by previous rheumatic infection. In
the latter class, the association of irregular hearts with mitral stenosis has
long been recognized; and, on account of this association, the irregular pulse
is sometimes described as the ‘ mitral pulse ’, with which all clinicians are
familiar.

While senile and rheumatic hearts are those most frequently affected by
this condition, there are numerous cases in which auricular fibrillation occurs,
where there is no history of rheumatism, and at an age when senile changes
are not present in a marked degree. Auricular fibrillation is present in the
great majority of cases with dropsy, or dyspnœa due to heart failure, where
there is an irregular pulse. Thus, in Withering’s report of cases to whom
he administered digitalis successfully, published in 1784, where the symptoms
of heart failure were associated with an irregular pulse, and in whom digitalis
acted in a special manner, there can be but little doubt that these were
cases of auricular fibrillation. Other cases are found recorded as *delirium
cordis*. In those predisposed to auricular fibrillation, violent exertion may
induce the condition, and many of the recorded instances of *heart overstrain*
afford excellent examples of auricular fibrillation, and of the heart failure
which accompanies it.

Personal experiences in the recognition of auricular fibrillation.—
My attention was first directed to this condition as a separate and definite
entity about 1890. I had been endeavouring to discriminate between the
different forms of irregular heart action, and it occurred to me to employ the
jugular pulse as an aid. By this means I was able to separate the great
majority of irregularities into definite groups, according to the mechanism
of their production, as revealed by simultaneous records of the jugular and

radial pulses. There was one group which showed a distinct difference from all others, by the presence of the ventricular form of the venous pulse. I was at a loss to understand the nature of the heart's action in these cases ; and as I found them very frequently among people with a history of rheumatism, I determined to watch individual cases with rheumatic hearts, to see when this irregularity arose, and when the auricular venous pulse changed to the

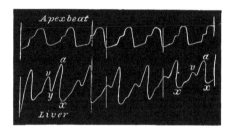

FIG. 119.   The liver pulse shows a well-marked wave (a) due to the auricle (Case 48.   1892).

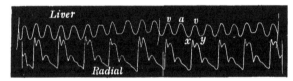

FIG. 120.   There is still a well-marked wave in the auricle (Case 48.   1897).

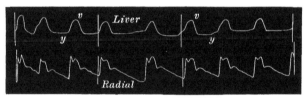

FIG. 121.   Showing the irregular rhythm, characteristic of auricular fibrillation. When compared with Fig. 119 and 120, it will be seen that there is no auricular wave in the liver pulse, and the heart's action is irregular (Case 48.   1898).

ventricular. The individual recorded as Case 48 came under my care in 1880, suffering from an attack of rheumatic fever. I examined her at intervals until her death in 1898. Up to 1897, her heart was regular, except for occasional ventricular extra-systoles. Her jugular and liver pulses were always of the auricular form (Fig. 119 and 120). There was a well-marked presystolic murmur. She became very ill in 1897, with a rapid and irregular heart. When the heart slowed down after a partial recovery, I found that the jugular and liver pulses were of the ventricular form (Fig. 121), that the presystolic murmur had disappeared, and that the heart was irregular ; in other words, all evidences of auricular activity had disappeared. From this date onwards, I was able to confirm these observations, and add to them other cases which showed waves due to the auricle, in jugular and apex tracings before the heart became irregular, and their disappearance when the heart became irregular. Thus, I established that all the positive evidences of auricular activity, capable of being revealed by clinical methods, showed the cessation of auricular action with the onset of this irregularity. For many years, I speculated as to the causes of auricular fibrillation. As the auricle was found distended and thin-walled at the post-mortem examination, I came to the conclusion that the disappearance of the signs of auricular systole was due to the auricle having become distended, atrophied, and paralysed. This view I put forward in a book on the pulse, which I published in 1902. Shortly after this was published, I had a series of cases, some of which I had watched for years, and at the post-mortem examinations the auricles were not thinned, but were hypertrophied. With this fact before me, I saw that my previous explanation could not be correct; for the fact that the auricles were hypertrophied, indicated that they must have contracted during the years that I had watched them, and when there had been an absence of all signs of auricular activity. As it was clear that the auricles could not have contracted during the normal period—that is to say, immediately before ventricular systole—the only alternative I could see was that they contracted during ventricular systole. As, in the meantime, I had studied several hundreds of cases and had seen this condition start under a variety of circumstances, particularly in individuals with frequent extrasystoles, I put forward the view that ventricles and auricles contracted together, and assumed that the stimulus for contraction arose in some place that affected auricles and ventricles simultaneously. As at this time I could not conceive of any other possibility to explain the facts, I suggested that the stimulus for contraction arose in the auriculo-ventricular node; and I called the condition ' nodal rhythm ', under which name the clinical aspects of auricular fibrillation are described in the two editions of this book, the first being published in 1908.

With the advent of the electrocardiograph, we obtained a more accurate method of recognizing the contractions of the chambers of the heart. When electrocardiograms were taken of the cases that I had called nodal rhythm, my clinical observations were verified, inasmuch as no evidence of the normal auricular systole was found. In cases where the heart periodically became disorderly in its rhythm, and where I was able to demonstrate that the auricular form of venous pulse was present with the regular heart action, and the ventricular form during the period of irregular action, the electrocardiograms also showed evidence of auricular contraction during the normal period of the heart's action, and a disappearance of the normal auricular activity during the period of irregular action, fully confirming the observations I had made on nodal rhythm.

The attention of other observers had also been arrested by some of the clinical features of this condition. Thus Hering, in 1903, separated from among other irregularities the irregularity peculiar to auricular fibrillation, and called it the *pulsus irregularis perpetuus*. He was mainly concerned with the physiological aspect of the subject, and did not recognize the full clinical picture, with the disappearance of all signs of auricular activity. Many other observers had noted the ' positive ' venous pulse, and in attributing it merely to tricuspid incompetence they had failed to appreciate its real meaning, and so missed the significance of its appearance.

Although the disappearance of the auricular contraction was the feature that puzzled me in these cases, I realized that my explanation of it, as being due to synchronous contraction of auricles and ventricles, was far from being established; and I endeavoured to interest others in the subject, who might investigate the matter by experimental methods, and find out, if possible, what the auricle was doing. Cushny was the first to suggest that auricular fibrillation might be a factor of clinical importance; and in 1906 he and Edmonds drew attention to the resemblance of the radial tracings in a case of paroxysmal irregularity in the human subject to the tracings from a dog, in which they produced experimental fibrillation of the auricles. Ou reading this communication, I was struck with the idea; and on a visit Professor Cushny paid to me in Burnley in 1906, he discussed with me the probability of auricular fibrillation being the cause of the irregular heart action in certain cases of ' nodal rhythm ', and he agreed that certain small waves, which I had recognized in the jugular pulse of one case (Fig. 122), were due to the fibrillation of the auricle.

I published, in 1907, tracings with this explanation, but I failed to appreciate the real significance of what auricular fibrillation was; I thought it only a passing event; and I practically gave up the idea that it was at the bottom of these cases that went on for years. Lewis had been pursuing an inquiry clinically and by experiment into the nature of cardiac irregularities, and had produced experimental fibrillation in the dog. In 1909 he took graphic records of the venous and arterial pulses. With the onset of fibrillation, he found that the arterial pulse became irregular, and the venous pulse changed from the auricular to the ventricular form. Pursuing his investigations further, Lewis was able to detect in the electrocardiogram of experimentally produced fibrillation, certain oscillations during ventricular diastole, which were induced by the fibrillating auricle. Examining more critically the electrocardiograms of typical cases of nodal rhythm which I sent to him, he found these oscillations also present, and demonstrated their correspondence with the small fibrillation waves I had noted in the jugular pulse.

When Lewis placed these facts before me, I had no hesitation in abandon-
ing my views, and accepting the fact that these cases owed their abnormal
action to auricular fibrillation ; and I now recognize that the reason those
evidences of auricular activity, to which I have referred, disappear, is because
the auricle ceases to act as a contracting chamber.

Rothberger and Winterberg had independently, in 1909, drawn attention
to the fact that in *pulsus irregularis perpetuus* the electrocardiogram corresponded to that of auricular fibrillation experimentally produced.

In the investigation which I have been carrying on for so many years,
I was not content merely to discover the mechanism by which the irregularities were produced, but I always kept before me the bearing these
symptoms had on the patient's present and future state, and what indications they gave for treatment. To this end, I made careful notes of all
attendant circumstances, such as the patient's history, the size of the heart,
the degree of heart failure, the response to treatment, and the future progress
of the case. The result is, that though I failed to recognize the nature of the
altered rhythm of the heart, yet from my notes of a great number of individual
patients, many of whom I had watched for a number of years, I had been
able to study many of the characteristics of this group and to recognize the
clinical features.

Up till 1908, these observations were carried on in my work as a general
practitioner. Since 1909 I have reviewed the whole subject, first at the
Mount Vernon Hospital, and then at the London Hospital, with the assistance of my colleagues, and we have verified the main features I had
previously recognized, and extended our observations. Although we can
recognize many salient features of the condition, there is still a great deal
of work to be done, before a full knowledge of the change in the heart's
action under this new rhythm can be acquired.

What is auricular fibrillation ?—The term ' fibrillation ' is applied
to a curious condition of the muscle fibres of the heart, where the individual
fibres, in place of contracting in an orderly and simultaneous manner during
systole, contract rapidly and independently of one another. The auricle,
when in a state of fibrillation, presents an entirely different aspect from
what it does during its normal action.

' The walls of the auricle stand in the diastolic position ; systole, either
complete or partial, is never accomplished ; the wall, as a whole, is stationary,
but careful examination of the muscle reveals an extremely active condition ;
it appears to be alive with movement ; rapid, minute, and constant twitchings or undulatory movements are observed in a multitude of small areas
upon its surface ' (Lewis).

When the ventricle passes into fibrillation, the circulation is at once
brought to a standstill ; and McWilliam has suggested that this is probably
the cause of sudden death in the human subject. When the auricles pass

into fibrillation, death does not ensue, for the fibrillation cannot pass along the bundle which connects auricle with ventricle.

Conditions inducing auricular fibrillation.—In experiment, auricular fibrillation can be produced by electrical stimulation of the auricular wall. In the human heart it is found to arise under a variety of conditions. It is probable that it is produced by altered nutrition of the muscle. Thus, I detected it in 1892 in a patient recovering from a mild attack of rheumatic fever, and there was no other evidence that the heart was affected. The attack passed off after some hours, and the youth has grown up into healthy manhood with no evident lesion of the heart. I have seen it appear in the heart in pneumonia, during the attack and during convalescence, with disastrous results in both cases. Digitalis can induce it in predisposed cases. I have known it occur intermittently in a fatal case of infective endocarditis, and Price has shown its occurrence in a fatal case of diphtheria, and G. A. Sutherland in a severe attack of rheumatic fever. Post-mortem examination in these cases showed that marked changes of an inflammatory nature had occurred in the walls of the auricle.

Effort, sometimes slight, and sometimes violent, may provoke auricular fibrillation. This occurs most frequently in the middle-aged or elderly, or in those with some old rheumatic affection. Thus, a healthy and vigorous member of our profession at the age of 50 years ran rapidly for 200 yards, and was seized with an attack which lasted for two hours. This was ten years ago, and he is still well and actively engaged in his work. In many cases, these attacks lasting for a short period are apt to recur with increasing frequency until they become permanent. While they are occurring intermittently, they are often easily provoked by effort, though they may not infrequently arise from no apparent cause. Thus, in one man under my care at the Mount Vernon Hospital, the heart would be detected beating irregularly several times a day, the irregular period lasting from half an hour to two hours. This irregularity was due to auricular fibrillation, as shown by records by the polygraph and electrocardiograph. He himself was not conscious of the altered rhythm, nor was there any recognizable cause for the onset.

We are not yet in a position to decide, with sufficient accuracy, the nature of the changes in the heart-wall which favour the occurrence of auricular fibrillation. In the hearts which I have had examined, which showed auricular fibrillation during life, there has been found in the auricle and ventricle, an increase of fibrous tissue and of nucleated cells in the muscular walls (see Cases 48, 49, and 51). In most cases, there is probably some definite change which predisposes to this condition, and it only needs an adequate stimulus to provoke it. This stimulus may be of a varied kind, for while the onset can frequently be traced to violent bodily effort, it often occurs when there is no excessive effort. At present, we can only say that one predisposing condition is certain organic changes in the muscle wall of the auricle.

Duration of auricular fibrillation.—In the majority of cases when auricular fibrillation sets in, it persists for the remainder of the individual's life. I have watched individual cases for over thirteen years, in whom it was constantly present (see Case 43). In many cases, it may appear for a few hours, and may never recur, or it may recur at infrequent intervals for some weeks and months, and then disappear. Many cases of paroxysmal tachycardia owe the paroxysms to auricular fibrillation, and in such cases it may last for a few seconds, a day or two, a few weeks, or even months (see Case 51). As a rule, however, when it is intermittent in its appearance, the tendency to its recurrence becomes greater, till finally it becomes permanently established.

Effect on the ventricles.—In fibrillation of the auricle, the stimulus for contraction arises no longer in the sino-auricular node, but in the fibrillating fibres of the auricle, and is transmitted to the auriculo-ventricular node in an irregular manner. It is probable that the manner in which the ventricle is affected, depends on the power of the node and bundle to receive and transmit the auricular stimulations; for I found that in some of my cases the ventricular rate varied very much, sometimes being rapid and sometimes slow (see Cases 44, 51, and 54). It might be suggested that with the onset of auricular fibrillation the ventricle takes on a rhythm of its own, and indeed at one stage of my investigations I had suggested an idio-ventricular rhythm. But, in experiment, if after fibrillation has been set up, the bundle is cut, the ventricular rate at once alters, and the ventricle assumes its own peculiar slow rhythm.

Rate.—Changes in the rate and rhythm of the ventricle, and in the size of the heart, are very common with the onset of auricular fibrillation. In several cases, I have detected these changes shortly after its inception. I have found the greatest difference in rate, ranging from 40 to 130 beats per minute. It is but seldom that we get the opportunity of seeing auricular fibrillation start, as the patient is frequently unconscious of the change in the heart's rhythm, though some recognize the curious sensation of fluttering. The patient may consult us because of the distress which may sooner or later appear, and then we usually find the rate remarkably increased, generally between 110 and 140 beats per minute and over. I have met with a number of cases, in which the rate has become slower on the inception of auricular fibrillation. When fibrillation has arisen as the result of the administration of digitalis, the rate has been infrequent (Case 92). If digitalis slows the heart in fibrillation through its action on the vagus and the auriculo-ventricular bundle, we might assume that the slowing occurs in consequence of some affection of the auriculo-ventricular bundle. In support of this view, I have observed a case for many years, in which there was persistent increase in the interval between the auricular and ventricular systoles, and in which at one time there was partial heart-block. When the patient's auricle started to fibrillate, the ventricular rate fell from 60 to 40 beats per minute, and has continued at this rate for nine years. Cases 80 and 81 show a slow pulse-rate, but in these there was present complete heart-block. In Case 79, the heart fell suddenly to 40 beats per minute and was quite regular ; the slow rate persisted for a fortnight, when it suddenly increased in rate and the auricle resumed its normal action. In this case, during its normal action, there were no evidences of heart-block.

Rhythm.—When the auricle passes into fibrillation, the ventricle usually becomes irregular in its action. The alteration is sudden, as shown not only by experiment but by clinical observations, in cases in which I have actually observed the change in the heart's action. The cessation of fibrillation can be recognized by the return to a regular rhythm ; occasionally the return is accompanied by a few irregular beats, due to extra-systoles. Though many speak of this condition as the *pulsus irregularis perpetuus*, I have seen a number of cases where the rhythm of the ventricle was regular (Fig. 61). In the majority of such cases, the rate was under fifty beats per minute. In several instances, the slow regular action has been induced by digitalis. In a case recently under observation, the rate under digitalis fell from 110 to 70 beats per minute. Prior to the administration of digitalis, the rhythm was very irregular, but when the rate fell to 70 beats per minute it was quite regular. The patient had no jugular pulse, but by the electro-cardiograph, Lewis demonstrated that auricular fibrillation was present.

The character of the irregularity as seen in the pulse is a completely disorderly one, in the sense that the interval between the beats is ever varying, two successive beats being seldom of the same length. Although, as a rule, there is a distinct relation between the size of the beats and the length of the preceding pause, the longer pauses being followed by bigger beats, not infrequently this is not so, big beats sometimes following very short pauses.

Many other conditions produce continuous irregularities, so that we have to be careful not to form our opinion on the irregularity by itself.

The size of the heart.—In the great majority of cases, a considerable enlargement of the heart follows the inception of auricular fibrillation. Though the auricles are often greatly distended, it is not possible to tell from clinical examination, how much of this enlargement is due to the auricles, and how much to the ventricles.

With the onset of fibrillation, the increase in size does not take place at once, though, in a few cases of periodic fibrillation, I have seen the heart increase greatly in size within a few hours of the onset, and the enlargement would disappear within a few hours after the cessation of the fibrillation. As a rule, little change in the size of the heart takes place at first, and if the heart is capable of maintaining an efficient circulation little increase in size may be detected for years. In the majority there is an inability to do the work efficiently, so that gradually the heart's strength becomes exhausted, and an increase in its size follows. With appropriate treatment, a considerable diminution may take place, but this is by no means constant. I have been surprised at its persistence in cases of old-standing auricular fibrillation, in whom a very striking improvement of the heart's condition has taken place as the result of treatment. In most of the cases we have carefully studied at the Mount Vernon Hospital, and at the London Hospital, we have failed to detect any decrease in the size of the heart, in patients who had suffered from extreme failure, and who had made a surprising recovery.

The jugular pulse in auricular fibrillation.—The size of the jugular pulse is extremely variable, in different cases, and in some individuals at different times. This is in a great measure due to the amount of distension of the right side of the heart and of the great veins, and also to the rate of the heart. In some slow-acting hearts, great waves can be seen extending up the neck with each contraction of the ventricle, and there is no difficulty in recognizing their nature (Fig. 59 and 60). In other hearts beating at more rapid rates, these waves are also evident ; one cannot be always sure of their nature from inspection alone, but a tracing will show them to be of ventricular form. When the veins are less full, and the rate frequent, it is utterly impossible to differentiate the waves that may appear in the veins. Even in a graphic record some difficulty may be met with, but if the time of the waves be accurately placed in the cardiac cycle in the manner already described (p. 155), as a rule the features of the tracing can be recognized. In many cases, the character of the ventricular waves shows a curious difference. Thus some slow beats will show a high wave at the same time as the carotid pulse (marked c in the tracings), and a great fall during the mid-systole of the ventricle, with a wave towards the end of systole, which ends as usual with the opening of the tricuspid valves (perpendicular line 6). With the more rapid beats the fall during mid-systole disappears, the characteristic wave of the ventricular venous pulse is shown. The fall is due to the dragging down of the auriculo-ventricular septum during ventricular systole.

Fibrillation waves.—There is an additional feature, which is also of value in recognizing the presence of auricular fibrillation, and that is the presence of the small waves caused in some way by the fibrillating auricle. They are not present in every case, nor always perceptible in those cases that show them. When present, they are most evident during those long pauses of the ventricle which are so frequent in auricular fibrillation. These fibrillation waves are of a variable size, sometimes very minute, as in Fig. 122, and sometimes very coarse, as in Fig. 123. In Fig. 124, they will be found to vary in size and duration at different times.

The electrocardiogram in auricular fibrillation.—While the normal electrocardiogram shows features similar to those in Fig. 16, a great number of differences can be obtained, each due to some abnormal action of the heart. So far as the electrocardiogram of auricular fibrillation is concerned, in addition to the irregular action of the ventricles, the records show some very characteristic signs, the chief being a total disappearance

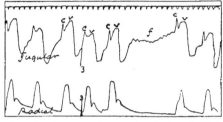

Fig. 122. A tracing from a patient with auricular fibrillation, showing small fibrillary waves (*f*) in the jugular tracing (Case 44).

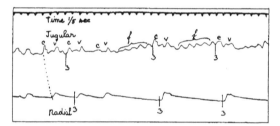

Fig. 123. The jugular tracing shows coarser fibrillary waves (*f*).

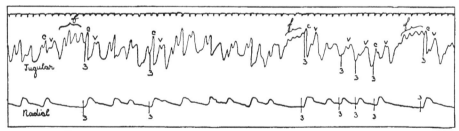

Fig. 124. The jugular tracing shows fibrillary waves (*f*) of different sizes.

of the peak, P, due to the auricle (Fig. 20). The variations R and T, due to the ventricle, maintain their characteristic form. Between the ventricular beats, the records may show a series of small movements, which we now recognize as being due to the fibrillating muscle of the auricular wall. This absence of the auricular movements and the presence of the movements during ventricular diastole are the means, by which auricular fibrillation can be recognized in the electrocardiographic record. Further, there is also the characteristic disorderly rhythm.

Dr. Lewis tells me, that the small movements shown in the electrocardiogram are not constant, but in every given case they come and go for no apparent reason. In this they differ from the movements in auricular flutter, which are constant. There appears to be some relation between these movements and the fibrillation waves found in the jugular tracing, and as these come and go, in an unaccountable way, it is probable that they are both due to the same factor.

Changes in the heart's murmurs.—I have already dealt with the evidences of auricular activity, obtained by graphic and electrocardiographic methods. The evidence of auricular activity obtained in the clinical examination, apart from the graphic records of the jugular pulse, is limited to the murmurs of mitral stenosis. We must bear in mind that stenosis of the mitral valve is a gradual process, at first not recognizable until a certain degree of narrowing has arisen. This narrowing obstructs the flow of blood from auricle to ventricle, and gives rise to a murmur on the contraction of the auricle. A presystolic murmur is evidence of a contracting auricle, and is usually an indication not only of an obstruction to the flow of blood from auricle to ventricle, but also of gradually progressing fibrotic changes in the valves and around the mitral orifice. With progressive narrowing, the presystolic murmur becomes louder and longer, while a new murmur may appear after the second sound. This diastolic murmur is due to the obstruction of the flow of blood through the mitral orifice at the end of ventricular systole. It is faint and short at first, but with further narrowing of the mitral orifice it increases, till it fills up a great portion of the diastolic period of the cardiac revolution, and may run up to the presystolic murmur. When this happens, the diastolic period is filled up entirely by murmurs. We may take it that the appearance of this diastolic mitral murmur is always an evidence, that the progressive narrowing of the mitral orifice has reached an advanced stage. But the fibrotic changes that cause mitral stenosis are not limited to the valvular orifices, but are also present in the muscular walls of the heart. These changes in the auricular wall predispose to auricular fibrillation, and this may arise at different stages. With the onset of fibrillation, a change takes place in the character of the murmurs.

If a presystolic murmur, due to the auricular systole, was present prior to the onset of the fibrillation, it at once disappears when the pulse becomes irregular. If a diastolic murmur, due to mitral stenosis, has been present, it persists, because it is caused, not by the systole of the auricle, but by the inrush of blood from the auricle into the ventricle when the ventricle relaxes after its systole. I wish to emphasize this change in the character of the murmurs in mitral stenosis with auricular fibrillation, for even those who detect the clinical symptoms of auricular fibrillation do not seem to have grasped the significance of the change in the murmurs. I have carefully studied a large number of cases of mitral stenosis with fibrillation, and many of them have come to an autopsy, and in none of them have I detected a presystolic murmur of the crescendo type. Where a murmur has preceded the first sound, it has filled the whole diastole when the rate was rapid. When the heart's rate is rapid in auricular fibrillation, this diastolic murmur often fills up the whole space between the second and first sounds, and it may simulate, and is often taken for, a presystolic murmur due to the systole of the auricle. If, however, this murmur be noticed during one of the long pauses, which occur frequently in most cases, or when the heart's rate

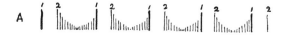

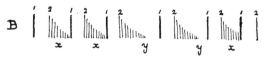

FIG. 125. Diagram illustrating the change in the murmurs in mitral stenosis when auricular fibrillation occurs. The perpendicular lines 1 and 2 represent the first and second sounds of the heart, and the shading between the second and first sounds represents the diastolic and presystolic murmurs with a regular rhythm (A). In B auricular fibrillation causes the rhythm to be irregular, and when the diastolic period is short as at x, x, x, the diastolic murmur fills up the whole interval. When, however, the diastolic period is lengthened as at y, y, the diastolic murmur does not fill up the whole period, and there is then a silence before the first sound when the presystolic murmur was heard before fibrillation set in.

becomes slow, it will be found that this murmur follows the second sound, but pauses some little distance before the first sound, and there is a silence immediately before the first sound in the place where the crescendo presystolic murmur due to the auricle should appear.

This is brought out in the diagram in Fig. 125, where A and B represent the sounds and murmurs in mitral stenosis before and after auricular fibrillation. In B it will be seen that there is no presystolic crescendo murmur, and that the diastolic murmur fills up the whole of the space between the second and first heart sounds, when the interval is short (x, x); but when the interval is long (y, y) the diastolic murmur does not reach the first sound, and there is a silence before it.

From these considerations, we can, in the great majority of cases, conclude that auricular fibrillation is present when there is a diastolic mitral murmur without a presystolic murmur. As a rule, the irregular action of the heart is also suggestive, but in many cases of mitral stenosis with auricular fibrillation, when the patient is under digitalis, the heart becomes slow and almost, or even quite, regular.

The explanation given here occurred to me in 1897, as an outcome of the study of the features of Case 48. Since that time I have continued the observations and verified it repeatedly ; but I have found the greatest difficulty in convincing physicians of the clinical facts. The murmur filling up the interval between the second and first sound is invariably looked upon as presystolic, while the long diastolic murmur present when the heart is slow (see Fig. 192), is not infrequently taken to be aortic ; on sundry occasions I have heard physicians express surprise that at the post-mortem examination there has been no aortic lesion, but mitral stenosis in cases with the long diastolic murmur. Quite recently Dr. Lewis has taken records, by means of the electro-phonograph, of cases of auricular fibrillation, and his results have confirmed the explanation given above.

Auricular fibrillation and digitalis.—Not the least in importance of the discoveries resulting from the recognition of auricular fibrillation as a clinical entity, is the light that is thrown upon the action of drugs of the digitalis group. I can only here refer, briefly, to a few points which I have been able to elucidate. I think every one who has carefully studied the description usually given of the effects of digitalis on the human heart, cannot but be struck with the absence of agreement among the different writers, as to the manner of its action, its dosage, and the best preparation. In some instances, some peculiar reaction which the observer may have noted is looked upon as the characteristic effect of digitalis, but the mechanism of this peculiar reaction has not been understood. It is a good many years since I was struck with the varied reactions, which I obtained from the use of digitalis. I collected a great number of cases ; in some I got a definite reaction on the heart, while in others no reaction was obtained. When I separated these into groups, I saw that the probable reasons for the varied reactions in the human heart were, that digitalis gives a reaction according to the nature of the lesions from which the heart is suffering. It will be observed that if this is found to be correct, we can at once understand how the physiologist and experimental pharmacologist have missed the most important effects of digitalis, for, so far as the heart in experimental work is concerned, they cannot reproduce the conditions under which the physician has to employ the drug.

It is not only in auricular fibrillation that digitalis acts beneficially, for there are many other conditions which benefit by it ; but cases of fibrillation stand apart from all others in regard to their response to this drug. All cases of auricular fibrillation are not responsive ; for there are factors which render certain hearts unsusceptible, as the presence of fever or extensive fibrous degeneration. It is in certain cases, where there is a fair amount of healthy muscle that its almost specific action is seen. It is some ten years, since I realized this peculiar response to digitalis. When I was appointed to the Mount Vernon Hospital and London Hospital, I seized the opportunity to start a series of observations under conditions, which permitted a degree of accuracy unattainable in private practice. In these observations, the same drug and the same dose were given to patients with and without auricular fibrillation. With only rare exceptions, all the cases that showed a marked effect upon the heart were cases of auricular fibrillation; for, although the other cases might exhibit some benefit from the use of the drug, they never showed the same tendency to slowing of the heart's rate.

The slowing effects of digitalis are shown in a very striking manner in those cases of auricular fibrillation, where heart failure set in with a great increase of rate of the heart. The chart (Fig. 126) is a good illustration of these types. The patient from whom the chart was obtained, suffered from extreme heart failure, and the rate of the heart was 140 per minute and very irregular. She was given 1 drachm of digitalis per day, and after five days the pulse-rate fell in the manner shown in the chart. At the same time, there was a remarkable improvement in the patient's general condition.

The difference in the reaction of hearts affected with auricular fibrillation and those with the normal rhythm is well brought out by the chart in Fig. 127, where the average heart-rate from six cases of mitral stenosis with auricular fibrillation is compared with six cases of mitral stenosis with the normal rhythm. The record begins with the rate on the day previous to administration of the drug; and it will be seen that the rate in the cases with auricular fibrillation is greater than the rate in cases with the normal rhythm. This, I may remark in passing, is a point of some interest; for cases of heart failure with mitral stenosis with the normal rhythm, rarely, have as rapid a pulse as those with mitral stenosis with auricular fibrillation.

In each case the tincture of digitalis was given, 1 drachm per day, and was continued till nausea or vomiting ensued.

Digitalis in some hearts induces auricular fibrillation. When this occurs, the rate of the ventricle becomes greatly decreased (see Case 92).

Effect on the heart's efficiency.—A great many patients in whom auricular fibrillation had occurred, suffered from lesions of the heart, which impaired its efficiency. In all these, the occurrence of fibrillation at once increased the impairment, and the symptoms of heart failure became intensified. In others, where there had only been a slight impairment of the cardiac efficiency, the onset of auricular fibrillation speedily provoked symptoms of extreme heart failure, while in others little difference could be detected. In a few cases, the onset of auricular fibrillation has only slightly embarrassed the heart in its work.

To a great extent the symptoms of heart failure arise most markedly in those in whom the change in the auricular action has affected the ventricle, particularly in increasing its rate. In a few cases, marked limitation of the heart's powers of response to effort has followed, with relatively slow acting hearts.

The symptoms of heart failure commonly produced are of the same kind as arise in heart failure from other causes; for example, shortness of breath

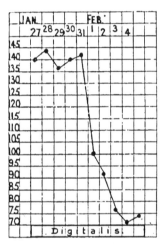

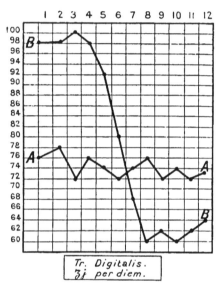

FIG. 126. Chart showing a typical reaction of digitalis in a case of auricular fibrillation with severe heart failure. The administration of the tincture of digitalis began on January 27, in doses of 15 minims four times daily.

FIG. 127. Chart showing the effects of similar doses of tincture of digitalis on six cases of mitral stenosis with the normal rhythm (A) and six cases of mitral stenosis with auricular fibrillation (B). The figures at the side represent heart-beats; those at the top, days. In each case the digitalis was continued till the heart became slowed, or until nausea or vomiting occurred. The average quantity before an effect was produced was 7 drachms (1 drachm per diem). This had little or no effect on the heart-rate in the patients with the normal rhythm (A), while there was a rapid decrease in the rate in the patients with auricular fibrillation (B).

on exertion and consciousness of the heart's action, particularly when some effort is made. With increase in the failure, œdema of the legs and lungs sets in. The face becomes livid, the patient cannot lie flat in bed, but has to be propped up. The liver becomes enlarged, while the veins in the neck may become engorged, and the pulsation in them becomes extremely marked. With these changes, dilatation of the heart and great increase in the rate may be detected. As a rule, the onset of these symptoms is slow and gradual, but occasionally they may set in with great rapidity ; they quickly disappear if the heart reverts to its normal rhythm.

Cause of heart-failure in auricular fibrillation.—However it may be brought about, the onset of fibrillation embarrasses the ventricle in its work, and in all probability the degree of heart insufficiency that results depends upon the extent of concomitant damage of the ventricles, and the amount of embarrassment caused by any valve lesion that may be present. There can be little doubt that the orderly action of the auricle in regulating the supply of blood to the ventricle, and in stimulating it in a normal manner, results in a more efficient action of the ventricle than the variable and irregular stimulation to contraction. When the ventricle is rapidly and irregularly stimulated to contraction, there results a gradual exhaustion of the strength of the ventricle, and evidences of heart failure supervene. In cases that have drifted and died, where I have had a post-mortem examination, there has been found extensive fibrous degeneration of the heart muscle (Cases 49 and 51). On the other hand, I have seen so many individuals with auricular fibrillation who have led strenuous lives, engaged in hard manual labour, that I infer that in them the muscle of the ventricle had not been seriously damaged (Case 44).

Clinical characteristics. *The patient's history.*—The conditions which induce auricular fibrillation vary ; but there are two classes among whom it is very frequent—namely, patients with a heart affection following upon rheumatic fever (frequently associated with mitral stenosis), and elderly patients with fibrous degenerative changes, usually spoken of as ' senile '. It may be found in the young and middle-aged, with no history of infection. It is customary in rheumatic hearts to take into account only the valvular changes, while as a matter of fact the really serious element is the slow, insidious change in the muscle that has started during the attack of rheumatic fever, and which finally provokes fibrillation of the auricle.

The patient's sensations.—Many people become conscious of the heart's action when it departs from its normal rhythm. Thus, extra-systoles are sometimes recognized by the individual's consciousness of the long pause, or of the big beat which follows the pause. The patients liable to paroxysmal tachycardia, are conscious of the attack by the feeling of a gentle fluttering sensation in the chest. When the attacks of tachycardia are due to auricular fibrillation, this fluttering is also present ; but usually it is not a continuous fluttering sensation, but is interrupted by thumping sensations, due to the occasional occurrence of bigger beats. This consciousness of the heart's action is frequent in cases of auricular fibrillation, the patients being conscious of the fluttering and irregular action of the heart. In many cases, where the heart does its work efficiently, these sensations are not perceived, unless the heart is submitted to over-exertion, or when it begins to fail.

Character of the pulse.—The symptom by which the clinical observer can most readily recognize this condition, is by the character of the pulse, the rhythm usually being irregular, and the irregularity of a very disorderly kind. Irregularities, apart from those due to auricular fibrillation, usually have a distinctive character, as the irregularity in the heart of the young, where variations in rate coincide with phases of respiration, as the intermittent pulse, or the irregular heart due to extra-systoles, the irregularity breaking in on an otherwise regular rhythm, unless it occurs alternating with a normal pulse-beat. In auricular fibrillation, as a rule, the pauses between the beats are continuously changing, and two succeeding beats are rarely of the same strength, or the pauses between the beats of the same duration. The character of the irregularities will be better recognized from the radial tracings, as shown in Fig. 59, 60, 64, 122, 123, and 124.

Symptoms of heart failure.—The sign which usually calls attention to auricular fibrillation is the patient's consciousness of his limitation. The signs of this limitation, however, are not peculiar to or characteristic of auricular fibrillation, but are common to heart failure induced by other conditions. These signs of heart failure may range from a slight breathlessness on exertion, to dyspnœa of the most severe kind, accompanied by dropsy, enlarged liver, and the symptoms associated with extreme heart failure.

As a rule, the onset of symptoms of heart failure is slow and gradual, due in a measure to the individual's persisting in living in his usual manner, though the heart is hampered by the abnormal action. On the other hand, the onset of heart failure may be very rapid. Within a few hours of the occurrence of auricular fibrillation, the distress of the patient may be very severe, the countenance dusky, the heart dilated, orthopnœa, and a feeling of distress is experienced. I have seen these phenomena arise rapidly in cases, where the fibrillation occurred intermittently, and the relief experienced by the patient, when the heart resumed the normal rhythm, was as remarkable and striking as the onset of the suffering. At once the patient knows that the heart's action has altered, and he breathes easier, and the feeling of distress disappears. Within a few hours, the heart and liver have become reduced in size, the lividity of the face has gone, and the tenderness of the chest-wall and over the region of the liver speedily disappears.

In many cases, the persistence of heart failure is accompanied by wasting, the patient sometimes losing a good deal of weight in a few months. Accompanying this, there is usually a certain amount of flushing of the cheeks, usually of a dusky colour, and occasionally a slight sallow tinge of jaundice. These symptoms with an enlarged liver may be mistaken for sarcoma of the liver.

Auricular fibrillation and angina pectoris.—Amongst the more common signs of heart failure, there is one which I have but rarely seen— namely, definite attacks of angina pectoris. As I have already stated, pain and hyperalgesia are not uncommon in the heart failure associated with auricular fibrillation, while I have met with typical attacks of angina pectoris in only a few cases. In quite a number of cases where the patient had angina pectoris, the attacks ceased with the onset of the fibrillation. Needless to say, the onset of auricular fibrillation in those cases induced such embarrassment to the heart's action, that the patients all drifted, and only lived a few months after its onset. The onset of fibrillation may be associated with angina pectoris (Case 50).

Prognosis.—We must bear in mind that auricular fibrillation is in reality a symptom of some myocardial change, and that, to be logical, we should only consider it from the point of view of a myocardial affection. We are at present so ignorant of myocardial disease, that we are forced to put one symptom forward as if it were in itself a disease. Illogical as this seems, it has its use, for the occurrence of auricular fibrillation induces such a profound change in the heart's action, affecting its efficiency, reacting on the ventricle, and modifying its behaviour to drugs, that we are compelled to look upon it as a condition apart. Considering the variety of conditions that induce auricular fibrillation, it is difficult to state briefly its prognostic significance. In referring to the pathological lesions associated with it, I showed that they were of a very diverse kind in nature and in degree. It is in all probability the extent of these pathological changes which determines the prognosis of auricular fibrillation, and an attempt should be made to estimate their extent. If we look upon the inception of the new rhythm as in itself embarrassing the heart in its work, then the maintenance of an efficient circulation depends on whether the heart is able to do its work, when hampered by the new rhythm. That this is the fundamental question will be recognized, when we study the effect of fibrillation in certain individuals. I have repeatedly seen individuals in whom fibrillation occurred for a short time, and in whom heart failure set in with an extraordinary rapidity, the patient becoming breathless, having to sit up in bed, the face becoming livid, the heart dilated, and the liver swelling, within a few hours after the onset of fibrillation. With the restoration of the normal rhythm, these symptoms quickly disappeared. When fibrillation became permanent in such individuals, the signs of heart failure persisted sometimes in spite of all treatment, till death supervened in a few weeks or a few months (Cases 51, 52, and 53).

On the other hand, I have repeatedly seen fibrillation set in, and the individual be altogether unconscious of its presence. These cases may go on for years with little inconvenience ; but the majority after some years gradually show signs of a limitation of the field of cardiac response, and their future depends upon how they respond to treatment, and on their ability to diminish the amount of their bodily work, and to live within the limits of the heart's strength (Cases 43, 44, and 45).

Much more frequently there is a considerable limitation of the heart's power of response to effort ; and if the usual life of the individual be pursued, without appropriate treatment, there is a great tendency for the heart gradually to fail. There is no doubt that the onset of fibrillation can lead directly to a fatal termination, or, rather, can be associated with conditions that lead to death. Thus, one of my patients died suddenly a few days after the inception of auricular fibrillation. Another one fell down dead six months after its inception. I have seen a number of other patients die suddenly, who had auricular fibrillation, but some of these suffered from a considerable degree of heart failure. It has appeared to me probable that in these cases the ventricle has passed into fibrillation, as McWilliam suggested. This view is probable also from the fact, that the histological changes in the ventricle were similar to those in the auricle in some of the cases of sudden death.

The usual mode of death in auricular fibrillation is a steady advance of the heart failure, as shown by the breathlessness on exertion, orthopnœa, dropsy, and enlargement of the liver, &c., sometimes with an absolute failure of response to all forms of treatment. Thus, I have seen death ensue in this manner a few weeks after the inception of fibrillation (Case 52), and others have drifted on for a few months (Case 50 and 51), while some have led a somewhat chequered career for a number of years, seldom fit for much bodily exercise.

In giving a prognosis in cases of auricular fibrillation, it is necessary to appreciate a good many other things, besides the mere presence of the fibrillation. It is necessary to form an opinion of the extent of the changes that have led up to the fibrillation, and in many cases to find out how long these changes have been going on ; as, for instance, the date of an attack of rheumatic fever ; and how the patient comported himself before the onset of fibrillation ; if, for instance, he was liable to attacks of heart failure, in which case such attacks point to a tendency to exhaustion which may be aggravated by the fibrillation. Amongst valvular lesions, cases with affections of the aortic valve are usually seriously embarrassed, particularly in aortic regurgitation, when, prior to the onset of fibrillation, there had been evidences of failure. The character of the murmurs present in mitral stenosis will shed light upon the progress of the disease as already described. When auricular fibrillation sets in, it is necessary to observe the accompanying changes in the heart, and the way in which it maintains the circulation. Thus, an increase in the size of the heart, or a rate over 120 beats per minute, usually leads to a speedy exhaustion of the heart's strength. I have occasionally met with an individual with a heart-rate of 100 and 120 per minute, with no increase in the size of the heart, who suffered little inconvenience ; but as a rule any rate over 90 beats per minute tends to induce dilatation and consequent exhaustion. On the other hand, when there is little increase in rate, or even when the rate is somewhat slower than normal and the response to effort good, the prognosis is usually very favourable.

In those with symptoms of manifest heart failure, prognosis depends to a great extent on the way in which they respond to treatment. I have already described the action of drugs of the digitalis group in patients with fibrillation, and I will show later, more fully, the action of other drugs in these cases, and the response of the heart to them, and what an important bearing it has upon prognosis.

I have already said that there are a great many individuals with fibrillation who lead useful and energetic lives, and whose capacity for work is little, if at all, impaired by the new rhythm. In such the prognosis is distinctly good.

There are, however, so many exceptions to these details, that a clearer insight may be gained, by looking at each case from a broader standpoint, of how the heart responds to effort, not, however, ignoring the details, but giving them their due consideration. It is in estimating this reserve power that we get the most valuable information. It may be taken for granted that if distress is induced by exertion, so long as the exertion is persisted in, it will ultimately lead to serious heart failure. On the other hand, when individuals with fibrillation are able to undertake the work equal to that done by a perfectly healthy man, there is proof of such a degree of healthy heart muscle and freedom from valvular or muscular embarrassment, that a good prognosis can be given.

We meet, however, with such varying degrees of exhaustion, that an estimate must be acquired of the amount, though it is impossible to describe with accuracy what that amount may be. Even with distinct limitation of the heart's power, as shown by the response to effort, the prognosis may still be favourable, so long as the patient lives within the limits of his powers, avoiding such efforts as cause him distress or exhaustion.

In transient attacks of auricular fibrillation, the attacks usually tend to become more frequent, until auricular fibrillation becomes permanently established. The prognosis of such cases depends on the way the circulation is maintained, this to be estimated in the manner already described. Transient attacks may appear for a short period and then disappear entirely. In two of my cases, I detected a transient attack of auricular fibrillation twenty years ago, and the patients still lead vigorous and active lives. From the recognition of such cases, we can conclude that auricular fibrillation is not of necessity a sign of extreme damage.

A most valuable aid in prognosis may be found in observing how the patient responds to treatment. In sudden attacks of severe heart failure, when the heart's rate is over 120 per minute, it will be well to suspend judgement, until the reaction to digitalis is found out. Many such cases respond speedily to digitalis, and with the resultant decrease in the heart's rate a remarkable degree of recovery may ensue, so that the patients may be able to undertake laborious work, so long as the rate is kept down by the digitalis. This would seem to imply that the exhaustion is mainly brought about by the ventricle being stimulated to too great an activity, and that the slowing enables the ventricle to get more rest, and so regain a measure of strength. From this result, we can also gather that the ventricular muscle must be fairly healthy, and we can estimate, within certain limits, the amount of healthy muscle by the degree of recovery.

Treatment. *General.*—When any individual with heart failure presents himself for treatment, it may be taken for granted that the individual has been undergoing a greater amount of exertion than the heart has been capable of performing without undue exhaustion. Hence the exhaustion of the heart's strength has been brought about in the first place by overwork. It may be that the amount of work has been small, as measured by what a healthy heart can perform, but when a heart is hampered by an inherent defect, such as auricular fibrillation, and the organic changes in the valves and muscle so commonly associated with this condition, the heart may be capable of a very limited amount of effort. With this conception of the cause of heart failure, the first and obvious course to pursue is to ease the heart of its work. In doing this much discrimination is required, and a thorough inquiry into the patient's mode of life has to be made in order to find out what circumstances, such as overwork, sleeplessnees, digestive trouble, pain or work, may have provoked or aggravated the heart failure. These have to be attended to in every case, and relief may be at once afforded with the removal of the disturbing or exhausting cause.

The use of digitalis.—While it is important to attend to such circumstances in heart failure with auricular fibrillation, as in all other forms, there are circumstances in cases of heart failure with fibrillation which when appreciated help greatly, not only in the restoration of the heart's strength, but in the prevention of heart failure. I have already dealt with the reaction of hearts affected with auricular fibrillation to digitalis from a physiological standpoint; it is in treatment of auricular fibrillation that we find the great value of this drug, and I cannot speak too highly of its therapeutic action.

It is seldom that I have been able to say that I have saved a patient from immediate peril by the use of drugs; but this I can say with confidence, that I have repeatedly seen patients in evident peril of death removed rapidly from danger, and restored to a condition of comparative health, and fit for work by the judicious use of digitalis. The manner of its application needs, however, very careful attention, for it is a drug that needs to be applied on certain definite lines, if full benefit is to be obtained from its action. I think it necessary to insist upon this point, for the somewhat 'rule-of-thumb' methods of its use, so generally employed, fail to get the full amount of benefit which this drug is capable of bestowing.

To understand the action of digitalis, it is necessary to appreciate the manner in which heart failure progresses in cases of auricular fibrillation, and the way it is controlled by digitalis. It may be taken for granted that when a patient with auricular fibrillation has a pulse-rate, or, to be more accurate, a ventricular rate, of 90 beats per minute and over, he will in course of time gradually lose strength, his heart will become more feeble, and the evidences of heart failure will become more severe. This process may be very gradual, but it is very sure. On the other hand, heart failure may set in rapidly, more especially when the heart's rate rises to 120 and 140 and over. The severity of the failure, however it is brought about, compels the patient to seek rest, and we generally find such patients in bed, sitting up and breathing in a laboured fashion, with considerable distress, the heart usually dilated and the face of a bluish tinge, and possibly with dropsy and pulsation of the liver. In all such cases the prompt administration of digitalis is urgently called for, and, if given in sufficient doses, relief may be obtained in a few days, the relief being accompanied by a remarkable slowing of the pulse-rate. When this is accomplished, or when there are other signs of a sufficiency, the digitalis should be stopped for a few days, and resumed in small doses when the rate begins to increase. The rate of the pulse should be watched, and the quantity sought for which keeps the heart about 70 beats per minute. It is seldom advisable to keep the rate under 50 beats per minute, although in some cases the patient feels fittest when it is at a rate of about 50 beats per minute. In this, we must be guided by the patient's sensations, and the manner in which he responds to effort.

Even when patients suffer from only a moderate degree of heart failure, and are able to go about, it is well to place them under the influence of this drug if the pulse-rate is over 90 beats per minute, and in some cases if it is over 80 per minute. My usual procedure in such cases is to attend to any circumstance that may aggravate the heart failure, and then to give the patient digitalis until the pulse-rate is reduced. If the failure is of some severity, I put him to bed until the proper effect is obtained, but where it is less in degree I permit him to go about his affairs.

In all cases where the heart has been sufficiently reduced in rate, I find out the quantity of the drug that is necessary to keep the heart at the rate, at which it can perform its work with the greatest efficiency. In doing this, the patient's sensations are of the greatest help, whether he is confined to bed or attending to his affairs. He readily appreciates the change in his response to effort, and some such symptom as a disagreeable action of the heart or breathlessness, can be employed as an indication that the heart's strength is being exhausted. Once the patient understands the meaning of these sensations, he is generally quick to perceive what digitalis does for him, and its administration can usually be left quite safely in his hands. On such lines, I have seen many people lead useful lives for long periods of years with no bad effects, except when they have not taken the drug in sufficient quantities to keep the heart at the required rate.

The foregoing line of treatment is applicable chiefly to cases in whom auricular fibrillation has arisen recently, or where the heart failure is of recent date. In more advanced cases, when the condition has induced from time to time periods of heart failure, and there has appeared the change that accompanies chronic heart disease, such as persistent shortness of breath, enlarged liver, and dropsy more or less continuous, the persistent use of digitalis may still tend to restore a measure of strength to the heart and give relief, enabling the individual to lead a useful life, though at a lower level, for an indefinite period.

In the search for an appropriate line of treatment in old-standing cases, I have used many methods and many drugs, often with little or no benefit, but in a certain proportion of apparently hopeless cases I have seen extraordinarily good results following the use of digitalis, pushed until a reaction was obtained, and then stopped for a time, and again resumed, time after time. Not infrequently, after it has seemed useless to continue the drug, I have seen the individual acquire such an amount of strength as would scarcely have been anticipated.

As the conditions preceding auricular fibrillation and producing it, are all due to changes in the heart muscle of a slowly progressive nature, it is easy to recognize that the heart's strength cannot always be restored, and that as the amount of efficient muscle becomes reduced, a period is reached when no method of treatment is of avail.

Method of administration.—A great diversity of opinion is to be found in regard to the form in which digitalis should be given, and also in regard to the dosage. So far as I have worked out the subject in regard to auricular fibrillation, I see no reason for giving the preference to any particular preparation. The best and most assured way, in cases of marked failure, is steadily to push the drug, whichever form be employed, until a reaction is observed. Usually the digestive system is the first affected, loss of appetite, nausea, vomiting, or diarrhœa being set up, the patient usually feeling ill and miserable. If the digitalis is effective on the heart, as a rule a marked slowing of the pulse is found at the same time, or even before any digestive disturbances arise. In some cases, a slowing of the pulse is the first sign of a sufficiency. When this stage is reached, I always stop the administration of the drug for a few days. In a day or two, patients feel remarkably well and bright, and if nausea was present, it disappears. The heart-rate is carefully observed, and when the rate shows signs of increasing, half-doses of the drug should be given, and the dose increased or diminished according to the manner in which it affects the rate, the object in view being to give just the amount which enables the heart to carry on its work with the greatest efficiency. As I have previously stated, the patient himself by his own sensations speedily acquires the knowledge of how much of the drug is needed, and by attending to his own experiences, he will soon find out the smallest dose which is needed to give the best results.

A good deal of my work has been done with the tincture of digitalis ; and I may say that I have used this preparation for over thirty years, and have never yet come across an ineffective preparation, my standard being the reaction in susceptible individuals.   Professor Cushny has tested experimentally a number of samples from the Mount Vernon and London Hospitals, and has found each sample effective.

The quantity I usually start with, where the failure is marked, is 1 drachm of the tincture per day, in doses of 15 to 20 minims.   This is steadily pushed until a reaction is obtained ; then it is stopped and employed in the manner already described.   Usually a reaction is obtained within a week, sometimes in a few days.   Where there is great distress and more urgency, I give as much as 2 drachms of the tincture daily, and then get a reaction in two or three days.

I have frequently used Nativelle's digitalin granules, and find them also very efficacious.   I have found that one of these granules is equal to 15 minims of the tincture.

Other drugs, such as strophanthus and squills, have the same effect as the digitalis, and in some cases they may cause less digestive disturbance ; but in the majority of cases I have found that when the digitalis is ineffective, so also are these drugs.   In many cases, the effects of digitalis are less disagreeable than these other drugs.

In some urgent cases, it may be necessary to produce a reaction more speedily, though I have rarely failed to get a reaction in good time by digitalis by the mouth.   In order to obtain a speedy reaction, strophanthin or strophanthone may be injected into the veins.   In a series of observations which have been carried out at the Mount Vernon Hospital and at the London Hospital, it has been found that in auricular fibrillation with a pulse-rate of over 140 per minute, intravenous injections of strophanthin ($\frac{1}{250}$ gr.) can reduce the rate and give relief in five or eight hours, but I am of opinion that it is only in very exceptional and urgent cases that this method is required.

Danger in the administration of digitalis.—For a long while, I was at a loss to understand the warning of authorities as to the danger of sudden death from administration of digitalis.   Of recent years I have obtained an inkling into the cause of sudden death.   I have been shown tracings of the slow pulse with characteristic coupled beats that occur under digitalis with auricular fibrillation, and have been informed that the patient died suddenly.   On inquiry, it was found that, notwithstanding the evidences of a sufficiency, the drug had been continued in large doses.   I was once asked to see a man who was said to be dying from heart failure.   He had to sit up in bed and breathed heavily ; his face was livid. He had dropsy, an enlarged liver, and a large and irregular heart beating at the rate of 130 to 140 per minute (auricular fibrillation). I told his doctor to push the digitalis till he showed evidences of a sufficiency, either by the slowing of the heart or nausea, and then to stop it. After five days he telephoned me that the patient was wonderfully free from distress, could lie flat, was a good colour, and the dropsy had almost gone, the pulse-rate being between 70 and 80. I told him to stop the digitalis for a few days, and if the pulse then increased to give smaller doses, and find out the exact quantity which kept the rate about 80. Three days later, he telephoned to say that the patient had been going on well, but that morning, during the doctor's visit, the patient fell back and died. I asked the doctor if he had stopped the digitalis, and he replied in the negative, saying that, as it had done him such a lot of good, he had continued it, in spite of my directions.

On making inquiries in a few other cases where I had heard of sudden death, I had no difficulty in recognizing that they were cases of auricular fibrillation, in which digitalis had been pushed after it had affected the heart. Seeing that I have been following this line of treatment by pushing the drug till I get evidences of its action, then stopping it and resuming it later, for over fifteen years, and have never had a sudden death, I am disposed to think that just as we recognize the danger of pushing chloroform beyond a certain stage, so there is danger when digitalis is pushed too far, whereas if the indications I have given are followed, such a catastrophe as death need not occur.

CHAPTER XXXI

Auricular Flutter

Definition of the term 'auricular flutter'.
Auricular flutter as a common clinical condition.
Conditions giving rise to auricular flutter.
The symptomatology of auricular flutter.
Jugular pulse with auricular flutter.
Radial pulse in auricular flutter.
Auricular flutter and fibrillation.
Auricular flutter and paroxysmal tachycardia.
Auricular flutter and digitalis.
Prognosis.
Treatment.

Definition of the term 'auricular flutter'.—The term 'auricular flutter' was first used by MacWilliam to describe a mode of contraction of the auricle in response to an electric stimulus. MacWilliam showed that if a weak stimulus was applied to the auricle of a dog or cat, the auricular contractions became greatly increased, attaining a speed of 300 or 400 per minute. This rapid action he called flutter. If the strength of the electric stimulus be increased, the auricle passed into fibrillation. The close connexion between flutter and fibrillation, shown in experiment, is also found to occur in man as a result of disease. The term 'flutter' was first adopted clinically by Jolly and Ritchie in describing a case of complete heart-block, where the auricle attained a speed of 300 per minute. Several isolated cases have been described of this condition, notably one by Hertz and Goodhart which I had an opportunity of seeing and of which Fig. 128 is a tracing, but it was not recognized until recently as a common clinical condition.

Auricular flutter as a common clinical condition.—My recognition of it as a fairly common clinical condition, arose as a result of the reports by Dr. Lewis on the electrocardiograms of a series of cases I sent him. These cases presented certain features which I could not recognize from physical examination, or from tracings of the radial and jugular pulses. Dr. Lewis has included some of these cases in a paper recently published by him, and his description, as well as that of Rihl and Ritchie, deals in such a convincing manner with the electrocardiographic evidence, that the recognition of this condition as a clinical entity may be considered to be established. It is imperative, however, that its recognition should be made on other evidences than that of the electrocardiogram, for there is no opportunity of examining the vast majority of cases by this method. I have examined a series of over 30 cases, in order to ascertain the more readily recognizable clinical features ; I give an account of 15 cases in which the diagnosis was confirmed by the electrocardiograph, while the remainder leave little doubt as to their nature. When I look back over my notes and tracings of cases, I find a considerable group in which the condition was probably present. Some of them I had mistaken for auricular fibrillation, while others I had put on one side as being insoluble.

Conditions giving rise to auricular flutter.—It is too soon yet to speak of the morbid state that induces auricular flutter. That it is due to some lesion, resulting in a fibrosis irritating the auricle, similar to that which occurs in auricular fibrillation, seems probable, especially as one condition may alternate with the other. It is likely that it will also be found to follow rheumatic affections of the heart, for it is certain that some of those attacks of paroxysmal tachycardia with regular rhythm, which occur in people with a rheumatic history, are really due to auricular flutter. As in auricular fibrillation, there is a tendency to the occurrence of auricular flutter in the elderly, particularly in those with extensive fibrotic degeneration of the heart muscle, while it seems that it may not infrequently be a terminal process in many diseased hearts. It is also possible that it may arise from an acute infection of the heart, as in Case 64.

The symptomatology of auricular flutter.—The evidences which this condition produces are extraordinarily varied, and it is doubtful if there is any other affection of the heart so protean in its manifestations. It is only in rare instances that the auricular movements can be recognized without the aid of mechanical means, and then it is by seeing the extremely rapid movements in the veins of the neck. By means of graphic records we can get these movements registered, but here again we are often baffled by the curious results which are recorded. As these graphic records may often be the only means by which we can detect the condition, I enter very fully into the interpretation of some of the anomalous forms the tracings may take. The most accurate of all methods is the electrocardiographic, but it is obvious that only a small proportion of cases can be investigated by this method, for many individuals are too ill to be moved to the instrument. For this reason it behoves us to study the ordinary graphic records, for they can usually be taken with little trouble.

The ventricular contractions are dependent on the ability of the bundle to receive and transmit the stimulus, and as this is sometimes varying, certain peculiarities of pulse rhythm arise, which, in the absence of other evidences, may indicate the presence of auricular flutter.

Apart from the direct evidences of auricular flutter, as shown by the movements in the jugular veins, we get other evidences depending on the diminished output of the heart. This may lead not only to the more common evidences of heart failure, as shortness of breath, but in many cases to a deficient supply of blood to the brain, inducing certain cerebral symptoms, which, taken along with other signs present, may lead to the recognition of this complaint.

From the history of the cases cited, it will be seen that the condition may last for a great many years, or it may appear as a terminal condition in certain diseases of the heart. If would seem also that before it becomes permanently established, it may appear intermittently, as attacks of paroxysmal tachycardia. When I look back over the records of my cases, I find a very considerable number who suffered from transient attacks of rapid and irregular action of the heart, which I had mistaken for auricular fibrillation, but which I now think were really cases of auricular flutter. Some of these have fallen unconscious, others were not inconvenienced by its presence, although aware of the unusual action of the heart, while some have been totally unconscious of anything amiss, while the attack is actually on (Case 61).

The patients usually complain of a distinct limitation of their powers when auricular flutter is present. In many cases, they are conscious of its onset by the peculiar nature of the heart's action, and this knowledge may have a depressing effect upon the patient's mind. They are also conscious of its cessation, and experience a sense of relief when this occurs, just as happens with attacks of paroxysmal tachycardia from other causes.

With the persistence of the attack, a gradual exhaustion of the heart's strength sets in and the patient becomes conscious of increasing limitation. This failure of the heart's strength may proceed so far as to endanger the life of the individual, and there are present the usual signs of extreme heart failure, as orthopnœa, dropsy, and enlargement and pulsation of the liver.

Peculiar features may arise, dependent, to a certain extent, on the manner in which the ventricle responds to the auricle. As a rule, the ventricle does not respond to each auricular contraction, though it may be greatly accelerated and attain a speed of 150 or more, the ventricle then responding to every second auricular beat. In many cases, the ventricle responds to a varying number of auricular beats, and we get a pulse rhythm of great variety.

The interference with the supply of blood to the organs produces certain peculiar symptoms. If the ventricle should respond to every auricular beat, the output may be so small that the blood supply to the brain may be so slight as to render the patient unconscious. From the cases recorded, it will be seen that attacks of loss of consciousness are not infrequent with this complaint. Sometimes the attacks do not produce loss of consciousness, but extreme giddiness. In one patient whom I saw when the ventricle attained a speed of nearly 300 beats, there was extreme collapse approaching loss of consciousness. The sensation experienced was difficult to describe, but it caused the greatest dread of these attacks, which at certain periods could be easily provoked by slight exertion, as by the bowels being moved, or by unpleasant dreams.

A frequent symptom is Cheyne-Stokes respiration, usually accompanied by a good deal of mental torpor. This does not arise at once, but after the condition has been present for some time. Should the heart revert to the normal action, the brain speedily clears up, and the Cheyne-Stokes respiration disappears.

Jugular pulse with auricular flutter.—The jugular pulse is the only direct source of information we get of the action of the right auricle in this condition. In some cases we may detect the presence of the rapid successions of waves in the jugular veins, or in the curious distension of the jugular bulb when the jugular valves are competent during certain phases of the ventricular systole. In analysing the waves thus seen, or when recorded by graphic means, it is necessary to recognize the variations in pressure, to which the venous blood near the heart is subjected. To understand the extremely varied results, we must bear in mind that the venous pressure is remarkably inconstant, not only in different individuals but in the same individual under different circumstances.

By the usual method of taking a tracing, when the cup or receiver is placed over the root of the neck above the inner end of the clavicle, the receiver covers not only the vein but a portion of the carotid and subclavian arteries (see Fig. 46). In normal acting hearts, if the vein be very empty, the only record obtained is that of the arterial pulse ; if there is a slight fullness of the veins, a small wave due to the auricle may be found preceding the arterial pulse (Fig. 57) ; while if the vein be very full, the waves present may be nearly or all due to the variations in the jugular veins, and these variations may be due to ventricular action as well as auricular, so much so indeed that with great engorgement and marked tricuspid incompetence, only one wave due to the ventricular systole may be present.

The simplest and most demonstrable form of jugular pulse with auricular flutter is that where the ventricle beats at an infrequent rate and the auricular waves are well marked in the veins, as in Fig. 128. In Fig. 129, the carotid beat c is distinct and is preceded by a number of waves due to the auricle, a. Here the auricle is beating at a rate of 275 beats per minute, and the ventricle 32 (Case 62). A similar condition is seen in Fig. 130, where the ventricular rate is slow and irregular, between 30 and 40, while the auricular waves (a) occur at the rate of 250 per minute. The wave c at the down-stroke 3 corresponds to the radial beat. Here it will be seen that after c the tracing is not sustained, but after an abrupt rise there is a sudden fall, while the wave is scarcely perceptible. It is important to recognize how these curves come about in order to appreciate the variations in other curves. If we look at a normal tracing from the neck, as in Fig. 52, it will be seen that after *c* there is a great fall. This fall is due to the dilatation of the right auricle emptying the jugular vein. This dilatation in a normal case, as in Fig. 52, is due to the relaxation of the auricle after its systole, but more particularly to the dragging down of the septum between the auricles and ventricles, while the ventricle is emptying itself of its contents. When the auricle is contracting at the rapid rate, the contractions during this period fail to affect, or affect very slightly, the blood in the jugular veins, hence the

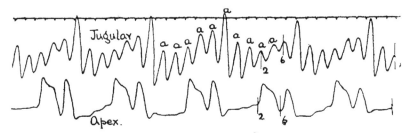

Fig. 128. Simultaneous tracings of the jugular pulse and apex beat, from Hertz and Goodhart's case of auricular flutter. The auricular beats (*a*) are 250 per minute, and the ventricle 60. The smaller beats of the ventricle are probably of the nature of extra-systoles.

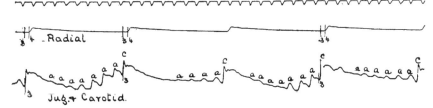

Fig. 129. The radial tracing shows a ventricular rate of 28, and the auricular traces (*a*) a rate of 280 per minute (Case 62).

absence or faint appearance of the wave *a* during this period. In Fig. 130, it will be noticed there is an increase in size of the wave marked $v + a$, appearing at the end of ventricular systole. This wave is a composite wave due to the auricular contraction falling at the same time as the normal *v* wave.

If these various factors in modifying the pressure in the jugular veins, with the knowledge that the method of taking a record is affected by the presence of the carotid and subclavian arteries, are recognized, we can analyse and appreciate such apparently hopelessly confused looking tracings as Fig. 131, particularly if we bear in mind that the sucking in of the structures at the root of the neck during inspiration, is a process which modifies the size of the waves.

With greater engorgement of the right side of the heart and fullness of the veins, we may get no direct effects, except those due to the auricular contractions, slightly modified by the effects of ventricular systole. This

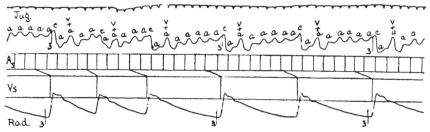

Fig. 130. Shows an auricular rate (*a*) of 220. The radial pulse is irregular, due to the ventricle responding to a varying number of auricular impulses, as shown by the intercalated diagram.

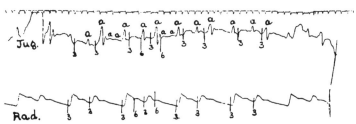

Fig. 131. From a patient during an attack of paroxysmal tachycardia, probably due to auricular flutter. The variations in the size of the auricular beats are due to the period of ventricular action during which they occurred (Case 68).

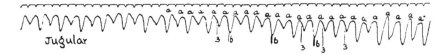

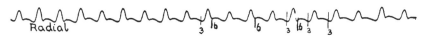

Fig. 132. The auricular rate (*a*) is about 240, and the ventricular one-half of this (Case 64).

is seen in Fig. 128, where the auricular waves are only slightly modified by the ventricular systole. In Fig. 132, there are two auricular beats to one ventricular, and a greater fall at the end of the downstroke 6 is noted, for this is the period of ventricular relaxation immediately after systole, when the blood begins to pass into the ventricle. In Fig. 133, the auricular rate is

270 and the ventricular 90. The large waves in the jugular occur during the ventricular systole, so that not only has the inflow into the ventricle ceased, but the auricle contracting at this time sends all the blood back into the veins. That these waves are auricular in origin, can be recognized by the fact that they continue uninterrupted, during the irregular periods of the ventricular contraction in Fig. 134. Fig. 129, 133, and 134 were taken from the same patient at different times and the interpretation verified by the electrocardiograph.

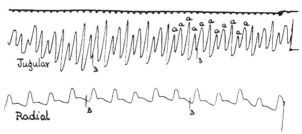

FIG. 133. The auricular rate is three times that of the ventricular = a, 270; v, 90 (Case 62).

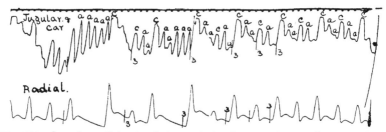

FIG. 134. Irregular radial pulse during auricular flutter. The auricular waves (a) are only perceptible during the long ventricular pauses (Case 62).

Where there is great tricuspid regurgitation, and the ventricular systole forces large waves of blood back into the auricle, all appearances of the auricular waves may be lost, and we get only the ventricular form of pulse in the jugular and in the liver as in Fig. 135 and 136. This patient (Case 68) had frequent attacks of paroxysmal tachycardia, and during one long paroxysm I obtained a large number of tracings. He was able to modify the ventricular rate for a short time by swallowing and belching air, by which means he evidently stimulated the vagus. This changed ventricular action is shown in Fig. 131. An analysis of the tracings shows that, during the rapid and regular period, the jugular and liver pulses were of the ventricular form (Fig. 135 and 136), while during the slow and irregular period (Fig. 131), the auricular waves appeared in the jugular, but modified in size, according to the phase of ventricular systole during which they fell.

Fig. 137 shows an irregular radial pulse with the ventricular form of the venous pulse. From the tracing one would infer that there was auricular fibrillation present, but the electrocardiogram (Fig. 138) shows that there was auricular flutter.

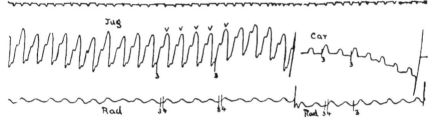

FIG. 135.   Tracing taken during an attack of paroxysmal tachycardia.   The jugular pulse is of the ventricular form.   Compare with Fig. 131 (Case 68).

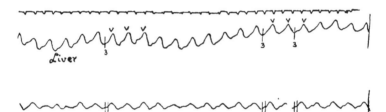

FIG. 136.   Tracings of the liver and radial pulses during an attack of paroxysmal tachycardia (Case 68).

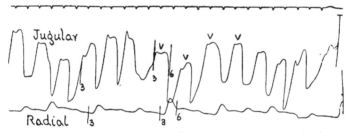

FIG. 137.   Tracing of the jugular and radial pulses during an attack of paroxysmal tachycardia, due to auricular flutter, as revealed by the electrocardiogram (see Fig. 138). The venous pulse is of the ventricular form.

In many cases, it is scarcely possible to recognize clearly the individual factors which modify the jugular pulse, and we may get a hopelessly confused series of movements, as in Fig. 139 (Case 58).   This tracing shows a regular pulse with rhythmical variations, when a large beat is always followed by a smaller ; the tracing from the neck shows a series of waves which I fail to understand, though I have marked certain of them with *a*. The electrocardiogram from this patient, taken on the same day, showed that there were two auricular beats to one ventricular beat.

The radial pulse in auricular flutter. When the ventricle responds to every auricular beat, we get a pulse of extreme rapidity which is uncountable except by graphic methods. The pulse at the same time becomes extremely weak, and is accompanied by evidence of diminished blood-supply to the brain. Fig. 140 and 141 show the greatly increased rate.

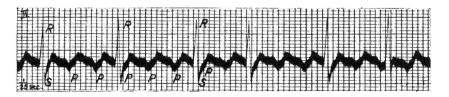

Fig. 138. Electrocardiogram taken during the same attack of paroxysmal tachycardia, as shown in Fig. 137. The auricular movements (P) are 310 per minute, and the ventricular (R) 120.

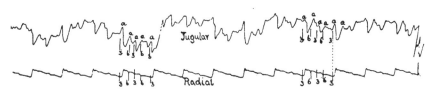

Fig. 139. Tracing of the jugular and radial pulses during an attack of auricular flutter. The auricular rate as revealed by the electrocardiogram was 200, and the ventricular 100 (Case 58).

In the vast majority of cases, the ventricle does not respond to each auricular beat, and as a consequence we get an extraordinary variety of rhythms. In many cases, the irregular rhythm seems so disorderly that it is impossible to bring out any reasonable interpretation. But when we know all these factors, then order comes out of chaos, and we can often clearly recognize a definite arrangement in the most disorderly looking tracing.

There are certain peculiarities which modify the size of the radial beat. The fact that a certain period of rest is required after a contraction, before the ventricle is able to contract with its full force, has already been dwelt upon. If the ventricle is stimulated too early, then the resultant contraction will be weak, as when the ventricle contracts at a great rate in response to auricular impulses. If there is a varying delay in the ventricular contraction, then within certain limits the ventricular beats will vary in strength, according to the length of the preceding pause.

But there is another factor which modifies the size of the beats, of whose origin we are still ignorant, although several explanations have been put forward, and that is, the factor which gives rise to the pulsus alternans. I shall point out later its significance with the normal rhythm, and its frequent association with degeneration of the heart muscle. It has long

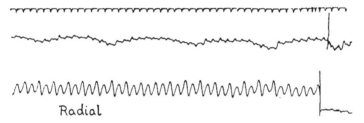

Radial

FIG. 140. Tracing of the radial pulse, and of the pulsation in the neck (probably carotid) during an attack of auricular flutter. The electrocardiogram revealed an auricular rate of 290-300 per minute, with the ventricular contractions at half this rate. Occasionally for short periods the ventricular rate equalled the auricular, and during one such period this tracing was taken. Note the pulsus alternans in the radial tracing (Case 55).

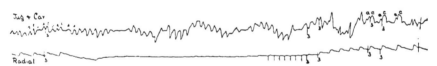

Jug + Car

Radial

FIG. 141. Tracings taken during a short attack of auricular flutter, during which the patient lost consciousness. From the character of the radial tracing it can be inferred that the ventricle contracted at a rate of 200, but the output was so small as to barely affect the radial pulse (Theodore Thompson).

been known to be a frequent event in paroxysmal tachycardia of abnormal origin, while infrequent in greatly increased rate with the normal rhythm. Its presence in tachycardias of abnormal rhythm may not necessarily be associated with degeneration of the heart muscle, at least to any serious extent. But this tendency to its appearance modifies the character of the pulse, as shown in such tracings as Fig. 139 and 142, and when associated with an irregular rhythm, introducing a confusing element into the interpretation.

The irregular rhythm of the beats is almost entirely due to the variation in the transmission of the stimulus from auricle to ventricle. Except in rare cases where there is complete block, due to disease of the auriculo-ventricular bundle, the ventricular contractions are in response to the auricular stimulus. The conduction of stimulus may be so constant that the ventricle responds to every second auricular beat, or every fourth, when we get a pulse with a regular rhythm. But frequently the conduction varies in a most inexplicable manner, so that we get ventricular responses and pulse-beats in irregular rhythms of great variety, as can be seen in the radial tracings given in this chapter.

These variations in the response of the ventricle to the auricle are due to some unknown cause. While disease in the bundle may account for a great many cases of delayed transmission, yet a study of some cases would show that there must be other factors at work apart from disease process. We sometimes find cases of complete block, suddenly relieved, and the heart's contraction continues in a normal fashion for years. In one peculiar case, I found partial block occur only after an extra-systole. In auricular flutter,

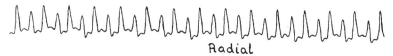

Radial

FIG. 142. Pulsus alternans during an attack of auricular flutter. The electrocardiogram from lead II in Fig. 143 was taken while the attack was on (Case 61).

some influence must be at work in producing, in the same case, such remarkable variations in the transmission of the stimulus which we may find at one examination.

Auricular flutter and fibrillation.—I have already remarked on the close relation between auricular flutter and auricular fibrillation in experiment. The same relation is found clinically. Thus I have seen a patient with auricular flutter ultimately develop auricular fibrillation. Under the influence of digitalis, as will be shown later, the flutter may pass into fibrillation, while in one case I found the heart's action vary every few minutes, passing from the normal to the fibrillation, and back to the normal, and then into flutter (Case 61, Fig. 142, 143, 144).

Auricular flutter and paroxysmal tachycardia.—From the history of the cases given in the appendix, it will be seen that the attacks of auricular flutter are the real cause of the condition that goes under the name of paroxysmal tachycardia. I am coming to the conclusion that the great majority of cases of paroxysmal tachycardia with a regular rhythm, or with the pulsus alternans, are really due to auricular flutter. In support of this view, I would refer the reader to Cases 55 and 61. That this is not so in all cases, is shown in Chapter XXIX, where a tachycardia from rapid auricular action may arise in a manner different from flutter.

Auricular flutter and digitalis.—In studying the effects of digitalis on the human heart, I had perceived the curious susceptibility of cases of

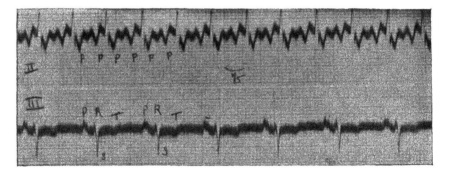

Fig. 143. When the upper record (lead II) was taken auricular flutter was present—the auricle (P) contracting at the rate of 300 per minute, and the ventricle at half this rate (see Fig. 142). A few minutes later the lower record was taken (lead III), and the heart had now resumed its normal action—auricle and ventricle beating at the rate of 96 (Case 61).

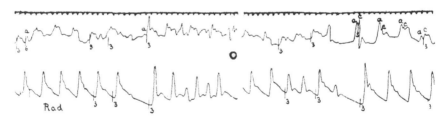

Fig. 144. Tracing of the radial and the pulsation of the neck, showing the beginning and end of a short attack of paroxysmal tachycardia, due to auricular fibrillation. The first six beats and the last three in the radial are regular and due to a normal contraction of the heart. The beats between occur during a period of auricular fibrillation. At o a portion of the tracing has been cut out. The attack lasted twenty seconds, and at o a period of fifteen seconds has been cut out. These attacks varied with periods of auricular flutter (Figs. 142 and 143) (Case 61).

auricular fibrillation to digitalis. Amongst the cases I had reckoned as auricular fibrillation (or nodal rhythm, as I then called this condition), I found some which, in view of later knowledge, were cases of auricular flutter. In some observations I published in 1904, I included a case where there was a rapid heart, which became slow and irregular, with the features characteristic of auricular fibrillation. When the digitalis was stopped, the heart speedily became rapid and regular, and after some time the normal rhythm became re-established (Case 69). Since that date, I have had similar instances, and recorded another experience in 1911 (Case 55). This case is now recognized as being originally auricular flutter, and the auricle while under the influence of digitalis passed into fibrillation, and with the cessation of digitalis reverted to the normal rhythm. A similar experience is recorded in Case 56, published in detail by Turnbull.

When we began to recognize the cases of auricular flutter, the question arose, could we cure them by giving the digitalis on a definite principle? We have tried this line of treatment in several cases, but with varying result.

In another patient of mine this line of treatment was pursued, and Dr. Lewis carefully studied the effects both by graphic and electrocardiographic records. The result was, that after a preliminary period in which the ventricular rate was slowed by an increase of the heart-block, the auricle passed into fibrillation, and when the drug was stopped, the heart reverted to the normal rhythm.

A similar test was made in Case 57, but the only effect was to increase the heart-block. Lewis records two other cases where, under digitalis, auricular fibrillation occurred and was succeeded by the normal rhythm.

In a case recently under observation the auricular flutter passed into fibrillation after 10 granules of digitalin and seems permanently established.

Prognosis.—From the perusal of the cases given in the Appendix to illustrate this condition, it will be seen that the prognosis is as varied as the symptomatology. We can, however, draw this conclusion, that auricular flutter, though it may impair the functional efficiency of the heart, is not in *itself* a dangerous condition. Where danger arises, it is in a heart which is already the seat of somewhat extensive disease, especially when affecting the ventricle or valvular disease with impaired ventricles. Hence, the already weakened heart is unable to cope with the burden thrown upon it by the abnormal rhythm. In giving a prognosis, each case must be carefully studied by itself, and the condition of the ventricle and the valve defects estimated, particularly the manner in which the efficiency of the circulation is maintained, before and after the inception of the abnormal rhythm, and the response to digitalis. There is danger when attacks of loss of consciousness arise, due to the rapid and inefficient action of the ventricle, with grave signs of heart failure. One patient whom I saw had an attack with congestion of the lungs, and died 24 hours later during a second attack.

Treatment.—The treatment of the transient attacks is discussed under the heading of paroxysmal tachycardia (p. 253).

When the condition is permanently established or persists for a long time, a course of digitalis should be tried, the digitalis to be pushed in the manner already described in the chapter on auricular fibrillation, and stopped as soon as there is evidence of a sufficiency, as shown by the slow pulse or nausea. The slowing of the pulse may be due to an increase of the heart-block, and with the stoppage of the digitalis, the rate may only gradually increase. If it is possible, the dose which will keep the ventricular contractions at a moderate rate (70 to 90 beats per minute), should be found, and the drug given as required. If this line of treatment be pursued, not only may it keep the patient in a better condition, but it may lead to auricular fibrillation and the restoration of the normal rhythm, while if there be extreme heart failure, it may restore a more efficient circulation.

When auricular flutter is present and there is a tendency for the ventricle to follow each auricular contraction, the quieter the patient can be kept the better, and sedatives and the bromides should be given to ensure sleep and to prevent mental disturbances, dreams, excitement, etc. (Case 55). As in auricular fibrillation, we know of no remedy which will of certainty stop this abnormal rhythm.

CHAPTER XXXII

Definition.
Symptoms.
Prognosis.
Treatment.

Definition.—As we get a clearer insight into the mechanism of the heart's action, we are able to identify more clearly the nature of any case which we were wont to include under some general term. Paroxysmal tachycardia is a term used to indicate the starting of the heart's contraction, in an abnormal place, with a sudden increase in the rate of the heart, and a sudden cessation of the rapidity on resumption of the normal rhythm. Analyses of a great many cases show that the cause of these attacks, in a considerable number, is due to a transient fibrillation of the auricle when the rhythm is irregular, or to auricular contractions from an abnormal source occurring at a great rate, from 150 to 300 per minute, when the rhythm is regular. In the Appendix, I quote a series of cases to show how diverse are the conditions which give rise to this abnormal action of the heart. Thus I have seen a large number of cases, in which the abnormal auricular rhythm ranged from a few beats of what we recognize as multiple auricular extra-systoles to short paroxysms (Fig. 115), or to long periods of hours and days (Fig. 116). The rate in these cases varied from 150 to about 300 per minute. It is only rarely that the ventricle accompanies the auricle at the higher rates, responding frequently to every second auricular contraction. It will thus be realized that there are cases of rapid abnormal auricular contractions which it is impossible to separate from the condition called auricular flutter, which is described in Chapter XXXI. There are cases, however, where it is not possible to state with certainty the nature of the attacks. The cause provoking the attacks is too subtle for detection, although effort, mental excitement, or poisoning from the intestines or some focus of infection may cause the attacks in those predisposed.

Symptoms.—The heart suddenly takes on a rapid action, and this may last for a few beats, or it may go on for minutes, hours, days, and weeks. When the attack stops, it does so suddenly, not gradually as in palpitation. The rate is usually increased, sometimes greatly. Sometimes the rate is not markedly increased. An individual may have but one attack ; or the attacks may come on at frequent intervals in the course of ten or twenty years; or they may be of great frequency, occurring every few weeks or days; or there may be several attacks on one day. After one or two attacks, the heart may settle down permanently with the fibrillation of the auricle, or auricular flutter.

The sensation felt by the patient when this rhythm is first started may be so slight as to pass unnoticed. Usually he is conscious of a curious fluttering sensation inside the left chest. This sensation is very characteristic and almost pathognomonic. It may be described variously according to the literary gift of the sufferer, but the essential feature is the soft and gentle movements, not rhythmical, but varying softly in intensity, in striking contrast to the sensations that may arise from stimulation of the heart during a normal rhythm, as in palpitation. Frequently this sensation is so disquieting that the patient rests, or walks about cautiously and quietly. About the same time the patient remarks a distinct limitation in the field of cardiac response, the exertion that he was wont to undertake with comfort now inducing breathlessness.

The associated heart failure may be so extreme that in a few days, or even in a few hours, evidences of imminent peril are shown. The patient has to keep in bed, the dyspnœa being so great that he cannot lie on his back, but must be propped up. If the patient survives, œdema of the legs quickly supervenes, the lips become livid and the face swollen. The pulse is small, rapid, and sometimes irregular, the beats varying remarkably in strength. The veins of the neck are often full and pulsate with great rapidity. The heart dilates in a few hours, sometimes extending two inches in the transverse direction. The sounds alter, becoming short and sharp, and if the heart's action is rapid, often no murmur may be detected. The liver becomes enlarged, and may be found pulsating two or three inches below the ribs. The tissues covering the heart and the liver often become extremely tender on pressure.

With the sudden reversion of the rhythm to the normal, the change in the patient's condition is even more remarkable than the rapid onset of the symptoms of heart failure. At once the patient heaves a sigh of relief, and in a very short time, within half an hour, all abnormal signs in the lips, face, and enlarged liver disappear, while in a few hours the heart may be found beating within its normal limits.

In others, the paroxysmal tachycardia may occur for a day or two, with no marked change in the size of the heart. In these, the patient is generally conscious of the heart's abnormal action, and instinctively avoids active exertion, either keeping in bed or resting in a chair, or walking about very quietly. The attack usually lasts for a few hours, but may occasionally last for many hours, or even one or two days. At the end of this time, no increase in the size of the heart is detectable, and there is no sign of dropsy or enlarged liver. This condition may be found at all ages over ten years.

Lewis has called attention to a feature which distinguishes paroxysmal tachycardia due to an abnormal rhythm from a period of rapid heart action, such as occurs in palpitation or from temporary excitement, namely, that effort has no effect on the rate in paroxysmal tachycardia, while in other conditions the rate increases with effort.

Prognosis.—The prognosis in these cases is one of considerable difficulty. The symptoms during an attack may be so alarming. that the inexperienced are apt to look upon the patient as hopelessly stricken. I remember being called one night to a woman 80 years of age. I found her heart extremely rapid and irregular, her face swollen and livid, and she was gasping for breath. I told the friends the end was approaching, but, calling to see her next morning, I found her walking out in the street. After that she had several attacks, and finally died during one. Other patients I have watched for years, when the symptoms have not been so extreme, some-times only giving rise to a slight uneasiness in the chest. In these, the heart has not dilated, though the rate may have reached nearly 200 per minute. Others have had but one attack, and I have watched some of these for over twenty years, and they have had no other.

In some the change from being transient becomes permanent, and here lies the danger. If the extreme form of heart failure persists and the dilatation cannot be reduced, then the patient drifts to death (Cases 51, 67, and 72).

The prognosis also depends on the degree of dilatation. If the heart does not increase in size and the attacks are transient, then on the whole the prognosis is good, though in many cases the patient's life is greatly crippled, because of the fact that the attacks recur in spite of treatment. When there is dilatation with the accompanying symptoms of dropsy and enlarged liver, then the outlook is bad.

Treatment.—Absolute quiet is needed during the attack—a suggestion scarcely necessary, for the patient usually seeks rest, though he may move about quietly with little distress. A great many suggestions as to the arrest of these attacks may be found scattered through medical literature. As the attacks are commonly but transient, some remedy employed oppor-tunely seems to the inexperienced onlooker to restore the heart to its normal action. Many patients themselves have a knack of doing something that seems to change the rhythm. Sometimes attacks can be stopped by the patient simply taking a series of deep breaths, by slapping the chest, by the sudden application of cold water to the chest, or by vomiting (see Case 68). Drugs of the most diverse character have been cited as active agents in stopping attacks, such as nitro-glycerine and adrenalin. In my early days I, too, thought I knew how to stop attacks ; but more extended experience has shown me that when they stopped, it was from some cause unknown to me, and which was independent of any means I employed. I have tried intravenous injections of strophanthin, with no satisfactory result.

When signs of heart failure appear, and the abnormal rhythm becomes permanent, and is found to be of the nature of auricular fibrillation or flutter, then the treatment, as described in Chapters XXX and XXXI, should be employed.

CHAPTER XXXIII

THE PULSUS ALTERNANS

Different forms of alternation.
Conditions producing the pulsus alternans.
Cause of the pulsus alternans.
Differential diagnosis.
Prognosis.
Treatment.

THIS term is applied to an irregularity which is due to a variation in the force of the beats of the pulse, each second beat varying in strength, a strong beat alternating with a weak one. The rhythm of the pulse, however, is perfectly regular (Fig. 145). In the great majority of cases, it can only be recognized by graphic records of the radial pulse. As a rule, the variation in the strength of the beat is too slight for the finger to detect, but in rare cases the finger can perceive the variation. It is also but seldom that we can detect a difference in the loudness of the sounds of the heart, although where there is a systolic murmur, particularly if it is musical, the difference in intensity is very distinct. Until recent years, different forms of irregularity were included under this term, but chiefly owing to Wenckebach the term is now restricted to one form, namely, where the pulse is perfectly regular in rhythm, but where every alternate beat varies in size, a large beat and a weak one alternating. In the most typical forms of this irregularity, all the chambers of the heart act in a normal manner, so far as sequence is concerned, and it is only the effects of the left ventricular systole in the radial pulse by which it is detected.

Different forms of alternation. When a large number of cases are examined which show alternation, it will be found that the conditions producing it are not always the same. I have said that in the most typical forms all the chambers of the heart act in a normal manner, but there are other forms of pulsus alternans where the chambers of the heart do not act in a normal manner. In paroxysmal tachycardia, the starting of the heart's contraction is at some place other than the normal. Thus in attacks of tachycardia, as in Fig. 117, 140, and 142, the heart's contraction arises in an abnormal manner.

In cases of auricular flutter (described in Chapter XXXI), the pulsus alternans is very apt to appear when the ventricular rate is increased, and there seems to be something in the mechanism of the condition which predisposes to the production of the pulsus alternans (Fig. 142). The detection of a pulsus alternans in a non-febrile case with a pulse of 100 beats per minute or over, should always arouse the suspicion that we have to deal with an abnormal rhythm, such as auricular flutter.

Conditions producing the pulsus alternans.—Putting aside the pulsus alternans which arises in consequence of an abnormal action of the heart, we find that the vast majority are associated with degenerative

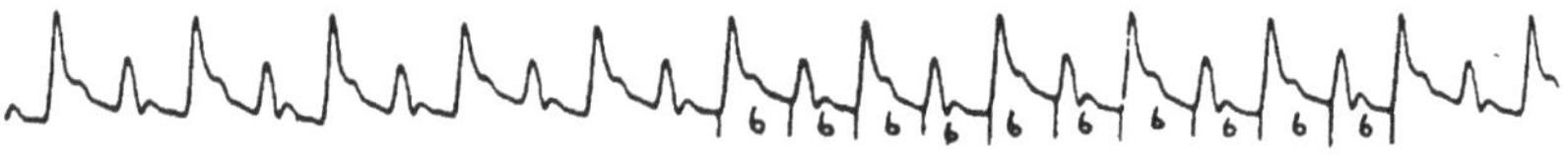

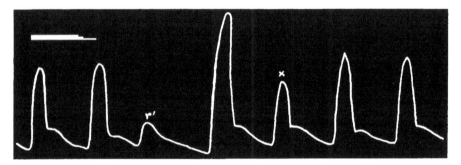

FIG. 145.   Radial tracing showing the pulsus alternans.   Each period is of exactly the same duration (six-tenths of a second).

FIG. 146.   Tracing from the carotid artery of a dog.   The heart was exposed and the ventricle directly stimulated to produce the extra-systole r'.   The long pause after the extra-systole is followed by a large beat and succeeded by one beat (×) smaller than the other beats. Its small size implies grave exhaustion of the contractile power of the left ventricle. Compare with Fig. 147 (Cushny).

changes in the heart muscle.   This occurs most frequently in people in the more advanced years of life.   It is occasionally found in younger subjects with evidence of extreme exhaustion of the heart muscle, though I have not had the opportunity of examining the heart muscle in the few fatal cases in which I have seen it occur in the young.   It may be present in an exhausted heart with chronic valvular disease, but the most typical examples have had no, or merely incidental, valvular affections.   I have found it occasionally in severe cases of pneumonia, and it possibly occurs in other acute exhausting diseases.

The pulsus alternans may only be called into evidence under special circumstances. Thus it may disappear entirely when the individual is at rest, and it is perhaps for this reason that it is detected more frequently in the consulting-room than in hospital wards. Where there is a tendency to its occurrence, some amount of bodily effort may suffice to produce it; or it may be brought about by some variation in the heart's rhythm, as when it occurs after an extra-systole (Fig. 146 and 147). Following an

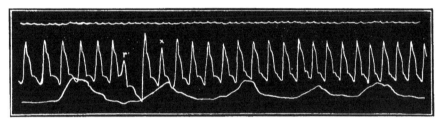

FIG. 147. The long pause after the extra-systole (r') is followed by a large beat; this in turn is followed by a small beat (×), and the succeeding beats are larger. The small beat (×) is an evidence that the contractility of the heart was greatly exhausted. Compare with Fig. 146. (From a case of advanced cardio-sclerosis.)

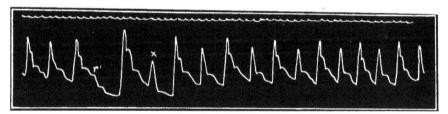

FIG. 148. The alternating character of the pulse is increased after the long pause following the extra-systole (r'); the second beat (×) following the pause appears at the normal interval, but is greatly reduced in size. (From a case of advanced cardio-sclerosis.)

extra-systole there is usually a long pause, succeeded by a series of normal beats. After the pause, alternation may arise and be continued for a varying period. Sometimes there is but one small beat (Fig. 147); at other times the alternation will last for a few beats, the beats gradually approximating and the alternation disappearing. If pulsus alternans be constantly present, it becomes marked after an extra-systole (Fig. 148). Where there are frequent extra-systoles a very confusing arrhythmia may be detected, consisting of extra-systoles and the pulsus alternans, especially after exercise. Other clinical peculiarities in the appearance of the pulsus alternans have been studied by Windle in his papers on the subject, which are well worth reading.

MACKENZIE   S

Cause of the pulsus alternans.—F. B. Hoffmann attributed the production of alternation to an impairment of the function of contractility, the contractions which produce the large beat being so long that the period of rest of the following beat is encroached upon. In consequence of the shorter rest, the second beat is smaller and shorter in duration, so that the rest preceding the next beat is large and gives rise to a stronger and longer beat, and so the alternation goes on. Muskens, Hering, and others suggested that all the muscle fibres do not contract in the production of the smaller beat, that there is an intermuscular block, so that some fibres only contract with each second beat. Einthoven and Lewis, examining

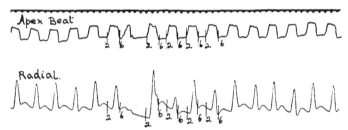

Fig. 149. Simultaneous tracings of the apex and radial. After an extra-systole the alternating character of the radial pulse becomes more marked. Notwithstanding the marked difference in size of the radial beats due to the alternation, there is no difference in the size or duration of the apex beats—in marked contrast to the apex beat caused by the extra-systole.

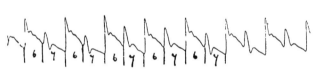

Fig. 150. Tracing of the pulsus bigeminus due to extra-systoles. The period between the big beat and the small is six-tenths of a second, and the period between the small beat and the big is seven-tenths of a second. (Compare with Fig. 145.)

cases of alternation by means of the electrocardiograph, could find no evidence of a variation of the duration of the systole, nor any change in the electric discharge which would indicate a variation in the amount of the muscle fibres participating in the contraction. Moreover, tracings of the apex beat show no difference in the character or duration of the beats (Fig. 149). It would seem, then, that so far, the real cause of this irregularity has escaped detection.

Differential diagnosis.—There are some pulses which bear a surprising resemblance to the pulsus alternans. The one for which it is most commonly mistaken is the pulsus bigeminus, already described in Chapter XXVII. Here the smaller beat is due to an extra-systole and is always premature, and is followed by a prolonged pause. The difference is well brought out by comparing Fig. 145 and 150. In Fig. 150 the interval between the big beat and the small beat is $\frac{6}{10}$ of a second, while between the small beat and the big beat it is $\frac{7}{10}$ of a second. In the pulsus alternans, in Fig. 145, the time between the large and the small beat is the same as that between the small and the large beat. Another somewhat rare form of resemblance is found in Fig. 151. This was taken from a healthy, vigorous man of 50, who complained of some dyspeptic symptoms. I had known for twenty years that he had a slow pulse, but I was surprised to see the apparent alternating character when taking a tracing. Listening to the heart, I detected, after each big beat, two short sharp sounds, characteristic of an extra-systole, and the explanation, therefore, was that an extra-systole occurred after every second normal beat, but of such weak force that no wave reached

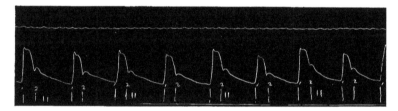

FIG. 151. Radial tracing simulating the pulsus alternans. On auscultation there were heard two short sharp sounds characteristic of extra-systoles after the large heat, but not after the small. These sounds are represented by the short lines in the tracing.

the radial. But the occurrence of the extra-systole had in some way caused a weakening of the following normal beat. Wardrop Griffith describes a somewhat similar experience.

Prognosis.—Before giving a prognosis in cases showing the pulsus alternans, we must have clearly in our minds the condition which produced it. Should it occur in the course of a persistent or paroxysmal tachycardia, it does not seem to have any very serious import. Thus the tracing in Fig. 117 was taken four years ago from a man with frequent attacks, yet they have not interfered with his following his work as a carpenter, during the intervening years, and he shows no signs of heart failure.

It is in cases where it arises with a normal action of the heart that it is of the most significance. It is invariably associated with some degree of heart exhaustion, and usually this is very considerable. In the great majority, the exhaustion is the outcome of such extensive degeneration and enfeeblement of the heart muscle that it must be looked upon as of very grave significance. This is particularly so where attacks of angina pectoris or Cheyne-Stokes respiration are also present ; the combination of such phenomena being invariably associated with such exhaustion of the heart muscle that a fatal issue may occur at any period.

The pulsus alternans may appear in less advanced cases, and with appropriate treatment, especially rest, a wonderful amount of recovery may take place, and the patient may lead a useful life for an indefinite number of years. But these individuals are always in peril, as a slight febrile attack is apt to put a greater strain on the heart than it can bear.

The pulsus alternans need not be present in any marked degree, for some of the most speedily fatal cases have only shown its presence for one or two beats after an extra-systole.

I was led to the recognition of the gravity of the prognosis in pulsus alternans by the following circumstance. In differentiating the different forms of irregularity, I had placed in a group a number of cases where the rhythm was regular, but the size of the beat varied in a regular manner, and I published a certain number of tracings in my book on the pulse in 1902. In 1905, Wenckebach called attention to these tracings, and pointed out how they differed from other forms of irregularity. When I saw his account, I started to re-examine all my patients who had shown this condition (about a dozen), and I found they were all dead. From this time I began to keep more careful records of the life history of those showing this irregularity, and now have records of over 100 cases, and it is upon the results of these cases I have based the prognosis given. In a recently published paper, Windle has described how he watched cases of pulsus alternans, and the majority died within two years of its detection, and his results agree with mine.

Treatment.—As the pulsus alternans is but a sign associated with other conditions, the treatment should be guided by those conditions. When not associated with an abnormal rhythm, its chief indication is a careful regulation of the patient's manner of life, so that he lives well within the limits of his heart's strength.

CHAPTER XXXIV

AFFECTIONS OF THE CONDUCTING FUNCTIONS OF THE AURICULO-
VENTRICULAR BUNDLE (HEART-BLOCK, ADAMS-STOKES DISEASE,
VENTRICULAR RHYTHM)

Definition.
Methods of recognizing depression of conductivity.
The intersystolic period (*a–c* interval).
Depression of conductivity without arrhythmia.
Missed beats due to depression of conductivity.
Independent ventricular rhythm due to heart-block.
Effect of the auricular contraction on the radial pulse.
Ætiology.
Significance of the milder forms of depression of conductivity.
Symptoms associated with heart-block.
Prognosis.
Treatment.

Definition.—The different forms of irregular action of the heart described in the previous chapters, have been due to the contraction starting at some place other than the normal pacemaker (the sino-auricular node), because the abnormal place started the contractions at a more rapid pace. In this chapter, the abnormal action dealt with is due to the stimulus from the pacemaker failing to reach the ventricle. The stimulus for contraction reaches the ventricle from the auricle, by passing along the bundle that connects the auricle and ventricle (Fig. 2 and 3). This bundle may be so affected that (1) the stimulus is delayed ; (2) the stimulus is at times prevented from crossing over ; (3) the stimulus may be completely blocked beyond the auriculo-ventricular node, and the ventricle then contracts in response to a stimulus that arises in the uninjured remains of the auriculo-ventricular bundle (heart-block, ventricular rhythm).

Methods of recognizing depression of conductivity.—Apart from suitable tracings, the clinical evidence is limited to the recognition of an advanced affection when there is a slow radial pulse, or, better, a slow ventricular rate, while the veins in the neck pulsate more frequently, owing to the normal rate of the auricular contractions being maintained. If the ventricular contractions are over thirty-six per minute, these may have a distinct relationship to the auricular waves in the jugular pulse, the ventricle responding to every second, third, or fourth auricular contraction.

When the ventricular contractions are about thirty or under, they are usually independent of the auricle, and auricle and ventricle beat at independent rates and in response to independent stimuli. In many cases, the ventricular rate may be considerably higher (Fig. 165).

When there is a mere delay in the response of the ventricle to the stimulus from the auricle, the evidence is very scanty, apart from graphic records. I have, however, in cases of mitral stenosis been able to recognize this delay by a slight separation of the presystolic murmur from the first sound of the heart, what is sometimes spoken of as a mid-diastolic murmur. Occasionally 'missed beats', or pulse intermissions, are due to the auricular stimulus failing to provoke a ventricular contraction, and a suspicion of the nature of this irregularity may be aroused by observing that during the pause the ventricular sounds are absent ; this distinguishes it from most cases of extra-systole, in which, as has already been described, there are usually heard two short, sharp sounds, the result of the weak, short, premature contraction of the ventricle. As, however, extra-systoles may occur with no audible sound, this distinction is not reliable. In tracings of the radial pulse alone, Wenckebach was able to recognize the nature of the irregularity by an ingenious method of measurement. No difficulty is presented, as a general rule, when tracings of the radial pulse or apex beat are taken at the same time as tracings of the jugular pulse. The slighter forms of this affection are recognized by the delay that occurs between the auricular and ventricular systoles. In the jugular tracings, as has already been shown, there is usually present a wave (a), due to the auricular systole, followed at a short interval by the carotid wave (c). This interval between a and c, is of great value in estimating the condition of the con-ductivity in the primitive tissue.

The intersystolic period (a–c interval).—This interval is occupied by three events, namely, (1) the systole of the auricle ; (2) the transmission of the stimulus from auricle to ventricle ; (3) a minute portion of time during which the ventricular pressure is rising before opening the semilunar valves (Anspannungszeit, or presphygmic interval). As 3 is practically constant, it may for the purpose of this inquiry be ignored, and assuming that the stimulus for contraction starts on its way to the ventricle at the beginning of auricular systole, any variation in the length of the a–c interval is due to the variation of the rate of stimulus conduction.

In normal hearts, I have found that the a–c interval is fairly constant, lasting usually one-fifth of a second (as in Fig. 52). It is a little shorter in frequent action of the heart.

Depression of conductivity without arrhythmia.—While the a–c interval may be considered normal when it does not exceed one-fifth of a second, considerable increase of this interval may take place with no interference with the rhythm of the heart.

In Fig. 152, there is a tracing of the jugular pulse taken at the same time as the radial pulse. The radial shows a perfectly regular rhythm,

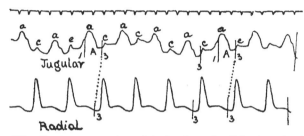

FIG. 152.   Simultaneous tracings of the jugular and radial pulses, showing a wide *a–c* interval (space *A*) due to senile cardio-sclerosis.

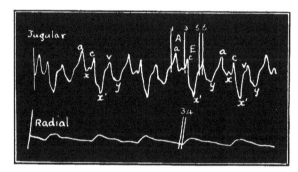

FIG. 153.   Shows a great increase in the *a–c* interval (space *A*) due to a delay in the stimulus passing from auricle to ventricle (Case 44, taken 1892).

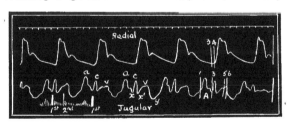

FIG. 153 A.   Shows an increased *a–c* interval, nearly two-fifths of a second in duration (space *A*). The shading shows the position of the murmurs—a short murmur due to the auricular systole, the loudest part of which is separated from the first sound by a brief interval, a murmur following the first sound, and another following the second sound running up to the presystolic (or auricular systolic) murmur (Case 44, taken 1903).

while the neck tracing shows a great increase in the *a–c* interval (space *A*). The heart may continue to beat perfectly regularly for years with the conductivity affected to this extent. Thus, Fig. 153 A was taken in 1903 from the same patient from whom Fig. 153 was taken in 1892, and the jugular tracing shows a like increase of the a–c interval (space A). Except for a short period in 1898, this patient's pulse was quite regular up to 1904.

Arrhythmia of a marked character arises when the conductivity is so grievously depressed that the stimulus occasionally, or frequently, fails to cross the auriculo-ventricular junction. How this occurs is well seen

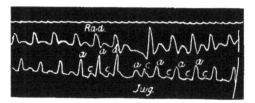

FIG. 154. Shows a gradual lengthening of the a–c interval till the stimulus from the auricle at a' reaches the auriculo-ventricular bundle before the latter has recovered from the previous stimulation, and finds it 'refractory'. The ventricle, therefore, does not respond to this stimulus, but remains quiescent till the next physiological stimulus comes from the auricle, and the conductivity being restored the ventricular beat (c) follows the auricular wave at a shorter interval. Note the increasing size of the a wave before the intermission. This is due to the auricular systole falling at the same time as the preceding ventricular systole, so that the auricular contents cannot be sent into the ventricle, but a bigger wave is sent back into the veins.

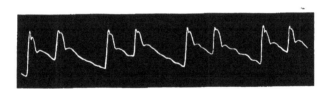

FIG. 155. Regularly intermitting pulse due to depression of conductivity
(Case 44, 1898).

in Fig. 154. There is a constant delay in the conduction of the stimulus here, the a–c interval being unduly prolonged. Before the intermission, there is a slight but gradual increase of the a–c interval. After the auricular wave a', there is no carotid wave c nor pulse-beat in the radial. The reason for this is manifestly that the auricular systole a' occurred so soon after the previous ventricular systole (as evidenced by the carotid wave c immediately before a'), that there was not sufficient time for the recovery of the function of stimulus conduction in the auriculo-ventricular bundle, and hence the stimulus failed to reach the ventricle, and a beat dropped out. By this means a longer rest was procured for these fibres, and when the next stimulus comes down from the auricle the longer rest has so restored the function of conductivity that the *a–c* interval, following the pause, is shorter than the average. This dropping out of ventricular beats may occur at regular intervals. Fig. 155 was taken in 1898 from the patient from whom Fig. 153 and 153 A were taken. For many years tracings from this patient showed constant depression of the conductivity. For some reason, in 1898, the conductivity became further depressed, so that at regular intervals a

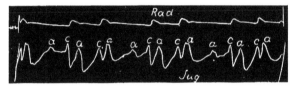

FIG. 156. Taken at the same visit as Fig. 155, and shows the venous pulse during the arrhythmia. The wave *a* is quite regular in its appearance. For the interpretation of this tracing see diagram, Fig. 157.

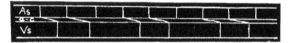

FIG. 157. Diagram constructed to show that the irregularity in Figs. 155 and 156 is due to a blocking of the conductivity at the fibres joining auricle and ventricle. Note the increased length of the *a–c* interval before the pause in the *Vs*.

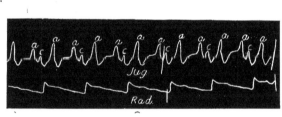

FIG. 158. The ventricle only responds to every alternate auricular systole—ventricular rate 48, auricular rate 96.

ventricular beat dropped out (Fig. 155). The true nature of this arrhythmia is shown in the jugular tracing (Fig. 156), where the auricle is shown to contract regularly (wave *a*), while the ventricle fails to respond to every third auricular systole. To demonstrate this more clearly, I reconstruct Fig. 156 in the form of a diagram (Fig. 157). The downstrokes in the upper division represent the auricular systole (*As*), those in the lowest the ventricular systoles (*Vs*), and correspond with the radial and carotid pulses in Fig. 155 and 156. The slanting lines represent the *a–c* interval. It will be seen that a ventricular beat drops out regularly after every third auricular systole.

Missed beats due to depression of conductivity.—Gaskell states that on applying a screw clamp around the auriculo-ventricular groove of a frog's heart, ' according to the tightness of the clamp the ventricle can be made to beat synchronously with the auricles, to respond to every second contraction of the auricle, to respond to every third, fourth, or other contraction, or to remain quiescent.' Hering and Erlanger have recently produced the same changes in the mammalian heart. All these varying results can be demonstrated to occur in the human heart.

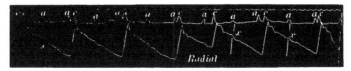

Fig. 159. Is from a slow, irregular pulse after influenza, and the jugular tracing shows that the slow pulse is due to the ventricle failing to respond to the stimulus from the auricle. Note that after the short pulse period in the radial, the a–c interval is much longer than at the other periods. This is because the fibres have had a short rest, and the conductivity has in consequence not been completely restored. Note also at x a slight depression in the radial tracing, due to the systole of the left auricle affecting the arterial column.

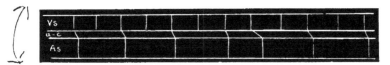

Fig. 160. Diagram of Fig. 159, showing the blocking of the stimulus after every second auricular systole, except in one instance when it gets through, with a lengthened a–c interval.

In Fig. 154, the ventricular systole is seen to drop out at rare intervals ; in Fig. 156, the ventricular systole drops out after every third auricular systole (3 : 2 rhythm) ; in Fig. 158, after every second (2 : 1 rhythm). In Fig. 159, the ventricular systole usually drops out after every second auricular systole ; but there is one short pulse period, and the a–c interval here is much longer than the a–c period after the longer periods, the lengthening being an evidence that the conducting power of the auriculo-ventricular fibres has not had time to recover as effectually, as after the longer pulse periods (see diagram, Fig. 160). In Fig. 161, there are three auricular contractions to one ventricular (3 : 1 rhythm), except during the last two arterial pulse periods, when there are but two auricular waves, and after the second of these the a–c interval is longer than the other a–c intervals in this tracing.

In Fig. 162, there are four auricular beats to one ventricular. This blocking may be so extreme that the auricle may beat ten or twelve times and the ventricle stand still.

In the tracings given so far, it has not been difficult to make out the feature in the tracing from the neck. When there is a large carotid pulse, as in aortic

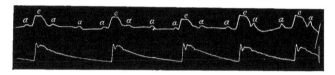

FIG. 161. Here the tracing from the neck shows sometimes three auricular waves (a) to one carotid wave (c). In the last two periods there are but two auricular waves, and the a–c interval is longer than in the periods when there are three auricular waves, because in the former case the conductivity has not had so long a time to be restored.

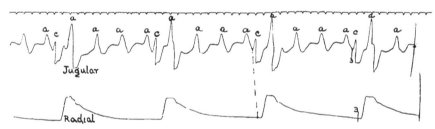

FIG. 162. Tracing from a case of heart-block. There are four auricular beats to one ventricular (4:1 rhythm).

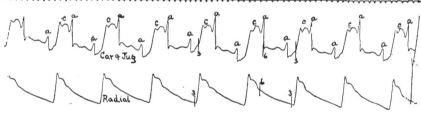

FIG. 163. Tracings from a patient with aortic regurgitation and partial heart-block. The waves a are regular, and the difference in their appearance is due to their time relation to the large carotid pulse (2:1 rhythm).

regurgitation, the feature of the tracing may be somewhat puzzling, as in Fig. 163, which shows two auricular beats to one carotid, the different position of the a wave depending on the period of movement in the carotid artery.

Independent ventricular rhythm due to heart-block.—In the tracings I have given so far, it could be shown that when the ventricle does contract it is in response to a stimulus from the auricle. When a ligature is applied in the auriculo-ventricular groove of the frog's heart, so that the stimulus can be conveyed no longer from auricle to ventricle, the latter beats, after a time, with a rhythm different from, and independent of, that of the auricle (complete heart-block). Wooldridge and Tigerstedt produced complete independence of the auricular and ventricular rhythms, by physiologically separating the auricles from the ventricles, while a similar result

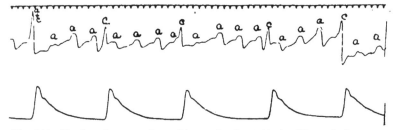

Fig. 164. Tracings from a patient with complete heart-block. The auricular waves, *a*, show a varying relation to the carotid waves, *c*, and to the radial pulse, due to the auricles pursuing one rhythm and the ventricles another (Case 78).

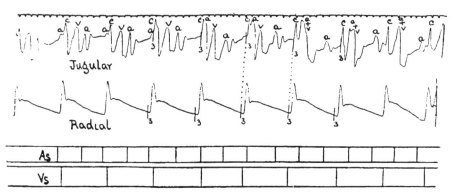

Fig. 165. Tracings from a man aged 22, with complete heart-block—the ventricular rate being 42 per minute. The diagram shows the independence of the auricular and ventricular rhythms (Case 77).

has been attained by His, jr., Hering and Erlanger, through compression of the auriculo-ventricular bundle. Erlanger has produced complete heart-block experimentally in dogs, and the dogs have lived for many months, with symptoms identical with those found in human subjects suffering from heart-block. This independent rhythm can be demonstrated as the cause of certain forms of a slow pulse-rate in the human subject. Fig. 164 is a tracing of the radial taken at the same time as the pulsation in the neck due to the jugular and carotid. The small waves, *a*, are due to the right auricle, and there are a varying number of these auricular waves to one carotid or radial pulse-beat. When one carefully analyses their relationship, it is found that the relationship of the auricular systole to the ventricular systole is a constantly varying one, sometimes at a distance, and then gradually approaching till they are synchronous. As a rule, in complete heart-block, as shown in Fig. 164, the rate is rarely above 32 per minute, but there are now on record a number of cases in which the ventricular rate has been as high as 60 beats per minute. In Fig. 165, the rate is 42 per minute (Case 77).

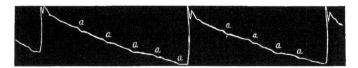

FIG. 166.   From Webster's case of heart-block, showing in the falling line of the radial tracing a series of interruptions (*a*) due to the left auricle.

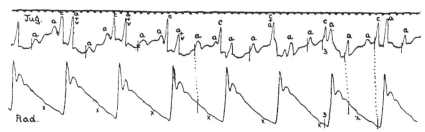

FIG. 167.   Tracing from a patient with complete heart-block, showing the effects of the auricular systole on the radial pulse (×).

Effect of the auricular contraction on the radial pulse.—The auricular systoles can sometimes be recognized in another way in tracings of the radial pulse, where, during a long ventricular pause, a series of notches can be seen occurring at regular intervals on the descending line of the radial tracing, as in Fig. 166. If a jugular tracing be taken at the same time, there will be found auricular beats occurring exactly at the same time as these notches, as is shown in Fig. 159 and 167. From this I suggest that those notches in Fig. 166 are due to the movement of the left auricle, the systole of the left auricle pressing against the aortic valves and temporarily affecting the arterial column. The sudden cessation of this pressure causes a slight but abrupt fall in the aortic pressure, giving rise to the notches in the radial tracing.

Ætiology.—Except in cases of complete heart-block, the anatomical changes have not been fully worked out. In the majority of the cases of heart-block examined post mortem, damage of the auriculo-ventricular bundle at or beyond the auriculo-ventricular node has been found, due to acute inflammatory changes, or to sclerotic changes, or to the presence of gummata. In the milder cases, one can only infer the cause. From Gaskell's experiments, we know that if the bridge of muscle connecting the auricle and ventricle be narrowed, the stimulus takes longer in passing. We know also that in rheumatic affections of the heart numerous deposits of cells occur in the muscle substance. As it is in rheumatic heart cases and hearts affected by degenerative changes in the muscle, that I have found most of the milder forms of depressed conductivity (Cases 44, 91, and 92), I infer that when such deposits occur, or when a slight cicatrization takes place, the bundle is injured, and so the function of conductivity is impaired. In other acute affections of the heart, we get evidence of the implication of this bundle in the diseased process. More and more is becoming known of heart-block in febrile affections of the heart, and a number of cases have been recorded of partial and complete block in such affections as influenza, pneumonia, rheumatic fever. In fibrous degeneration of the heart muscle, we may find evidence of impaired conductivity, and even heart-block in an individual who has shown extra-systoles and auricular fibrillation.

Several cases have been reported where the damage to the bundle was due to gummata, and the recovery of other cases, under anti-syphilitic treatment, indicates that syphilis may be an agent in the production of complete heart-block; and in Chapter XXXVII I refer to involvement of the bundle in sub-acute rheumatism and give illustrative cases (Cases 85–9).

In complete heart-block, the auriculo-ventricular node may be either destroyed or separated from the remainder of the auriculo-ventricular bundle. The remains of the bundle in the ventricle beyond the auriculo-ventricular node have been found perfectly normal, in a case described by Keith, in which there was a history of complete heart-block for eighteen years. Seeing that the bundle was healthy, it must have had some function during life, and as it did not convey stimuli from auricle to ventricle, it must have had some other function, which I suggest was stimulus production and the maintenance of the slow ventricular rate. This view is supported by the fact that the electrocardiograph shows that the stimulus for contraction enters the heart by the normal path.

There is a great defect in our knowledge of the condition leading up to heart-block. Before the slow ventricular rhythm becomes permanent, in many people there are periods in which, though the rhythm of the heart is normal, there is frequently an increased a–c interval; and ventricular systoles may drop out, at intervals more or less regular and frequent. Some people may have attacks of giddiness, or slight loss of consciousness on effort, due to a transient block, one of the early stages of this complaint.

Dr. Lewis has called my attention to a peculiar condition in a few patients whom I had sent for electrocardiographic examination, in which

I had recognized a delay in the transmission of the stimulus from auricle to ventricle. From the character of the electric record, he found that the contraction of the left ventricle had preceded that of the right (normally the right ventricle starts before the left). From this he inferred that the right branch of the bundle was destroyed. When he asked me for particulars of the clinical condition, I found that I had noted a reduplication of the first sound and an increased a–c interval.

The possibility of vagal stimulation taking part in the production of heart-block must be borne in mind. Stimulation of the vagus can produce a similar action of the heart, as Chauveau pointed out. I give tracings (Fig. 258 and 259) where a mild form of heart-block was produced by a reflex stimulation of the vagus by swallowing (Case 91). Digitalis may also produce it (see p. 373).

Significance of the milder forms of depression of conductivity.—It must not be thought that the foregoing facts are merely of academic interest. Their recognition and appreciation clear up many obscurities surrounding heart affections, and are of practical importance in treatment. As will be shown, in acute and subacute affections of the heart, the presence of the irregularity due to this cause, indicates that the muscle is being invaded by the disease. When it occurs without any irregularity, the increased a–c interval is of importance in the administration of such drugs as digitalis. I have rarely failed in such cases in increasing the a–c interval, and causing the dropping out of ventricular systoles by the administration of digitalis; and the recognition of this form of irregularity produced by digitalis is of importance, as an indication that a sufficiency of the drug has been taken. But it must not be assumed that in producing this slight increase in the heart-block, danger has been incurred, or that the heart-block is a contra-indication to the use of digitalis.

Symptoms associated with heart-block.—Apart from the characteristic irregularity, and the slow ventricular rhythm with its associated syncopal attacks, there are no characteristics. Patients with a pulse-rate of thirty to forty beats per minute may go about their affairs, but quietly—the field of response being distinctly limited. The manner of limitation is varied; in some it is a sense of weakness, in others it is breathlessness on exertion, the feet feeling heavy and the knees stiff. In some, exertion induces giddiness. These symptoms are due to the ventricle not responding to the exertion, as already explained, and therefore not pumping enough blood to the organs. The picture given by the late Sir W. T. Gairdner, a sufferer from heart-block, of his own experiences, is very characteristic of some cases. ' I am wonderfully free '—he wrote me four years after the slow rhythm began, and two years before his death at the age of 82, his pulse-rate then being 30 per minute—' from all the symptoms that usually go along with organic heart-disease. My sleep is almost always undisturbed, and I get abundance of it, both by day and night, nor is there the slightest trace of angina pectoris, severe dyspnœa, dropsy, or any of the usual accidents of prolonged cardiac disease.' He wrote later: 'Although a little uncertain in my gait, I can go from one room to another or even up a simple stair, taking plenty of time and assisted by the railing ; but for the last two years at least, if not more, my position has been, with few exceptions, recumbent, or at most sitting, and repeated attempts have shown me that it is practically impossible to cross the street or to go into the garden opposite the house except in a wheeled armchair ; and along with this there is a feeling of perpetual weariness which never leaves me even after the soundest sleep, and which is not explained by any pain or suffering, though in itself it often tends to fits of yawning and even exclamations which would sound to others as if I was suffering inwardly.'

The syncopal and epileptiform attacks, due to cerebral anæmia, induced by the slow action or temporary stoppage of the ventricles (Adams-Stokes syndrome), have been described on p. 49. This tendency to infrequent action may appear in affections of the bundle at two stages, namely, before the permanent establishment of the independent ventricular rhythm and after its establishment. While there are intermittent periods of complete heart-block, there is a certain liability to these syncopal attacks, and the following appears to me to be the reason. After a Stannius' ligature is applied between auricle and ventricle, the ventricle stands still for a longer or shorter period before it starts on its own rhythm. The principle under-lying this is that when a rapid rhythm ceases and is replaced by a slower rhythm of a different origin, the slower rhythm remains quiescent for a brief period before it takes up its own rhythm (see Chapter XXIX). In certain cases of heart-block, the stimulus to contraction passing from auricle to ventricle may suddenly stop, and the ventricle pause for a brief period before it starts its own contraction. It is during this period that the syncopal attacks occur. Thus Sir W. T. Gairdner noticed that his attacks always came on with the sudden dropping of his pulse-rate : ' These cardiac and cerebral attacks were at one time so frequent that I think from twenty to thirty of them were numbered in twenty-four hours.' His pulse-rate would be 70 per minute, and after his syncopal attack he invariably found it at or below 30 per minute. When the pulse subsided to a permanent rate of 20 to 30 per minute, the cerebral attacks disappeared. My reading of this description is that while the block was partial, the stimulus at times got through from the auricle, and the rate of the pulse rose to 70 ; then the stimulus suddenly failed to get through, and the ventricle paused for a brief period, as it does on first applying the Stannius' ligature, anæmia of the brain resulted, and the patient fainted. On the ventricle starting its own rhythm, the circulation of the brain was restored, and the patient, recovering, found his pulse at the rate of 30 per minute. When, however, the block became permanent, the ventricle went on at its slow, independent rate, with no pauses, and therefore with no syncopal attacks. As a rule, before the block becomes complete and the ventricle takes up its own rhythm, there is a period of partial block during which the ventricle may fail to respond to several auricular beats. Thus in Fig. 168, there is a long ventricular pause during which there are seven auricular beats. Previous to this there had been no attacks or loss of consciousness, and I warned the patient's doctor that they might occur. Two days later she fell unconscious in the street. Sometimes the attacks arise with greater frequency than mentioned from Sir W. Gairdner's experiences. One patient, for instance, had attacks for ten days coming on every few minutes. Thus I sat by his side taking tracings continuously for one hour and a half, and during that time he had fifty attacks of loss of consciousness, and fifteen slight epileptiform seizures. When the ventricle stood still for about 10

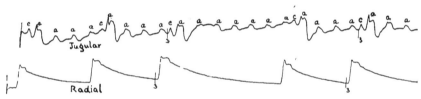

FIG. 168.   Shows partial block with a prolonged standstill of the ventricle. This was taken two days before the patient's first attack of loss of consciousness.

seconds, he became unconscious, and when it stood still for 16 seconds, he had convulsive movements. The standstill rarely exceeded 20 seconds at one time.

While these attacks were on, the patient's condition was very characteristic. He would be talking quietly, when he suddenly ceased and shut his eyes, and his breathing stopped. With the return of the pulse he would recover, slightly confused, and would resume the conversation. If the ventricle stood still a little longer, the muscles of the face would begin to twitch, then the arms, and he would breathe heavily, so that with the previous stopping of the respiration and the subsequent heavy breathing, a sort of Cheyne-Stokes respiration would appear. If the ventricle started off after 18 seconds, the patient would at once return to consciousness and seem confused. When he recovered after the convulsive attacks he was conscious of twitching of his face.

Syncopal attacks may appear when the rate is constant at 30 and under. In such cases, there may be a greater infrequency of the heart's action, the rate falling sometimes as low as 5 beats per minute, or there may be multiple extra-systoles for a period during which the output is insufficient to maintain consciousness. During this time, they may go from one convulsion into another and the face becomes dusky, and if the ventricle stands still too long, they die.

From the patient's sensations of an attack, I quote the following letter, written by an old friend of mine who suffered from Adams-Stokes syndrome due to auricular fibrillation and heart-block, the pulse-rate usually being 30 per minute (Case 81):

' At your request I try to give you a description of an extraordinary swoon I had whilst suffering under heart trouble. It happened in the middle of the night. I awoke from a quiet sleep feeling a most curious creepy sensation ; my functions all seemed to be stopping, and in front of me, about two feet from the floor, appeared a circular light about two inches in diameter, and brilliant beyond anything I had ever seen before. I thought the period of my dissolution had arrived. I was perfectly calm, and I began to reason with myself whether I should waken my wife (I don't know whether I should have had strength ; I was turned from her at the time), in which case she would be greatly alarmed, or leave things to take their course. Before my mind was made up what to do, the light began to contract, and when it was reduced to about half its original size suddenly went out, but before entirely losing consciousness I had such a feeling of peace and restfulness as I never experienced before, and had just time to say to myself, " There is no after-life anyway."

' How long I lay in that condition of course I don't know, but when I did come to, I felt it utterly impossible to move : I might have been a leaden image, I felt such a weight. For a long time I persevered in trying to move a limb. At last I got a little life in one of my feet, and then gradually the use of all my limbs.'

Cheyne-Stokes respiration may appear in patients suffering from heart-block.

A curious feature in cases of heart-block is that circumstances that usually excite the heart to rapid action, have little effect upon the independent ventricular rhythm. Causes of excitement, and the administration of alcohol or chloroform, have very slight or no effect on the ventricle, though the auricular contractions may be rendered much more frequent.

Prognosis.—In the milder cases, where there is a delay in the stimulus passing from auricle to ventricle, or where there may be occasionally the characteristic irregularity caused by the dropping out of a ventricular systole, no grave conditions arise. Its recognition, however, warns us that myocardial changes are involved, and the prognosis must be based on other evidences of myocardial degeneration, and especially on its functional efficiency. By itself partial heart-block has little bearing on the cardiac efficiency (see Case 44). Patients with mild forms of heart-block, even where the pulse is continuously about 30, may lead quiet, uneventful lives for ten or twenty years. But in these cases, one can reasonably infer that the rest of the heart muscle has escaped damage. When there is marked impairment of the heart's efficiency before the onset of complete heart-block, then the prognosis becomes grave. When there is a tendency to syncopal attacks, at the stage between partial and complete heart-block, the danger from a prolonged standstill is not great unless there is advanced degeneration of the heart muscle. But with recurrent syncopal attacks in complete heart-block, then the patient's life is uncertain, as such patients usually die in one of these attacks, often being found dead in bed or elsewhere. Death may arise from muscle failure due to degenerative change in the heart muscle, preceded by objective symptoms of heart failure, as œdema of the lungs and dropsy. The condition of the heart muscle, as shown by its efficiency, is the chief element in prognosis. Case 78 had a very limited field of cardiac response.

Treatment.—We occasionally meet with cases where, after repeated attacks of syncope and long-continued slow pulse, the conducting power is restored and the rate becomes normal. But considering the pathological change producing these cases, it will be realized how futile it is, except in syphilitic cases, to attempt to give remedies to cure. Not infrequently partial heart-block of varying degree may be present in acute and subacute affections, and it may completely disappear with the recovery of the patient from the affection (Case 87). In chronic cases, as the milder forms of heart-block imply degenerative change in the heart muscle, the treatment is guided by that condition more than by the lesion in the bundle. When the heart-block begins to interfere with the functional efficiency of the heart, then care should be taken not to expose the heart to too great a strain. If attacks of syncope appear, the patient must be kept at perfect rest till the tendency passes off, and until time has shown that they have ceased the patient should not go about without an attendant. In a few cases, the attacks seem to be brought on by vagal stimulation, and then the administration of atropine (1/50 gr. hypodermically) may be used to diminish their frequency. We must recognize our helplessness, as a rule, in preventing the attacks of loss of consciousness during the periods of frequent occurrence and in restoring a patient during a long attack. I have for years been trying to find a means which would increase the rate of the ventricle in heart-block or diminish the liability to the attacks, but I have failed. Sometimes I have fancied one thing helped and then another, but when carefully tested they have failed me, so that when the attacks cease, the cessation is due to circumstances which we do not control. I mention this failure in order that we may prosecute inquiries with the specific object of finding a remedy which will stimulate the ventricle to action in heart-block.

If a history of syphilis is obtained, and if there is a positive Wassermann reaction, then the energetic use of antisyphilitic remedies should be tried.

When the heart-block becomes permanent, the heart muscle may be so efficient that the patient may live for a great many years, and such patients

T 2

should be enjoined to live within the limits of their strength, being guided by the ease with which they can undertake effort. Heart failure with dropsy may occur, and then the treatment should follow the lines indicated in the chapter on treatment. Here I may say that the heart-block is not a contra-indication to the digitalis group of remedies; rather does it indicate them, for they act in strengthening the muscle and do not slow the ventricular rate.

(Cases of auricular fibrillation and heart-block seem not to be infrequent, and a series of cases are recorded in the appendix (Cases 79, 80, and 81). The relation between auricular flutter and heart-block has been dealt with (Chapter XXXI).)

CHAPTER XXXV

ACUTE FEBRILE AFFECTIONS OF THE HEART

Manner in which the heart is affected in fever.
The febrile heart.
Acute febrile affections of the heart.
Symptoms in myocarditis.
Symptoms in endocarditis.
Symptoms in pericarditis.
The heart in rheumatic fever.
The heart in pneumonia.
The heart in diphtheria.
Septic infections.
Prognosis.
Treatment.

Manner in which the heart is affected in fever.—In considering the state of the circulation in febrile conditions, it is necessary to bear in mind three facts, viz. that the heart's action is modified by an increase in temperature, that the heart reacts differently according to the toxins produced by the agent causing the fever, and finally, that the heart itself may be the seat of the conditions causing the fever. Recent researches demonstrate conclusively the invasion of the heart by the specific organism in rheumatic fever, pneumonia, typhoid fever, diphtheria, erysipelas, influenza, and various septic infections. The results of such invasion are shown in the occurrence of endocarditis, myocarditis, and pericarditis. The symptoms evoked in such invasions are not always distinctive, and may resemble the symptoms induced in the heart by febrile conditions alone, or by toxins produced from other sources in the body. I dwell upon this because an attempt should always be made in febrile conditions to judge rightly the effects on the heart. One cannot but be struck, for instance, by the fact that people with previously seriously damaged hearts may pass scatheless through severe attacks of pneumonia or typhoid fever, while the young and vigorous may succumb after a few days' illness on account of the implication of the heart in the disease.

Another point to bear in mind is that in the invasion of the heart the specific organism rarely affects one tissue alone. In order to be exact and methodical, writers usually describe separately the symptoms of endocarditis, myocarditis, and pericarditis. But if one reflects on the nature of the symptoms, such as the condition of the pulse, its strength, rate, and rhythm, the size of the heart, and the præcordial distress—symptoms which are usually included in the description of endocarditis and pericarditis—it will be realized that they are not really the manifestations of endocarditis or pericarditis, but are the signs of a myocardial affection. One must consider carefully the murmurs arising in the course of a febrile attack, even in rheumatic fever, for the presence of a murmur may not necessarily mean the invasion of the mitral valves by the inflammatory process, but may be due to the tonicity of the poisoned heart muscle failing and giving rise to incompetence of the mitral orifice—due, therefore, not to an endo-cardial, but to a myocardial affection. Endocarditis and pericarditis, both acute and chronic, bulk so largely in medical literature only because an abnormal sound invariably impresses the mind more than an abnormal sign perceptible by the other senses, and the easy recognition of the valvular murmur and the friction sound has led to the associated symptoms being ascribed to the same lesion.

The febrile heart.—By this term, I mean the changes induced by the rise in temperature. The whole circulatory apparatus is remarkably sensi-tive to alterations in temperature, whether arising from external sources or due to changes within the body. The most striking of these is the change in rate—a rise in temperature increasing the rate, and a fall diminishing it. In the more simple febrile affections, there is a certain correspondence between the height of the temperature and the rate of the heart's con-traction. Roughly speaking, there is an increase of from eight to ten beats with a rise of temperature of one degree F. This does not hold universally, but any considerable departure from this rule should always arouse watch-fulness and suggest the possibility of other complications, such as the involvement of the heart in the infection.

In the simple febrile heart, the radial artery enlarges and the pulse remains of good strength, particularly during the diastolic phase of the cardiac cycle. The heart itself shows little change at first, beyond having its rate abnor-mally accelerated by exertion. The sounds are clear and distinct, and there is no increase in size. With long continuation of the fever, a certain amount of dilatation may arise. This most readily occurs on the right side of the heart, particularly if the pulmonary circulation is interfered with, as by a pneumonia or a pleuritic effusion, or by lying a long time on the back, as during the course of typhoid fever. The sounds may become feeble, or systolic murmurs may develop at the tricuspid and mitral orifices, and the characteristic pulsation of the right heart in the epigas-trium become visible (Fig. 33). In many of the minor febrile attacks, the course is modified by the nature of the toxins generated. A rise of a few degrees of temperature may provoke an undue frequency, 120–140, and with the subsidence of the temperature the rate may speedily fall to normal, leaving no ill effects. A slight rise of temperature may even be accompanied by a fall in the pulse-rate, sometimes, if the patient's pulse is normally a slow one, below 50 per minute. I have found remarkable variation in rate with the same temperature at different times, in the same individual, due probably to a difference in the agent producing the fever. The effects produced by agents other than a rise in temperature cannot perhaps be better illustrated than by those occurring during an attack of ague ; here in the course of twenty-four hours, with a continuously high temperature, we have a remarkable series of changes in the pulse. During the cold stage the pulse becomes small and scarcely perceptible, on account of the contraction of the peripheral arteries. The blood driven from the surface and from the arterial system accumulates in the venous system and in the internal organs. Then the lips and fingers become blue, and the congestion of internal organs may reach such a degree that capillary hæmorrhages occur within them. Within a few hours, the temperature still being high, the arterioles relax, the arteries become larger, and the pulse itself is of considerable force.

Acute febrile affections of the heart.—The lesion induced by the invasion of the heart by specific organisms is rarely limited to one structure or tissue, so that it would be better to use the term carditis than to employ such misleading terms as endocarditis and pericarditis. This will be brought out more clearly when an analysis is made of the symptoms present in any given case ; and I shall endeavour briefly to summarize the symptoms and try to apportion them to the particular tissues affected. I do this here, because by the appreciation of the nature of the primary lesion we are better able to understand the conditions found many years after, when the cicatrizing process has wrought other changes.

Symptoms in myocarditis.—The rate and rhythm are the most easily recognized. Seeing that a rise of temperature alone induces an increased frequency, it is impossible to apportion the relative influences of this and of the myocardial infection. But many cases of moderate fever have a heart-rate greatly accelerated, and then we can infer there is some other factor at work than the rise in temperature. It would be of great interest to know the mechanism by which increased rate is brought about by myocardial lesions, whether through nerve stimulation arising reflexly from the inflamed tissue, or from the increased irritability of the muscle, particularly of the tissue in which the stimulus for contraction arises. But here such an inquiry would be purely speculative.

Changes in rhythm come under a different category, and in irregularity we often get a clue to the changes that are going on in the muscle. The arrhythmia, due to purely nervous influences, is generally abolished during the excitation of the heart by the fever—the chief exception being the arrhythmia, due to vagus stimulation in affections of the brain (as in tubercular meningitis).

The myocardial irregularities have not been as carefully worked out in acute conditions as their importance demands, and the slight advance I have made in the study of the subject shows it to be of the utmost importance if we would understand the pathology of the living heart.

The most characteristic evidence of direct damage done to the muscle of the heart is the irregularity or pulse intermission, due to the dropping out of ventricular systoles, because of the damage done to the auriculo-ventricular bundle by the lesion. There are now on record a considerable number of cases, where the damage to the bundle has been recognized during many forms of acute infection (rheumatic fever, diphtheria, influenza, septic infection).

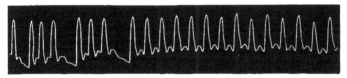

Fig. 169. Irregular pulse in the course of a pneumonia, showing the pulsus alternans in the latter half of the tracing. The intermissions may be due also to failure of contractility.

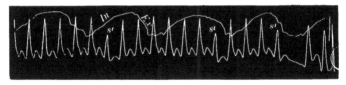

Fig. 170. Tracing of the respiratory curve and of the irregular pulse in the course of a fatal case of pneumonia. The small beats s^1 are probably due to exhausted contractility.

In acute affections of the heart, writers usually content themselves by mentioning irregularity as one of several symptoms, but the instances cited show that if graphic records were taken this condition would be found fairly frequent.

Towards the later stages of fatal pneumonias, I have frequently detected a missed beat or an irregularity. Analysis of a number of these cases has shown that it has probably been due to failure of the power of contraction. Thus a typical example is seen in Fig. 169, where towards the end of the tracing there is shown a marked pulsus alternans. The missed beats in the earlier part of the tracing, I think, are due to the contraction having been so feeble that it failed to propagate a wave into the arteries. Thus we see in Fig. 170, from another case of pneumonia, how the small beats s' arise at the normal interval, but the exhaustion of the heart is so great that it only sends out a small quantity of blood, and after the last small beat it fails altogether to send out a wave. Such signs in pneumonia, I have found always to be of the gravest significance. John Hay has shown a similar arrhythmia in a patient suffering from septic poisoning.

Extra-systoles are of rare occurrence in severe infectious febrile hearts ; but Fig. 171 shows the occurrence of extra-systoles in the course of a fatal attack of rheumatic fever. As there is no compensatory pause, the premature beat is probably of auricular origin.

I have seen in several instances the sudden inception of auricular fibrillation in pneumonia, and always with disastrous results. In one patient whom I saw in consultation, everything seemed to be progressing favourably, but while talking to the doctor in attendance we were suddenly summoned to the bedside of the patient, and found that the heart's action had, in the interval since our seeing him, taken on this abnormal rhythm, and the pulse had become rapid and irregular. The patient died a few hours after. In another case I was called to see, the doctor told me the patient had passed well through an attack of pneumonia terminating by crisis. The day following the fall of temperature the patient suddenly became

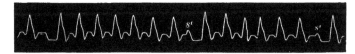

Fig. 171.   Extra-systoles occurring in the course of a fatal attack of rheumatic fever.

weak and ill, and the doctor being summoned found him collapsed. I saw him shortly after and found auricular fibrillation present ; the doctor assured me that he had gone through the pneumonia with a good and regular pulse. He also died a few hours after.

G. A. Sutherland has shown me records of a case of rheumatic fever in a child aged 5, in whom there was auricular fibrillation. The child died, and on examining the heart, Carey Coombs found extensive inflammatory changes in the auricular muscle. In a case of diphtheria, F. W. Price obtained tracings showing the presence of auricular fibrillation and heart-block, and in the post-mortem examination, Ivy Mackenzie found extensive inflammatory changes affecting the auricle and the auriculo-ventricular bundle. The history of Case 64 shows that auricular flutter may arise in acute affections of the heart.

Evidences of myocardial affections can be found in the changes in the size of the heart. The symptoms of dilatation are described in Chapter XXXVIII, but it is well to remember that the size of the heart may very speedily become greatly increased in the course of a febrile affection of the heart, as in rheumatic fever, diphtheria, etc. In such cases, the sounds often become very faint, and soft murmurs may arise at the mitral and tricuspid orifices, and simulate valvular changes.

Symptoms in endocarditis.—The only direct evidence of acute endocarditis is the presence of murmurs at one or other orifice of the heart. For practical purposes there are only two murmurs which need to be considered here, viz. a mitral systolic murmur and an aortic diastolic. It is not always easy to tell whether the appearance of a murmur during a febrile attack is due to involvement of the mitral valve in an endocarditic process, or to the relaxation of the muscle supporting the orifice. A diastolic aortic murmur is, as a rule, diagnostic of the involvement of the aortic valve in some destructive process. At first this murmur is so faint that one is simply conscious of the fact that the sound does not end with sufficient abruptness. Gradually, however, this passes into a very soft short whiff at the end of the second sound, becoming day by day more marked.

In the vast majority of cases, the murmurs due to endocarditis are not definitely recognized until some time after the subsidence of the fever— when the sclerosis sets in. This is particularly the case with presystolic mitral murmurs, which are never recognized during the acute condition that induces the lesion, unless there is narrowing of the mitral orifice on account of vegetations. The formation of vegetations at the mitral and aortic orifices may give rise to murmurs, indistinguishable from those due to destruction of the cusps. The presence of a musical murmur may generally be assumed, particularly in acute cases, to be due to a vegetation. An attack of hemiplegia during an acute febrile condition may generally be ascribed to an infarct from a valvular vegetation, and infarcts in any other organ may be assumed to arise from the same cause.

Symptoms in pericarditis.—Until the introduction of auscultation, dry pericarditis was a disease only discovered on the post-mortem table. The only evidence we have of its presence is the characteristic superficial to-and-fro murmur produced by the movements of the heart. Its discovery is usually accidental, and made when the heart is examined as a matter of routine. There is no other distinctive sign associated with it, and, in marked contrast to dry pleurisy, it is essentially a painless complaint. When pains are associated with its presence, it will invariably be found that there is evidence of a myocardial affection. This curious painlessness of pericarditis compared with pleurisy is one that has long puzzled me, and I have only a dim perception of how it may arise. I merely call attention to this fact in passing.

Pericarditis may arise in the course of a number of chronic complaints, as in diabetes and Bright's disease, or in the course of an acute disease, as pneumonia or rheumatic fever. Sometimes one comes across it quite accidentally—the patient, not feeling quite well, consults his doctor, and in the course of an examination this is detected. Such patients may go quietly about their occupation for many weeks with a well-marked to-and-fro murmur, and suffer no further trouble.

When effusion takes place into the pericardial sac, there is an increase in the area of the cardiac dullness, which assumes a somewhat characteristic shape. It reaches up to or above the second rib, and if the area be mapped out, it will have a somewhat pear-shaped character. There is an absence of the heart's movements at the lower point to the left, and this should always arouse the suspicion of effusion where there is an increase in the heart's dullness. Ewart describes a small area of dullness behind at the base of the left lung. This is important to remember, for an increase in the size of this area may cause an extensive pericardial effusion to simulate fluid in the pleural cavity. I have tapped a pericardial purulent effusion in mistake for an empyema, and my mistake arose from not ascertaining the position of the heart's movements. Had the case been one of pleural effusion, I should have found the heart beating to the right of the sternum ; but the whole left chest was dull, so that the idea of it being pericardial never crossed my mind.

The question of pericardial effusion embarrassing the work of the heart, has arisen on account of the results of experimentally distending the sac with fluid. I have never found any very serious embarrassment of the heart from extensive pericardial effusion, the reason being probably that while the normal pericardium is a more or less inelastic bag, with the inflammatory invasion it becomes distensible, and therefore able to accommodate an enormous amount of fluid with little embarrassment to the heart.

The heart in rheumatic fever.—The real nature of the changes that take place in acute affections of the heart are being gradually revealed ; and it is now possible to connect many of the obscure signs observed during life with the disease process in the heart. Many workers have contributed to our present knowledge, but the following description is taken more particularly from the observations of Cowan and of Poynton and Paine, as they have sought, with some degree of success, to correlate their pathological findings with clinical and experimental data. These observations have been worked out more particularly in rheumatic affections of the heart ; but similar changes have been found in other acute affections, as in pneumonia, diphtheria, influenza, septic poisoning.

According to Poynton and Paine, the heart trouble starts with the invasion of the heart by the specific organism of rheumatic fever—the *Diplococcus rheumaticus.* (Many later investigators have failed to isolate this organism.) They reckon to have isolated this organism from vegetations found on the valves of the heart and pericardium in acute rheumatism, have cultivated it, and produced changes in animals identical with rheumatic endocarditis, myocarditis, and pericarditis. The invasion of the endocardium usually affects first the base of the valves, and produces swelling and infiltration of the margins. The swollen edges may break down and ulcerate, or vegetations may form. The course of the disease varies greatly, from the simple endocarditis which recovers, to extensive ulceration of the valves, associated with the severe symptoms characteristic of malignant endocarditis.

The myocardium rarely escapes, and the changes in it are of great importance, both for the acute condition and for the subsequent integrity of the heart muscle. Fatty degeneration and breaking down of the muscle-fibres are fairly common, while the specific organism has been found accompanied by cellular infiltration. There may be congestion of the blood-vessels, exudation of the leucocytes, and swelling of the connective tissues. Aschoff describes the occurrence of numerous cellular foci.

During the acute attack extreme dilatation may occur, due probably to a toxæmic poisoning of the heart muscle, as no microscopic change may be present. This poisoning is probably also the cause of the extreme weakness and irritability of the heart, which persist for some time after the subsidence of the fever. The pericardium is also liable to invasion, and here the changes may vary from a slight transient pericarditis to an extreme inflammation, which does not entirely subside, but lingers on, forming adhesions to the tissue outside the pericardium and penetrating to the heart itself.

A process of slow cicatrization often follows, producing changes in the valves, heart muscle, and pericardium that seriously embarrass the heart in its work in after years.

Symptoms.—Attacks of rheumatic fever may complete their course with no affection of the heart. In some instances, the heart may be affected and give rise to no positive sign ; and it may be only after months or years that a murmur or irregular action indicates that there must have been some affection of the heart which the symptoms of the subsequent sclerosing process have revealed.

Generally, however, we can recognize certain changes in the heart's condition, chiefly in an increase in the size and the presence of a murmur. These cardiac changes may go on with very little increase of temperature, and little or no evidence of joint trouble. Sometimes in these milder cases, I have detected evidence of involvement of the auriculo-ventricular bundle by signs of interference with its power of conveying the stimulus from auricle to ventricle.

With more serious involvement the dilatation of the heart may be extreme, and it may be mistaken for pericardial effusion. At first, the full extent of the enlargement may not be realized, because it is partly masked by the lung. When the lung is pushed aside, the greatly enlarged heart can then be readily recognized. The rate of the heart is usually greatly increased, beyond what might be expected, from a mere rise in temperature. The pulse becomes soft and compressible, and sometimes shows irregularities whose nature in all cases I have not been able to make out. With subsidence of the fever, the patient enters on a long and slow convalescence. Other cases do not terminate so favourably, especially if the heart has been damaged by a previous attack. Complications, as pneumonia, are apt to arise. In severe cases there may be a considerable amount of præcordial distress. The breathing becomes shallow and rapid. The patient feels easiest with his shoulders well raised. The face becomes dusky, the lips dark red, sleep is broken and fitful, and the patient is continuously altering his position. The mind wanders and mental delusions arise.

From such a state as this the young during their first attack may recover, but in the middle-aged the condition is very serious. Attacks of syncope may appear, and the patient may die in one. Frequently they gradually sink, in spite of all treatment, and die.

In the recurring attacks of rheumatic fever, this question of previous damage to the heart is a very important one. Patients with damaged aortic and mitral valves may pass scatheless through serious attacks of rheumatic fever, presumably where the heart is not involved in these later attacks. When, however, the process lays hold on the heart, the patient's life is in great danger, and after a period of extreme suffering the struggle frequently ends in death.

While the foregoing description gives briefly the main points of the heart affection in rheumatic fever, it also holds good for the condition in other infectious diseases, apart from the recurrent attacks. As, however, the presence of other lesions has a modifying effect upon the course of the disease, it is necessary to refer to them. Unfortunately, the reference can only be brief and in the main unsatisfactory, the analysis of the symptoms in these cases having been very imperfectly carried out.

The heart in pneumonia.—The invading organism may assail the heart as well as the lungs, and the course of the illness be rapid and severe. It is difficult to distinguish between the changes due to invasion of the heart and those due to the general infection. In severe cases, the evidence of the heart affection is very prominent. Within a few hours of the initial rigor, and before there is any pulmonary sign, the evidence of the heart affection is all too apparent. The patient may be young and, prior to the attack, a perfect specimen of youthful health and vigour. A few hours after the rigor, the temperature may be over 102° F. The condition of the pulse is the best guide to the state of the heart at this stage, and shows ominous signs of what is to follow. It is greatly increased in rate, 115–130 per minute. It is soft and compressible, and offers no resistance between the beats. The peculiar manner in which it impinges against the finger— sharp and short, then quickly subsiding, indicating an absence of sustained pressure—is always to me a serious sign. It is usually associated with greatly relaxed arteries, and a sphygmogram shows little or no sign of a dicrotic wave (Fig. 172–6), indicating great lowering of the pressure during the diastole of the heart. The heart itself shows little definite sign. The sounds are short and sharp at first, becoming later somewhat muffled. A certain amount of dilatation occurs, detected more particularly to the

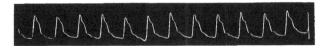

Fig. 172. Febrile pulse of low arterial pressure, T. 103°, P. 116, R. 36. This was taken eight hours after the rigor at the beginning of a pneumonia. This and the four following tracings show a type of asthenic pulse.

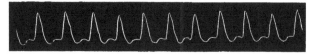

Fig. 173.   T. 101·5°, P. 96, R. 28—second day.

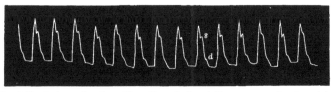

Fig. 174.   Asthenic type of pulse with well-marked systolic wave *s*, and only a faint indication of the dicrotic wave *d*—third day.

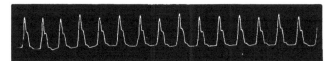

Fig. 175.   T. 130°, P. 124, R. 48—fourth day.

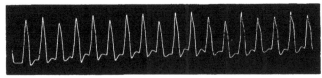

Fig. 176.   T. 102°, P. 148, R. 52.   The irregularity and rapidity of the pulse heralded the
fatal end on the fifth day.

right of the sternum. Usually in these cases the end comes with tragic suddenness ; the rate of the pulse increases, irregularities appear, and the patient succumbs within three or four days of the initial rigor. Fig. 172–6 show the characteristic features of the pulse in acute fatal pneumonia in a young, previously strong and healthy adult.

There are two conditions I have come to look upon as signs of grave complications in pneumonia—the occurrence of an occasional irregularity before the crisis, and a pulse-rate over 140 per minute. Neither of these is necessarily a fatal symptom. I had pointed this out in my book on the pulse, and John Hay, analysing 200 cases of pneumonia, found a small number recover who had shown an irregularity preceding the crisis. I, therefore, went into the matter more carefully, and found that the occasional irregularity might be due to more conditions than one, and in all my fatal cases, the irregularity was due to exhaustion of the contractility, as shown in Figs. 169 and 170 ; but this subject needs further elucidation.

The heart in diphtheria.—The complications here are so varied that danger may arise in several quarters. The heart muscle itself may be the seat of profound changes, the symptoms somewhat resembling those in rheumatic fever. But in diphtheria, more than in any other acute disease, there is a tendency to fatal syncope, and I do not understand how this is brought about.

Septic infections.—There are a great many septic infections that injure the heart, either from toxæmia or by a specific organism invading the heart. In the latter case, the endocardium is frequently attacked, and the disease is then described as septic endocarditis. In these cases, there is also invasion of the myocardium, and it is the profound depression of the heart muscle which is often the grave element.

In an account of 150 cases of infective endocarditis, Horder states that in 90 per cent. of cases a culture of a pathogenic organism can be obtained. The following table gives the analysis of forty positive results of blood culture during life :—

Number of Cases.					Micro-organism isolated.
26	.	.	.	.	Streptococcus
5	.	.	.	.	Bacillus influenzæ
5	.	.	.	.	Pneumococcus
2	.	.	.	.	Gonococcus
1	.	.	.	.	Staphylococcus albus
1	.	.	.	.	Unclassified

The illness in these cases usually begins insidiously, and at first may be mistaken for some trivial febrile complaint, or for influenza. Soon, however, the extreme prostration of the patient, the recurrence of rigors, and the patient's own sensation of illness, show that the condition is of a more serious nature. Usually, also, there is excessive perspiration. If the heart be watched, it will be found to dilate and a systolic murmur appear. The true nature of the condition may not be revealed until the detachment of a vegetation produces hemiplegia, or an infarct in the spleen or kidney or elsewhere, and death may speedily supervene (malignant endocarditis).

Other cases may linger on with indefinite febrile attacks, the patient sick, pale, and ill, and the real nature of the illness be a mystery. In some of these cases, very little change takes place in the heart. I have seen a case after confinement have slight fever for nine weeks with no change in the size of the heart, the rate generally about 80 per minute, a rough systolic mitral murmur the only abnormal sign, until an attack of hemiplegia led to the recognition that the rough mitral murmur was due to vegetations on the valves. Osler has recently published an account of ten cases of chronic infectious endocarditis. In addition to the irregular fever, he gives the following as the most suggestive features which help to identify the nature of the disease : (1) A knowledge of the existence of an old valve trouble ; (2) the occurrence of embolic features, sudden swelling of the spleen, sudden attack of hæmaturia, embolism of the retinal arteries, hemiplegia, or the blocking of a vessel in one of the limbs ; (3) the onset of special skin symptoms, purpura, and more particularly the painful erythematous nodules, in all probability due to minute emboli ; (4) the progressive cardiac changes, the gradual increase in the dilatation of the heart, the marked change in the character of the mitral murmur, the onset of a loud rasping tricuspid murmur, or the development under observation of an aortic diastolic bruit.

In pyæmia and puerperal septicæmia, we get conditions of profound gravity caused by certain organisms. The pulse in these cases gives the most trustworthy information. It is small, soft, and easily compressed, not necessarily very rapid, and the temperature need not be high (101–2°). The heart shows little change except that the sounds are feeble, the patient is lethargic, the face is slightly sallow or pale and sunken. The aspect of the patient, taken with the rate of the pulse, affords assistance in recognizing the condition. I dwell upon this because, happily, some of the younger members of the profession have little experience of dangerous forms of puerperal fever, but, having heard of the terrors surrounding them, are not infrequently unnecessarily frightened at the occurrence of a post-partum rise of temperature of trivial significance, while others do not recognize the significance of the heart symptoms when danger actually arises.

Prognosis.—In acute disease due to some infective agent, the prognosis depends upon the nature and intensity of the infection. So far as the heart is concerned, judgement must be suspended till the cessation of the active lesion. As these effects may linger on for some time, it is manifestly impossible to do more than lay down certain general rules. After acute affections, such as rheumatic fever, and after subacute affections, no prognosis should be given until all the symptoms of the original affection have disappeared. If the heart has resumed its normal aspect, in size, rate, and rhythm, we may gather that the damage has been slight and that the future is hopeful. The presence of the youthful irregularity may be a further guarantee of the integrity of the myocardium (see Chapter XXVI).   If some evidence of damage persists, then we must recognize this, lest it be due to the persistence of some low inflammatory condition which leads to the formation of fibrous changes, in which case it may be a long while before the changes are sufficiently stationary to permit of an opinion.

Treatment.—When the real nature of the trouble is appreciated in acute affections of the heart, it will be realized how powerless we are directly to modify the diseased process.   In vaccine or serum therapy, there is a promise of a specific remedy in each case to meet the special organism causing the mischief.   But so far our efforts have been attended with little success.   Horder states that of thirty-nine cases treated in this way only one recovered, and unfortunately in this case no micro-organism was demonstrated in the blood.   He says, ' I have given the treatment most thorough trial in several cases, and occasionally seen temporary improvement result, but never any permanent good.'

In rheumatic fever, the salicylates have an undoubted action on the course of the disease in many cases, and it may be that the drug can modify the heart affection.   Their employment is so frequently of use that it should always be tried, and given in such doses that a physiological reaction is obtained.

Apart from the probably specific action of salicylate in rheumatic cases, the employment of cardiac or other drugs is of little avail.[1]   The heart is already in possession of a poison far more powerful than the drugs at our command, and these in medicinal doses are without effect.   But on this account it must not be supposed that all treatment is useless ; rather should it direct our attention to the consideration of other means of treatment.   The man who puts his faith in drugs exclusively neglects too often the most useful methods.   Recognizing that the heart muscle is greatly embarrassed in its work, the endeavour should be made to give it as little work to do as possible, and to save it from all sources of irritation ; in fact, to place it in a condition of rest, as far as rest is possible for such an active organ as the heart.   To this end the general condition of the patient should be carefully studied ; the position he assumes should be one that gives the heart least work to do ; the food should be so administered that while nourishing him

---

[1] Horder says : ' " Blood antiseptics " seem doomed to failure in dealing with pyogenic blood infections, because it is not possible to get the drugs into the blood in a nascent or active condition.   Combination with the proteids of the blood-cells or the plasma takes place before the drug comes into contact with the micro-organism.   Quinine, mercury, arsenic, carbolic acid, formalin, and many other reputed remedies, all fail, whether administered by the mouth, subcutaneously, or intravenously.   The sulpho-carbolates which have had a special vogue are equally disappointing ; I have used them in very large doses in several cases without any results.   Silver salts in combination with nuclein have been highly spoken of in the treatment of septicæmia, but here again I have never seen any good results in infective endocarditis. The same remarks apply to yeast and its active principle.'

it does not lead to abdominal distension: his bowels should be so regulated as to act freely without straining. As fidgeting and restlessness keep the heart irritable and variable in its action, everything should be done for his bodily comfort—sponging, and arranging his pillows and the bedclothes, and the many little things that a deft and intelligent nurse can suggest. Above all, sleeplessness, which is so often present, or the sleep that is broken and disturbed, should have most careful consideration, and suitable hypnotics be given as described in Chapter XLVI.

When there is reason to suspect that the heart muscle has been affected by the illness, great care should be taken during the convalescence to give the heart muscle time to recover. Any cause, effort or excitement, that accelerates the heart's action, should be avoided, and exertion only permitted when the dilatation has subsided, and effort ceases to call forth any disagreeable sensation. It may be weeks or months after the fever before the heart muscle recovers.

CHAPTER XXXVI

POISONED HEARTS

Symptoms.
Associated symptoms.
Prognosis.
Treatment.

ANOTHER group of cases of muscle affection stands out prominently. We have already seen that acute, subacute, and chronic processes may arise and by impairing the structures of the heart provoke definite lesions. The muscle of the heart may be impaired by agents which affect it in the manner of a poison, without producing structural changes, unless the poison is long continued, when by its persistent action it may lead to structural changes.

In the reaction to certain agents which injuriously affect the human organism, and which we may call 'poisons', there are many individual peculiarities. The same poison and the same amount given to two individuals often produces different phenomena. So far as the heart is concerned, we get an extraordinarily different reaction among different people. To illustrate this, I need but refer to the different effects of tobacco and alcohol on different individuals. My attention was drawn to the effects of another poison on the heart during a number of years preceding 1894, when the beer in certain districts of Lancashire was contaminated in the process of manufacture by arsenic. During these years, peripheral neuritis was very common amongst the beer-drinkers. Certain cases of heart failure were also fairly frequent, and Graham Steell pointed out that these cases were due essentially to 'muscle failure'. With the discovery and prevention of the arsenical contamination, all these cases suddenly disappeared, and I saw no more of this type of heart failure.

But in recent years, I have had the opportunity of seeing other cases which presented features similar to those I found present in alcoholic and arsenical poisoning, associated with microbic infections, apart from infections of the heart itself, and these I now recognize as due to toxic agents produced by the microbe (see Cases 83 and 84).

A great many people who have got some derangement of the digestive apparatus (dilatation of the stomach or of some other portion of the gut, gastric ulcer, colitis), often exhibit evidence of a cardiac impairment, or of abnormal rhythm, as extra-systoles and attacks of paroxysmal tachycardia, and the cure of the digestive affection is often followed by the disappearance of all signs of cardiac trouble.

Symptoms.—(a) *Subjective sensations.*—The poisoned heart invariably gives rise to those sensations which I have already described as due to the exhaustion of the heart muscle ; a sense of exhaustion and breathlessness on exertion being the most frequent. Consciousness of the increased rate is often a disagreeable sensation and is a frequent complaint. While these distressing sensations are generally occasioned during effort, sometimes they do not appear till some hours later. Thus a young man who suffered from intestinal stasis was capable of considerable effort and experienced no discomfort until two or three hours after some strenuous exertion, when the heart became rapid in rate, and this was accompanied by a disagreeable sense of exhaustion. Sensations referable to other organs may accompany the cardiac sensation, as the morning nausea, the sinking sensation, and loss of appetite of the alcoholic.

(b) *Increased rate.*—A persistent increase in rate, in the absence of fever and of such apparent diseases as exophthalmic goitre and pernicious anæmia (even in these cases the probable cause of the increased rate is poisoning), should always lead to an examination for a possible poisoning. The cause may be so obscure that it may be months before its nature is discovered, and in many cases we may never be able to find out the real source. One of my earliest experiences was in the case of a woman who complained of great weakness, and breathlessness on exertion. Repeated examinations and a consultation with a distinguished physician revealed only a persistent increase in the heart's rate, from 90 to 120 per minute. After several months, she was seized with a severe hæmoptysis, and died after a few weeks from acute pulmonary tuberculosis. In another case, a girl of $15\frac{1}{2}$, the same complaint, weakness and breathlessness on exertion, was made, and I could detect nothing definitely wrong, save a pulse-rate of 130 to 140 per minute. I tried many remedies to lessen the rate, pushing the digitalis on two occasions till nausea and vomiting occurred. After several months' useless treatment, the true cause was revealed by the pointing of a psoas abscess. Other infections, as from the colon bacillus, may stimulate the heart to greatly increased rate, with little or no increase in the size of the heart.

(c) *Dilatation of the heart.* In some cases the muscle wall is so profoundly affected by the poison that the heart dilates. In such cases there is always an increase in rate and great exhaustion of the heart's strength. This is not infrequent in people who indulge in drinking bouts, lasting for several weeks (see Cases 82 and 83).

(d) *Venous and liver engorgement.* In addition to the increased size and rate of the heart, the jugular veins may become greatly distended, and pulsate, and the liver may increase in size and the tissues covering it be extremely tender on percussion. Cases 83 and 84 illustrate this condition, where the poison in one case was due to arsenic and beer, and in the second case to a streptococcus infection.

Associated symptoms.—So far I have referred to the condition as it affects the heart, but almost invariably there are present phenomena arising from the toxæmic condition. Discoloration of the skin, as in the axilla, abdomen, and the face, is frequently present, especially in those with intestinal toxæmia. General weakness is often complained of, and when associated with palpitation or irregular action of the heart, is often put down to some heart trouble. In these cases the exhaustion is of that type referred to on p. 97, as vaso-motor in origin, and the exhaustion is a feeling spread more or less over the body, as distinct from the definite symptoms which arise from heart exhaustion pure and simple. Curious attacks may occur, evidently vaso-motor in origin, when the patient becomes very chilly and the hands and feet go cold and a rigor occurs, sometimes with partial loss of consciousness or attacks of angina pectoris.

Prognosis.—It is manifest that the prognosis really depends on the cause of the infection, and on the persistence of the poisoning. If the alcoholic will mend his ways in time, he may escape any permanent injury, but with a continuance of his evil ways, organic changes may be set up (Case 82). Notwithstanding the severity of the heart failure, the power of the heart to recover is remarkable, with the cessation of the poison (Case 84). The prognosis therefore depends more on the nature of the agent and its effect on the organism as a whole, than on its specific action on the heart muscle itself. The effect on the heart may have given a clue to the nature of the case, as in the persistent increase in rate in cases of tubercular infection.

Treatment.—The appropriate treatment is to get rid of the poison. Simple as this proposition seems, yet it is wonderful to find how often it is neglected, or, if not neglected, how attempts are made to cure the heart condition as if it were something apart from the intoxication. Thus I have seen a woman who suffered from a bacillus coli infection for some years, in whom the heart had become rapid in rate and easily exhausted. She was submitted for six months to most elaborate methods of treatment. She had cure after cure of Nauheim baths, movements and exercises, digitalis and strophanthus and hypodermic injections of strychnine ; all without the slightest effect. The whole cardiac condition ceased eighteen months later with the disappearance of the coli infection, brought about apparently by the use of vaccines. Case 84 was sent me by Sir Almroth Wright for treatment, because of the profound degree of heart failure ; but I sent it back to him with the opinion that if his methods in removing the poison were ineffective, my attempts would be unavailing. This opinion was based on a long investigation I had made in private and in hospital on the effects of cardiac remedies in hearts affected by an acute infection or poisoning.

I had found that these cases were quite unsusceptible to drugs and methods, which might affect the heart when free from these influences.

That the same resistance to treatment is present in alcoholics may be gathered from the following experience, which illustrates more than one moral. Some years ago, while visiting a spa whose waters were supposed to have special effects in curing all sorts of cardiac complaints, one of the physicians told me that he could cure tachycardia. I asked him what form of tachycardia, but he replied that he would show me a case. This he did, and the patient confirmed his claim that he had come there the previous year with a pulse-rate of 140, and under the treatment the rate had fallen to normal, but that a relapse had taken place, and he was again in the process of being cured, his pulse-rate having fallen from 140 to 110 beats per minute. Meeting the patient in the garden afterwards, he dilated upon his complaint till I interrupted him and asked him to tell me truthfully the cause of his heart trouble. He hesitated, and then said there would be nothing the matter with his heart if he could leave the whisky alone. At home he was nipping all day long, and he came to the spa to avoid the temptation, and was ashamed to give the real reason and pretended it was to get his heart cured. ' The doctor thinks he is curing me with his baths and exercises ; I have cured myself many a time by being teetotal.'

CHAPTER XXXVII

AFFECTIONS OF THE MYOCARDIUM

Introduction.
Evidences of the impairment of the myocardium.
Acute affections of the myocardium.
Subacute affections of the myocardium.
Progress of myocardial disease.

Introduction.—I have already dealt with the prime importance of a healthy muscle in the maintenance of an efficient circulation. When we come to consider the conditions causing impairment of the heart muscle, we are confronted by such a variety of circumstances that it is very difficult, in a great many cases, to determine the real nature of the impairment. Thus, microbic invasion, malnutrition, poisoning, organic changes due to fibrous and fatty degeneration, the result of old infections or of arterial disease or of those changes which we call senile, all tend to impair the functional efficiency of the organ. Inasmuch as the symptoms provoked by the various conditions are merely those of an impaired muscle, we get little help in differentiation from the study of these symptoms. The clinical evidence is restricted to certain alterations in the size, rate, and rhythm of the heart, or to evidence evoked by its functional inefficiency. It is only in recent years that our methods have enabled us to recognize those abnormal rhythms, while the evidences of functional impairment have been hitherto to a great extent ignored. Seeing that the symptoms produced by myocardial affections are common to many different forms of disease, we have to search for information as to the nature of the impairment from other sources.

In dealing with the principles of heart failure, the importance of the heart muscle, on whose integrity the efficient circulation depended, was dwelt upon. The manner in which exhaustion arose, and the nature of the symptoms which were evoked, were described (Chapter IV). In this chapter I attempt to deal with some of the more common causes producing inefficiency of the heart muscle, and to apply the principles of heart failure so as to correlate the diseased conditions with the symptoms. But at the outset, I am conscious of the great limitations under which we labour, in dealing with a subject on which so much of our knowledge has to depend on inference rather than on demonstration. Great as our limitations are, yet the very recognition of these limitations is an element of profit, because when we know where we are ignorant, we are provided with a subject which calls for research and observation. Our limitations are in a measure due to the fact that the vast majority of cases of impaired myocardium do not die during the early stages, so that we do not have an opportunity of recognizing the nature of the changes which cause the impairment. Moreover by the time death supervenes the original changes have become greatly modified, either by intensification or by the introduction of subsidiary changes. so that it is mere guesswork to attempt to picture the conditions which existed during the early stages of heart failure. Moreover, the gross organic changes detected post-mortem, give but little clue to the altered functions which were present during life.

Evidences of the impairment of the myocardium.—It is manifest that the impairment of any organ will lead to some degree of functional inefficiency. In the case of a muscular organ, such as the heart, the inefficiency will be shown by a failure of the blood-supply to certain organs, and these organs will manifest the cardiac inefficiency by exhibiting their peculiar phenomena. The principle of this inefficiency has been dealt with in Chapter VI, and here I just mention that inefficiency, in the first instance, is shown by a limitation of the field of cardiac response, and that the evidence is purely subjective.

Rate.—The rate of the heart in myocardial affections is extremely variable, and as the variation of rate depends on so many factors it is not always easy to recognize the actual factor in any given case. In some febrile cases, a persistent increase in the rate may be taken as indicating the presence of some agent which either weakens the myocardium by injury (as the fibrotic changes in rheumatic affections) or poisoning (as alcohol and the toxins of infectious diseases). In great exhaustion, increased rate is frequently present, but it may be that it is the increased rate which induces the exhaustion. With extreme degeneration of the heart muscle, the rate may not be altered.

Rhythm.—The different abnormal rhythms and their relation to diseases of the myocardium have already been described. Suffice it here to say that extra-systoles, auricular fibrillation, auricular flutter, irregularities and abnormal rhythms due to injury of the conducting system and the pulsus alternans, may all be the expression of an injured or impaired myocardium.

The size of the heart.—When the heart is hypertrophied, it may be assumed that some factor is present which has thrown more work on the heart, and naturally the significance of the hypertrophy depends on the nature of this factor and the ability of the heart to overcome the obstacle to its work. It may be stated that a hypertrophied heart is always an impaired heart, and however complete the compensatory hypertrophy may be, there will always be found a limitation in the field of response.

The evidence of hypertrophy is mostly limited to the forcible thrust of the apex beat. But though this is often a marked sign, we not infrequently meet with a large forcible apex in very inefficient hearts, with very extensive degeneration of the left ventricle. The electrocardiograph shows a modified form when associated with hypertrophy of the different chambers.

Dilatation of the heart. This is a very striking evidence of a purely muscular affection, and particularly of a functional origin. In acute conditions, it is due to a poisoning of the muscle, affecting the function of tonicity. This may be the case also in chronic affections. As dilatation is so frequently accompanied by other evidences, dependent upon the dilatation and the inefficiency brought about by the dilatation, the subject is fully dealt with in Chapter XXXVIII.

Acute affections of the myocardium.—As acute diseases can rarely be found to exist without the presence of disease affecting other structures of the heart, or from the heart being inflamed by fever, they are discussed in the chapter dealing with acute febrile affections of the heart (Chapter XXXV).

Subacute affections of the myocardium.—There is also a great deal of obscurity surrounding the symptoms produced by less acute affections of the myocardium. In acute febrile cases of infective origin, a certain progress has been made, as the opportunity of studying them during life and comparing the symptoms with the results found post mortem, are unfortunately not infrequent. But in milder affections of a less severe nature, the symptoms are less obtrusive, and often pass unrecognized, while there is no opportunity for studying the lesion, as death occurs so long after the inception of the disease that it is not possible to correlate the symptoms during life with the causal affection. We repeatedly see individuals suffering from some serious cardiac affection, but in the absence of any characteristic manifestations, it is not possible to recognize the nature of the trouble. From among a number of such obscure conditions, I have been able to select some which presented certain features in common, so that it is possible to place them in distinctive groups. The minute study of the symptoms present affords reasonable grounds for recognizing the nature of the lesion, and the seat of at least a portion of the mischief; and with this knowledge we can refer other phenomena, with approximate certainty, to a myocardial origin.

I give an account of five cases where the evidence of a subacute affection of the myocardium is fairly conclusive (Cases 85-9). I have seen a number of other cases with similar symptoms and histories, but in these there was no evidence of injury to the bundle.

Four, if not five, of the cases cited suffered from ' muscular rheumatism ', shown by pain and stiffness in the movement of certain muscles (as in lumbago). This condition has lately been the subject of a good deal of study by Stockman and others. Stockman has detected in the affected muscles small tender nodules ; these he has excised, and found that they consist mainly of fibrous tissue with proliferating cells, which originate in a fibrositis of the muscle-fibre sheaths, nerve sheaths, and tendons. In a number of individuals who have suffered from this form of rheumatism, I have found also present distinct evidence of some coincident cardiac trouble. The analysis of the symptoms presented by these patients revealed phenomena which give a fairly clear indication of the nature and situation of a portion of the lesion ; for in all these cases, there was distinct evidence of an injury to the auriculo-ventricular bundle. This was shown in some by a delay in the transmission of the stimulus from auricle to ventricle, and in others by the dropping out of ventricular contractions. This evidence leaves little doubt that the rheumatic affection had invaded the heart, and that in all proba- bility a lesion, similar to that which affected the skeletal muscles, had also affected the heart muscle. If this assumption is correct, we can infer with fair certainty the origin of the other symptoms that were present. The symptoms evoked in these subacute cases are in the first instance purely subjective, the individual being conscious of his limitations by sensations of discomfort or distress, when he undertook such effort as he had hitherto been able to perform with ease and comfort. Some of these sensations were referable to the heart itself, as throbbing and violent action of the heart, while there was also breathlessness and pain. At times, such sensations may arise when no bodily effort is made. The ease with which the distress is provoked, is indicative to a certain extent of the severity of the affection. In the cases quoted, varied degrees of distress were present, as palpitation only on exertion, violent attacks when at rest, and pain sometimes of great severity.

In all the five cases, heart-block of varying degree was present—a mere delay in the conduction of the stimulus from auricle to ventricle, the dropping out of beats at infrequent intervals, the dropping out of every third ventricular beat ; 3 : 2 heart-block ; the dropping out of every second ventricular beat, 2 : 1 heart-block.

Another noteworthy point is that four of the cases made good recoveries ; in four cases, apparently complete, and in one, with some persistent ineffi- ciency of the heart muscle (Case 86). The treatment which seemed most effective was rest. In some of the cases, many forms of treatment were tried ; various drugs, the waters of Buxton, Harrogate, and Nauheim were all equally ineffective.

Progress of myocardial disease.—After the subsidence of the symptoms provoked by the acute or subacute process, there may be a long period of seeming quiescence, when the individual may pursue a strenuous life with no evident impairment of his powers. In certain cases, we can detect evidences of damage long before any noticeable failure of the heart appears, as in the persistence of a wide a–c interval, evidence of a myocardial affection which has invaded the auriculo-ventricular bundle (Case 44). The damage done to valves by an acute endocarditis is often progressive, as shown by the gradual alteration in the character of the murmurs in aortic regurgitation and mitral stenosis. In many such cases, the myocardium is affected at the same time, and here also the damage is not stationary but progressive. Probably in every case of myocardial disease, there is from the beginning a slight impairment of the functional efficiency of the heart shown by a limitation in the response to effort. Unaware of this impairment, the individual attempts to lead the life of a healthy person, and the early symptoms of exhaustion are ignored. The increasing ease with which these symptoms are produced, directs attention ultimately to the cardiac impairment. This recognition of the impairment may follow long after the original damage, the time of its appearance depending naturally on the extent of the damage and the rapidity of its progress, and the amount of effort to which the individual is subjected. In addition to the changes induced by acute affections, there are a series of cases where we cannot recognize the origin, but find them associated with other conditions, such as high blood-pressure, kidney disease, sometimes with a history of alcohol or syphilis. These cases all pursue a similar course and show the same phenomena.

It is almost universally acknowledged that cases of heart disease with valvular murmurs, resulting from infection, such as rheumatic fever, are cases of chronic valvular disease, and these are separated from cases of heart failure with no murmurs and no history of infection, which are usually spoken of as cases of chronic myocarditis. This distinction is scarcely justified.

The morbid conditions most frequently found in the damaged heart muscle are fibrous changes, affecting chiefly the left ventricle. In looking over the notes of a number of cases whom I have watched for long periods, and where I have seen the gradual onset of heart failure and the final result, I find a remarkable correspondence in the symptoms of those cases which are usually described as chronic valvular disease, and those in whom there was no valvular disease. In like manner, the post-mortem examination revealed a remarkable resemblance in the state of the myocardium in the cases of valvular disease, with cases with no valvular disease (compare Cases 22, 24, 35, 49, 51).

These cases are typical of the more common conditions found post mortem, where the heart failure has been the primary cause of death. Sometimes similar changes are found in the hearts of old people who may die from intercurrent diseases. Other morbid conditions than fibrotic degeneration may be found, as extensive fatty degenerative changes, or atrophic changes in the heart-wall, due to some obscure arterial disease or to the plugging of an artery. All these changes may appear in the hearts of the elderly, and as we know little about their origin, it is customary to speak of them as ' senile changes '.

CHAPTER XXXVIII

AFFECTIONS OF THE MYOCARDIUM (*continued*)
DILATATION OF THE HEART

The cause of dilatation of the heart.
The function of tonicity.
The symptoms of depression of tonicity.
Evidence of dilatation of the heart.
Functional murmurs and dilatation of the heart.
The effects of dilatation of the heart, and how they are brought about.
Dropsy.
Dropsy and dilatation of the heart.
Enlargement of the liver.
Œdema of the lungs.
Urinary symptoms.
Prognosis.
Treatment.

ALTHOUGH the matter of the ' tone ' of the heart is frequently present in the minds of physicians, nevertheless I venture to doubt if ever it is more than a vague conception. Some writers have described certain conditions associated with it, yet it has not received that consideration its importance merits. The recognition of depression of tonicity will be found to be of the greatest service in appreciating the nature of the heart failure, and the remedies appropriate for the restoration of the heart's power. For some years now, I have been inquiring into this function, and although many important features have been revealed, I am far from comprehending its full significance.

The cause of dilatation of the heart.—Before considering the symptoms produced by depression of tonicity, it is necessary to appreciate the cause of the most prominent of these symptoms, namely, dilatation of the heart, and one cannot fail to be struck with the inadequacy of the explanation usually given for this condition. The prevalent idea seems to be, that it is due to an increasing pressure within the chambers forcing the walls outwards. But if it be asked, Whence comes this distending force? the inadequacy of such an explanation is at once apparent. During systole, the increased pressure within the chamber is produced by the contraction of the wall of the chamber itself, and one can scarcely assume that in the process of contraction dilatation is produced. Dilatation of an auricle, it is true, might be produced by the forcible regurgitation of blood from a powerful ventricle, but such a thing can only happen when there is a lesion of the auriculo-ventricular valves. Regurgitation, apart from valvular lesion, can only occur after the muscle fibres surrounding the auriculo-ventricular orifices have become relaxed—that is to say, dilatation of the auricle from such a cause would be produced after dilatation of the ventricle.

That neither the resistance opposed to a chamber during the systole, nor the distending force during its diastole, is the cause of dilatation becomes evident when the conditions observed in certain hearts are carefully studied. Thus hearts whose walls are thinned, and whose muscle fibres are degenerated, may continue to work against an abnormally high arterial pressure, and never show any signs of dilatation. In fact, the wall of the left ventricle may be so thinned that it actually bursts in its effort to overcome the aortic pressure, yet the walls show no signs of dilatation. Professor Keith, who has especially looked into this matter of ruptured hearts, informs me that such hearts may show no sign of increase in the size of their cavities. In a patient under my care, the heart was so enfeebled that he could scarcely walk fifty yards without an attack of angina pectoris coming on, but no enlargement of the heart could be detected. He died suddenly from rupture of the heart, and I found that part of the heart-wall was so thinned as to be made up of little except the endocardium and pericardium, yet, notwithstanding this enfeeblement of the heart-wall, there was no sign of dilatation of the cavity.

Dilatation of the left ventricle may occur even when the diastolic force filling the ventricle is greatly diminished, as in cases of pure mitral stenosis. Here the quantity of blood reaching the ventricle, and the force with which it enters the ventricle, are so greatly diminished, that we must look for some other cause for the dilatation of the left ventricle that is found in advanced cases of mitral stenosis.

Taking dilatation as being due to the depression of the function of tonicity, we have seen from experiment that certain substances modify the activity of this function. It was shown that antiarin and digitalis increased the tone, while muscarin and lactic acid tended to depress the function and caused dilatation. Various agents are known to have this effect on the human heart, such as arsenic, alcohol, and the toxins of infective microbes. It is necessary, therefore, in any given case of dilatation of the heart, in the absence of organic disease, to search for a possible poison. In all the poisoned cases I have seen, there was always present marked evidence of functional impairment accompanying the dilatation.

The function of tonicity.—In default of this mechanical explanation we turn naturally to the functions of the normal heart, to inquire what maintains the fibres in health in a position short of their extreme relaxation. In this way we may succeed in obtaining a more definite conception

of what occurs in dilatation, even if we fail to elucidate altogether its
ætiology.

This power of maintaining a position short of extreme relaxation
is not peculiar to the cardiac muscle, but is also met with in the ordinary
skeletal fibres, and in both cases it is due to the possession by the fibres of
the function of tonicity.

The symptoms of depression of tonicity.—These symptoms are
threefold : (1) those due directly to the changes in the heart, viz. increased
size of the heart, alterations in the position and in the character of the
movements of the heart, and the presence of murmurs ; (2) those due
to functional inefficiency of the heart, and manifested by symptoms due
to the failure of the circulation in remote organs and tissues, as
dropsy, enlargement of the liver, and breathlessness ; (3) certain reflex
sensory symptoms mainly shown by regions of hyperalgesia affecting
the skin, mamma, and muscles of the left chest and axillary fold, and sometimes also the left sterno-mastoid and trapezius muscles.

Evidence of dilatation of the heart.—The evidence of dilatation
of the heart is made out by marking out the increased size of the heart.
I need not dwell upon how this is done, for the methods for percussing out
the heart's dullness are described in sufficient fullness in every handbook
of physical diagnosis. For practical purposes, the transverse dullness at
the level of the fourth interspace gives on the whole the best estimate of
the size of the heart. In exceptional cases, the whole area of deep dullness
may be with advantage mapped out, as when dullness is found extending
to the left above the third rib. In such cases, the possibility of pericardial
effusion should be kept in mind.

It is very difficult to tell with certainty what share each chamber of
the heart takes in the production of the increased size, on account of the
displacement of the whole organ. The manner in which the heart is fixed
above, by the aorta, pulmonary artery and veins, and superior vena cava,
and below by the inferior vena cava, keeps fixed an axis on which the
heart to a certain extent rotates in the enlargement of its various cavities.
The tendency when the right ventricle dilates, is for it to push the left
ventricle to the left and behind, with the result that, in the great majority
of cases, we get evidence of an extension of the dullness to the left. When
the right auricle becomes greatly distended, it may push itself to the front
of the chest, and, as Keith's dissections show, compress the right ventricle
to a remarkable degree. When there is extension of the dullness beyond
the right border of the sternum, it may with certainty be put down to the
right auricle, except in aneurysm or other intra-thoracic tumour.

The manner in which the right heart pushes over to the left side, is well
brought out in Fig. 177 and 178. These are typical of the dilatation
secondary to mitral stenosis with auricular fibrillation. If a comparison be

made with the position of the chambers in the normal heart (Fig. 22), it will be observed that the increase to the right side, notwithstanding the great dilatation of the right heart, is very slight, whereas the great increase in the size of the heart is to the left—sometimes with only a slight depression of the apex (Fig. 177), sometimes with considerable depression (Fig. 178).

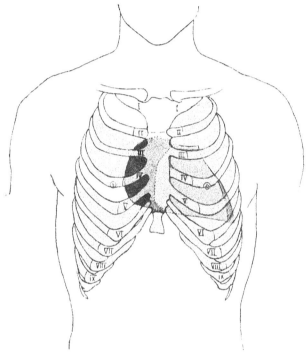

Fig. 177.   Position of the chambers of the heart in extreme dilatation, as in the late stage of mitral stenosis with auricular fibrillation.   The portion of the heart on the right of the sternum shaded deeply, together with that behind the sternum up to the dotted line, represents the right auricle, while the small strip to the left shaded deeply, represents the left ventricle. The part between is the right ventricle (Harris).

Note also how the right auricle pushes into the second left interspace.   So long as the lungs cover a portion of the heart, the perceptible movements will be entirely due to the right ventricle ; but when the lung is pushed from the front of the heart, the real apex will be found at the extreme left.

In seeking for the cause of the increased dulness, the character of the impulse should always be studied, not only to determine the nature of the heart's enlargement, but to distinguish it from pericardial effusions and displacement of the heart by such conditions as aneurysm, pleural effusion, and so forth. Another point to bear in mind is that, in the early stages of enlargement of the heart, the lung may still cover a part of its left border, but with persistence of the enlargement the lung is compressed, and if non-adherent, recedes from the anterior surface of the heart, altering altogether the characters of the apex movements.

The large diffuse apex beat with the out-thrust or impulse during ventricular systole, is characteristic of hypertrophy of the left ventricle. When

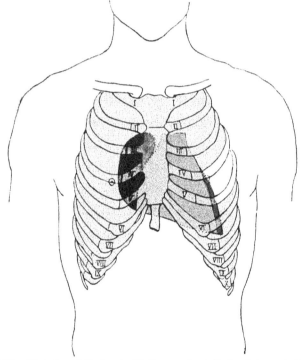

Fig. 178. Dilatation of the heart with the apex beat displaced downwards. The shading is the same as in the preceding figure (Harris).

the apex is diffuse, but the out-thrust or impulse diastolic in time, then it is due to the right ventricle, and indicates great enlargement, usually dilatation of the right ventricle (see Fig. 30). This will be revealed by the study of Fig. 177 and 178, where the small portion of the left ventricle that is in front may scarcely be apparent during life, and especially if covered by the lungs.

Functional murmurs and dilatation of the heart.—Functional murmurs have hitherto been looked upon as a consequence of simple dilatation of the heart, but this explanation is far from being sufficient. Thus we may have considerable dilatation of the heart without a murmur. Again, we may have very little dilatation with marked systolic murmurs at apex and base, and with great regurgitant waves in the veins. The explanation of these apparent anomalies seems to be in the condition of the muscles supporting the auriculo-ventricular orifice. If their tonicity be depressed, regurgitation ensues, and gives rise to the functional murmurs, but functional murmurs can arise apart from dilatation.

The effects of dilatation of the heart, and how they are brought about.—Before describing in detail the results that follow dilatation of the heart, it is necessary to consider the manner in which these symptoms of heart failure are brought about. The maintenance of the circulation is due to the contractile force of the heart, and normally the factors concerned are so balanced that everything is done to facilitate the work of the heart. It is reasonable to assume that the chambers of the heart are normally of the size that enables them to contract with the greatest efficiency. The dilatation of these chambers will therefore embarrass the heart muscle, with the usual result, a limitation of the reserve force. At first, this limitation may only call forth disagreeable symptoms when it is exhausted, the exhaustion occurring much sooner than normal. The degree of exhaustion depends on the integrity of the heart muscle. If the contractile force is embarrassed by inherent defects of the muscular wall, or by other causes, such as irregularity of action, or valvular defects, then the heart failure corresponds to the degree of embarrassment and inability of the muscle to overcome it. For this reason we find all degrees of heart failure associated with dilatation. In the milder cases, there may be only the subjective symptoms of breathlessness, palpitation, and weakness. In the more extreme cases, dropsy (more or less extensive), diminished secretion of urine, effusion of fluid into the serous cavities, enlargement of the liver, lividity of the face, may be present. The rationale of the production of this extreme heart failure seems to be as follows : So long as the contractile force of the heart is able to maintain a degree of arterial pressure sufficient to supply the organs and tissues, the heart failure will be limited to those subjective symptoms involved in a great reduction of reserve force ; the patient is comfortable at rest, for the heart is then able to maintain the circulation, but is distressed by exertion, for the heart has so little reserve force that it is unable to meet the extra demand. When the force of the heart fails to maintain the arterial pressure at the height necessary for the tissues, then we get the symptoms in the remote organs and tissues (dropsy, ascites, enlarged liver, etc.). In certain cases of extreme heart failure, especially with auricular fibrillation, the regurgitant wave sent back by the right ventricle distends the liver and causes the liver to pulsate.

I have endeavoured in a number of ways to demonstrate the relationship between dilatation of the heart and these evidences of extreme heart failure, and I give a few instances where the association of these symptoms with dilatation of the heart is clearly marked.

In advanced cases of myocardial degeneration with a blood-pressure continuously high, between 180 mm. Hg. and 200 mm. Hg., the heart may be of normal size, or only very slightly enlarged. There may be great limitation of the field of response, exertion readily inducing attacks of angina pectoris or breathlessness. Cheyne-Stokes respiration may occur also, and attacks of cardiac asthma or severe dyspnœa at nights. There may be large pulsation in the veins of the neck, but no dropsy. Patients may gradually weaken and die, and the heart remain unchanged in size. On the other hand, in the course of a day or two, one may be struck by a great change. The patient seems easier ; the blood-pressure has fallen to 150 mm., or lower ; attacks of angina pectoris, cardiac asthma, and Cheyne-Stokes respiration disappear. But the legs begin to swell, the urine becomes scanty, the jugular pulse disappears, the breathing is continuously hurried, and the patient has to be propped up in bed. He may begin to expectorate blood-stained mucus, and there is evidence of œdema of the base of the lung. If the heart be examined, it will be found to extend one or two inches further to the left, and it may be a mitral murmur has developed.

Even more striking, because more sudden and violent, are the changes that take place in certain cases of paroxysmal tachycardia. In describing this condition (Chapter XXXII), I pointed out that the symptoms varied in patients according to the condition of tonicity,—if the heart remained unaltered in size during an attack, the symptoms were less marked and the condition less grave than if the heart dilated. In the cases recorded in the Appendix (Cases 51 and 72), the heart dilated, and in the course of a few hours symptoms of extreme heart failure set in. I have seen these cases on several occasions shortly before an attack, and watched the steady progress of the change. The hearts were nearly normal in size, but in three hours' time the transverse diameter had increased by two inches, the face had become livid and the lips swollen. The veins of the neck, which had shown little movement, now pulsated largely. In the course of twenty-four hours, œdema of the legs appeared, and the liver became large, and in one case pulsated. After some days, the dropsy extended up the legs, the abdomen became distended and the urine scanty. With the cessation of the attack of paroxysmal tachycardia, the patients at once experienced relief, and in a few hours every vestige of heart failure had disappeared, and the heart itself returned to a normal size and rhythm. I give these instances because, owing to the sudden change of appearance, one could account fairly satisfactorily for the symptoms. In various modifications, they will be found associated with extreme heart failure from all forms of cardiac disease. I have seen many cases in which the inception of auricular fibrillation was followed by these changes, and when it persisted a partial recovery only followed. In certain alcoholic hearts—especially in those of Graham Steell's group of ' muscle failure '—these phenomena can also be recognized, as well as in other conditions.

Dropsy.—Œdema of the subcutaneous tissues is a common feature in heart failure with dilatation. It is apart from my purpose to discuss the various theories propounded to account for its occurrence, it being sufficient here to note that its appearance is often a definite sign of heart dilatation, and its disappearance an equally definite sign of restoration of the heart's tone. It begins first in the most dependent parts : in people not confined to bed it is found first about and above the ankles ; in people lying in bed, across the sacrum. It may linger in the legs for years in some folks— worse towards night, better in the morning. In extreme cases, it invades the thighs and abdominal wall. The loose cellular tissue of the scrotum, penis, and vulva becomes infiltrated, and may attain an enormous size. Before marked effusion takes place into the abdominal cavity, the bowels often become greatly distended with flatus. The effusion may finally invade the pleural cavities, producing hydrothorax. The distended abdomen and the hydrothorax add to the embarrassment of the breathing. If the patient leans more to one side than to the other, in extreme cases, the arm and cheek of that side may become greatly swollen.

Associated with dropsy, there is usually a diminished urinary secretion, and disappearance of the dropsy usually coincides with an increased flow of urine.

The significance of œdema is extremely varied. Many elderly people, especially if they are stout, may for years have their legs more or less swollen, even if their hearts present no particular abnormality beyond a slight dilata- tion, though it is more common amongst those with the auricular fibrillation. It may be present in attacks of heart failure to an extreme degree, with ascites and hydrothorax, and notwithstanding the patient may make a good and lasting recovery. These are found more particularly in cases of rheumatic affection of the heart of some duration, starting in some with the auricular fibrillation. If the heart reverts to its normal rhythm, the disappearance of the dropsy is more speedy than its onset. If the heart reacts to digitalis, the disappearance of the dropsy accompanies the other beneficial effects of the drug. When all attempts to restore the heart fail, the dropsy increases, embarrasses the heart and the respiration by effusion into the serous cavities, and adds much to the suffering of the patient, who drifts to a fatal issue.

In extreme heart failure, we may find a localised œdema of one arm. This results from the patient lying on that side. If it is not on the side on which the patient lies, then it is due to a blocking of the superior vena cava from a clot. So extensive may such clotting be that it will be found extending high up into the jugular vein, and along the subclavian into the brachial.

In such cases, there will be no jugular pulse on that side, while it may be very marked on the opposite side.

Dropsy and dilatation of the heart.—One of the reasons inducing me to include dropsy as a symptom of dilatation of the heart, is that I am doubtful if it is possible for dropsy to occur from heart failure, without dilatation. I see, not infrequently, cases of dropsy and enlargement of the liver diagnosed and treated for heart failure because there was a valvular murmur. In these cases, there has been no increase in the size of the heart, and I have therefore assumed that the dropsy was not cardiac in origin. The subsequent progress of the cases revealed that there were other causes for the dropsy (as cirrhosis of the liver, myxœdema).

Enlargement of the liver.—Another result of the failure of the circulation secondary to dilatation of the heart, is swelling of the liver from passive congestion (Chapter XXII). It may not appear in the earlier stages in the first instance, but when a patient has once recovered from an attack of heart failure with enlargement of the liver, every subsequent attack induces this symptom, sometimes before any sign of dropsy sets in.

There may be associated with the enlargement a certain amount of jaundice, and the combination of enlarged liver and jaundice, with the wasting that sometimes accompanies long-continued heart failure, may raise the suspicion of malignant disease of the liver. The dilatation or irregular action of the heart should direct attention to the real nature of the trouble.

There may be a considerable degree of pain and discomfort associated with the enlargement of the liver, and the painful contracted muscles may embarrass the respiration.

Œdema of the lungs.—A symptom of great value is found in the careful auscultation of the bases of the lungs, in cases threatened with some forms of heart failure. I carried out for some years an extensive observation on all kinds of people—healthy, and with failing hearts from a great variety of causes—and I was able to anticipate attacks of heart failure in a great number of cases. If one systematically examines the bases of the lungs in elderly people who are perforce confined to bed, as in consequence of an operation or a fractured leg, in a certain proportion, the earliest symptom of heart failure will be found in the appearance of fine crepitations in this region. The same experience will be met with in patients confined to bed from any exhausting complaint, particularly if the heart muscle be involved in the ailment, as in typhoid fever. Many patients with mitral lesions have no dropsy, but suffer from severe attacks of heart failure with great breathlessness. In such cases, the bases of the lungs will be found to show signs of œdema at the early stages of the breakdown.

It has been my habit in these cases to begin the examination of the patient by asking him on which side he lies, then make him sit up, and while I auscultate the base of that lung on the side he had lain, I ask him to take in one full and deep inspiration. This opens up the alveoli at the base, and if there is any abnormal moisture it is manifested by numerous fine crepitations. Healthy people show no sign of this. Slightly weakened hearts may show it with the first deep inspiration only; if there is distinct cardiac enfeeblement, the crepitations do not disappear at first, but persist. I have seen cases where the first sign was the crepitation during the first deep inspiration, and gradually the crepitation became more persistent until the resonance of the bases of the lung became impaired, even to complete dulness, with no breath sounds; and at the post-mortem examination the lungs at the bases have been sodden and airless. In some instances, there have been patches of inflammation (catarrhal pneumonia—the hypostatic pneumonia, in addition, of the feeble).

I have also seen this hypostatic congestion disappear, and as the patient improved the crepitations gradually disappeared, the last sign being the crepitations with the first deep inspiration.

I have found this method of observation of the greatest practical use. In the elderly it governs the position which the patient should occupy— lying down or propped up. In typhoid fever, it is a prognostic sign of the very greatest value—the absence of œdema indicating that the heart has escaped infection; its presence and gradual increase, a sign of great gravity. In heart disease, it is likewise one indication of the heart's condition, and in the complication of pregnancy and heart disease it is one of the most important guides in the management of these cases.

It is of no less importance in treatment, as will be realized when the reason for its appearance is appreciated. It invariably accompanies dilatation of the right heart, and the manner of its production is as follows: The factors that move the blood through the lungs are twofold—first and most important, the right ventricle; and second, the movements of respiration. In healthy hearts, the first of these is so powerful that the second is scarcely appreciated. When, however, the right ventricle is enfeebled, the assistance of the respiratory movements becomes necessary. When the patient lies in bed on one side, the pressure of the ribs on the mattress restrains their movements, so that the flow of blood through this part of the lung is retarded and œdema results. This can be shown in the early stages, for when the patient breathes deeply the whole of the crepitations may disappear.

From this account will be realized the part that can be played in suitable cases by placing the patient in a position to breathe freely, avoiding the restraint exerted by pressure on the ribs, and by making the patient deeply inspire. In addition, the importance of recognizing the nature of the symptoms due to the enlargement of the liver is here apparent, where not only the abdominal muscles, but the intercostals also, may be tender and contracted. In thus ceasing to act as respiratory agents, while exercising

their primitive function of protection, these contracted muscles further add
to the embarrassment of the heart in its work.

Urinary symptoms.—I doubt if ever we get the characteristic urinary
symptoms of heart failure in the absence of dilatation of the heart. These
symptoms are a scanty secretion and increased specific gravity, and
frequently the presence of albumen. A diminished supply of blood to the
kidneys may cause a large quantity of albumen to appear in the scanty
urine, as can be observed in heart-block, when the heart's rate becomes
very infrequent. The diminution of the quantity usually goes hand in
hand with the dropsy. The cause in the main is a fall in arterial pressure
and a rise in the venous, with consequent venous stasis in the kidneys.
Other conditions may co-operate, such as the chemical constitution of the
fluid in the tissues and changes in the secreting cells of the kidney. It is
often a difficult point to determine whether the albuminuria has been
pre-existent, or whether it is induced by the venous stasis and subsequent
inflammatory changes in the kidneys. This history of the patient will help,
and the presence of arterio-sclerosis and retinitis point to a pre-existent
Bright's disease. It may be necessary to suspend judgement until a recovery
of tonicity of the heart restores the circulation, as with the increase in flow
of urine the albuminuria may entirely disappear.

It is often useful to direct the patient's attention to the urinary secretion,
as its diminution may give the first warning of an impending breakdown,
and the increase in the flow is often the first sign of recovery of heart power.

Prognosis.—It is a confident belief that dilatation of the heart is a
frequent occurrence even in healthy people, who may have been subjected
to some severe bodily effort ; and it is supposed to be particularly common
in young people who indulge in strenuous games. Such dilatation is supposed
to be of a grave nature, and many physicians indulge in gloomy forebodings
unless strenuous efforts are made to combat the dilatation. Yet it is a curious
fact that in dilatation, with a healthy heart muscle, there is not on record
a single case of any harm following the neglect of these conditions, even
when it has been recognized and some suggested treatment rejected. While
I recognize that the size of the heart, especially in the young, may vary
slightly in size from time to time, I am perfectly certain that the variation
has no grave significance, that it is a perfectly normal occurrence, and needs
no treatment. I have seen in some cases, as in poisoning after a drinking
bout, or after the onset of paroxysmal tachycardia and auricular fibrillation,
marked dilatation, accompanied by evidences of heart failure ; but in these
cases the heart muscle was either poisoned or suffered from some disease.
From my experience, I am aware that there is a widespread belief that
dilatation of the heart is a very common affection, and I have little hesitation
in saying that there is really very little justification for this belief, and that
error in diagnosis is the chief cause of its existence. We hear, for instance,

of cases in which the heart has been detected out in the axilla, while the patient was scarcely conscious of any limitation in his powers, and that after some fanciful exercises or baths, there has been a speedy withdrawal of the heart within normal limits.

For some years, in the Mount Vernon and London Hospitals, my colleagues and myself have been carefully investigating all the perceptible changes in hearts during heart failure and during recovery. In a great many of these cases, the hearts were greatly increased in size. Many of the patients when they came under our care suffered from extreme heart failure. A good number of them were sufficiently restored to be able to follow somewhat strenuous occupations, but we could detect, in the majority, no appreciable difference in the size of the heart.

The prognosis, therefore, should not be based on the presence of an increase in the heart's size, but on other evidences. Even with the presence of objective signs of heart failure, as dropsy or enlargement of the liver, the prognosis will depend on the condition that has induced the dilatation, and in any case, the prognosis must be suspended until a period of treatment has been given, and especially till after the effect of digitalis has been noted.

Treatment.—As dilatation is invariably secondary to some other condition of the heart, the treatment has to take into consideration other factors. I may point out, however, that, unless in the acute febrile stage, dilatation is an indication for the prescription of digitalis in all rheumatic hearts. In other conditions it should be tried, especially if there is dropsy and deficient secretion of urine. The treatment of such associated symptoms as dropsy and diminution of urine, should consist in the attempt to restore the heart's strength. When dropsy becomes a distressing symptom, special means have to be undertaken for its removal. As free diuresis is the most effective way of getting rid of it, a great many agents are recommended which effect this purpose. The virtues of many a prescription can be established by the recital of illustrative cases, in which its exhibition was followed by an extraordinary discharge of urine, and speedy disappearance of all dropsy. These preparations will be found to vary from the mixtures containing every conceivable drug that is supposed to have diuretic properties, to some recent synthetical preparation. The fact of the matter is, that in many of these cases the secretory activity of the kidneys seems to be in temporary abeyance, and some slight adventitious aid gives it the necessary stimulus. This auspicious moment, coinciding with the administration of the drug, results in a profuse diuresis. This aid need not be a drug. I have seen a patient, who had to sit up in a chair for three weeks on account of his breathing, become extremely dropsical, passing very little urine. The mere return to bed was followed at once by a profuse diuresis, and the rapid disappearance of the dropsy. It is, however, necessary in many cases to try various agents, and happily here the digitalis group is most effective, the combination of digitalis, squill, and calomel being particularly useful, not only from its action on the heart and kidneys, but also from its effects on the bowels. When these drugs fail others may be found to act, such as theobrominæ sodii salicylas (diuretin) or theocin-sodium acetate.   In some cases, the elimination of common salt from the food helps to reduce the dropsy.   In all cases of dropsy, the bowels should invariably be kept well moved.

Special efforts to give relief are often necessary.   In certain cases, when the patient can go about, an elastic bandage skilfully applied is beneficial, particularly in those hard, swollen legs when the skin threatens to give way. Massage also is of assistance.   When the legs or genitals become greatly distended, deep pricks with a needle will often be followed by a free flow of serum and a great diminution of the swelling.   The utmost cleanliness should be observed in carrying out this simple procedure.   The employment of Southey's tubes, inserted into the legs or abdominal cavity, will often drain off a large quantity of fluid.   The abdominal and thoracic cavities may need to be tapped ; such tapping invariably gives temporary relief. In some advanced cases, where the penis is greatly swollen (ram's horn), there may be inability to void urine.   In using a catheter, there may be some trouble in finding the meatus, the glans penis being buried in the scrotum under the swollen prepuce.   If the swollen foreskin be gently but firmly grasped in the hand and compressed, the fluid is driven out, and the glans can then be exposed.

The employment of judicious breathing exercises in œdema of the lung is often beneficial, the patient sitting up and breathing slowly and deeply. In severe cases, this is limited at first to a few movements.   If the patient bears the exercise, these deep respirations should be employed at regular intervals every two or three hours when awake.   In the intervals, the patient should be propped as high as he can bear with comfort.

Where fluid accumulates in the thoracic and abdominal cavities, in such quantities as to embarrass the respiration of the heart, if it is not diminished by drugs, then it should be drawn off by tapping.

CHAPTER XXXIX

THE SENILE HEART

Introduction.
Conditions inducing degenerative changes in the arterial system.
Obliteration of the capillaries.
Symptoms.
Prognosis.
Treatment.

Introduction.—There are certain changes, which we recognize as accompanying and giving rise to the features characteristic of advancing years. These changes may be detected in every tissue and organ of the body; and they can be recognized in the bald scalp, white hair, or tortuous artery. The changes in the arteries and capillaries may modify the structure and functions of the various organs, but not all organs equally. Arterial degeneration may in one person be more advanced in the brain, in another in the kidneys, in another in the limbs, in another in the heart. In many, these changes are merely those associated with advancing years, and give rise to what we understand by senile changes. When affecting the heart, they are usually accompanied by some fibrous or fatty changes in the heart muscle. If these changes are considerable in extent, then we get a train of symptoms which we recognize as due to ' senile changes '.

There are two main circumstances that induce degenerative changes (fatty and fibrous) in the heart, namely, the cicatricial changes that follow acute affections, as after rheumatic fever, and the changes that accompany arterial degeneration. Both these conditions affect the muscular structure as well as the valves, and the resulting heart failure is often the outcome of the invasion of both tissues by the sclerotic process. Although it may be convenient to follow conventional lines and describe separately the valvular affections, it must be borne in mind always that, in the serious cases, there is a widespread condition of which the valvular lesion is but a part.

The changes due to rheumatic fever have a certain resemblance to those due to arterial degeneration. In both instances there is a replacement of the muscular fibres by fibrous tissue, and a shrinking of the valvular apparatus, and as a consequence both conditions present identical symptoms. Though there is this resemblance in ʻprogress and symptoms, there are other differences which have an important bearing on prognosis and treatment.

The consideration of the rheumatic and other inflammatory forms of sclerosis is included in the chapters on valvular disease. Here I wish to draw particular attention to the changes in the heart, that are associated with arterial degeneration and senile changes. The causes of arterial degeneration are still not clear, and it is difficult to say of the complications in any given case, showing arterial degeneration, which are the cause and which the consequence. Clifford Allbutt rightly protests against arterio-sclerosis being considered a disease ; it is the outcome of processes which we imperfectly understand, and may arise as the result of high blood-pressure, toxic conditions, or senile changes. I do not enter into the, at present, hopeless task of distinguishing the causes of the changes in the arterial system. A little of the truth may be present in each of the many competing theories at present holding the field, but no one of them can be considered wholly satisfactory and convincing.

In the meantime, an appreciation of the changes as they affect the heart gives us great assistance in the treatment of our patients.

Conditions inducing degenerative changes in the arterial system.— It is usual to attribute the changes to some earlier process that has affected the blood or the arteries, of which kidney disease, syphilis, over-exertion, are the most striking examples. But it will be found frequently that extensive arterial degeneration may be present, for which one can find no definite cause.

There can be no doubt that affections of the kidneys tend to induce these changes. But in many people, the kidney lesions are undoubtedly secondary, and patients may show well-marked and extensive arterial degeneration many years before there is the slightest evidence of kidney ailment. In such instances, it is but reasonable to assume that the renal degeneration, like the cardiac and cerebral, is secondary to the arterial degeneration.

Obliteration of the capillaries.— One of the most striking changes that take place in the progress of arterial degeneration is the diminution of the capillary field. This obliteration of the capillaries is likely to be found of the greatest importance, not only in the production of the degenerative changes that occur in the heart itself, but by narrowing the communication between the arterial and the venous system, it entails more work on the heart in forcing the blood through the constricted area.

If one notes the changes in the skin that occur with advancing years, how it loses its velvety thickness, becomes shrivelled and attenuated, so that in advanced conditions the scalp may be found denuded of hair and plastered to the underlying bones, the extent of the diminution of the capillary field may, to a certain extent, be appreciated. A still more striking evidence of the diminished capillary field in the old is the absence of free bleeding in a freshly-made wound. In the young, the abundant oozing of bright red blood is a source of satisfaction to the surgeon, for it is a testimony to the healthiness of the subject and to the recuperative power, and is in striking contrast to the bleeding from a wound in the aged, where the bleeding is mostly from some cut vein or from the persistent spouting of a degenerated artery, indicating an impoverished blood-supply rendering the healing process less satisfactory.

This diminution of the capillary field, so easily recognized in the external body-wall, also occurs in the heart, and the results are shown in a variety of ways. It leads to malnutrition of the tissues and degeneration of the heart muscle. The character of the degeneration varies according to the structure affected, but in all it leads to impairment of function. The first structures to show evidence of the capillary obliteration are those that have the smallest blood-supply, and it may be partly for this reason that it is early marked in the cornea (arcus senilis), the valves of the heart, and the elastic tissue of the arterial walls.

In the heart muscle, the effect of these changes in the arteries and capillaries is a degeneration, fibrous or fatty. In the production of this myocardial degeneration, we get the diminished capillary field complicating the consequences of the degenerated artery—a degeneration at times so extreme that little blood can penetrate the coronary arteries or their branches. If it be borne in mind how dependent the muscular structure of the heart is upon an abundant supply of blood, it will be easy to recognize the fact that such changes must have a profound effect upon the efficiency of the organ.

Accompanying the arterial degeneration, there may be a great increase in the muscular coat of the smaller arteries. This hypertrophy implies during life abnormal contraction (hypertonus of Russell). This is bound to raise the blood-pressure and embarrass the heart.

The diminished capillary field has also probably a further complicating effect in so far as it introduces an obstruction to the heart's contraction. The narrowing of the outflow necessitates a greater force to send the blood through the tissues ; consequently, the ventricle has to contract more strongly to raise the arterial pressure, and thus produce a further embarrassment to the degenerated heart.

Symptoms.—The symptoms arising from such changes are extremely varied, and at first sight hopelessly confused ; but there is good reason to expect that, with a better knowledge of the functions of the different parts of the heart, a more satisfactory appreciation of all the symptoms may be obtained ; and, in turn, a more accurate understanding of the symptoms during life will guide the pathologist in his post-mortem examination. I have submitted to Professor Keith a large number of hearts affected by the changes associated with arterio-sclerosis, from patients ranging from 42 to 77 years of age, and in all the post-mortem appearance had such a close resemblance that it might have been assumed that during life the symptoms would have been identical. A study of these symptoms showed, however, a wide diversity, some patients suffering from angina pectoris, others with no pain ; some with severe cardiac asthma, others with no respiratory trouble ; some had very irregular hearts, due to auricular fibrillation, others frequent or infrequent extra-systole, while some had marked pulsus alternans, and in others the heart was perfectly regular till the end. Some patients had extensive dropsy, other patients showed no sign of œdema. Some had aortic or mitral murmurs, others had no murmurs. It will thus be seen that the symptoms of well-authenticated cardio-sclerosis exhibit every phase of cardiac symptoms, and the superficial observer might think that each case presented a different form of heart disease. Instead of this, while the organic or fundamental lesion is the same, the variety of symptoms is due to the different parts or functions particularly affected.

The earliest result of these degenerative changes is a diminution of the reserve force of the heart, manifested by a limitation of the field of cardiac response. The patient rarely presents himself before the physician until this exhaustion of the reserve force has produced some distressing symptom, it may be breathlessness, cardiac asthma, angina pectoris, or ' bronchitis '. In every case, it will be found to be preceded by a history of an ever-diminishing area of cardiac response. At the beginning, the individual will not acknowledge that his powers are being curtailed—indeed, the patient may be proud of his virility—but it may be taken as a certain sign that when a middle-aged man boasts of his strength he is trying to hide from others his own consciousness of a limitation of his powers. As he continues to work as hard as he did before these degenerative changes made their appearance, the exhaustion of the reserve force, though slight at first and scarcely perceptible, in the long run reaches a stage when the suffering or discomfort entailed compels the patient to consult his physician. When this occurs, the changes in heart and blood-vessels are well established. The skin of the hand has already lost its velvety thickness, and the arteries show a varying degree of change, as tortuosity, slight or considerable thickening of the radial ; sometimes one can detect pieces of peculiar hardness, fine and granular, or patches like small beads, or the artery may be thickened like the characteristic pipe-stem, the surface being slightly nodulated.

Even in the absence of any of these signs in the superficial arteries, it must not be inferred that the degenerative process is absent in the visceral arteries. Arterial degeneration is often very irregularly distributed, affecting different regions in different patients. It is for this reason that in this affection the symptoms of its progress may be more marked ; now in the cerebral arteries, giving rise to cerebral apoplexy ; now in the arteries of the leg, giving rise to gangrene ; now in the arteries of the heart, giving rise to the symptoms here described.

The blood-pressure measurements show, in many cases, a great rise. In the earlier stages, when the patients are first seen, there is seldom much enlargement of the heart unless there has been long-standing Bright's disease. Usually the heart's dullness does not extend beyond the nipple line. The sounds of the heart may be clear and well struck, often with some accentuation of the second sound. In some, an aortic murmur may be present, most frequently systolic in time, though occasionally there may also be a diastolic murmur, usually of very short duration. The heart's action, though frequently perfectly regular until the end, may show irregularities, the most common being of the nature of extra-systole. In advanced cases, we may find good examples of the pulsus alternans. The heart may be continuously irregular (auricular fibrillation), and sometimes of great rapidity. Not infrequently this continuous irregularity, with or without excessive rapidity, comes on in intermittent attacks lasting for a few minutes, a few hours, or a few days (paroxysmal tachycardia). In rare cases, the degenerative process may affect the auriculo-ventricular bundle and give rise to heart-block.

The subjective phenomena vary. In the early stages, there may be no symptom beyond a limitation of the field of cardiac response, shown by breathlessness on moderate exertion. In more advanced cases, there may be a slight tightness across the chest on exertion, or on going into the cold air, as on going from a warm room into a cold bedroom, or going into the open air on a winter's morning. This sensation is usually ignored until it is accompanied by pain, sometimes of such severity as to be recognized as an attack of angina pectoris. In rare cases, the pain may never arise, but the gripping sensation felt in the chest may be so severe that the patient feels his chest fixed, and has to stop and draw several deep breaths to relieve the spasm.

In many cases, it is only breathlessness on exertion that arrests the patient, the breathing being short and hurried on such exertion as he used to undertake in comfort. In extreme cases, the mere turning over in bed induces the hurried respiration. The breathlessness may seize him in the night—in attacks of cardiac asthma, or Cheyne-Stokes respiration may appear.

The symptoms described so far arise from the heart, while the tonicity is still good. In a great many of these cases, a stage is reached when the heart dilates. In addition to the increased size of the heart, a number of symptoms disappear, while others come into prominence : the arterial pressure falls ; dropsy sets in, and œdema of the lungs, sometimes with the expectoration of blood or blood-stained sputum, in short, all the symptoms already described under failure of tonicity (Chapter XXXVIII).

If the cause of the symptoms in cardio-sclerosis is appreciated, it helps one to understand the reason of the great variety of phenomena present in this affection. The variations in symptoms are, in all likelihood, due to the parts invaded by the degenerative process. As the presence or absence of aortic murmurs depends on whether the disease affects the aortic valves, so the presence or absence of various irregularities (with the exception of the pulsus alternans) depends on the invasion of the myocardium. The position and character of the invasion determines whether it terminates in auricular fibrillation or in heart-block. In like manner, the degree of exhaustion of the function of contractility determines the nature of the subjective phenomena, the breathlessness, anginal symptoms, and the cardiac asthma. On the other hand, with exhaustion of the tonicity, we get the transformation in the character of the symptoms, resulting in the dilatation of the heart, dropsy, œdema of the lungs, and so forth.

Prognosis.—Prognosis depends to a great extent on the nature of the symptoms, and the manner in which the heart responds to treatment. If, for instance, a patient has an irregular pulse due to extra-systole, while in other respects the response of the heart to effort is such as would be expected under normal conditions at his time of life, then the prognosis, in the absence of other evidences of disease, is very favourable. When graver symptoms are present, as the tightness across the chest, slight or severe attacks of pain, then, if the previous history of the patient points to worry, sleeplessness, and overwork, a prognosis should be deferred to see how he responds to treatment. If these signs speedily disappear under treatment, the prognosis is favourable ; on the other hand, the prognosis becomes the more unfavourable the more the symptoms refuse to yield. But even here comparative freedom from suffering may be enjoyed by a patient who pursues a life that exposes him to little effort, and many patients may live a useful though crippled life for years. Where there are attacks of cardiac asthma occurring in the night, or attacks of Cheyne-Stokes respiration, or when the pulsus alternans is present, the condition may be considered far advanced, and though the patient may live for months or a few years, it is with very limited powers, and he is liable to a serious breakdown at any time. When the pulse is continually irregular, the prognosis depends on how well the heart maintains the circulation. If dropsy supervenes and steadily increases in senile degeneration, it is not very susceptible to treatment in contrast to the parallel condition due to rheumatic sclerosis. But apart from this, many patients may lead a fairly active existence with auricular fibrillation for many years, though exposed to frequent attacks of ' bronchitis '.

It must be borne in mind that the sudden inception of auricular fibrillation is not infrequently the direct cause of death in the elderly.

The rather rapid dilatation of the heart, with accompanying dropsy, is usually a sign of approaching dissolution.

I doubt if the blood-pressure measurements prove of much use as a guide in prognosis. I have watched, for a number of years, individuals glide past 70 years of age with a blood-pressure from 180 to 200 mm. Hg., and I could not see that their condition was materially worse in consequence.

Treatment.—In treating chronic myocardial affections, it should always be borne in mind that the condition is often progressive, and we cannot stay it, because the changes are those which are inseparable from advancing years. It usually proceeds very slowly, so that a man may show signs of arterial degeneration and irregularity of the heart from the age of 50 to 60 years, but may live in fair health for twenty years afterwards, ending his days without any marked failure of the heart. The early stages are generally recognized in the examination of the patient for some other condition, when the distinctive signs may be found in the tortuous arteries, raised blood-pressure, and the occasional occurrence of an extra-systole. Medical men often attempt to combat these signs by some treatment more or less energetic, and, as many people are frightened by the evidences of advancing years, they readily comply with the proposals that are supposed to put back the hands of time ; hence the great variety of drugs, methods, and modes of life we find current.

It is rare that one has occasion to treat the milder symptoms in the working-man—not that they are not frequently present, but because he has not the time to consider his complaints, and he seems in no way to suffer from the neglect. It is the well-to-do who are most concerned about some trifling symptom incidental to these changes, and when their attention is called to such a symptom as an extra-systole, either by their own sensations or by their medical attendant, they believe that some calamity is impending, and readily submit to any suggestion that promises to stave off the evil day.

When the patient is aware of the irregular action of his heart, and when we find by examination that there are no changes beyond what would be expected at his time of life, he should be strongly reassured that the irregularity is a trivial symptom and of no vital importance. When the symptoms are unpleasant and are aggravated by his mode of life—for example, by too close application to a sedentary occupation—certain rational suggestions as to the manner of living are obligatory.

In cases presenting these milder signs, no further treatment is necessary, beyond insisting that the patient should lead a well-regulated life, avoiding over-feeding, over-drinking, and taking as much exercise in the open air as can be reasonably obtained. Some of the symptoms, as extra-systole, come on for periods and disappear for longer and shorter intervals. In these cases, I have frequently seen the patient get much benefit from a holiday with healthy open-air exercise. Several of my patients, for instance, were conscious of the occurrence of extra-systoles, and when they felt them they indulged in a game of golf two or three afternoons a week, or took a short golfing holiday, and invariably experienced relief. In like manner, judicious hill-climbing and walking are of benefit. In some cases, the bodily exertion may, in the first instance, increase the frequency of these extra-systoles, but the exercise should not be given up on that account ; rather should it be continued with moderation till a recovery of the reserve force takes place by training, when the irregularities will become less frequent or disappear.

The amount of recovery depends on the stage which the degeneration of the heart muscle has reached. We know of no method which can restore a better blood-supply by removing the arterial degeneration, and without this it is impossible to arrive at any process that would restore the degenerate muscle of the heart ; so that when a considerable degree of recovery has taken place, it is foolish to imagine that the favourable result has come to pass because the treatment has restored the degenerated muscle fibres. All we can say in such cases is, that the treatment has increased the reserve force of the muscle fibres. Recovery means the retention of a certain amount of active muscle fibre, and the greater the recovery the less the degeneration, and the less serious the prospect for the patient.

Another most important factor in treatment in all these cases is sleep. Many suffer from troubled and broken sleep, and when they begin to suffer from attacks of heart failure, the occurrence of sleepless nights almost invariably precipitates the exhaustion. Attacks of angina pectoris may be directly induced by this want of refreshing sleep, and may be stopped by measures taken to induce sleep. The means best adapted to this object varies with different individuals. In some, it may be found that their former habits in the matter of their food are no longer suitable for their condition ; it is sometimes enough for them to take some light nourishment, as milk or biscuit, on going to bed or during the night, to induce a restful sleep. Most require some form of hypnotic, and the bromides—20 grains of bromide of ammonium thrice daily, for instance—may induce a degree of drowsiness that is very beneficial. Again, the safer hypnotics, as veronal or sulphonal, prove very useful in the milder cases. When, however, the nights are disturbed by attacks of distressful breathing, oxygen is of great service in some cases, and in others opiates or chloral must be resorted to. On the whole, I find chloral the more useful drug. But the cases are so variable that sometimes one drug is more efficacious than the other, so that it may be necessary to try each of them, or a combination of both. As regards contra-indications, I do not prescribe opiates when there is exudation in the bronchial tubes with duskiness of the face, as I have seen serious results follow, probably from the secretion not being got rid of, and thus inducing a certain amount of suffocation, which further impairs the enfeebled heart.

Iodide of potassium is supposed generally to be of service in the relief of many of the milder symptoms, associated with arterial degeneration. In many people, the symptoms are not constant, but are manifested occasionally in attacks of dizziness, dull headaches, inability to walk as far as usual on account of breathlessness, slight attacks of angina pectoris, and even more violent attacks ; these all seem to benefit by the use of iodide of potassium. I am not at all sure that the good results attributed to the iodide may not have been due to the accompanying change in the food and mode of life. The action of iodide of potassium is not understood.

CHAPTER XL

SOUNDS AND MURMURS, NORMAL AND ABNORMAL

Introduction.
The attitude of the profession to abnormal sounds.
Variations in the sounds of the heart.
The cause of functional murmurs.
The quantity of blood thrown back to cause a murmur.
The differentiation of functional and organic murmurs.
The significance of functional murmurs.
The significance of organic murmurs.

Introduction.—Before entering on the study of valve affections, it is necessary, in order to understand the significance of murmurs, to appreciate the following clinical facts :

1. That murmurs may appear in hearts with no damage to the valves (functional murmurs), and in hearts with damaged valves (organic murmurs).

2. Individuals with functional murmurs may be in perfect health, and lead strenuous lives, and never show the slightest sign of heart failure. From this we can conclude that murmurs may be a physiological and normal event, and indicate neither impairment of the heart's efficiency nor fore-shadow the oncoming of heart failure. Functional murmurs may be present in debilitated individuals, and in these the murmur is not necessarily indicative of disease ; nor is the valve incompetence the cause of the debility.

3. Functional murmurs may be associated with heart failure of a grievous kind. In such cases, it will be found that though the murmur is associated with the heart failure, the valvular incompetence is not the cause of the heart failure, but is one of the changes which have arisen in consequence of impaired functional efficiency of the heart muscle.

4. Individuals with organic murmurs—the result of damaged valves— may lead vigorous lives, being engaged in strenuous occupation, and never show any signs of heart failure. From this we can conclude (a) that valve lesions of themselves are not necessarily of serious significance, (b) that the affection which causes the valve lesion has ceased to progress, (c) that little or no embarrassment to the heart results from the damaged valve, and (d) that no coincident damage has occurred to the heart muscle, or at least not so marked as to impair its efficiency.

5. That heart murmurs may be associated with heart failure.

The attitude of the profession to abnormal sounds.—As a general rule, the more obtrusive a symptom is, the more it impresses the mind of the observer, and much more importance is attached to it than to less conspicuous phenomena. This is particularly noticeable in signs which are detected by auscultation. To the human mind, sounds arising from obscure causes have always been a source of mystery, and the human imagination, when dealing with the mysterious, invariably associates it with something malign. This peculiar trait is shown by the attitude of the profession towards murmurs and abnormal sounds of the heart. Within a few years of the discovery of the stethoscope, it was found that people who died from heart failure often exhibited murmurs of different kinds, and hence it occurred to the physician of that day that murmurs were manifestations of diseases of a serious nature. This notion was taught at a period when the cause of the sounds of the heart, and much less the cause of the murmurs, was not understood. As years went ou, and investigation into the sounds of the heart ultimately brought out the true origin of some of these, the inquiry into the cause of the different murmurs was diligently pursued, and their origin at the different orifices gradually established. Time after time, physicians were able to indicate at which orifice a murmur was generated, and confirmation of their predictions was found repeatedly at the post-mortem examination. It came to be looked on by the profession that murmurs were an evidence of disease of the valves. As, however, many cases showed murmurs during life, particularly systolic murmurs, and the valves were found intact at the post-mortem examination, a ' functional ' murmur was recognized. But although these functional murmurs were not considered evidence of disease, they came to be regarded as evidence of impairment of the heart's efficiency, and as such to be indications for treatment and a restriction of the life of the individual.

So deep an impression have murmurs made in the minds of the profession, that a large proportion deems them invariably an evidence of an unhealthy heart ; the result of which is that we find every form of murmur looked on as an evidence of impairment, if not of disease. It is true that many physicians recognize and acknowledge that some functional murmurs may be harmless, but when they attempt in their writings to deal with this problem, their words convey so confused an impression, that it is evident that they have but a hazy conception of the manner in which a harmless functional murmur is to be distinguished from a murmur, which may be an indication of, or associated with, heart failure.

Variations in the sounds of the heart.—The first sound is produced by two factors, the contraction of the ventricular muscle and the sudden stretching of the mitral and tricuspid valves. Composed of these two elements, it is subject to many modifications, according to changes in the muscles or valves. Consequently, alteration in the character of the first sound is frequent, and satisfactory explanations for these variations are not forthcoming. Moreover, experience has shown us that little can be made out of these modified sounds alone, and while the modification should be noted, the real opinion of the heart's condition should be based on other evidences, which are never lacking. A certain number of modified first sounds have gained a place in the terminology of cardiac affections, and therefore need a brief reference.

Feebleness or absence of the first sound may indicate extreme exhaustion of the heart muscle, in the presence of other signs of heart exhaustion. A 'flapping' first sound is sometimes spoken of as indicative of a thin-walled ventricle, but we must be chary of trusting to such a sign.

A reduplication of the first sound may be due to a slight difference in the time of contraction of the two ventricles, or at least to a minute difference in the times of the closure of the mitral and tricuspid valves. Recently it has been found that a reduplicated first sound may indicate damage to the branch of the auriculo-ventricular bundle leading to the right ventricle, thus giving a lack of synchronism in the times of the contraction of the two ventricles.

The second sound is valvular in its production. An accentuation of the aortic sound is present when the aortic pressure is raised, and the pulmonary second sound may be found slightly accentuated when there is engorgement of the lungs ; its cause is possibly due to increased pressure in the pulmonary artery.

Reduplication of the second sound is loudest usually at the mitral area. It is not clear how it is produced, but it is so often present in mitral stenosis, that its detection should always arouse the suspicion of stenosis of the mitral valve in the absence of more reliable evidence.

A curious modification of the sounds of the heart is found when there appears a third sound, interpolated between the first and second sounds. The triple heart sound or gallop rhythm has been the cause of a good deal of controversy. There appear to be different conditions producing it ; one of those is the reduplication of the first sound as already mentioned, due to a lesion of the right branch of the auriculo-ventricular bundle. Some have looked upon it as a grave sign, and no doubt it occurs towards the end of heart failure in such conditions as kidney disease ; but I have found it in individuals who were free from any cardiac lesion, and who have lived for many years with no evidence of heart failure.

Muffled sounds seem to be of little significance ; sometimes they change into murmurs.

The cause of functional murmurs.—There are some murmurs whose nature is so obscure that they are still the subject of discussion. The majority of murmurs can now, with fair certainty, be referred to definite orifices of the heart. Organic murmurs are due to lesions affecting the valves, and these can often be identified by certain peculiarities of the murmurs. There are, however, murmurs which arise when there is no lesion of the valves ; these are spoken of as functional murmurs. The functional murmur usually occurs during ventricular systole, and may be heard in various regions of the heart. When heard loudest at the apex, it is assumed to be mitral in origin ; when loudest over the middle of the sternum, it is supposed to be tricuspid in origin. These murmurs are not infrequently heard loudest towards the base of the heart, and it is difficult to determine in which particular region, tricuspid, aortic, or pulmonary, they are heard loudest, and it is even suggested they are cardio-pulmonary in origin. It is not possible, in all cases, to distinguish them from organic murmurs. Much study has been devoted towards finding out if the mitral functional murmur could not be distinguished from the organic murmur, because of its character and the regions into which it is propagated. While many organic murmurs do show very characteristic features, others resemble functional murmurs so closely that it is not always possible to speak with certainty.

Functional murmurs are usually assumed to be due to dilatation of the heart, rendering the orifices so wide that the valves fail to close them. This is not entirely correct, for while it is true that we may find a murmur with dilatation of the heart, we may often find great dilatation and no murmur. Further, we find murmurs come and go when there is no perceptible change in the size of the heart, the murmurs appearing only when the heart is excited or when the individual stands, and disappearing when the heart quietens or the individual is at rest. Again, murmurs which we find when the heart is acting quietly with the body at rest, may disappear on exertion or excitement.

From this it can be inferred that there is some special mechanism, apart from that involved in the dilatation of auricle and ventricle as a whole, and this obscure mechanism varies under circumstances which we are still unable to appreciate. The importance of this is seen in connexion with the heart of the young, where it is probable that the heart has a peculiar power of adapting itself, which is gradually lost in adult life. It must be remembered also that free regurgitation can take place at the mitral and tricuspid orifices without murmurs. We frequently get evidence of marked tricuspid regurgitation in the veins of the neck and in the liver, with no tricuspid murmur.

The quantity of blood thrown back to cause a murmur.—Seeing that the chief importance attached to regurgitant murmurs is that they are evidences of blood escaping back from the contracting chamber, and that the regurgitation has been assumed to be the chief factor in producing heart failure, according to the back-pressure theory, it is desirable that we should form some idea of the quantity of blood which is actually thrown back. Unfortunately, there are few accurate data upon the subject, and we are forced to estimate the amount by indirect methods.   I have been able to keep under observation, for twenty or thirty years, individuals with loud, rasping systolic mitral murmurs, and who gave a history of rheumatic fever, so that I could safely conclude that the murmurs were due to some damage of the mitral valves.   These patients never suffered from heart failure ; and I venture the conclusion that, in them, the leak was small and the damage slight, so that one may say, within certain limits, that in regard to mitral murmurs the narrower the orifice the louder the murmur. Where there are functional murmurs, the leak, if this be present, causing them is also slight and never such as to embarrass the auricles in their work, apart from cases where there is grave damage done to the heart muscle.   The small quantity of blood thrown back does not alter appreciably the size of the auricles, for we often find murmurs in hearts of the normal size.   A better method of estimating the quantity of blood thrown back in tricuspid regurgitation, is to measure the size of the v wave in cases with the auricular form of venous pulse.   I have sought for evidences of the amount in a large number of cases with a tricuspid systolic murmur, and was unable to find any perceptible increase in the size of the v wave.   Now if the regurgitation had been extreme, the appearance of these waves would have been earlier in the period of ventricular systole.   I have noted their size in individual cases where the tricuspid systolic murmur was present and where it was absent, and could detect no change in the size of the wave.

It may be stated that I was mistaken in thinking the murmur tricuspid in origin, for a great many people are under the impression that tricuspid regurgitation occurs only in the last stage of extreme heart failure—a fallacious notion which is the outcome of the back-pressure theory of heart failure.   I have examined cases where the tricuspid valve was damaged, so that tricuspid regurgitation was bound to occur, and even in these cases the v wave was no larger than that we find in normal hearts (Fig. 49).

Nor does it appear that in aortic disease the loudness of the diastolic murmur is any measure of the amount of regurgitation.   I have watched patients for years with a loud diastolic aortic murmur, and they never showed any trace of heart failure which might be referred to the effects of regurgitation.   Moreover, the experimental work of Henderson has shown that a slight damage to the valve, permitting the leakage of only a few drops of blood, will cause a marked diastolic murmur and the collapsing pulse.   In aortic regurgitation, there is often great dilatation of the smaller arteries, and it is concluded that the collapsing pulse is not entirely due to the regurgitation, but due, in part at least, to some reflex causing a dilatation of the arterioles and capillaries, which takes place when the aorta is damaged.

The differentiation of functional and organic murmurs.—It is not always easy to distinguish between functional and organic murmurs.   As a rule, functional murmurs are systolic in time, and arise usually at the tricuspid or mitral orifice. They are usually soft and blowing, but these characteristics do not distinguish them from some organic murmurs. Much has been written to determine the different features; but while the character of the organic murmur may often be characteristic, organic murmurs, both in their character and propagation, resemble functional murmurs so closely that it is not possible in all cases to differentiate them. A very rough murmur, especially if accompanied by a purring tremor or a musical note, is indicative of a valve lesion. In the early stages, however, of an endocarditis the murmur is usually soft and blowing, resembling a functional murmur. It is necessary to distinguish between these two murmurs, and to do this the whole circumstances of the case must be considered. In the first place, it is necessary to bear in mind that a murmur may be a normal event. When we find a murmur occurring in an individual in robust health, and if we can safely assume it to be functional, we may consider it as indicative neither of impairment nor disease. On the other hand, when we find a murmur occurring in debilitated persons, search should be made for conditions which account for the debility, as anæmia, imperfect nourishment and rest, or disease of other organs. It is of importance to differentiate these murmurs in febrile cases, or after the subsidence of an acute febrile attack, as after rheumatic fever. The question then arises whether the heart has been affected by the disease process. Here it is necessary to bear in mind, that fever alone may produce changes in the heart's action, such as increase in size and murmurs, so that during the febrile stage of such acute illnesses judgement should be suspended until more definite signs of an organic lesion are forthcoming. The persistence of a murmur after a febrile attack, or its appearance, should be considered along with the other evidences. Thus, after the subsidence of the fever, if the rate becomes slow and the youthful type of irregularity is developed, it may be assumed that the heart has escaped infection, and that the murmur is merely functional (Chapter XXVI). If, on the other hand, the rate is persistently increased, then the fear is that the heart has become infected, and that active changes are going on. The importance of this aspect of the subject is more fully dealt with in Chapter XXVI.

The significance of functional murmurs.—Seeing that individuals with functional murmurs may be in perfect health, leading strenuous lives, and never show any sign of heart failure, we may conclude that murmurs may be a physiological and normal sign, and indicate no impairment of the heart's efficiency, nor foreshadow the oncoming of heart failure.

I wish to insist upon this fact, for the possibility that a healthy heart may present a murmur is so opposed to the views of a great many of the profession, teachers and practitioners, that much harm is done to people who have to be examined for life insurance or for entrance to the services.

I base my views on the fact that I have watched numbers of healthy young people, who exhibited this murmur, grow up into manhood and womanhood, and lead healthy and vigorous lives, and never show the slightest sign of heart failure. Moreover, if we consider how little we know of the causation of murmurs, it will be realized how little justification we have for treating them as abnormalities. Even if they were due to regurgitation, it is quite conceivable that the regurgitation might be an essential to a good functioning heart. We might reason as follows. A chamber of the heart will contract most efficiently when it has reached a certain degree of distension. If circumstances should arise, as during effort, when a chamber was overdistended, then the conditions would not be favourable to a good contraction. But if a mechanism were present, which relieved the chamber which was distended, a slight regurgitation might take place, a murmur might arise and the contraction be effective. I have already pointed out that the fear of regurgitation has attained the dimensions of a bogy in the medical mind ; further, I have already pointed out that, even with organic disease, the amount of regurgitation required to produce a murmur is very slight. Functional murmurs may be present in debilitated individuals, and in these cases the murmur is not necessarily an indication of disease or impairment, nor is the valve incompetency which its presence indicates the cause of the debility. Manifestly, the murmur is then but one of the many symptoms which the individual may exhibit, and the diagnosis of such cases will necessitate a search for other evidences which may throw light on the cause of the debility. A functional murmur may be present in cases of grave heart failure, but in such cases the murmur is but an associated symptom ; for the valvular incompetence is not the cause of the heart failure, but is merely one of the changes which have arisen in consequence of impaired functional efficiency of the heart muscle.

The significance of organic murmurs.—Organic murmurs have a varied significance, and it is necessary to grasp the idea that, though murmurs are associated with heart failure, the valve lesions which they indicate are not the cause of it. It is also well to bear in mind that individuals with murmurs, due to damaged valves, caused by some infective disease, such as rheumatic fever, may lead vigorous lives and be engaged in strenuous occupations, and never show any sign of heart failure. From this we can conclude that valve lesions in themselves may not necessarily be of serious significance. As, however, murmurs are often associated with heart failure, the presence of organic murmurs should be considered from the following standpoints : (1) as an indication that the heart has been invaded by a disease process ; (2) whether the damage done by the disease process is stationary or slowly progressive ; (3) whether the disease process has affected and impaired the heart muscle at the same time ; and (4) whether the damage to the valve is such that it obstructs the work of the heart, so as to embarrass the muscle sufficiently to impair its efficiency. In acute illnesses, it will not be possible to answer these questions, for there the immediate question concerns the acute affections. In chronic cases, that is to say what is called chronic valvular disease, it is absolutely necessary that these questions should be considered and answered, if a rational conclusion is to be obtained. The manner of obtaining the knowledge necessary to answer these questions, will be dealt with in the description of the different valve lesions.

The estimation of the significance of functional murmurs is not based on the murmur itself, but on the functional efficiency of the heart, and on the presence or absence of other signs of cardiac affections (size, rate, and rhythm). If we find in a heart of normal size and rhythm (or with the 'youthful type' of irregularity) a systolic murmur with absence of any sign that would indicate that it is definitely organic in origin, and with a good functioning organ, then we may conclude that the heart is perfectly normal. If there be evidence of weakness, or other signs of abnormal conditions present, then the opinion should be based on these other signs, and not on the murmur.

CHAPTER XLI

VALVULAR DEFECTS

The manner of heart failure with valvular defects.
Mitral stenosis.
    Conditions inducing heart failure in mitral stenosis.
    The murmurs present in mitral stenosis.
    Progress and symptoms in mitral stenosis.
    Occasional symptoms.
Mitral regurgitation.
    Murmurs due to mitral regurgitation.
    Conditions inducing heart failure in mitral regurgitation.

The manner of heart failure with valvular defects.—It is manifest that valvular defects can embarrass the work of the heart in two ways : first, by narrowing the orifice and thereby impeding the outflow ; second, by imperfect closure so that leakage occurs.

The defects are recognized clinically mainly by the presence of murmurs ; but it must not be assumed that absence of murmurs implies an intact valvular apparatus, for great widening of an orifice and large regurgitation may take place when no murmur can be detected. As valvular lesions are produced by a variety of conditions, it might have been more logical to discuss them under the heading of these conditions. As, however, they are presented to us at a stage when all immediate symptoms of their causal condition are in abeyance, it is more convenient to describe them at the time that the heart-changes evoke symptoms of exhaustion. Years may elapse after the mischief has been done to the valves, before symptoms arise that call attention to the heart trouble. In the acute condition producing the valvular lesion, the matter is presented in an entirely different aspect, for the febrile state and the symptoms associated with the cause of the fever predominate. In chronic valvular affections, the subjective symptoms of heart failure only arise when exhaustion of the heart muscle sets in. The symptoms due to exhaustion appear at varying periods, after the damage has been done to the valves; and the time of the appearance of these symptoms depends on the degree of embarrassment offered to the heart's work by the damaged valve, on the condition of the muscle-wall, and on such accessory factors as tend to exhaustion, as over-exertion, excessive food, drink, and so forth.

In organic lesions of the valves, it must always be borne in mind that the sclerotic process causing the lesions may be progressive, and that there may also be present advancing changes in the heart muscle.

Generally speaking, the symptoms of heart failure show little that is distinctive of the particular valves affected. In the aortic cases, the reflex sensory phenomena are more prominent, and the ashen colour of the face is sometimes characteristic. Where there is a mitral lesion, the pulmonary symptoms are usually more prominent, and the face may be ruddy with a dark tinge. Apart from such differences, there is a great similarity in the symptoms of heart failure produced by all kinds of lesions.

MITRAL STENOSIS

Conditions inducing heart failure in mitral stenosis.—This is, perhaps, the most common of valvular defects with which heart failure is associated. It arises generally in consequence of rheumatic endocarditis, though it may be found in people with no rheumatic history, and a previous history of erysipelas, or some other febrile complaint, may give a possible clue to its origin.

The condition is never recognized during the acute process which induces it, for the reason that it is not produced till the cicatrizing process following the inflammation narrows the orifice, and on account of its origin in scar-formation it is often a progressive lesion. Once the stenosis is present it may remain moderate in amount, and offer so little embarrassment to the heart that patients may reach extreme old age with no heart failure. As a rule, however, the cicatrizing process goes on with varying rapidity until in some cases the mitral orifice is reduced to a mere slit, and the valves resemble a thickened calcareous diaphragm. It is important to bear in mind the progressive nature of the lesion, for it accounts for the varying changes in the symptoms. It should also be borne in mind that the cicatrizing process may be going on in the muscle, causing contraction of the chordæ tendineæ, impairing at other places the functional activity of the heart muscle, and affecting the auriculo-ventricular bundle, depressing the conductivity or producing the conditions which lead to auricular fibrillation, thereby profoundly affecting the efficiency of the heart and modifying the nature of its rhythm.

From this, it can readily be understood that the manner in which heart failure is brought about in many cases is somewhat complicated. In some, embarrassment may not ensue until the narrowing of the orifice has become extreme. In others, there may be a fatal issue while the narrowing is yet moderate. In the latter cases, the muscle-wall will inevitably be found to have been damaged.

The murmurs present in mitral stenosis.—*The presystolic murmur.* The presystolic murmur—the auricular systolic murmur of Gairdner—is due to the contraction of the left auricle forcing blood through the narrowed mitral orifice. With the varying changes in advancing cicatrization, the murmurs of mitral stenosis alter, and present peculiarities that have hitherto not been sufficiently appreciated. In the very early stages,—some years before the appearance of a murmur,—I have detected a slight presystolic thrill. The first murmur to appear precedes, or runs up to, and seems to terminate in the first sound, and is audible over a small area around the apex. At first it may not be always present. This murmur may vary in duration, being usually short and abrupt, but it sometimes begins earlier and is somewhat prolonged. It is of a crescendo character, rising in pitch till it ends in the first sound.

The mid-diastolic murmur.—Although this is the usual position in the cardiac cycle of the presystolic murmur, I have found a few cases, in which it did not terminate abruptly in the first sound, but was separated from it by a very brief interval (see Cases 44 and 92). In some of my cases I asked a number of my colleagues to mark out on a tracing of the radial pulse the exact position of the murmur in the cardiac cycle, and every one without hesitation indicated the position where the loudest part of the murmur is separated by a minute interval from the first sound. When a jugular or an apex tracing was taken, it was seen that the position was identical with that of the auricular systole. In other words, there was a delay in the transmission of the stimulus for contraction between auricle and ventricle. This delay can sometimes be increased by digitalis, and the position of this murmur in its relation to the first sound moves in the same way; such a murmur has hitherto been described as ' *mid-diastolic* '.

I mention this not only to enforce the evidence of changes in the auriculo-ventricular bundle in mitral stenosis, but because some clinicians deny that the auricular systole causes the presystolic murmur in mitral stenosis.

The diastolic murmur.—With advancing stenosis of the orifice, another murmur makes its appearance, namely, one occurring immediately after the second sound, heard only in the immediate neighbourhood of the apex beat. At first it is very faint, and not very constant, but it usually increases in duration until the whole diastolic period may be filled up by it. This diastolic mitral murmur diminishes in intensity from the beginning—differing thus in its diminuendo character from that of the presystolic. Frequently we can detect a continuous murmur during the diastole of the heart, beginning loudly, falling away, then increasing in intensity. The first or diminuendo portion of such a murmur is the diastolic mitral murmur, while the terminal crescendo portion is the presystolic. The cause of the diminuendo diastolic mitral murmur is the flow of the blood that has been accumulated in the auricle, during the ventricular systole, through the narrowed mitral orifice ; this begins as soon as the mitral valves open, that is, when the pressure in the ventricle falls below that in the auricle.

The disappearance of the presystolic murmur.—The next change in the character of these murmurs is the sudden disappearance of the presystolic crescendo murmur, while the diastolic murmur persists. Usually this change occurs with the onset of grave symptoms of heart failure, the heart's action becoming rapid and irregular. At other times, the change takes place with no serious symptom, but the heart invariably becomes irregular. I have explained this fully in Chapter XXX, as being due to the fact that the rhythm of the heart starts no longer with an effective auricular systole, but the auricle is standing still in the condition we call fibrillation.

When the heart's action is slow, there is no difficulty in recognizing the diastolic murmur, and the absence of the presystolic. The diastolic murmur is sometimes of great length, starting immediately after the second sound, and when the heart's action is rapid, it may fill up the whole diastolic pause, and it might hastily be assumed that the murmur was presystolic. But if it be carefully auscultated, it will be found that it is not crescendo in character ; when a longer pause occurs, it will be found that the murmur stops short before the first sound, so that there is a silence between the end of the murmur and the first sound (see Fig. 125). In these cases, the jugular and liver pulses are invariably of the ventricular form.

Progress and symptoms of mitral stenosis.—From the progressive nature of the lesions in the valve and in the heart muscle, it will be realized that the symptoms are not constant.

The patient comes first into consideration, mostly in early or middle adult life. The complaints then are shortness of breath, a sense of suffocation, and palpitation on exertion. In some the face is ruddy, with a hue a shade darker than is compatible with the ruddy countenance of robust health ; in others there is pallor. At this stage, there is little or no increase in the size of the heart and no dropsy. A presystolic murmur can usually be detected. The patient's complaints may be the only evidence we have of the heart failure, and these point to an exhaustion of the reserve contractile force. After a period of rest, this exhaustion may disappear, and the patient may go on for years with but little further trouble. After a time, however, some again break down, and the symptoms complained of may be of the same nature. Frequently, however, a change is found in the character of the murmurs—a diastolic murmur usually being perceived, and there is sometimes a longer duration of the thrill, these signs implying an increased narrowing of the orifice. On the other hand, in those in whom no further narrowing takes place, the murmur does not change, and the patient may go on for many years, and, if a female, may bear children, with no breakdown. In these cases, we can infer that there is no progressive muscular or valvular sclerosis. With the increased narrowing of the orifice, as indicated by the appearance of the diastolic mitral murmur, the heart becomes much embarrassed, the symptoms become much more distressing, and finally dilatation of the heart (failure of tonicity) may set in. But even without the progressive narrowing, dilatation may appear early, and then it may be inferred with certainty that the rheumatic process has permanently injured the heart muscle.

The rhythm of the heart may become continuously irregular, from the cicatrizing process affecting the auricle, and with the onset of auricular fibrillation further embarrassment arises, as described in Chapter XXX. If there be no change in the size of the heart with auricular fibrillation, and no great acceleration of rate, the heart failure may be very slight in degree; but if the heart dilates, especially if the rate is accelerated, then all the extreme symptoms of heart failure follow (dropsy, enlargement of the liver, &c.).

In the vast majority of cases, the heart recovers from its first breakdown, and usually from many subsequent attacks. Indeed, after one attack, I have known patients go on for twenty years and more, with no further trouble beyond a slight limitation of the field of response to effort.

After repeated attacks, the patient's life becomes one of great limitation. The future depends often on the rapidity of the advance of the sclerotic process of the valves and the heart muscle. If the rate of advance be slow, and the heart muscle capable of responding to treatment, the patient may go on for many years with a crippled existence. Sometimes we find in the young, about 20 years of age, at the post-mortem examination, the orifice narrowed to a mere slit. In others we find the mitral orifice not much contracted, but the heart-wall greatly dilated, and evidence of fibrosis of the muscle. Hence it will be seen that the progress of these cases is largely dependent on the rate of change in the muscle as well as in the valve. The final issue is usually by great extension of the dropsy and exhaustion.

There are several complications which may arise.

Occasional symptoms.—*Paroxysmal tachycardia.*—In place of the auricular fibrillation being permanently established, it may appear intermittently, as attacks of paroxysmal tachycardia. Other conditions may produce these attacks of paroxysmal tachycardia, notably auricular flutter. These attacks are of varying importance. Some patients may have them for more than twenty years and seem little the worse. Others may have them occasionally, and then the heart settles down with the rhythm permanently altered. In such cases, the future depends on whether the heart slows down or remains at a greatly increased rate, as already described.

Hæmoptysis.—At various stages, patients may be seized with great bleeding from the lungs. Here doubtless the cause is engorgement of the pulmonary circulation and rupture of the blood-vessels. As a rule, this is a grave sign, the patient dying sometimes shortly after an attack, although in auricular fibrillation the patient may make a good recovery, especially if the heart is susceptible to digitalis.

Cerebral embolism.—Vegetations may exist at the mitral valves, with no certain sign of their presence until a small portion is detached and impacted in some vessel, giving rise to a hemiplegic attack, or an attack of aphasia. Usually, recovery takes place speedily, and may be permanent, but cases have been recorded in which the aphasia or hemiplegia has remained complete for many years. Clotting may occur in the auricular appendage, during auricular fibrillation, and be a source of embolic infarct.

Attacks of angina pectoris.—Although very rare, these may occur in mitral stenosis. In the few cases I have observed, they were all secondary to some excessive exertion, and the patients had only one or two attacks, remaining perfectly free from them for years afterwards.

MITRAL REGURGITATION

Mitral regurgitation may be the result of a damaged valve, or of dilatation of the orifice, from depression of the tonicity of the muscles supporting the valves.

Murmurs due to mitral regurgitation.—The murmur of mitral regurgitation is systolic in time, heard loudest at the apex. It may be soft and blowing, of little intensity, and heard over a very limited area, or propagated into the axilla ; or it may be rough and loud, and heard over the whole heart and round to the back of the chest. It is not always possible to tell whether it is due to dilatation of the orifice, or to damage of the valves. The rough loud murmur with an accompanying thrill is always a sign of damaged valves.

Conditions inducing heart failure in mitral regurgitation.—When the muscle is unimpaired, little or no bad effect may follow damage to the mitral valves. Even where the regurgitation is due to ' functional ' dilatation of the orifice from depressed tonicity, the contractile power of the muscle may maintain a good and efficient circulation. The really serious trouble in connexion with mitral regurgitation arises when the muscle is impaired and the regurgitation is due to a complication of the dilated orifice and diseased valve. The subsequent results depend on the degree of the exhaustion of the muscle of the heart. The backward pressure resulting from the regurgitation embarrasses the left auricle. The exhaustion also affects the right ventricle and so adds to the embarrassment of the pulmonary circulation. While back-pressure is a factor of importance and may be a predisposing cause, yet it produces comparatively few symptoms until the tonicity gives way, which is manifested by dilatation of the heart. The dilatation is generally looked upon as the result of the regurgitation, the back-pressure ultimately producing yielding of the walls of the right heart. This is not quite correct, for long before there is any back-pressure we may find evidence of a dilated right heart. If we examine carefully the condition of the heart when the valves have been damaged by rheumatic endocarditis, during one of the slight attacks of heart failure which are liable to occur after over-exertion, we may find the heart slightly dilated, the right ventricle being in front so that the left ventricle is pushed to the left behind the lung ; the apex beat is then due to the right ventricle, which gives a negative cardiogram (Fig. 38). After a few days' rest and treatment, the right heart may retreat and the apex beat is then due to the left ventricle ; the cardiogram now presents the normal characters, rising during systole. In such cases, there is no evidence whatever of pulmonary engorgement and back-pressure. In fact, in the majority of cases, as Graham Steell says, ' the change in the valves is altogether inadequate to explain the evidently free regurgitation that occurred during life, and the disastrous dilatation of the heart. The muscle-failure factor, it may be presumed, was the essential one.'

The damage to the valves is most commonly the result of rheumatic endocarditis, and, as we have seen, the process is rarely limited to the endocardium, but invades the myocardium. Septic endocarditis may also damage the valves. In all cases of mitral stenosis, there is mitral regurgitation, but the amount of the regurgitation is never so marked as to be the serious factor in the case.

Serious regurgitation occurs through the mitral orifice with the valves uninjured in the latter stages of many affections, but more particularly in renal disease and cardio-sclerosis. Here the condition is brought about by the failure of the muscle to support the orifice, and this is too often the sign of a final and fatal exhaustion of the heart muscle.

It will thus be seen that the symptoms produced by mitral incompetence are only of gravity when there is also muscle failure, and this is dealt with in sufficient detail in the chapter on dilatation of the heart (Chapter XXXVIII).

CHAPTER XLII

Valvular Defects (*continued*)

Affections of the tricuspid valves.
    Tricuspid incompetence.
    Tricuspid stenosis.
Disease of the aortic valves.
    Ætiology.
    Aortic stenosis.
    Aortic regurgitation.
Prognosis in valvular affections.
Treatment.

AFFECTIONS OF THE TRICUSPID VALVES

Lesions of the tricuspid valves are rare, and are nearly always associated with similar lesions in the mitral and aortic valves. The heart failure associated with these lesions is never due to the tricuspid lesion alone.

Tricuspid incompetence.—Although actual disease of the valves is rare, incompetence of the tricuspid orifice is extremely common—so common, indeed, that I am inclined to look upon the valves as being barely able to close the orifice perfectly. This view is based upon the observation of many patients, in whom I have been able to detect a tricuspid systolic murmur with no appreciable increase in the size of the heart. The murmur in many cases is very fugitive, being present in the first few minutes of an examination, and disappearing when the heart becomes quieter. A consideration of the size of the orifice and the size of the valves led John Hunter to doubt their competency, while Mayo declared that the tricuspid valves never perfectly close the orifice. Experimentally, it has been found impossible to raise the pressure in the right ventricle, on account of the ease with which regurgitation takes place through the tricuspid orifice.

The slighter forms of tricuspid murmurs are limited to a small area over the middle of the sternum. With increase in the size of the right heart, they may be heard over the whole anterior surface of the heart. They are often associated with mitral systolic murmurs, but one can usually detect a difference in quality in the mitral murmur heard beyond the left nipple line and in the axilla, from the tricuspid murmur heard over the middle of the sternum.

It should never be concluded that no tricuspid regurgitation occurs because of the absence of a murmur, for it is of frequent occurrence to find evidence of tricuspid incompetence in the character of the jugular and liver pulsation (ventricular form), and in the greatly widened orifice post mortem, while during life there was no systolic tricuspid murmur. A weak muscular wall and a wide orifice may give rise to no murmur.

I dwell at some length on these points, not because the tricuspid regurgitation is of much practical value, but because misunderstanding of its symptoms has led to a wrong construction being put on the effects of tricuspid regurgitation, and to the real significance of the ventricular form of the venous and liver pulse being missed. I have already pointed out that slight regurgitation in a normal heart would add to the accumulating blood in the right auricle during ventricular systole, and would, therefore, be a factor in the production of wave v in the jugular pulse. Now most writers overlook the fact that a dilating auricle is interposed between ventricle and jugular, and have assumed that as soon as tricuspid regurgitation takes place a wave appears in the jugular at the beginning of ventricular systole. They have, therefore, regarded the ventricular form of the venous pulse as only a sign of tricuspid regurgitation, and have missed the real significance of this very important symptom. That it is a sign of tricuspid regurgitation there is no doubt, but it is a sign of far greater significance, namely, that the auricle does not precede the ventricle in the cardiac cycle.

Tricuspid stenosis.—In the majority of cases, tricuspid stenosis is not recognized during life, as the symptoms produced are not always distinctive. It is only rarely that a presystolic tricuspid murmur is heard ; I have only heard it in three cases, in which it was present in a very limited area over the middle of the sternum. There is usually present also a mitral presystolic murmur at the apex ; but as each murmur is confined to such limited regions I have had no difficulty in distinguishing them. In one case, the auricle had become so greatly hypertrophied that it sent back a large wave into the jugular, and that with such force that it caused the valves in the jugular and subclavian veins to close with a snap, which I could hear over these veins as a clear, sharp sound preceding the first sound.

As a result of the stenosis of the tricuspid orifice, the right auricle hypertrophies, and on this account sends a wave back into the vein with such force that it distends the liver, and I, therefore, look upon pulsation of the liver with a marked wave due to the auricle, as an evidence of possible tricuspid stenosis.

DISEASE OF THE AORTIC VALVES

Ætiology.—By far the greater number of cases of affection of the aortic valves owe the lesions, primarily, to rheumatic or syphilitic endocarditis and the sclerotic process accompanying arterial degeneration. Under rare circumstances the valves may rupture, but here there is usually some antecedent disease of the valve. Congenital defects may, in rare cases, give rise to great embarrassment of the heart.

It is the lesions induced by the first-named conditions that require most consideration. The condition is usually well established before it is found out. In many cases, the presence of aortic changes is discovered accidentally, when a systematic examination is being made for other ailments, or for life insurance or a health certificate.

The heart failure in aortic valvular disease is rarely due to this lesion alone. In the majority of cases, changes impairing the power of the muscle have been proceeding at the same time as those that induced the valvular changes.

In the rheumatic cases, there is frequently present a complicating lesion of the mitral valve.

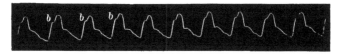

Fig. 179.   Anacrotic pulse, from a case of aortic stenosis.

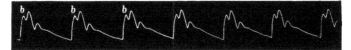

Fig. 180.   Pulsus bisferiens, from a case of aortic stenosis.

When the valvular disease embarrasses the heart's work by the extent of the lesion, as by great incompetence, and the heart muscle is healthy, the latter responds to the obstruction to its work by hypertrophy, and this may proceed to an enormous extent, giving rise to one of the largest of human hearts—the cor bovinum.

Aortic stenosis.—Aortic stenosis is often associated with aortic regurgitation, and the symptoms of the latter usually dominate the situation. When there is little or no regurgitation, the symptoms of aortic stenosis, being less prominent, are often only detected accidentally in the routine examination of the patient.

The sign most characteristic of aortic stenosis is a murmur systolic in time, heard loudest over the second right costal cartilage, and propagated into the carotids. It may be faint—a mere whiff, or it may be prolonged, and accompanied by a thrill perceptible over the upper part of the chest-wall. The heart's rate is often slow, between fifty and sixty beats per minute. The radial pulse is sometimes very characteristic. It impinges against the finger in a slow, leisurely fashion, and a sphygmographic tracing may show a slanting upstroke with a slight interruption near the summit (anacrotic pulse, Fig. 179), or even a double wave at the top (pulsus bisferiens, Fig. 180). Graham Steell and Lewis state that they have been able to detect this double beat by the finger, and Graham Steell says he has perceived it on one side only. Its real nature is yet obscure.

Beyond these signs, there is little that is characteristic in aortic stenosis. There may be symptoms of angina pectoris, but these are due to associated changes in the heart muscle, and other evidences of heart failure can be referred to the same cause.

Aortic regurgitation.—The aortic valves being contracted are no longer able to support efficiently the column of arterial blood during the diastole, but permit a backward flow into the heart, and as a result we find certain alterations in the character of the second sound and of the arterial pulse. The closure of the valves no longer gives to the second sound the characteristic snap, but the sound ends in a murmur sometimes long drawn out, sometimes so brief as to be scarcely perceptible—as if the second sound terminated not abruptly but with a faint sigh. The diastolic murmur is usually propagated down the sternum, but sometimes it is heard loudest at the apex. Foster has suggested that this variation in the propagation of the murmur depends on the direction given to the backward flow by the position of the retracted cusp. This seems plausible, but I have not been able to verify it, and the explanation is ignored in recent textbooks.

The regurgitant murmur is usually associated with the murmur of aortic stenosis, and we get the characteristic double aortic murmur (bellows murmur). There is frequently dilatation of the smaller arteries, and this, combined with the effect of the regurgitation on the arterial pulse, causes the artery to become emptier than usual towards the end of diastole. This means a fall of pressure, and in order to maintain a normal mean pressure, the heart increases the force of its contractions, raising the pressure during systole, so that there is a great increase in the systolic pressure and a great fall during diastole, thus giving rise to the characteristic collapsing pulse (Corrigan's pulse, the water-hammer pulse, Fig. 181, 182, 183). The collapsing character of the radial pulse may be intensified by raising the arm above the head. At times, the arterial pulse is conveyed through the capillaries into the veins, and G. Gibson has obtained a graphic record of such pulsation of the veins on the back of the hand. If the forehead be rubbed so as to produce redness, the flush is seen to wax and wane with each beat of the heart (capillary pulsation).

The double aortic murmur may be detected without any history of a heart affection. In many cases, there may be little or no dilatation, and the individual may be able to indulge in games and in occupations requiring considerable exertion with no discomfort. In such cases, it may safely be

z 2

assumed that the damage to the valves has been slight, and that the heart muscle has escaped serious injury.

In other cases, the heart is greatly enlarged, and the apex beat is diffuse and forcible. The systole and diastole of the heart may cause movements of the liver that simulate pulsation of that organ, but analysis of its graphic records show it to be merely the dragging up and pushing down of the liver by the changes in the size of the heart (Figs. 31, 32). Even under these circumstances, the individual may for years pursue an active vocation, but he is always liable to attacks of heart failure. The condition is often

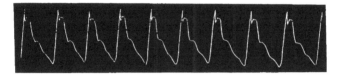

FIG. 181.   Pulse of slight aortic regurgitation with good heart muscle.

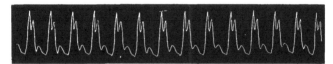

FIG. 182.   Pulse of slight aortic regurgitation with great cardiac failure.

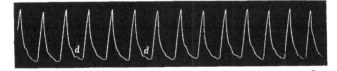

FIG. 183.   Pulse of extreme aortic regurgitation with great cardiac failure.

associated with affection of the mitral valves; and this is one of the factors participating in the production of the heart failure that finally terminates these cases.

The most frequent sufferers from aortic valvular disease are the middle-aged. In them the sclerotic process has been gradually advancing, and the early symptoms of exhausted reserve force have been neglected until symptoms of distress command attention. There may have been a history of rheumatism, of excessive drinking, of hard bodily exertion, of syphilis, but, on the other hand, no definite causal condition may be discovered. The facial aspect is frequently pale grey (earthy countenance), though in others it may be full-blooded and ruddy. The complaints are varied. Shortness of breath on exertion, violent throbbing in the neck, attacks of pain over the chest on exertion, are amongst the most common symptoms of which the patient complains in the first instance. For a varying period, under suitable treatment, a certain store of reserve force is gained, and he may go on for months or years, sometimes in fair comfort, but his existence is usually more or less crippled.

A feature strikingly characteristic of aortic regurgitation is the susceptibility to nerve stimulation. The heart and blood-vessels are readily stimulated, the former to rapid action, the latter to variation in the calibre of the vessels. The recognition of this peculiarity is of importance; for I have repeatedly seen individuals in whom the heart became rapid in action, and with consequent exhaustion, when they were first informed they had got an affection of the heart. Moreover, these cases are very susceptible to a mental stimulus, which may increase the heart-rate, and also raise the blood-pressure and induce attacks of angina pectoris (Cases 38 and 42). The difference of the blood-pressure in the arteries of the arm and leg has been commented on (p. 138), and also the susceptibility to attacks of pain (p. 71).

The end of these patients is very varied. Many aortic cases suffer from extreme exhaustion, and others show no objective signs of heart failure, such as dropsy. Where there is dilatation and dropsy, it is generally because there is present some disease of the muscle-wall, as shown by the presence of auricular fibrillation. Some of the most intractable cases of auricular fibrillation are those where there is also aortic regurgitation, so that I look upon the appearance of auricular fibrillation in aortic cases as a somewhat grave event, more so than when it occurs with mitral stenosis. Those who suffer from angina pectoris may die suddenly. I have seen a few cases die during a sudden attack of dyspnœa of the greatest severity.

Prognosis in valvular affections.—Let it always be remembered that frequently sound and healthy hearts may show a murmur, and that it is necessary, therefore, to seek for other evidences on which to base a prognosis. The heart failure which may be present depends upon so many and so varied conditions—as the extent of the valvular lesion, its progressive nature depending on the cicatrizing process affecting the valves, the coincident changes in the muscle and in the auriculo-ventricular bundle, the conditions of life of the individual—that no rule applicable to all cases can be made. If, however, an attempt be made to appreciate the value of the symptoms present, on the lines I have laid down, an approach to a true prognosis may be made in each case. There is just one point I again wish to insist upon : let no single symptom be the ground for forming an unfavourable prognosis. In this respect, the presence of a murmur has so oppressed the profession that a vast amount of positive harm is continually being done to patients, by taking too seriously the prognostic significance of this sign. The field of cardiac response is the only true and safe guide in these cases. Even if for the time being it is limited, judgement should be suspended until an opportunity has been obtained for ascertaining to what extent the heart muscle can regain a store of reserve force.

Treatment.—As heart failure with valvular defects touches every phase of the subject, the matter of treatment must be discussed from a very wide aspect. The special chapters on treatment, therefore, include the full consideration of this subject.

CHAPTER XLIII

Ætiology.
Symptoms.
Prognosis.
Treatment.

Ætiology.—The adherent pericardium, secondary to rheumatic pericarditis, rarely gives rise to any sign. In these cases the pericardium is not adherent to structures outside the heart. On the other hand, certain obscure inflammatory affections, probably of a tubercular nature, such as occur in ' polyserositis ', give rise to very marked phenomena. There is an extension of an inflammatory process which affects all the structures in the mediastinum, welding together the heart and pericardium, and firmly binding these to all the surrounding structures. The heart becomes anchored to the spinal column behind and to the chest-wall in front. As the spinal column is unyielding, the contracting heart pulls on the ribs in front, and as they yield to a greater or less extent we find the ribs drawn in during systole and springing back during diastole. This embarrassment of the heart leads to great enlargement in its size, and some of the biggest hearts met with are due to this disease.

Symptoms.—The patients are always very short of breath, and usually have to be propped up when in bed. As a rule, little or no pain is complained of, but in one case I found that attacks of angina pectoris of the most severe form were easily provoked. A slight effort would bring on an attack, especially if the patient laughed. Attacks could sometimes be induced by pinching the skin under the left nipple, or by applying the stethoscope.

The adhesion of the heart to the lungs, blood-vessels, and other surrounding structures produces a great variety of symptoms, the cause of many of which is obscure. The chief symptoms are great enlargement of the heart—so great sometimes as to cause a marked difference between the two sides of the chest—and retraction of the structures surrounding the heart during ventricular systole. The systolic retraction alone is not distinctive, as I have shown that it occurs when the anterior surface of the heart is made up of the right ventricle (Fig. 37). During the ventricular systole, there is often an indrawing of the lower intercostal space on the left side behind (Broadbent's sign, Fig. 184). Tallant and Cooper have shown that this may arise in enlargement of the heart (with compression of the lungs) without pericardial adhesion. In such cases, however, the interspaces affected vary with respiration, and Cooper suggests that when they do not vary with respiration the sign is, as Broadbent states, an evidence of pericardial adhesion. When the chest-wall is thin and the heart is not covered by lung, the systolic retraction of the different interspaces can be seen in a peculiar wave-like rhythm.

Though various murmurs and modified sounds are often heard, no distinctive sign can be found on auscultation. The veins of the neck may sometimes be seen to swell up during inspiration. A very curious symptom

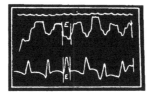

FIG. 184. The upper tracing was taken from the 9th left intercostal space behind from a case of adhesive mediastinitis, and shows ' Broadbent's sign ', which is seen to be an indrawing of the intercostal space during ventricular systole (space *E*).

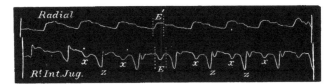

FIG. 185. Simultaneous tracings of the radial and jugular pulses, showing a great depression (*z*) occurring during the ventricular diastole. (From a case of adhesive mediastinitis.)

is a sudden collapse of these veins at the beginning of diastole, which Friedreich has explained as due to the springing back of the ribs after the ventricular systole has dragged them down, the cavity of the thorax being thus suddenly enlarged and expediting the flow from the overfilled veins. This is well seen in the jugular tracing, Fig. 185, where the fall *z* is due to the diastolic expansion of the chest.

The radial pulse may show a diminution in size during inspiration—the pulsus paradoxus. It is now recognized that a respiratory variation of the pulse may occur in a great variety of conditions, but I think that in adhesive mediastinitis it presents certain distinctive features. Curiously enough, no tracings have been given, so far as I know, showing the pulsus paradoxus in adhesive mediastinitis along with the respiratory curve, except in two instances taken by Nicholson from Gibson's cases. The study of these tracings, compared with some I have taken, leads me to think that the variations point to very different causes. As, however, my observations are few in number, I do not enter into the subject, but call attention to a field that needs exploring.

There is usually associated with these signs enlargement, and sometimes pulsation of the liver, which in Wenckebach's case was of the auricular type. The spleen also may be greatly enlarged, and there may be considerable dropsy.

Prognosis.—The future of these cases is bad, though they sometimes show periods during which they make remarkable progress towards recovery from serious symptoms. But these are only temporary, and they gradually drift to a fatal issue.

Treatment.—The treatment of these cases has so far been unsatisfactory, and one can only advise the principles usual in extreme heart failure. Attempts have been made, following the suggestion of Brauer, to free the heart by resecting the ribs. This has been done in several cases, and Wenckebach describes marked improvement in a case in which the operation was performed.

CHAPTER XLIV

Congenital Affections of the Heart

Ætiology.
Symptoms.
Prognosis.
Treatment.

Ætiology.—Congenital heart affections are due to the persistence of certain fœtal forms of the circulation, such as persistent patency of the foramen ovale or ductus arteriosus, or to some interference with development leading to deformation of the valves, or narrowing and obliteration of the large arterial trunks. They may also arise in consequence of fœtal endocarditis. The conditions are incompatible with life in many cases.

It is only in exceptional instances that the symptoms permit of a recognition of the nature of the cardiac defect.

Symptoms.—The most characteristic symptom is cyanosis, which is present in a great number of patients. Clubbing of the fingers is a common accompaniment of the cyanosis. The size of the heart is often greatly increased. This may be due to hypertrophy of the left ventricle, when there is an obstruction to the outflow of the blood through the aorta, or to dilatation of the right heart, when there is interference with the pulmonary circulation or a patent foramen ovale. Murmurs are usually present, almost invariably systolic in time, but it is difficult to detect their origin except in the case of the patent ductus. Here the communication between the aorta and pulmonary artery persists, and as the pressure is much higher in the aorta a continuous stream passes during the whole cardiac cycle from the aorta, to the pulmonary artery, and, as Gibson has pointed out, this leads to a murmur which, beginning with great intensity at ventricular systole, extends over ventricular systole into diastole, fading away towards the end of diastole. This murmur is loudest over the second and third left interspaces, and here also a well-marked thrill synchronous with the murmur can be felt.

Prognosis.—If there be no cyanosis, little or no enlargement of the heart, and the development of the child good, with a fair field of cardiac response,.then the prognosis is good ; otherwise the outlook is bad, though the child may lead a crippled existence for many years.

Treatment.—If the heart maintains the circulation well, no treatment is required. In more serious cases, beyond attending to the child's comfort and nourishment, special treatment for the heart is of little benefit, digitalis being rarely of value unless there is dropsy.

CHAPTER XLV

Responsibility of the medical profession.
Basis for prognosis.

Responsibility of the medical profession.—In addition to recognizing the meaning of any abnormal sign or symptom, we should endeavour to acquire a knowledge of what bearing it has upon the future history of the patient. This knowledge can only be obtained by watching how patients, exhibiting the abnormality, meet the storm and stress of life. This has been a special object of my work on the heart for over a quarter of a century, and in the following observations I am culling from my own personal experience, and in each deduction I give, I have in my mind a number of cases from which it has been drawn.

I am rather afraid that our profession as a body does not recognize sufficiently its responsibility in regard to prognosis. When an individual submits himself for an opinion, he does so with such implicit confidence that the verdict given may alter the whole tenor of his life. He may be, for instance, seeking to enter some profession, when a preliminary medical examination reveals what the medical man takes to be an abnormality. An imperfect knowledge of its nature may, and unfortunately often does, lead to its being regarded as presaging possibly grave consequences, and the candidate is rejected. He is thus shut off from the prospect of his chosen calling, and, knowing the reason of his rejection, passes through life uneasily conscious that some disaster is always impending, while all the time the supposed abnormality may be a sign of little or no consequence.

If we look at an insurance paper, we realize the hardships to which an applicant is exposed. Is the pulse regular ? Are the sounds pure ? If either question is answered in the negative, the applicant is either rejected or is penalized for life by having to pay a higher premium, and, in addition, is burdened with the painful consciousness of infirmity.

I dwell on this matter with some insistence, because I have known of so many instances in which gross injustice has been done to individuals, not only in the pecuniary aspect, but in having imposed upon them great expense, unnecessary treatment, and mental disquiet, because the meaning and prognostic significance of some simple symptom, as a murmur or an extra-systole, have not hitherto been recognized. I sometimes wonder whether the use of auscultation has not been the means of doing more harm than good. That it is not an unalloyed blessing is too painfully evident, for not only have totally incorrect conclusions been drawn as to the bearing of murmurs on the future of the patient, but so much time has been spent in investigating the physics of their production, that more important matters have been lost sight of. It is so easy to recognize a murmur, that other less obvious but more significant signs have too often been neglected.

A serious responsibility is thrown upon every practitioner at times in advising upon other questions. 'Should a man give up his business?' This is a question on which advice is constantly sought; and whether the individual be a statesman or a labourer the greatest care is necessary in formulating the answer. 'Should a woman with some heart affection marry, or, if she is pregnant, should the pregnancy be allowed to proceed?' These are problems that every general practitioner at one time or another will have to meet; and if he seeks for guidance in the text-books, he finds merely general views which he cannot apply to the individual case. This fact alone should arrest the attention of the profession, and make it conscious how inefficient the teaching of heart affections has been.

Basis for prognosis.—A rational prognosis must be based on a clear idea of the manner in which any given symptom is produced. Knowledge never dispelled the terrors of darkness with more effect than in showing the true meaning of the symptoms in affections of the heart. So impressed are the public and profession with the suddenness with which death may take place, that an unnecessary fear lays hold of them when the heart shows any sign out of the common, lest this should be the thing that slays. It is because of this, that I have entered with such fullness into the explanation of so many symptoms. I confess there are still many which I do not understand; but I have endeavoured to find out their value by watching individuals who exhibited them, and to find a basis on which their value can be estimated.

In estimating the value of any abnormal sign, or in determining the condition of a heart, the most reliable guide is the manner in which the heart responds to exertion. This, again, is but an attempt to estimate the amount of reserve force. If the individual can with comfort make such exertions as we would expect at his time of life, then the abnormality may with certainty be assumed to be of little real significance.

If there be a complete breakdown, the decision should not be made until time has shown to what extent recovery takes place. The amount of recovery enables us to judge the condition of the muscle of the heart, for it is on its capability to renew its reserve force that the future of the patient depends. An axiom, applicable to a great many cases, is that patients usually recover from their first attack of heart failure, however extreme it may be. The reason for this is that the patient has persistently been giving a crippled heart more work to do than it was fit for, so that a period of rest is sufficient to restore a measure of strength to the exhausted muscle.

Even cases that never show a complete restoration of function, and in which attacks of extreme failure are frequent, may go on for many years, and the individuals lead sometimes fairly useful lives, though in time the progressive changes become so great, or the muscle so exhausted, that the possibility of even temporary recovery is precluded.

In individuals in whom there is a distinct limitation of the field of cardiac response, a close scrutiny should be made into the cause. It should be borne in mind that if a heart is not properly exercised its field of response becomes more and more restricted. Thus a man who for a long time leads a sedentary life, is often startled by the fact that he is rendered extremely breathless, by undertaking some exertion that he was wont to make with ease a few years previously. But with moderate training, there is soon restored sufficient reserve force to enable him to perform his task without distress. Therefore, in all cases, even when there is an abnormal symptom— as a murmur or an irregularity—this question of the nature of the exhaustion should be borne in mind. It must not be forgotten, also, that the supposed abnormality may have nothing to do with the symptoms of exhaustion. This is particularly the case in the young, in whom syncopal attacks are not infrequent. I have repeatedly seen grave alarm aroused because a boy or girl has fainted, and has had an irregular pulse when quiet in bed. This irregularity has been of the youthful type, and if it had any connexion with the syncopal attacks it was merely incidental, and in no sense added any gravity to a trivial affection.

While the lines on which prognosis is based can be fairly well recognized in regard to the more common affections of the heart, we often meet with patients who show symptoms whose nature is too obscure for us to identify. A prognosis in these cases is often required and difficult to give. The plan I have adopted is to exclude the possibility of degenerated muscle by an examination of the condition of the heart muscle, and particularly its efficiency as laid down in Chapter V. We should always consider how far the subjective complaints may be nervous in origin. Having satisfied myself that the muscle is sound, I give a favourable prognosis, at the same time indicating the obscurity of the case. I do this because, as a matter of experience, I have found that these exceptional cases, particularly in young adults, always tend to recovery to a greater or less degree. This, unfortunately, is not the usual plan ; for some signs are too often taken to be more serious the more obscure they are. In many cases, the physician must be prepared to back up his opinion by taking a grave amount of responsibility. For instance, I have on several occasions seen patients kept in bed and put through elaborate forms of treatment after some such ffection as influenza. The patients have complained of obscure signs, to them alarming, and a certain amount of abnormality has been present, as frequent pulse or extra-systoles. Having satisfied myself that there was no serious mischief, I have had no hesitation in making the patients get up and resume their ordinary life, even when the medical attendant has shrunk from the responsibility. I have never yet had cause to regret such a procedure; and it is better to run a little risk in a rare case than to have a patient drifting on to invalidism, because of our ignorance and fear of responsibility.

CHAPTER XLVI

TREATMENT

What to treat.
Difficulty in estimating the effects of remedies.
Principles of treatment.
Remedial measures.
Rest.
Diet.
Exercises.
Massage.
Venesection.
Baths.
Spa treatment.
The Nauheim baths.
Cause of the efficacy of the spa treatment.

What to treat.—Before entering upon the consideration of the treatment of affections of the heart, it is necessary to have a clear idea of what we aim at in treating any given individual. This is all the more necessary if we desire to treat the patient on a rational system ; for it will be found that the careful analysis of the symptoms in each case, and of the circumstances that have led to heart failure, vary so much that no two patients present the same conditions, and, therefore, each patient has to be treated with reference to his special requirements. Moreover, there are many phenomena whose nature is obscure which nevertheless are often the object towards which the treatment is directed, though in themselves these phenomena are not the signs of disease nor suitable indications for treatment. We are, therefore, bound to search for some general principle that will guide us in appreciating the peculiarities of each individual, and to recognize the necessity for treatment of any given symptom whose nature we may not understand.

Before setting forth the indications for recognizing the significance of symptoms, and their relation to heart failure and to treatment, it is necessary to point out that many prevalent ideas as to the need for treatment have to be materially modified. Until late years, so very little was known of the mechanism by which many cardiac phenomena were produced, and of their bearing upon the heart's efficiency, that the conception of heart failure and the manner of its production have been imperfectly realized. As practising physicians, we constantly meet patients being subjected to strenuous and irksome treatment because of the presence of some symptom which, being considered abnormal, becomes in consequence a suitable object towards which treatment should be directed, but which in reality may have indicated no harm in the present nor foreboded any danger in the future ; while, in some instances, the supposed abnormality may actually have been an indication of a sound and healthy heart.

From such considerations as these, it has been necessary to watch individuals for years in order to ascertain the significance of many heart symptoms, and to find out the bearing of the abnormal symptoms (whether their mechanism be understood or not) upon the patient's future, and what indications they may give for treatment. Hence the determination of the value of symptoms plays a very important part, in seeking for some definite principle on which to base a line of treatment. In order to give a clear idea of what the principle may be, it is necessary to understand what heart failure is, seeing that the necessity for treatment is in many cases due to the fact that the heart cannot maintain an efficient circulation. I would refer to the conception of heart failure, which I have given in Chapter II ; for only by the due appreciation of what heart failure is can a rational therapy be given.

Difficulty in estimating the effects of remedies.—While the description in Chapter II deals with actual failure of the heart, it is necessary to recognize the fact that the majority of ' heart ' patients whom the physician has to treat suffer, only to a slight extent, if at all, from heart failure. Disagreeable sensations may arise, due to, or associated with, some circulatory condition, as palpitation, irregular action, feeling of weakness and faintness, or nervous sensations of various kinds. There may be found a certain limitation of the field of cardiac response, with some more or less distinct cardiac abnormality, as a murmur, irregular action, or an increase in size, and, in consequence, the heart is considered the organ at fault, and towards its restoration active means are taken. The remedial measures may result in the restoration of the patient to a more healthy condition, with the disappearance of disagreeable sensations. If care be not taken to recognize the nature of the complaint, and the part played by the various agencies employed, some particular agent may come to be reckoned as valuable in the treatment of all sorts of heart affections. It is, therefore, necessary, before entering more particularly on the consideration of the agents usefully employed in treating cardiac conditions, to glance briefly at certain factors which influence patients and physicians in the selection of cardiac remedies.

The most potent of these factors is suggestion, which is so subtle in its action that neither patient nor physician realize its activity. I have just referred to the fact that, in many cases, the symptoms of the supposed heart affection are dependent on the state of the patient's nervous system, and the treatment, by improving the health of the patient, dispels these symptoms. In the course of treatment the patient's mode of living may be materially modified, as in restricting his diet or indulgences, or the amount of effort, or in seeking change of scene, &c. To these changes may be added some drug, or exercise, or bath, and the resultant improvement is attributed to the special means. In this way, numerous special agents have obtained a reputation as being efficacious in treatment. But, in addition to this doubtful source of obtaining remedial measures, another occurs, due to the nervous condition of the patient. There are many people who imagine they have a cardiac affection, and are in consequence peculiarly apprehensive, and any circumstance which removes that apprehension will at once relieve the patient; but, some remedy being applied at the same time, the patient fancies that the relief has been obtained by the specific action of the agent on the cardiac trouble. To discriminate the real from the seeming is a matter of extreme difficulty, particularly when there is a certain degree of heart failure, due to some organic lesion of the heart. It has been said, with a great deal of truth, that the cardiopath tends to become a neuropath. And it is this fact which, not being recognized, misleads the profession in regard to the value of remedies.

As an illustration, I may quote the following experience: I have seen at intervals an intelligent man who suffered from advanced cardio-sclerosis, and frequent attacks of angina pectoris. Relief from these attacks was always obtained by one-hundredth of a grain of nitro-glycerine. He also had at times attacks of dyspnœa which were rather distressing. He told me that relief from the dyspnœa was always obtained by the use of the nitro-glycerine, although it took half an hour to act. I had ascertained that his attacks of dyspnœa would sometimes stop, if he became deeply interested, or if he talked. I reasoned with the patient that I was in doubt whether the nitro-glycerine could give him relief, stating that the action of the drug was very speedy, and I would have expected relief in a few minutes after taking it. However, he was so confident of its good effect that he promised to keep a diary for me of the attacks of dyspnœa. This diary I have before me now, and I need only say that it recited the occurrence of two attacks, which were duly relieved half an hour after taking the nitro-glycerine. Then a third attack was described, for which only a peppermint lozenge was taken, and in a quarter of an hour complete relief was obtained. When next I saw the patient and talked over the experience, he remarked that he had great faith in the efficacy of peppermint. It is scarcely necessary to point out that the infinitesimal quantity of peppermint could only have acted when accompanied by the faith in its activity.

This effect upon the patient of measures plus faith is well recognized though not sufficiently discounted. Nay, more; it can be affirmed that the medical profession too often shares the same unconscious deception.

I have marvelled that men, trained in the exact sciences, and who can reason logically, appear to lose all sense of proportion and reality when they come to deal with remedies that are supposed to affect the organism. The readiness with which statements are accepted, and the entire absence of the critical spirit, have introduced so many so-called cardiac remedies, that it is possible for one individual to determine the efficacy of only a small number. When the evidence on which many of the remedies are recommended is examined, it is found that it is impossible to put the evidence to a test. If one inquires into the proof, it will be found that the proof depends on inferences drawn from the improvement in the condition of certain patients, when the remedy has been applied. The careful reader can seldom tell the exact nature of the complaints of such patients ; and it will often be found that, at the same time, other agencies were employed, or that the individual was susceptible to suggestion. If, for instance, we inquire into the administration of such a drug as digitalis, whose potency no one can deny, and whose action on the heart and blood-vessels can be accurately measured by various mechanical means, we find the drug recommended in doses so small that we can get no evidence of its action. The digitalis is recommended in doses of 2 to 5 minims of the tincture, and its result is said to be detected by some in a few minutes after the dose, and by others after a few hours. When it is pointed out that neither the rate, nor the rhythm, nor the size of the heart, nor the blood-pressure is affected. by such doses, the answer is that the finger can detect some change in the character of the pulse or of the artery. This being purely personal evidence cannot be contested, for the observer claims a delicacy in perception denied to ordinary mortals. In like manner strychnine, camphor, and caffeine have of late years come to receive such an amount of commendation, that the belief in their efficacy amounts almost to a superstition. Yet, given in medicinal doses, they are absolutely without detectable effect upon the heart or blood-vessels, experimentally, or in the human subject. No great harm might accrue from these beliefs, were it not that it leads to the perpetuation of methods of treatment which are vain and valueless. Positive harm can actually occur ; for, in cases of serious heart failure, the belief in these ineffective remedies leads to their employment and to the neglect of more efficient measures, so that the patient's life may be put in jeopardy, if not sometimes sacrificed. I have repeatedly been called to see patients *in extremis* from the heart failure, following after fibrillation of the auricle, where for long periods small ineffective doses of digitalis, or frequent hypodermic injections of strychnine, were given. The immediate prescription of effective doses of digitalis has in many cases improved the patients' condition, so that in a few days they have been out of danger. I shall again revert to this matter in speaking on the value of drugs.

This aspect of the subject is of further importance, in so far as it concerns the advances to be made in the treatment of heart affections. There are many forms of heart trouble for which our present methods are of no avail ; but, to a great extent, the profession is prevented from realizing its deficiency because of the faith in the ineffective procedures, so that, in place of realizing our limitations, and striving to perfect our methods, writers are too often content to recapitulate an array of methods and remedies which the practitioner, in attempting to employ, finds to be absolutely useless. If the profession were more impressed by their impotence, there would be more hope for advance in treatment.

Principles of treatment.—If we bear in mind the view that heart failure begins by an exhaustion of reserve force, and is perceived only when exertion is made to the full amount of which the heart is capable, the first duty in treatment is to ascertain what circumstances have induced the heart failure. To this end an inquiry is made into the patient's condition, to find out when he first became conscious of the limitations of his cardiac field of response. Then a searching examination into the circumstances preceding that period, as to the question of overstrain, worry, sleeplessness, possibility of infection. The inquiry next proceeds to the examination of the circulatory system, and any defect there must be considered from the point of view whether its presence embarrasses the heart in its work, and the failure has been due to a gradual weakening of the heart from this cause. If the physician is careful to bear in mind that an abnormal sign is not necessarily an evidence in itself of disease, and that it is not the sign which has to be treated, but that the essential aim in the treatment of heart failure is the restoration of the reserve force of the heart muscle, then he will have a sure guide in applying treatment to the diverse conditions, even when the symptoms are not fully understood. Before proceeding to treat the patient, then, we try to appreciate the value of his symptoms, subjective as well as objective. When we do find some abnormality, on physical examination, its bearing upon the subjective sensations has to be considered on the lines already laid down, and all attendant circumstances that may have contributed to the heart failure must be taken into consideration. When we detect some actual cardiac defect, and we do recognize that the heart failure is undoubtedly brought about by its presence, then, provided that we cannot remove the actual lesion, the object of treatment is to restore the exhausted muscle, and place the patient in such a position that he can lead a life useful and free from discomfort, though hampered by an obstacle to the heart's full efficiency. We should keep steadily before our view the fact that the heart is impaired, and it is vain to attempt to restore the irremediable. This suggestion may seem so self-evident as scarcely to need remarking, still less to be emphasized ; but, from practical observation, I feel the necessity of insisting upon it, for patients with an incurable cardiac defect are continually being subjected to treatment whenever they consult a physician, and they may be found going to health resorts, year after year, under the impression that in some way or other the defect needs treatment. If the patient had an ankylosed joint or a wooden leg, it would be recognized that baths or drugs can do little for him; but the thickened edges of a mitral valve are supposed in some way to need constant treatment. The object of treatment should not be to try to remove what cannot be cured, but to make the best of what power the heart still possesses. In the nature of things, it may be that only a partial restoration of the heart can be looked for; and when we recognize that the fullest amount possible is gained, judicious advice as to the future life of the patient may cause him to lead a life at a lower level, it is true, but still useful and interesting, and his years may be prolonged to the allotted span. Many individuals with a reserve force limited on account of inherent defects in the heart, may never suffer from heart failure of any serious moment, and where the lesion is not a progressive one, they may suffer little inconvenience, provided that their limitations be appreciated by themselves and their medical advisers. It is in these cases that the advice of a wise physician is of great service. The knowledge of how much an individual may do, the permission to do as much as his reserve force will allow him without inducing exhaustion, can only be acquired by the full and careful consideration of all the individual symptoms. Much inconvenience may be caused to the patient by taking too grave a view of his cardiac defect, and so limiting him far too strictly, and hampering him in his life work, and oppressing him needlessly with the supposed gravity of his condition. On the other hand, the pursuits of a man whose heart is embarrassed by a grave defect may imperceptibly call too frequently on the full extent of the reserve force of the heart, and, the period of rest being insufficient, exhaustion of the reserve force gradually proceeds, until heart failure of a more or less serious degree is induced. The work of man has attained a rough and ready standard in most trades and professions, and the amount is fairly commensurate with the reserve force of the average healthy man. The man with a cardiac defect is handicapped in the race, and, if the handicap is too heavy, his endeavour to keep his place is made at the expense of his heart's strength. The inevitable result is exhaustion of the reserve force, which advances slowly but surely.

I put the matter in this way, and dwell upon it with some insistence, because, if the physician guides the sufferer in his work, he may give life and hope to many a stricken fellow. Thus in the early years, after some cardiac lesion following rheumatic fever or other infective complaint, the choice of a profession which will never entail severe bodily exertion, may enable the lamed individual to live a useful and contented life.

In more advanced years, the recognition of early stages of some progressive lesion, as cardio-sclerosis, may enable the physician to advise the patient to avoid certain deleterious influences in his work or mode of life, measures which may diminish the progressive exhaustion of his reserve force, and enable him to pursue a useful and comfortable existence for an indefinite number of years. So in the many other phases, in which a heart trouble may mar a patient's life, as, for instance, the question of pregnancy and its relation to heart trouble—a subject, indeed, of the first importance, but, unfortunately, too little considered.

It may reasonably be asked, what are the indications which should guide the physician in advising a restricted life ? No answer can be given of definiteness sufficient to be applicable to every case. It is in this respect that a wise judgement needs to be exercised. Many symptoms are so obscure in their origin, and there is such a tendency in the human mind to see evil in what is not understood, that a very urgent caution has to be given not to attach too grave a significance to any sign or symptom. The more common forms of these have been dealt with in their appropriate chapters ; here I would lay down the general proposition, let no abnormal sign of itself be the reason for giving a prognosis or for subjecting the patient to treatment. A careful search should be made for accompanying symptoms, and a careful inquiry into the condition of the reserve force and the reason for any exhaustion, and on the result of such an examination the final decision should be based.

When the heart lesion is not progressive, the best line of advice is that the patient should follow his trade or profession, so long as it does not involve over-exhaustion of the reserve force, and indulge in such exercise as he can in comfort, avoiding all forms of effort that induces distress. When effort that may involve strain has to be undertaken, a period of rest should follow, sufficient to permit full recuperation. By this line of conduct, the heart itself will benefit by the judicious exercise of its functions, and the patient will be freed from the restrictions of an invalid life.

Remedial measures.—When the heart failure persists in spite of restriction of effort and the removal of injurious influences, further measures must be adopted. The periods of rest must be increased, and remedies that may strengthen the heart administered. The administration of drugs of the digitalis group may be called for. In acute cases with fever, digitalis is ineffective, and treatment should be directed to the cause of the fever, and to giving the heart as little to do as possible. In like manner, when there is evidence of a progressive lesion of the heart, the amount of effort must be reduced to the lowest possible. When the heart failure is extreme, and the rest force is being exhausted, as shown by the persistence of objective symptoms of heart failure, such as dropsy, difficulty in breathing, &c., then absolute rest is indicated, the pushing of such drugs as digitalis, until their physiological effect is produced, and the treatment of special symptoms by appropriate remedies. Sleep must be obtained, if necessary by opium, or chloral, if the milder hypnotics fail. The food must be carefully regulated, the bowels must be carefully attended to, and aperients or enemata given if necessary. If there is much dropsy and congestion of the liver, a smart mercurial purge may be of use. If, however, the movement of the bowels induces extreme exhaustion, they had better be left alone for the time being.

Rest.—It may seem unnecessary to dwell upon such a well-recognized agent in cardiac treatment as rest, were it not for the fact that its effects are seldom fully appreciated. In a great many systems of treatment, rest is only one of the factors employed, and the resultant benefit is rarely attributed to the rest, but to some other agent that has been employed at the same time, such as baths, massage, drugs, movements, change of residence. Were the value of simple rest to body and mind sufficiently appreciated, we should hear less of the vaunted cures by special methods.

In the closer study of the heart, as revealed by graphic records, we cannot but be struck with the great difference in vigour with which the heart's functions are performed, according to the amount of rest that has preceded their exercise. It has already been dwelt upon that after a contraction of the heart, the power of contracting is for a brief period abolished. When the power begins to return, the resultant contraction is at first extremely feeble, but with increased delay, there comes an increase in the strength of the contraction. While this is true in regard to healthy hearts as well as diseased, it is much more readily demonstrated in the human heart when there is a certain amount of exhaustion.

In many cases, where the heart is continuously irregular, it will be found that the size of the beats has a definite relation to the preceding pause. The restorative qualities of rest can also be demonstrated in the case of the rate of passage of the stimulus from auricle to ventricle. In many cases, where the function of conduction is depressed, the slightest slowing of the heart's rate shortens the interval between the auricular and ventricular systoles. It is probable that the extraordinarily beneficial action of drugs of the digitalis group is, in some measure, due to the fact that they induce a marked slowing of the heart's action, so that more rest is obtained for the exhausted muscle.

When a heart is exercised to the exhaustion of its reserve force, it is absolutely necessary that a period of rest should follow, of sufficient length to permit the restoration of this reserve force. If the rest is not sufficient, the exhaustion gradually becomes more readily induced, and the signs of heart failure become more obtrusive. Recognizing thus the potency of rest in maintaining the working power of the heart, we can readily appreciate its beneficial effect in treating exhaustion. We have, therefore, to consider how best the necessary rest can be obtained. In many cases by diminishing the amount of the day's labour, a longer period of rest may be obtained, which is sufficient to restore the exhausted heart. Other means for obtaining rest for the heart can be employed in protecting the heart from undue excitement. Bodily effort is not the only cause of exhaustion; in many people, an irritable mechanism playing upon the heart induces a reaction that is peculiarly exhausting. In many sensitive nervous people, the readiness with which the heart responds to stimulation constitutes the real source of trouble, and in time leads to very marked exhaustion, especially if the heart is affected by some organic lesion. In some cases, more good can be done by treating the nervous element in the case, by finding out and removing the cause of the excitability, or by removing the patient to more congenial surroundings, as to an environment which will interest without exciting, or by dulling the nervous system with such drugs as the bromides.

Worry, business or domestic, plays an important part in depressing the heart's functions, and when it is not possible to free the patient from it altogether, steps should be taken to mitigate it as far as possible. Other forms of mental disquiet should also be inquired into and treated. Sleeplessness, disturbed sleep, and unpleasant dreams do much to hinder a patient's recovery, and aggravate the heart failure. It may be said with truth, that no heart can regain its full strength if sufficient sleep is not obtained. The various remedies for obtaining sleep will be considered later.

These suggestions have reference to rest, as applicable to the milder forms of heart failure. Rest is of far greater value in cases of extreme heart failure, where the reserve force is practically exhausted and the rest force encroached upon, that is to say, the exhaustion has become so great that the symptoms do not abate when the patient is laid in bed. While this condition demands the exhibition of other remedies than that of rest, yet rest itself is of the utmost value. In these extreme cases, it is not always easy to hit upon the position the body should occupy that is the most beneficial. As a rule, the patient's sensations are a very good guide. It may be that lying in bed causes such distress that the patient is not at ease, unless he assumes some position which he finds removes the discomfort, such as sitting in a chair, leaning forward on a support. Such individuals should be permitted to assume the position in which they find the most comfort, or, at least, the least discomfort, as it favours the circulation in regions which induce the distress, as in the lungs or brain, though it may militate against the circulation in other regions, as in the legs. When dropsy tends to increase in such cases, careful change in position, raising the legs as high as possible, deft bandaging and massage, may do much to diminish the swelling, other treatment being at the same time directed to the dropsy and heart condition. When the failure is not so extreme, and particularly if there is dropsy, complete rest in bed is of the greatest service, and many cases recover without other means. If necessary, the shoulders may be raised, by pillows or a bed-rest, to such a height as may prevent attacks of dyspnœa coming on during sleep. In all cases, mild or severe, every source of discomfort from other parts of the body should be attended to, such as an irritating skin affection, piles, frequent micturition.

Diet.—A pressing consideration that arises more particularly in the severer cases of heart failure is the question of diet. The subject is forced upon every physician, and many have elaborated special systems. Many dietaries are based on theoretical considerations, or on the physician's own personal experience. When it is borne in mind that we still know very little about the factors concerned in metabolism, and that, notwithstanding dogmatic assertions, every given dietary must be based upon a very imperfect knowledge of the intricate digestive processes, we should be chary of basing our practice on any special dietary. Moreover, we must be still more chary of drawing conclusions from our own personal experience. Repeatedly, patients are told to avoid this article of diet or that, and the only ground for the objection is that the article disagrees with the physician. It is very curious how many people imagine their own digestive organs to be the standard of perfection.

In prescribing a diet, we must be guided by common sense and a consciousness of our own limitations. In forbidding articles of food, we may be producing other effects than we imagine. Thus, when physicians fancy they can stop senile changes by eliminating chalk or common salt from the food of their patient, they must seriously consider not only the very doubtful result of such deprivation, but the effect the deprivations may have on the patient's mind. Thus, to carry out the instructions to have a salt-free diet, the food for the whole family may have to be rendered unpalatable, for many dishes cooked without salt lose their savour. Moreover, the patient is made conscious at every meal of his heart trouble, and if he travels, he may have to take food in which salt is an ingredient, and he then becomes morbidly anxious as to the result. Of course, it is foolish for the patient to have taken his instructions so literally, but the physician can seldom imagine the effect of his remarks on a mind made highly nervous because of some heart trouble. These remarks are made, because I have repeatedly seen patients and their friends made absolutely miserable on account of uncalled-for restrictions.

In cases of heart failure, a great deal of harm can be done by injudicious feeding. It must be kept in mind that in cases of extreme heart failure, and in febrile cases, the digestive functions are themselves greatly weakened, and that to pour food into a weakened stomach is not only to add to the discomfort of the patient, but it may produce flatulent distension of the stomach and bowels, which, pressing on the diaphragm, embarrasses the heart and respiration. The manifest weakness of the patient is often taken as an indication for more food to restore the strength, and satisfaction is felt so long as fluid is seen to disappear into the patient's interior. It is very curious how very prevalent the custom is, when the stomach is weak, to give it more work to do. The food is prepared in such a manner that the assistance of the mouth is dispensed with, and more work is thrown upon the stomach.

Bread and milk, a favourite food, is prepared so that no mastication is needed ; and the stomach burdened with the duty of getting rid of the load. The great importance of oral digestion is not sufficiently appreciated. Not only does the process of mastication in several subtle ways stimulate the digestive glands of other organs, but the juices from the mouth are so mixed with food that they not only assist digestion, but prevent flatulence, which is so often such a troublesome feature in the weakened digestion which accompanies heart failure.

In cases of extreme heart failure, with dropsy, the food should be limited in quantity—as a rule, small quantities of milk given at frequent intervals, in some cases, not more than one pint a day. The patient should be encouraged to take a small portion of biscuit, or a dainty sandwich, with fresh potted meat, chewed very thoroughly. The mouthfuls should be small, especially when there is laboured breathing. In febrile cases, or when the mouth tends to become dirty, it should be washed and sponged out, and immediately afterwards a small piece of solid food should be given to chew.

In less severe cases, the food should be more varied, but it should never be forced on the patient. The quantity he can chew is often a very good guide, because if he cannot be tempted to chew very much, it is manifest that his digestive organs are at fault, and it is a very bad practice in such cases to pour in beef tea and other easily eliminated fluids. The guiding principle should be food, tempting, needing mastication, with little fluid, and that chiefly milk, given in small quantities, and at fairly frequent intervals, these to depend on the quantity he is able to take. The kind of food should be that which the patient likes, so long as it does not disagree with him. Food which causes discomfort or distaste should not be forced. The doctor must be on his guard not to prescribe a dietary suitable to himself, but must bear in mind that what disagrees with him may agree with the patient. In selecting a dietary, the resources of an intelligent housewife will often be found to be of much service.

Individuals with heart trouble, but able to get about, should lead a life of abstemiousness, avoiding all excesses. The meals should be small in quantity, and of such frequency that all faintness is avoided. It often happens that they become faint in the night or early in the morning, as they have not broken their fast since the evening meal. A dry biscuit and a small cup of milk at bedtime, or in the early morning, will often prevent the occurrence of disagreeable sensations.

A class of people, for whom many dietaries have been evolved, are those who, with advancing years, show some signs of wear and tear. It may be that in their vigorous manhood they enjoyed and gratified excellent appetites, but as the years begin to tell, the pleasures of the table no longer appeal to them. Signs of the heart failing may manifest themselves, and the individual begins to take thought and seeks advice. Such a one readily

becomes the victim of a dietetic craze.   A course of life that seems to put
back the hand of time appeals to him.   As one who has watched many of
these patients over periods of many years, I have seen no evidence which
convinces me that the various abstemious dietaries that I have tried and
seen others try, arrest the progress of senility.   With advance of years, the
appetite diminishes as a rule ; and this is good, as the process of assimilation
also becomes enfeebled.   While moderation in all things is good, it is difficult
to tell what are its limits.

In some of my cardio-sclerotic patients, the appetite has been maintained
with remarkable |keenness.   I have seen such patients become seriously
crippled through failure of the heart, with auricular fibrillation, very high
blood-pressure, and swelling in the legs.   I have endeavoured to restrain their
appetite and to restrict their diet, but have only succeeded in increasing their
weakness and making them miserable.   With the resumption of their old
dietary, I have seen them improve, and glide gently past the threescore years
and ten, and well on to the fourscore years, before they passed away with
little suffering.   To the dyspeptic, asceticism may appear an ennobling
creed, but, as a practical physician, doing my best for my patients, I think
I would rather see my patients passing the declining years in comfort, even
though their chief pleasures were those of the table, than having their lives
made tedious and uninteresting, through depriving them of that which gives
them pleasure, in the hope of adding a few months to their existence.

Exercises.—It may be laid down as a general law, that every organ in
the body is benefited by the exercise of its functions.   The benefit does
not accrue merely by the exercise at a low level, but by periods of increased
effort followed by periods of comparative rest.   This is well seen in all muscular
organs where, in the nature of things, muscular effort is intermittent.   While
most muscular organs obtain periods of absolute rest, no such possibility
can pertain to the heart's action ; it has to be content with periods of comparative rest.   Nevertheless, it follows the law that periods of increased work
are beneficial to its well-being. · The beneficial effect arises not only from
the exercise of its inherent functions, but also from the fact that the more
energetic action causes the whole organ to be flushed by a large supply of
blood.   There is no agent so potent as exercise, for rapidly and thoroughly
producing a reaction on the heart.   This reaction, when carried to excess,
may do harm, but, when judiciously employed, it is an excellent and extremely
valuable help in treatment.

Considering that heart failure is induced by a disproportionate relation
between the work the heart has to do and the period of rest, it seems, at
first sight, paradoxical that exercise should be an agent in restoring the
heart's strength.   If, however, we bear in mind that there are limits which
may be transgressed, and that there are conditions when it is not wise to
exercise, just as there are conditions which benefit by exercise, we may

be able to determine which cases need or do not need this method of treatment. The conditions which contra-indicate exercise in treatment are acute and progressive affections of the heart, and when heart failure is so extreme that the rest force is being exhausted. All other conditions benefit by exercise judiciously employed, and no abnormal sign should be taken to forbid exercise unless it is accompanied by progressive exhaustion.

The manner of using this really potent therapeutical agent depends on the nature of the case. It is obvious that the same amount and the same form are not applicable to all cases, nor is there any necessity for the many elaborate methods which have been evolved, as none of them possesses any specific virtue, notwithstanding the assurance of their inventors. There is no harm likely to arise from their use, but the belief that only certain methods are efficacious tends to limit the employment of exercises as a general method of treatment.

When patients go out, their exercise should be in the open air, even though it is limited to certain gymnastic movements. If they can walk quietly, that in itself may be sufficient ; and, if the walk be taken systematically, a great amount of reserve force may gradually be acquired. As a rule, people benefit more by exercise when it has an object beyond medical needs ; hence the added interest of a game, or the study of objects of interest, as architecture, botany, etc., will add materially to the efficiency of the exercise. The particular taste of each patient has, therefore, to be studied, and the form of exercise prescribed that is likely to combine therapeutic with personal interest.

When patients are confined to the house or to bed, moderate exercise of the muscles proves useful, so long as it does not embarrass the heart. To this end, the various movements and gymnastics may be of use.

In the great majority of cases of serious heart failure, even after recovery has set in, the judicious employment of muscular exertion is beneficial. It may be a matter of difficulty to determine whether more serious cases are fit for exertion, and, if so, to what extent. There is a very simple rule I have been accustomed to follow for years with the greatest satisfaction—let the patient employ the form of muscular exercise which causes no discomfort. By discomfort, I mean when the various signs which are given by the heart when its reserve force is exhausted—breathlessness, palpitation, sense of exhaustion, pain. No fixed amount of exercise should be made, for an amount of effort that exhausts a patient one day may be undertaken with ease the following day. If the rule be followed that the amount of effort be determined by the ease with which it is accomplished, no danger will arise from over-exertion, while opportunity will be afforded for the heart to regain its full measure of strength. Discomfort may be experienced at first in the muscles exercised, when some particular group of muscles is more particularly employed, as certain thigh muscles in climbing, and certain arm muscles in playing golf—indications more of want of training of these muscles than of heart exhaustion. This form of discomfort need not prevent further exercise.

Massage.—To patients who are perforce confined to bed, but for whom absolute rest is not imperative, massage may prove helpful. It is particularly useful for patients who may be expected to regain sufficient strength to be able to resume an active life, as in the convalescence from febrile affections after the more urgent symptoms have disappeared, in all forms of extreme heart failure, in patients with angina pectoris when the heart exhaustion has for the time gone so far as to necessitate complete rest. In dropsical cases, the gentle but firm massage of the legs may prevent the dropsy reaching an extreme degree, and in some cases it accelerates its disappearance.

It is not necessary that a skilled person should apply the massage, for that would exclude its use among the majority of sufferers; the gentle but firm pressure intermittently applied to the muscles, systematically undertaken, is usually quite sufficient.

Venesection.—In a number of cases, the abstraction of blood from the patient affords very considerable relief. Unfortunately the relief is only temporary, and in extreme cases only delays the end. Although I have practised venesection in a great variety of cases, I cannot say I have seen it do any lasting good. The indications for its use that have been my guide have been distress in breathing, on account of great distension of the right heart, which has generally been recognized by the increase of the heart's dulness to the right. In cases of high blood-pressure (cardio-sclerosis), it has sometimes been difficult to detect much enlargement of the right heart, and the tense filling of the veins of the arm has been the indication. I have always bled at the usual place—at the bend of the elbow—and abstracted from twenty to thirty ounces of blood. The immediate relief given to the patient is often very striking, particularly in cases with auricular fibrillation, and cases with high blood-pressure and extreme failure of the heart.

Baths.—A very powerful influence can be exercised on the circulation by the immersion of the body in water; this may act in several ways, perhaps mainly depending on the temperature. Great therapeutic efficacy is claimed for certain waters, but it is very doubtful if the ingredients in these waters have any effect upon the heart, beyond their effect in stimulating the skin. My personal experience has been limited to observing the results in patients who have returned from the various spas; and I have seen nothing of their good effects to lead me to place hydrotherapy very high as a means of treating affections of the heart. The best results I have seen have been in patients who have bathed in the open sea. When I have had patients with heart trouble who were fond of sea-bathing, I have allowed them to indulge in it, warning them to be honest with themselves, and refrain if it brought on any sense of discomfort. In many cases, the result has been extremely satisfactory, the whole system of the patients has been braced up, and they have returned from the holiday greatly benefited.

Spa treatment.—Sea-bathing has, after all, only a limited sphere of usefulness, and many patients obtain great benefits from visiting spas, and the supporters of each claim for its waters some special virtue. In order to assess the value of these claims, it is well to bear in mind by what process benefit is obtained at the various spas. The vast majority of patients go there as much for a holiday as for treatment, and when a patient is sent there, it is often because the individual, in addition to his complaint, has been busy with his affairs, and his heart complaint has been thereby aggravated ; or a patient is convalescent, and a change of air, scene, and mode of life is often found beneficial. As the various spas cater for the more enjoyable side of existence, they attract large numbers of invalids who naturally desire the reputed benefits of the waters, and drink them enthusiastically, or, if they cannot drink them, at the least bathe in them. It will thus be seen that the benefits gained at such places arise from a variety of sources, and it is but human nature to attribute what benefit has accrued to the factors that most appeal to the imagination, such as hot gaseous waters from the bowels of the earth. Every practitioner of experience will agree with me that a large proportion of heart cases return from their holiday greatly improved ; and this improvement is not limited to those who went to some particular spa, but includes all sorts of places—spas, seaside and mountain resorts, sailing on sea and lake. It is evident that results thus obtained, cannot be due to the peculiar constituents of the waters of any single place.

The Nauheim baths.—When I began to write this book, the purpose was to give a faithful account of my own experience. It was no part of my project to enter into controversial matters, and in matters of dispute I have simply expressed my own views. But I feel it would be misleading if I passed in silence a method of treatment that has obtained a world-wide reputation which I consider out of proportion to its merits. Though I enter into this matter reluctantly, I conceive it none the less a duty to give my views on it, particularly as I am impressed with the injury done to individual patients, through the unmerited reputation of the Nauheim baths among the medical profession. Institutes have been started for the financial exploitation of the Nauheim waters ; and I must confess to a feeling of shame for my profession when I consider the manner in which it has been imposed upon. One reads in sober English medical journals accounts of cures effected that seem like the puffs of an empiric remedy. One writer will tell how a patient obtained no benefit from his treatment, but was cured by a visit to Nauheim. Another describes how he watched the patients enter into the bath-room feeble, tottering, and livid, and how they came out upright and brisk, with a glow of health on their countenances. It is little wonder that the stay-at-home practitioner is impressed by all this dithyrambic praise. The following painful experience resulted directly from this indiscriminate exaltation of the virtues of the Nauheim waters. I saw a man in consultation whose history was this : He was seized with symptoms of heart failure, and, not improving as he liked, his doctor advised him to go to Nauheim. An eminent physician was consulted later, who also strongly recommended Nauheim. Visiting another part of the country, he was taken ill, and the doctor who saw him there also told him to go to Nauheim. He was so impressed with the advice given independently by three doctors, that he made up his mind to follow it and go to Nauheim. His circumstances were such that he had to stop all his professional work, and to expend a sum of money that he could ill afford. He was only able to travel to Nauheim by easy stages, and took three days on the journey, arriving there spent and exhausted. He was put through the routine treatment of the baths, and had digitalis prescribed in addition. He returned to England worse than when he set out, though bearing with him a letter from the Nauheim physician saying that he had greatly improved by his visit. The patient himself shrewdly remarked that, seeing that he arrived there dead-beat from his journey, it would have been surprising if he had not picked up a little by the rest, but as to his condition he had gained no benefit, but the reverse, from his trip. When I saw him after his return, his was an undoubted case of advanced myocardial degeneration, with extreme exhaustion of the heart muscle. The organic changes were irremediable ; but the exertion of going to and from Nauheim had injuriously exhausted the heart, and no doubt hastened the end of the patient, in addition to exhausting his financial resources, for which those dependent on him had to suffer.

This is by no means an exceptional instance ; and one physician of experience tells me that every year he is called upon to treat a number of the ' Nauheim wrecks ', as he calls them, on their return. But I do not wish to seem to condemn a method without reason, and shall briefly recount my experiences in an attempt to appreciate the curative virtues of the Nauheim methods.

On arriving at Nauheim and interviewing several doctors as to how the efficacy of the cure was to be investigated, I discovered that in serious cases no practising physician believed the waters to possess sufficient curative properties, but that accessory means had to be taken if a good result was to be obtained. Nor could I find among those practising there, any agreement in regard to what was the best accessory means. One said the waters were good, when assisted by the additional movements attained by the machinery of the Zander Institute ; another derided the use of the Zander machinery, and said the best effects were obtained from the baths combined with his specially invented method of exercise ; while a third said the methods of the other two were of little avail, and that the best results were obtained when to the baths something extra was added—such as an electric current. When all these methods and baths were of little avail, every doctor prescribed in addition drugs of the digitalis group. It was hopeless for me to attempt to find out the efficacy of any given bath, or method, when such complications were introduced, so I did what little I could to understand the influence of the baths.

I found that twenty years ago, when the notion was prevalent that to have a good heart you must have a strong pulse, these baths had a remarkable effect in strengthening the pulse, raising the arterial pressure 20, 30, and 40 mm. Hg. But nowadays, the fashion being to soften a strong pulse, these waters are discovered to have a remarkable effect in lowering the arterial pressure. So remarkable are these waters that it is claimed that they can increase the pressure when it is low, and lower the pressure when it is high.

I found that these baths were so modified as to be of different strengths, and it was stated that the different baths were given according to the nature of the complaint. But I could find no evidence of any rule being followed. I found that people with nothing the matter with their hearts were having the same baths as those who were suffering from severe heart affection. I also found patients, with a weak frequent pulse, having the same baths as others with a slow hard pulse.

I saw nothing which, by the greatest stretch of imagination, could confirm the statement that patients are to be seen entering these baths bent and ill, and coming out of them straight and strong. In the patients I watched in the baths, I could discover no improvement from the single immersion. Certain effects on the heart, such as slowing of its action, did occur in several cases, notably in healthy hearts, as in my own case and in that of a friend whom I watched. This was in the strong 'Sprudel'-bath, when the temperature of the water was 89° F. But it seemed to me merely a temperature effect, and this was confirmed by the fact that when I returned home I found my pulse-rate and that of my friend slowed in exactly the same manner, when we lay in a bath of ordinary tap-water at the same temperature. I found this experience corroborated in a series of careful observations by Reissner and Grote, who compared the effects of the waters from these springs with those of plain water at the same temperature, and found the slowing of the heart entirely dependent on the temperature. This effect of temperature is practically never referred to, but is attributed to some specific effect of the waters on the skin. Thus in lying in the bath, the water being charged with carbonic acid, this gas comes off in innumerable small bubbles which can be seen adhering to the skin. At the same time the skin becomes red. These very simple phenomena are pointed out, as in some way bringing about a reflex stimulation of the heart.

Cause of the efficacy of the spa treatment.—It may be said, and truthfully, that large numbers of people flock to Nauheim, and many of them derive great benefit from the treatment. I recognize this, and have carefully endeavoured to find out the reason for the success of the Nauheim methods. When the cases that are cured and the cause of their cure are strictly analysed it will be found that, at Nauheim, what I call the essentials of treatment are carried out in an excellent manner. Everything is conducive to the restfulness of the patient. It is a pleasant place, sunny and well shaded, with beautiful gardens and an excellent band. People jaded with their cares and duties, find here that repose which is essential to the recovery of the heart. A very large proportion of them are somewhat neurotic, and there is consequently a very susceptible mental element that can be influenced. The patient comes to Nauheim buoyed up with the reputation of the place. When he consults a doctor, he is confidently told that the treatment will do him good—at once half the cure is effected in a great proportion of the cases.

Of wonderful cures I saw none. Pursuing my work in a remote manufacturing town, when I read of the wonderful cures performed at places like Nauheim, I imagined that these would be the class of cases that I failed to benefit. What was my surprise to find at Nauheim, that the so-called wonderful cures that were being effected, were identical with the cures that practitioners achieve at home.

I found at Nauheim that which I had also found at other spas, that the practitioners there were scarcely aware of what the human heart was capable. Those who, like myself, have practised largely among the better working class know what enormous capacity for recovery it possesses. Many of the ailments I saw at Nauheim would not keep a working man or woman from their work, and here they were going through elaborate methods of cure. I may frankly confess that I saw no patient get benefit at Nauheim, who would not have done equally well elsewhere.

The argument is used that cases that have been treated elsewhere without success, have obtained benefit at Nauheim. What doctor of experience has not the same to tell ? I have repeatedly had patients place themselves under my care who had been treated by other doctors, and they have benefited. But I trust I am not so foolish as to fancy the recovery was due to my skill. In many heart cases, the early stages of recovery are very protracted, and marked improvement often takes place with some slight change in the treatment, and the conclusion is often too hastily drawn that the recent change effected the cure, whereas the heart's power was being slowly restored by the treatment previously employed.

I have gone into the subject of the Nauheim treatment at length, so that the reader may appreciate the strength or weakness of the position I take up ; and I want each practitioner seriously to consider his responsibility in every case before recommending an elaborate and expensive treatment. If the individual is well-to-do, and there is not much the matter with him—well, Nauheim is as good a place to send him to as any other. But when it means crippling a man's resources, either by the outlay or by stopping his work, a grave responsibility rests upon his adviser.

In the case of growing boys and girls, I think Nauheim and the various methods are distinctly detrimental, when the heart's weakness is purely functional and the symptoms consist in occasional fainting and some supposed enlargement and irregularity of the heart. This class of patient is often sent there, and, in consequence of the elaborate ritual, they get the notion there must be something serious, and go through life under the impression that they have a weak heart, with the consequences seen in the *malade imaginaire.* I have seen numbers of these going through these elaborate methods, whom I would have sent out to the play-fields.

The assembling in crowds of neurotic people is a bad feature. They are so fond of detailing their symptoms to one another that they cultivate the habit of self-analysis. If this were done sanely, good might result, but it often ends in making the individual too self-conscious of what little infirmity he suffers from, so that I prefer to send my heart cases with a nervous element where they will associate as much as possible with healthy people, whose pursuits and tastes do not lean towards introspection.

CHAPTER XLVII

TREATMENT (*continued*)

Drugs.
Digitalis.
Preparation and method of administration.
Strophanthus.
Squills.
The nitrites.
Iodide of potassium.
Sedatives.
Oxygen.
Aconite.
Atropine.
Other drugs.

Drugs.—In entering upon this part of the subject of treatment of diseases of the heart, one is met by a great number of drugs, for which such potent effects are claimed, that it is not possible for one individual to appraise the value of all of them. When, however, the searcher after truth endeavours to find out on what grounds a great number of these remedies have acquired their reputation, he finds such an absence of evidence of value that many of these merit little or no consideration. In taking this line, it might be said that evidence is being wilfully ignored; but we must consider what is evidence. In regard to the heart, we get such unmistakable evidence of the effects of drugs that the proof of any active drug is easy to obtain. The manner in which a drug can modify the action of the heart, the rhythm of the heart, and the blood-pressure can be so readily registered, that it is easy to demonstrate the specific effect of any drug upon the heart or blood-vessels. Moreover, other phenomena, as the response to exertion, alteration in the size of the heart, generally go hand in hand with the more demonstrable effects, so that altogether we are in possession of many ways of demonstrating the action of remedies on the human heart. Nowadays, the statement of any authority, however eminent, should count for very little, unless he is prepared to give more definite proofs for the faith that is in him than his *ipse dixit*. We need only point to the widely prevalent idea that strychnine, camphor, and caffeine are active and valuable cardiac drugs. Yet there is not a single observation, clinical or experimental, of the slightest value to show that these drugs in medicinal doses have any effect upon the heart or blood-vessels. The whole evidence is based upon conclusions drawn from some extremely doubtful experiments, and upon the fact that patients have fancied they were better after their use. I have already dealt with this kind of evidence. The rule of thumb clinical methods of estimating the value of drugs so widely employed, lead to such inaccurate and unfortunate results, that it seemed to me, with the great advance that has been made in recent years in our diagnostic methods, and our more exact knowledge of the more common cardiac phenomena, that it was desirable that these advances should be used for the study of drugs which affect the heart.

For many years, while engaged in general practice, I had been carrying on an investigation on these lines, and had obtained many striking and instructive results. The subject is a big one, and it required more careful methods than one could apply in general practice. When I was given the charge of the cardiac wards at the London and Mount Vernon Hospitals, at the latter of which I was assisted by Professor Cushny, we carried out a definite series of observations on all sorts of cardiac drugs. As we desired above all things to make our observations of real practical value to the general practitioner, we employed the remedies in the form most commonly used in general practice. We elected to begin with the drugs administered by the mouth, as it is manifestly absurd to expect a busy practitioner to give his remedies by hypodermic or intravenous injections. The following description of the effects of remedies will, therefore, be based upon the results which were obtained in this way. Needless to say, many negative results are not included here.

When patients first came under our care, we put them to bed and allowed them a limited liberty, according to the degree of heart failure. Any incidental trouble from which they might suffer, as flatulence, constipation, sleeplessness, was remedied. Careful observations were made on their powers of response to effort, estimating the reserve force of the heart by noting how they performed some standardized exertion. Accurate records were made as to the heart's rate, rhythm, and size, the movements in the arteries and jugular veins, condition of the lungs and respiration, blood-pressure, state of the liver, the extent of dropsy, and other evidences of heart failure. The daily progress of the case, as measured by these phenomena, was carefully recorded. When the condition was urgent, drugs were given at once, but where there was no urgency the effect of rest alone was allowed to act, and so long as improvement continued no drug was given. When no further progress was made, we placed the patient upon such drug as seemed likely to improve his condition, and that drug was pushed until some physiological effect was shown. The drug was then withheld or diminished, according as the patient's condition seemed to warrant. If the result was not satisfactory, the patient was allowed to come out of the influence of the drug, and another remedy was substituted and the same process repeated. Professor Cushny took samples of the different drugs used, and submitted them to a physiological assay, while patients showing any doubtful or obscure action were examined by Dr. Lewis by means of the electrocardiograph. It will be understood that this method of observation was very laborious and time-robbing, and can only be undertaken by those who are familiar with the various mechanical methods employed in the clinical study of the heart, and capable of interpreting accurately the results. While these are still capable of improvement, they afford essential aids in this much-needed line of observation.

The description of Case 90 is an example of the manner in which we recorded our cases.

Digitalis.—The most valuable cardiac drugs we possess belong to the series which includes digitalis, strophanthus, and squills. These drugs have a remarkable similarity in their action on the heart. Of these, digitalis is the most useful; and it will be found that if digitalis fails to act, then the others will be of little value. Unfortunately, in some people, accompanying the cardiac action, other effects are produced, which are so disagreeable as to prevent a continued use of the drug. Under these circumstances, the same cardiac reaction can be obtained sometimes by strophanthus or squills, with less disagreeable effects on other organs.

One peculiar feature about the action of digitalis is the difference in its effects on different individuals. In some, there is quickly developed an intolerance of the drug, on account of nausea, vomiting, severe headache, diarrhœa; in others, it acts speedily upon the heart, and produces a different result in different people. In many, the effects upon the digestive and circulatory system are coincident, the first sign of nausea being accompanied by a marked reaction of the heart. In others, large doses could be taken for indefinite periods with little or no effect on the patient, the preparation employed being exactly identical with that which produced a reaction in others. This inconsistent reaction is a common experience, and has usually been attributed to variations in the potency of the preparation used, or to the capricious nature of the drug. As an outcome of the careful observations of the varied reactions, I have no hesitation in saying that the variability is not due to the drug, but either to the differences in the susceptibility of the individuals, or to the nature of the lesions by which they are affected.

Before prescribing such a drug as digitalis, we should have a clear idea of our object. In a great many individuals, there may be symptoms refer-able to the heart, such as a feeling of weakness or palpitation, and some abnormal sign may be found in the heart, such as a murmur or irregularity ; and therefore digitalis is supposed to be indicated, small doses (1 to 5 drops of the tincture) are prescribed, and any good results that may follow are attributed to the small doses of digitalis. While I am not prepared to say that the digitalis has not been of some use in such cases, I can, however, confidently assert that there is never shown any evidence characteristic of the action of the drug with small doses, until a considerable quantity of the drug has accumulated in the system. Even in severe cases of heart failure, where rest is enjoined, the good effect of the small doses, which have been given, has been in all probability obtained by the rest and the accompanying care to protect the heart from excitement. This conclusion has been forced upon me by careful observation of the effect of rest and small doses; and it needs to be commented upon for the reason that the faith in small

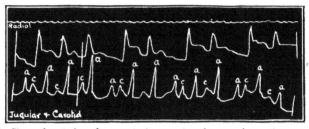

FIG. 186. Shows the missing of a ventricular systole at frequent intervals on account of the delay in the stimulus passing from the auricle. It will be noticed that the wave a is perfectly regular in its appearance, and that its relationship to the carotid and radial is variable (digitalis effect). Note the gradual increase of the size of the auricular wave, a, before the intermission. This is due to the gradual increase in the width of the a–c interval until the auricular contraction occurs before the preceding ventricular systole is completed (see also Fig. 252, 253, and 257).

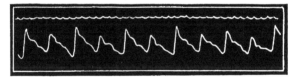

FIG. 187. Typical pulsus alternans due to digitalis (Case 52).

doses is so common in the profession, that much injury results from not pushing digitalis in really severe cases.

When there are undoubted signs of heart failure, such as breathlessness on slight exertion, dropsy, a rapid action of the heart, digitalis when indicated should be given in fair doses, and pushed until some physiological reaction is produced. This physiological reaction varies in different people, and in some its nature depends on the character of the heart lesion.

The most common sign of a sufficient dose is nausea, or even vomiting. In a great many cases, as soon as or before this happens, the heart will be found affected, usually by becoming slow in its rate, continually or at intervals, while at the same time there may be dropping out of ventricular systoles (heart-block) (Fig. 186, 252, 253, and 257), or the occurrence of

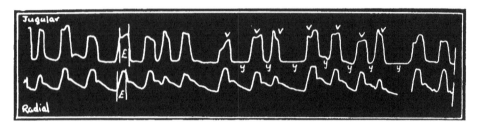

FIG. 188. Tracings from an old rheumatic case with auricular fibrillation, showing the characteristic irregularity and ventricular venous pulse. At the post-mortem examination there was both mitral and tricuspid stenosis. Before digitalis. (Fig. 189 is from the same patient.)

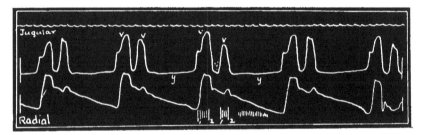

FIG. 189. Shows the characteristic effect of digitalis in old rheumatic hearts with auricular fibrillation. The figures 1, 2, represent the first and second sounds of the heart, and the shading represents the murmurs present.

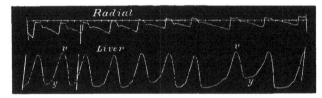

FIG. 190. Tracings of the radial and liver pulses before administration of digitalis from an old rheumatic heart, with great dilatation, and where the mitral valves were shrunken at the post-mortem examination. Fig. 190 was taken from the patient after the administration of digitalis.

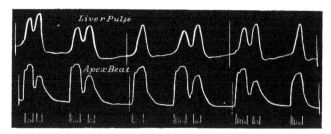

FIG. 190 A.   Simultaneous tracings of the liver pulse and apex beat, showing complete harmony in the rhythm of both ventricles.   The sounds and murmurs present are diagrammatically represented.   After digitalis.

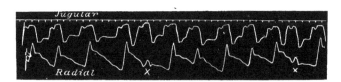

FIG. 191.   Simultaneous tracings of the jugular and radial pulses.   The jugular pulse is of the ventricular type, and the tracing shows complete agreement in rhythm between the right and left ventricles.   From an old rheumatic heart, in which, at the post-mortem examination, there was found great stenosis of the mitral orifice.   Before digitalis.   Fig. 192 was taken from the same patient.

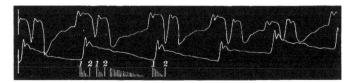

FIG. 192.   Simultaneous tracings of the apex beat and of the radial pulse from a case of mitral stenosis.   The coupled beats are well marked in the apex tracing.   The shading underneath shows the time of the murmurs.   After digitalis.

extra-systoles (Fig. 254 and 264), or the pulsus alternans (Fig. 187 and 254). In auricular fibrillation the slowing of the heart may be very marked—the rate falling from 130 or 140 to 60 or 70, sometimes with coupled beats (Fig. 188–92). When this phase is reached, the drug should be stopped for one or two days, or until the nausea has passed off. It very often happens that, as soon as the nausea has passed off, the patient feels remarkably well and is able to exert himself with less distress, and the aim should be to keep the heart at the rate at which he feels best. This is achieved by giving him half the dose at first, and watching to see if the pulse-rate alters, and increase and diminish the doses according as the pulse-rate increases or diminishes. After a time, the patient can tell by his own sensations when he has had enough and when he needs more ; and I have found these sensations invariably an excellent guide, and in many cases can leave the future administration of the drug to the patient. This is particularly the case when the patients suffer from old rheumatic affections of the heart, or when auricular fibrillation has occurred. I have watched patients who managed themselves with digitalis over long periods, twelve years and more, and have never seen anything but good result. The tendency to nausea or marked slowing of the heart-rate, should be the signal to stop, and thus act as prevention to an overdose.

In watching cases going under the influence of digitalis for the first time, and when the patient is going about or able to get out of bed, I have found the first effects of digitalis can be detected by observing the rate and rhythm of the heart after exertion. A patient makes some effort, as walking round the room or walking up one or two flights of stairs, according to his strength and condition. After he lies down, the rate and rhythm of the heart are graphically recorded, or the heart auscultated. After the rapid action in consequence of the exertion has subsided, if the heart is under the influence of digitalis, it will be found to become slower than it was before the exertion was made. The slowing very often occurs periodically, the slow periods separated from each other by ten to twenty beats. During the periodic slowing, extra-systoles are apt to occur, and in certain cases heart-block. This reaction only occurs when the normal rhythm is present ; that is, when the normal auricular systole is followed by a normal auricular systole. In auricular fibrillation, there is only a marked slowing of the pulse, sometimes with coupled beats, and sometimes with long pauses.

In discussing the physiological action of the digitalis, too much reliance has been placed hitherto upon the results of experiments, the supposition being that similar effects will be shown on the human heart, while little or no consideration has been given to the fact that the human heart, to which digitalis has been applied, is the seat of a disease process, which, by altering the physiology of the heart, as by inducing a new rhythm, may profoundly modify the heart's action and its susceptibility to drugs, and in consequence produce results which cannot be obtained by experiment. It is commonly asserted, for instance, that as digitalis acts upon the muscular wall of the arteries, it is useful to raise the blood-pressure, and is contra-indicated in cases of high blood-pressure. In all our observations made at Mount Vernon Hospital and London Hospital, as well as those made in private practice, we have only found rare instances where the blood-pressure was noticeably raised, and a great number in which it was lowered.

A great deal of good results from the slowing of the heart's action. I have already referred to the fact, that a pause of extreme brevity in the diastole of the heart is enough to increase greatly the strength of the following systole. This slowing by digitalis probably acts through stimulation of the vagus, and all the chambers of the heart take part in the slowing. In addition to this slowing of the heart as a whole, a still further slowing of the ventricle is sometimes found, due to the fact that the stimulus fails to reach the ventricle, after the auricle has contracted (partial heart-block). In many cases when this occurs, there will be found in the jugular tracing an increase in the interval between the waves due to the auricle, and the waves due to the carotid (a wide a–c interval, Fig. 256). It can, with fair certainty, be assumed that in such cases there is some damage to the auriculo-ventricular bundle, and this is one of the instances where the reaction due to digitalis is dependent on a lesion in the heart.

I have always found when digitalis slowed the heart in this manner, either with a slowing of the whole heart or with the occurrence of partial heart-block, that the patient was much better, could breathe easier, and do more exertion in comfort ; and in treatment the digitalis should not be pushed beyond this stage. If continued beyond this stage, disagreeable sensations are produced, such as oppression of the chest, distress, nausea, a feeling of malaise, sometimes with great mental depression. Before such sensations are produced, the drug should be stopped. I generally stop it a day or two, and then resume in smaller doses of sufficient strength to maintain the slow action, guided also by the patient's sensations of improvement.

While digitalis is of use in different forms of heart lesion, it is in cases with auricular fibrillation that it acts with almost specific efficacy. Where digitalis has been given to patients with extreme heart failure, where the patient is evidently in peril of his life, and where in a few days a great and striking alteration has occurred, all my cases have been those whom I have hitherto described as cases of ' nodal rhythm ', but which we now recognize as being due to auricular fibrillation. In searching the records in literature for the evidence of the good effects of digitalis, I feel fairly certain that it is in patients with auricular fibrillation, particularly when it is subsequent to rheumatic fever, that the extraordinarily good results have been obtained. If one reads carefully the records given by Withering in the first valuable account of digitalis in 1785, though he only used it as a diuretic, yet he noted its good effects in heart cases; and several of his successful cases had undoubtedly auricular fibrillation.

Preparation and method of administration.—As a result of my experiences, I prefer to push the digitalis until some physiological reaction occurs, such as nausea, diarrhœa, or slowing of the heart. I am confident that if an outlook is kept for such signs, there need be no fear of poisoning, or any other deleterious effect. The dose, therefore, in any given case, depends partly on the nature of the case. In giving the tincture to an adult, doses of 15 to 20 minims thrice daily usually produce the effect in three to five days. If the distress in breathing is great, and the pulse rapid, double the quantity may be safely administered, and the physiological effect looked for in twenty-four or forty-eight hours.

The form of preparation I have used as a standard, is the tincture, which I have never yet found to fail me. If it can be obtained of a guaranteed strength, well and good, but I soon find out for myself whether it is active. I use the tincture because it is handiest and most reasonable in price, a very important consideration to the general practitioner in practice amongst the working classes. A more elegant preparation may be used, and I have made a large number of observations with digitalin (Nativelle's Granules). Each of these granules containing $\frac{1}{240}$ grain, I find has the same effect as about 15 minims of the tincture. Many patients themselves buy the leaves and make an infusion of variable strength; but they get to know the physiological effect and treat themselves. One man whom I have had under observation for thirteen years with auricular fibrillation, uses as a standard the degree of swelling of his legs, his test being that when he cannot comfortably lace up his boots, it is a sign to take his home-made infusion of digitalis.

So far as I have seen, there is no special virtue in the various extractives obtained from the digitalis leaf; and I see no ground for according them priority over such a preparation as the tincture, which includes all the different glucosides.

In persistent dropsy due to heart failure, greater benefit may be obtained when the digitalis is combined with mercury and squills (as for instance, mercurial pill 2 grains, powdered digitalis leaves $\frac{1}{2}$ grain, squills 1 grain). This combination is often useful when digitalis by itself is without effect. One patient received much benefit from this preparation; but she was so salivated by the mercury that the medicine could not be used for a sufficient length of time. A number of other preparations of digitalis and strophanthus were used without effect. At last, the patient took the pills with her food, and for some reason she was not again salivated, and was able to keep the dropsy in check.

It is a common practice to seek a more speedy effect by hypodermic injections of digitalin; and we have tested this method in numerous cases, but failed to get any effect from this method of administration. Unfortunately, it is too often used when patients are dying from some grave affection, as pneumonia, as a last resort, probably more for the purpose of doing something than with expectations of great benefit. I have never seen much good follow the administration of digitalis in acute febrile states. The factors exciting the heart, such as high temperature, toxins, or the invasion of the heart by specific organisms exert, an influence over the heart which the digitalis cannot overcome. I think it desirable to mention this, as it is a waste of time and opportunity to apply remedies which are of no avail in urgent cases, while, by recognizing their uselessness, we may search for more helpful measures.

The recommendation of digitalis is usually accompanied by warnings as to dangers which may result from its use. It would be of great advantage if writers would state clearly what is the danger of which they are afraid. So long as vague statements are made that such a drug should be used cautiously, or sudden death may result, the reader is oppressed by some fear, which is all the greater because of the indefinite nature of the warning. If writers would even give the experience which has led them to make use of the warning, the value of their experience might be ascertained ; but when they limit themselves to obscure hints, they play upon the characteristic weakness of human nature, for the mysterious and the unknown inevitably provoke fear, whereas the bare citation of the writer's experience would very likely rob the whole statement of the mysterious, and therefore of the fearsome. I am certain that if the line of observation in each case be pursued, such as I have indicated, no danger will arise. I can imagine that danger might arise if the drug were pushed beyond the limits indicated by the first signs of its physiological reaction ; and I can only say that in over thirty years' familiar use of the drug, I have never seen any evil result from its use when given in the manner I have indicated. I have seen great distress arise from over-dosing, when others have given it, and neglected the signs of a sufficiency. I have already referred to one source of danger in auricular fibrillation (p. 235).

In the recommendation of the use of the drug, I have followed the results of my own experience and that of some other observers. It is but right to state that there are authorities who recommend digitalis in much smaller doses even in grave cases, and some find evidence of its good effects in the course of a few minutes, and others in the course of a few hours, but I have failed to detect these signs.

Strophanthus.—As in the case of digitalis, there seems to be a discrepancy between the experimental and the therapeutic results when applied to human beings.

' Strophanthus acts as a stimulant to the heart muscle and its ganglia, but does not slow the pulse by its action on the vagus as does digitalis ' (Hare). As an outcome of my own experience in private practice and researches at the Mount Vernon Hospital and at the London Hospital, no distinction can be made between the reaction of these drugs. Patients whose hearts are affected by digitalis in a peculiar manner, are affected in like manner by strophanthus. The slowing, which is accepted to be due to vagus stimulation, is produced by both, so that what I have written of digitalis applies also to strophanthus.

In some cases, there was not so marked an effect upon the digestive tract, although in other cases the reaction was just as severe. The headache, too. was found to arise from both drugs in the same individual.

Taking the B.P. tincture as our standard drug, we found in most cases about twice as much of the tincture of strophanthus was required to produce the same effect as of the digitalis. When Professor Cushny tested physiologically the two tinctures, he found in the exposed heart of the frog that the tincture of strophanthus was thirty times stronger than the digitalis tincture. From this we can infer, that the absorption of the tincture of strophanthus in the digestive tract is in some way interfered with.

The difference in the relative activities of the two drugs was impressed upon me several years ago by a young man whom I saw in consultation. His heart was affected by a rheumatic lesion; he had mitral stenosis and auricular fibrillation. For years, he had been accustomed to keep his heart fit by taking digitalis. When I asked him if he had tried strophanthus, he replied that it took twice as long to get as good a result.

In somewhat urgent cases of old rheumatic hearts, when there was auricular fibrillation I have seen remarkably good results follow big doses of the tincture of strophanthus, as much as three drams in one day. Within thirty-six hours sickness and nausea were experienced, but at the same time, the heart's action had become much slower and the patient's general condition improved.

In prescribing the tincture of strophanthus, it must not be added to a mixture containing water, for Professor Cushny found that if this were done, in a few days the preparation had become inert.

At the Mount Vernon and London Hospitals, we carried out a series of observations on the hypodermic injection of digitalin and the intravenous injection of strophanthin. The following is a summary of the results by Dr. Rowland, who made most of the observations.

An investigation was made into the relative value of digitalin and strophanthin, as immediate cardiac remedies. The purpose of the research was to compare the hypodermic and intravenous methods of administration, and also to find out exactly the type of cases that did or did not respond to these drugs. Continuous polygraphic records of pulse and respiration were taken for two or three hours after the administration, and the blood-pressure was measured every five minutes during the same period in cases of heart failure with regular rhythm.

It was found that digitalin, when administered hypodermically, had no effect upon the pulse or respiration rate in any form of heart failure, nor did it have any effect upon the blood-pressure, in cases of heart failure with a regular rhythm. The action of strophanthin, when administered hypodermically, was equally inefficient. Strophanthin, when administered intravenously, was found to have a most beneficial effect in certain cases of heart failure, namely, those with auricular fibrillation in which the pulse was extremely rapid.

In such cases, about half an hour after administration, the pulse-rate is reduced, and there is a great improvement in the general condition. The following case may be cited as an example of what occurred in many cases : A woman with auricular fibrillation, pulse-rate 120 to 130 per minute, marked dyspnœa, &c. Digitalin in doses of $\frac{1}{100}$, $\frac{1}{50}$, and $\frac{1}{25}$ grain, and strophanthin grain $\frac{1}{100}$, hypodermically, had no effect, during the three hours following the administration, upon the pulse or respiration rate, or general condition. Strophanthin, grain $\frac{1}{100}$, intravenously, caused the pulse to decrease from 122 to 68 per minute in 30 minutes, accompanied with marked improvement in general condition. Strophanthin acts by stimulation of the vagal nerve-endings, because its action can be annihilated by the hypodermic injection of atropine. In the above case, on the administration of $\frac{1}{30}$ grain of atropine sulphate the pulse-rate in 10 minutes became 135 per minute, and the patient complained of shortness of breath and palpitation.

In cases of heart failure with regular rhythm, strophanthin intravenously had very little effect upon general condition, and no effect upon the pulse-rate or blood-pressure.

Squills.—In a few cases where digitalis and strophanthin were not well borne, because of trouble with the digestion or headaches, we have obtained very satisfactory results with the tincture of squills, carefully pushed. Its physiological effect is identical with that of the other two drugs, and the reaction can be obtained in about the same time and in the same doses as with the tincture of digitalis.

The nitrites.—The principal effect of the nitrites upon the blood-vessels is to cause dilatation of the arteries and veins. It is now accepted that the cause of the dilatation is by the stimulation of the nerves and muscles of the vessel-walls. This effect is accompanied by an acceleration of the heart-rate and a great fall in the arterial pressure. When, for any reason, a sudden effect is wanted upon the heart, the nitrites are the most potent of drugs for the purpose. A few drops (3 to 10 minims) of nitrite of amyl inhaled produces its effect in a few seconds. The face becomes flushed, and the patient becomes conscious of throbbing in the head. If continued, the patient becomes faint and giddy and is forced to lie down. It should never be pushed beyond this stage. In a few minutes, the effect passes off and the blood-pressure, which has undergone a sudden fall, gradually rises, and may even become higher than it was before the inhalation.

Other nitrites, as nitro-glycerine (dose $\frac{1}{100}$ to $\frac{1}{30}$ of a grain in tablets or in alcoholic solution), erythrol tetranitrate (dose 1 grain in pills), sodium nitrite (1 to 2 grains in pills or solution), act in the same way as amyl nitrite, but slower, and the effect remains longer.

Spiritus ætheris nitrosi (sweet spirits of nitre) is a very popular remedy. It contains traces of ethyl nitrite, and is often prescribed in doses of 30 to 60 minims for its supposed effect in relaxing the blood-vessels. As it is usually prescribed in water, the nitrite which it contains rapidly evaporates and the resultant effect is due to the ether and alcohol.

The best therapeutic effect of nitrites is obtained in cases requiring a rapid action, as in angina pectoris. Some of the slower acting nitrites are recommended to reduce high blood-pressure, but I have had no satisfactory results from them when used for this purpose, nor does it seem a reasonable procedure to use them, when the increased blood-pressure may be due to some irritating substance circulating in the blood as in kidney disease.

Iodide of potassium.—The iodides, particularly the iodide of potassium, have obtained a reputation as a drug of great therapeutic value in cardio-vascular disease. The undoubted good results seen in syphilitic affections have led to its employment in such condition as aneurysms, and Balfour and Bramwell have particularly extolled the virtues of iodide of potassium in this affection. It is frequently used in all sorts of senile changes in the heart and blood-vessels, and remarkable virtue has been attributed to its action. It is difficult to understand, however, how it acts. It used to be held that it lowered the blood-pressure, but careful observations seem to indicate that it has little effect on the blood-pressure. Many suggestions have been made as to its action on the walls of the blood-vessels, but the proof is purely speculative. The fact that some observers say that it is necessary to give large doses (20 to 30 grains three or four times a day), while others claim equally good results from doses of 5 to 10 grains, seems to indicate that the resultant benefit is due to the alteration in the patient's habits which accompany the use of the drug, such as rest, change of diet, etc.

Sedatives.—Little benefit is likely to arise from treatment so long as a patient is worried or sleepless. I have already referred to the importance of rest, and it is often necessary to seek the aid of drugs to obtain rest and sleep and freedom from worry and other excitations ; and sedative drugs used with discrimination are of the greatest use.

The bromides are the most useful drugs in this respect. In all cases of mild degrees of heart failure, where the patient is able to get about, but where he is worried, sleepless, irritable, or apprehensive, the bromides are extremely useful, and of far more value than other cardiac drugs. I have for many years employed the bromide of ammonium, for I find patients state that they are not so depressed from its use as from the bromide of potassium. The drug should be pushed until a slight lassitude is induced, or even until the patient becomes torpid, particularly in severe cases of angina pectoris (Case 42). The doses employed are 20 grains, two or four times a day, according to the severity of the case.

For sleeplessness, the milder hypnotics may first be tried, the bromides, acetanilide, veronal, or sulphonal; but if these fail, resort must be had to chloral or opium. In great restlessness, due to dyspnœa, Cheyne-Stokes respiration, cardiac asthma, one of these drugs should be carefully pushed until the desired effect is obtained : 5 to 10 grains of chloral every two hours, or ¼ grain of morphin (⅓ grain hypodermically) repeated every two hours will often suffice. When there is œdema of the lungs or bronchitis, the opiates should be avoided, as they tend to check the free expulsion of the phlegm and danger may arise from this cause. Neither chloral nor opium should be continued for more than a few days, as the patients become sick and mentally confused and very troublesome.

Oxygen.—The administration of oxygen in affections of the heart has been followed for many years, but the results on the whole are disappointing, though there is a limited field where it seems to be of use. It is difficult, however, to describe the condition that calls for its use ; and I have given it in a great variety of cases, in some with excellent results, in the majority with no appreciable benefit, or only temporary relief. Even in patients suffering from apparently similar affections, the results have been very unequal ; for instance, a few patients suffering from cardiac asthma, have been greatly relieved, while others have experienced no benefit. This difference in effect caused me to look more carefully into the symptoms present, and I have found those who got benefit always had evidence of cyanosis.

The conditions in which I have found oxygen of benefit are in some cases with Cheyne-Stokes respiration, cardiac asthma, angina pectoris, and heart-block ; sometimes in cases of angina and cardiac asthma the patient has had a better night when the oxygen has been taken for a quarter of an hour before going to bed. In most cases, relief has occurred when the oxygen was taken during an attack of dyspnœa or pain, and, in cases of heart-block, during the attack of unconsciousness.

I have followed Leonard Hill's method of administration by giving the patient large doses. Hill employs a mask which encloses the patient's head, and the oxygen is poured into the mask from the cylinder, so that the patient breathes practically pure oxygen. I have used in many cases a lady's hat-box, in which a piece is cut for the neck, and the head enclosed in the box and the lid put on, and the oxygen given through a hole in the box. The head is then surrounded by an atmosphere of almost pure oxygen. By this method, Hill states a far greater amount of oxygen is taken up in the blood. The duration of an administration lasts from ten to twenty minutes. Parkinson has carried out a series of observations on the effect of oxygen given in this way to healthy people, and fiuds that it almost invariably reduces the rate of the heart, though only to a slight extent.

Aconite.—In medicinal doses, aconite is supposed to act upon the heart through vagus stimulation, and a very current impression is that it is a powerful drug in slowing the heart and in weakening its action, and the dose, when given frequently, is stated to be from 2 to 5 minims of the B.P. preparation. In a series of observations on its actions, we carefully increased the doses of the tincture in a number of patients, until 15 minims were taken every two hours for several days; but, though accurate records were kept of the pulse-rate, blood-pressure, and the patient's sensations, no effect was observed. Presuming that the preparation was not a good one, we tried others, so-called standardized preparations; and the same absence of result was experienced. We then tried aconitine, beginning with doses of $\frac{1}{600}$ grain, gradually raising the dose to $\frac{1}{300}$ grain every four hours. After a couple of days, the pulse-rate was, if anything, increased; the patients felt a good deal of dis comfort, a disagreeable pricking sensation in the throat with a sensation of choking, numbness of the limbs, a good deal of sweating, and, towards the end of the observation, painful consciousness of the heart's action, which at times would beat violently and rapidly. In cases of auricular fibrillation with rapid heart action, when digitalis produced slowing, no slowing resulted from the aconite.

I do not see what place aconite should occupy in treatment, as far as its effect upon the heart is concerned.

Atropine.—The principal effect of atropine upon the circulatory system is said to be due to its action in paralysing the cardiac inhibitory terminations. In practice, it has been found of use in rare cases of heart-block, where there has been difficulty in the passage of the stimulus from auricle to ventricle. When this occurs, an increase of the difficulty may result in the stoppage of the stimulus passing, and as it is well known that vagal action does produce this delay in the conduction of the stimulus, atropine, given in such cases, may cause removal of the heart-block. It should be given by hypodermic injection in doses of $\frac{1}{100}$ grain, or $\frac{1}{50}$ of the sulphate, and repeated in half an hour if necessary.

Other drugs.—A great number of agents are used in therapy, but it is doubtful if many of them have any real effect on the heart. Some undoubtedly can show evidence of a reaction, as alcohol and hot fluids; their activity in producing a dilatation of the arterioles can be employed with benefit when a rapid effect is desired, as in attacks of faintness or prostration. It is scarcely necessary at this time of day to add a warning as to the use of alcohol in milder forms of heart failure, and particularly in those with a neurotic tendency. The temporary benefit thus obtained may lead to a too frequent use, with the danger of a habit being created.

Other drugs, such as caffeine, strychnine, oil of camphor, act probably on the nervous system, and by producing some exhilaration prove useful in cases where a temporary exhaustion causes distress. But it cannot be too strongly insisted upon that, though they are commonly employed in cases of the most diverse kind—for instance, as where there is a rapid heart in pneumonia, and where there is a sluggish ventricle in heart-block—they are without any perceptible effect and their potency is very limited, and they should not be relied upon in cases of real heart exhaustion.

APPENDIX

CASE 1.—*Angina pectoris from overstrain.*

Male. Born 1889. Always enjoyed good health and led an active life till, at the age of 18 (September 1907), he went for a cycling tour, and one day after riding fifty miles in a rather hilly country, he felt very fatigued. Next morning he felt a suffocating feeling in his chest which came on with exertion, but which passed off towards noon. He started to cycle and was very well till he came to a hill, when the suffocating feeling returned. He rested a good deal this and the following day, but found that the hills always brought on the disagreeable suffocating sensation with pain across the chest. He also became conscious of his heart thumping, which rather frightened him, so that he returned home by train. I saw him on his return and could detect nothing wrong. I advised him to avoid any exertion which induced discomfort and to take things quietly. This he did, and suffered very little for a couple of months, when he began to play games, and the suffocating feeling returned, with difficulty of breathing, palpitation, and a good deal of pain referred to the region of the heart. These attacks also came on in bed, when he had not been exerting himself much during the day. When I saw him at this time, save for a very slight increase in the size of the heart, I could find nothing wrong. As he was evidently alarmed about himself, I gave him a very reassuring prognosis, told him to continue in work as an art-student, but in the meantime to avoid violent exertion, and take moderate exercise. This he did, and in a few months he was quite well, and has shown no tendency to recurrence, though leading an active and energetic life.

CASE 2.—*Angina pectoris from overstrain. Recovery.*

Male. Consulted me first on November 19, 1891, being then 42 years of age. He complained of a great pain which came into the left side of his chest when he attempted to lift any heavy object, or when he exerted himself, as in going upstairs. The pain was referred to a well-defined area covering the arm, the left breast, and extending up to the shoulder. The skin and subcutaneous tissues of the left chest were tender on pressure from the middle line to the anterior axillary line, and were very tender under the left breast. The second and third dorsal vertebræ were very tender on pressure. The pulse was quiet and regular, the heart normal in size, and the sounds clear, the second sound being accentuated in the aortic area. His work for the last few years had sometimes entailed great bodily exertion for a short time.

He was told to rest, which he did for a few weeks and then felt much better. He resumed his work, but after a few months he had to give it up, as the attacks of pain returned with increased severity. He got a job as caretaker in a school, and as this entailed but slight exertion he gradually improved. I saw him again on May 21, 1905. He had been working as a joiner for some years, and was free from pain unless he performed some violent effort, when it would appear and compel him to stop. The heart had increased in size, being dull to the nipple line, and the first sound was faint and muffled. Beyond this I could detect nothing amiss. He has still continued his work as a joiner (1913), and is now 64 years of age.

CASE 3.—*Attacks of angina pectoris. Complete cessation for nineteen years.*

Male. Born 1845. The patient was a healthy man leading a vigorous active life, but at times liable to periods of weakness from ill-defined causes. In 1884 I saw him recovering from an attack of syncope, into which he had fallen half an hour previously. He had been leading a somewhat strenuous life, and had been feeling out of sorts. I could detect nothing wrong, and he was better after a few days' rest. During the next few years he developed contractions of the tendons of the ring and little fingers of both hands, and tophi were deposited in his ears. In 1892, while in church one day, he was seized with severe pain on the inner side of the left forearm near the elbow. While the pain lasted, the perspiration poured off him. He consulted me on the following day, but I could detect no cardiac or other abnormality. Some months later I detected a transient irregularity of the pulse during a slight feverish cold from which he was suffering. After this he appeared to be quite well and able to take active exercise without discomfort. On March 11, 1894, he was again seized with the pain, and noted its exact site. It was situated on places exactly identical on inner sides of both forearms near the elbow. The pain held him for nearly an hour, and next day he consulted me, and I found the heart's action extremely irregular, due to the frequent occurrence of ventricular extra-systoles. The patient from being a bright, lively man had become haggard and careworn, with an ill-defined sense of oppression and discomfort in the chest. He remained in this state for ten days, when the pulse became quite regular and the oppression left him. After a holiday he quite regained his wonted vigour, and continued in active work until he was 59 years of age, when he retired from his more exacting duties, not because of ill health, and is at the age of 68 still very active. There has been no recurrence of the pain.

CASE 4.—*Pericarditis, angina pectoris. Recovery.*

Male. Born 1850. The patient was a cotton manufacturer who had lived an active, strenuous life, with a good deal of anxiety and worry in business affairs. Except for a feeling of faintness at times, he was in good health till the year 1891. On August 21 of that year he felt dizzy and not quite well, feeling languid and oppressed, with a sense of constriction across the chest, especially on walking. He went to bed at 10 o'clock and slept for an hour and a half, and then he woke up suffering great pain and difficulty in breathing and with a feeling of impending death. I was summoned to him in the middle of the night; he had severe pain across the middle of the chest in front and was gasping for breath; the respirations were 34 per minute. The pulse was of fair strength, 68 per minute. The size of the heart was normal, the dullness extending 3 inches to the left of the mid-line. The sounds were clear, but there was a soft to-and-fro murmur with each heart contraction, heard over the middle of the sternum. He was relieved by an injection of morphia. Next day he was better, but the to-and-fro murmur persisted. On the 23rd he felt much better and the murmur had disappeared. After this he made a good recovery and had no return of the trouble, and in 1913 he is still actively engaged in his business at the age of 63.

CASE 5.—*Angina pectoris with pericarditis. Pneumonia. Post-mortem report.*

Male. Born 1869. The patient came under my care on August 9, 1892, complaining of severe pain in the abdomen. He said he had had good health until the last few months, when he had been having attacks of shortness of breath and palpitation, occasionally during the night. There was no history of rheumatism or other definite complaint. I could find no definite cause for the pain. On examining the chest I found marked increase of the heart's dullness extending 2 inches to the right of the mid-line and 3 inches to the left. There was also marked pulsation in the veins of the neck, and the superficial veins of the thorax were full and pulsated visibly. On February 10, 1893, he had an attack of diarrhœa, and the heart's condition was as before.

On March 18, 1893, he came off work in the forenoon because he felt weak and exhausted, and he remained in this weakly state for two days, when he began to have pain across the lower part of his chest in front and became very short of breath. The pain struck round to the left shoulder-blade, and it gave him much pain in lifting the left arm. The pain also struck down the inner side of the left arm to the little and ring fingers. On the 22nd I found the attacks of pain came on while lying in bed with great severity and spread into the left arm. There was great tenderness of the skin and deeper tissues of the left breast. The pectoralis major and sterno-mastoid muscles of both sides were very tender on pressure. The temperature was 102°, and the pulse 112 per minute. This state continued till the 26th, when the temperature fell to normal and I detected the characteristic to-and-fro murmur of pericarditis. The pain had disappeared and there was only slight tenderness over the skin of the left breast. The pericardial friction persisted, and on April 7, 1893, there was still a very slight hyperalgesia of the skin over the third and fourth left ribs. On the 12th the pericardial friction had disappeared, there was no pain or hyperalgesia. From this date he made a good recovery and remained well till January 10, 1894, when he developed pneumonia of the right lung. There was at first hyperalgesia of the subcutaneous tissues over an irregular area embracing the lower part of the chest and upper part of the abdomen on the right side. After a few days the area of cutaneous hyperalgesia appeared in the lower portion of the left side of the chest. He died on January 15. At the post-mortem examination there was found pneumonia of the right lower lobe and recent pleuritic adhesions, also some recent pleurisy of the lower part of the left side. The pericardial sac was practically obliterated, the adhesions mostly giving way readily, but at some places the bands were thick and strong. The right side of the heart was found greatly dilated. The valves were intact, the mitral orifice permitted the entrance of two fingers and the tricuspid of four.

CASE 6.—*Angina pectoris from exhaustion. Recovery.*

Female. Born 1845. The patient up till the age of 44 had enjoyed good health, married and had six children. She began at that age to be more easily tired and to have a slight pain in the chest on exertion. In the notes I made of her condition in November 1891, when I saw her several times, she complained particularly of a severe pain seizing her after exertion, over the left side of the chest and in both arms, particularly down the inner side of the left arm to the elbow. The pain subsided when she was at rest. The skin and deeper tissues and mammary gland of the left side of the chest were very tender on pressure, particularly under the left breast and over the second and third ribs in the nipple line. After a period of rest and treatment she made some improvement, but she had a very worried and anxious life, and there were periods when these attacks of pain became easily provoked. At other times she would be comparatively free. She went on till she was about 58 years of age, when she gradually developed rheumatoid arthritis, so that after 60 years of age she became more or less a cripple, and the heart symptoms to a great extent subsided, and she is now (at the age of 68) practically free from any heart trouble

CASE 7.—*Angina pectoris from exhaustion. Recovery.*

Female. Born 1859, aged 48. Consulted me first on February 11, 1907, complaining of the heart beating violently and palpitation, shortness of breath, and attacks of pain in her chest. The patient was the mother of six children ; she had to look after the house and went to work at a mill, so that from 5 o'clock in the morning till 10 o'clock at night she had never any rest. She was pale, but fairly well nourished, the heart was slightly enlarged, and there was a systolic mitral murmur.

Lately she had noticed the symptoms of which she complained coming on very readily. The attacks of pain were sometimes of very great severity, and might come on while she was working at the mill. They started over the front of the chest and passed up to the left shoulder and down the inside of the arm to the little finger. They might hold her for a few minutes and then pass off, leaving her very weak and the finger so numb and useless that she could not hold the shuttle. On two occasions on coming home from work, she had been seized with such violent attacks of pain that she was forced to her knees and had to lean her head on a chair. The attacks lasted ten minutes, and after they were over she passed a large quantity of pale urine. She was sleepless, depressed, and cried easily. She was ordered rest and bromide of ammonium. She began to sleep better and felt much more comfortable with the bromide. The attacks of pain gradually diminished in severity till the month of June, when they ceased altogether. She remained better so long as she did not overexert herself. The last report I had of her, in March 1913, was that she was going on very well, and was able to attend to her household duties and occasionally work at the mill.

CASE 8.—*Angina pectoris.*

Male. Born 1857. The patient had always enjoyed good health, but noted that in 1904–5 he could not go uphill quickly without a sensation of tightness being felt across the upper part of the chest. This, however, was slight, and gave him no concern. On November 25, 1905, he visited some houses that were being built (he is a master builder); the day being cold, and feeling somewhat chilly, he seized a spade and for a quarter of an hour dug up earth and threw it into a cart. He did this with a good deal of energy. He then examined a few partially built houses, running up and down a great many steps. On his way home he became conscious of pain in the chest, and, as it continued to increase in severity, he called on me. I examined him carefully, and found a slight dilatation of the heart with an impure first sound. The blood-pressure was 130 mm. Hg. On his way home the pain increased in severity, and after he reached home it became very violent. My colleague saw him and prescribed opium, which relieved him. When I saw him next morning, he gave a graphic account of his sufferings. He said : ' In the tram coming home the pain got worse, and after getting home it became so severe that I felt I was going to die. The pain spread from my chest down my left arm to my little finger. You asked me, when I saw you yesterday, if I felt any gripping sensation, and I did not know what you meant, but, by George! I know now. When the pain was at its worst I felt my chest suddenly seized as in a vice, and I rolled on the floor in agony. The pain and the gripping eased off for a time and then came again. This continued till I got the opium. This morning I awoke all right, but at 10.30 that gripping sensation came on and held me tight for ten minutes. I dared not move for fear the awful pain should come on, and I felt every minute it was about to come, and I was in such terror of it that the sweat poured off me.'

For some weeks slight attacks continued to occur, but after treatment, mainly by rest, they gradually subsided, and in three weeks he was able to go about with comfort, except when going up a hill, when he felt a tight sensation coming into the chest and a curious feeling that the pain would come on if he did not stop. I kept the patient under observation for two years and repeatedly examined him, but, save for an occasional extra-systole, I could never detect anything abnormal. His blood-pressure was always about 130 mm. Hg. I have seen him at rare intervals, and in 1913 he reports that he keeps in fair health and has never had any return of the violent pain.

CASE 9.—*Attacks of angina pectoris kept away by less effort.*

Male. Consulted me on August 10, 1903, then aged 49. He complained of a pain which he felt most under his left breast. The pain first appeared eighteen months previously, and it was slight at first and infrequent. Lately it had been easily provoked by exertion, and frequently when at his desk after his mid-day meal. Fifteen months before he had two attacks during which he felt faint, and another in which he lost consciousness for a few minutes. He described the pain as coming on with great severity, compelling him to stand still if he should be walking. It started under the left breast and usually remained there, but sometimes it would spread down the left arm, on the inside, to the fingers. If he stopped, it would pass off in a few minutes.

He was rather stout, and had led a strenuous life and had a good deal of worry. He had abstained from alcohol all his life, and there was no history of any infective complaint.

An examination of the heart revealed nothing amiss. He was advised to rest for a fortnight and to lead a less strenuous life and to lessen the amount of his work. The pain gradually diminished and he resumed his work. He remained fairly free from attacks, but every now and again, when he worked too hard, they would recur. He reported himself personally from time to time until the end of 1903. I did not see him again until December 1905. He had been fairly free from the pain on the whole, and was able to take a good deal of exercise and enjoyed working in his garden. The heart was quite sound and his blood-pressure 120. He consulted me in April 1907 for an attack of pain which had come on while he was at his desk an hour after a meal. He had walked hurriedly after the meal. I gave some simple directions as to avoiding exertion after meals. I heard from him in March 1913 that he has been hard at work, though taking more holidays. The pain tended to recur at times when he worked too hard, otherwise he felt very well.

CASE 10.—*Angina pectoris with slowly advancing changes in the heart.*

Male. Born 1845. My first note of this patient was in 1889, when he complained of his heart thumping at times on exertion, and his sight became dim. The heart was irregular, and from a tracing of the radial pulse, the irregularity was either due to auricular fibrillation or auricular flutter. The attacks ceased after a few weeks. In 1890 I attended him for a protracted attack of typhoid fever, from which he made a good recovery. On December 31, 1892, he felt giddy when walking in the street, and suddenly lost consciousness. He recovered at once and came to see me. I could detect nothing to account for the attack. His heart was slightly increased n size, and there was a systolic murmur heard over the heart at the apex, and into the axilla, at the base and up along the carotids. From this date he lived an active vigorous life until the summer of 1904, when he felt rather ill and out of sorts, and went for a holiday, travelling on the Continent. He felt fairly well until one day while walking uphill he was seized with severe pain across the chest, which passed off after a few minutes. When returning home on July 22, 1904, after a long railway journey, he was seized in the train with an attack of pain of great severity, and the pain was felt on the left side of the chest. He described his sensation as if his heart ' was being wrung as women wring a wet cloth '. During the attack his hands and feet were very cold. After a quarter of an hour the pain abated, but continued to a slight extent for an hour after. He consulted me on August 3. He had been keeping very quiet, and the pain arose rarely and was not severe. He looked well. The arteries were large and thickened ; the pulse-rate was 64 ; the heart's dullness extended a little beyond the nipple line, and a systolic murmur was present at the apex and base, as in 1892. I advised him to lead a less strenuous life, and this he has done, and was able to attend to his business on four days a week, and save for breathlessness on moderate exertion, he remained free from distress till 1910, when he experienced pain and tightness across the chest when going up a hill. This tendency has become a little more marked of late, but he leads a fairly active life still. I saw him on June 18, 1913. There was now no attack of pain, but he was more breathless on exertion, and his heart was easily provoked to excited action. On examination I found the heart's size unaltered, but now t had the irregular rhythm characteristic of auricular fibrillation.

CASE 11.—*Angina pectoris.*

Female. Aged 54. Consulted me on August 14, 1903, for an attack of pain which came across her chest, at times with agonizing severity. The attacks were usually provoked by exertion, and on one occasion she woke up with great pain during the night. I had known this patient for a great number of years and had attended her in two confinements. After the last confinement in 1890, she had a long febrile illness from which she made a good recovery. She consulted me again on May 9, 1906, complaining of a return of the pain.

APPENDIX 391

She was a healthy-looking woman. The radial artery was slightly thickened, the pulse hard, the blood-pressure was 250 mm. Hg. The heart was slightly increased in size, the fat breast preventing an accurate delimitation of the dullness. The left breast was very tender on pressure, the heart-sounds were clear. The pain was felt most severely under the left breast and held her with great severity for five to ten minutes. Sometimes the pain was so severe and accompanied with such prostration that she felt as if she were going to die. Some days she would have five or six attacks n a day, and they would come on without any apparent cause, though exertion would provoke them. She was given chloral at night, and after a few days the attacks diminished, and the blood-pressure fell and varied from 190 to 220 mm. Hg. On July 2, 1906, she was put on bromide of ammonium, 20 grains three times a day, and from this date she steadily improved, and the attacks ceased after July 28, the blood-pressure on that date being 200 mm. After this she remained quite free, the blood-pressure varying from 210 to 180 mm., and she ceased visiting me on October 13, 1906. A year later, on October 7, 1907, she reported herself as feeling quite well and free from attacks, but rather short of breath on going upstairs. The blood-pressure was 200 mm. The last report I had of her, on March 1913, was that she kept well and was free from pain (aged 64).

CASE 12.—*Attacks of angina pectoris, with obscure action of the heart. Recovery.*

Female. Born 1849. I had known this patient since 1887. She consulted me in September 1897, being then 48 years of age, for weakness and breathlessness. I could find nothing wrong; she was stout and healthy-looking, and after some simple treatment, she went on all right till the spring of 1902, when she began to have attacks of pain in her chest, coming on at times independently of effort. She had a severe attack on the 5th of June and consulted me on the 8th. The pain was described as coming on suddenly and referred to a small region from the second to the fifth left costal cartilage, and the skin over these areas was distinctly hyperalgesic. The left breast was also tender to pressure, and tenderness was also elicited on lightly pinching the left sterno-mastoid and trapezius muscles. The skin over the middle of the scapula was also very tender on pressure. The pulse was regular, about 65 to 70 beats per minute, and an examination of the heart revealed no abnormality. After a period of rest the attacks ceased, and there were no other attacks till January 1903, when she had an attack similar to that she had in June. After this, went on well until the end of 1903, when she began to have curious attacks, in which she became dazed, at times nearly losing consciousness, with aching in the head and over the heart a feeling of tightness. After this she had several attacks, but I never saw her in one. On January 31, 1904, while sitting still, she suddenly was seized with great pain in the left chest which lasted for ten minutes. She then perceived that the heart was fluttering, and this fluttering sensation continued for twenty-four hours. I did not see her until three days after, when she told me that she had experienced the attacks of fluttering frequently, but thought nothing of them. Though I asked her to let me know when she felt them again, they were so slight that I never saw her in one. The heart was always perfectly quiet and regular when I saw her. After this the attacks ceased, and the last report I had of her in March 1913 was that she was keeping quite well, save for a little rheumatism in her feet, and that she looked well and stout (aged 64).

CASE 13.—*Angina pectoris from over-exertion. Recovery.*

Male. Born 1840. An active man accustomed to much exercise in the open air. In October 1908, while shooting, he felt very weak, but continued in spite of the weakness, until December 2, when out shooting, climbing a hill, he was seized with shortness of breath and pain of great severity, starting in the chest and passing down both arms. The pain passed off after a few minutes, but he felt very prostrate for a few hours. After this he experienced pain on the slightest exertion, as in going upstairs. He became very anxious about himself, as he was told that he had angina pectoris, of which his brother died at the age of 50, and he was advised to lead a restricted life and give up exercise. He consulted me in March 1909, and he was in a great state of nervous tension and looked anxious and worried. He described the pain as coming on only with exertion, and it was sometimes easily provoked, especially after a bad night's sleep. The pain was usually in the chest in the slighter attacks, but in the severer ones it went into his left arm. He was a man of spare habit, but well nourished. The arteries were soft and the pulse regular and full, about 60 or 70 per minute. The blood-pressure was 140 mm. Hg. The heart was dull to the left nipple and the sounds were slightly muffled.

Considering the attacks were induced by a man of 60 ignoring the evidence of his weakness, and climbing hills when he felt unfit, I reasoned that with rest and a mind relieved he would improve, and I gave a good prognosis and deterred him from giving up his shooting, as he had been advised. I also wrote to his medical attendant advising a course of bromide of ammonium when he was restless and sleepless. I told him also to stop the special diet he had been following, but to eat sparingly and not worry about his food. Following these directions he made an excellent recovery and resumed his ordinary life, living at a somewhat lower level. Since that t me he has had a few attacks, but always in consequence of violent exertion or excitement, and now at 65 years of age, four and a half years after his severe attack, he leads an interesting and useful life, free from distress.

CASE 14.—*Attacks of angina pectoris with remission for five years.*

Male. Born 1852. Consulted me in October 1907, complaining of a tight feeling across the chest. The patient was a well-nourished, healthy man. Up to 35 years of age, he worked as a mechanic and did hard manual labour. For the past twenty years he had not had much bodily exertion, his duties being that of a salesman for a cotton manufactory. His pulse was regular and his arteries soft ; the heart's dullness extended to the left nipple line ; the sounds were clear. The blood-pressure was 160 mm. He had been a temperate liver, but a heavy smoker. The attacks of pain in the chest had been coming on for a long while, for he remembered some slight attacks three years before, and they were very readily provoked at this time, especially after a long day's work on going to bed. The pain struck over the middle of the sternum and sometimes spread across the chest to each nipple. He had greatly diminished the amount of tobacco he smoked five weeks before he consulted me. I recommended him to limit his efforts strictly to his duties and to rest as much as possible. As he was often distressed by the pain on going to bed, I put him on 10 grains of chloral. After two weeks he began to sleep better, and the attacks got fewer and less severe. The chloral was stopped, but the pain returned, and it was again resumed, and in ten days the pain had again disappeared. On November 20 he still had the pain, and the blood-pressure was 150 mm. On November 27 he said he had no pain, and the blood-pressure was 190 mm. From that date he gradually resumed his old life, resting more and taking things easier, and he continued free from pain till 1913, when the attacks again returned, and he wrote me on March 18 saying that he was under treatment for them.

CASE 15.—*Angina pectoris due to some senile changes.*

Male. Born 1837. He had enjoyed good health and lived an active life till 1900. When 63 years of age he began to feel a sense of constriction across the chest, particularly after exertion. The distress varied ; at times he was quite free from it, but at other times it came on with little provocation. In 1901 the distress was induced with greater readiness, and the constricting sensation was accompanied by pain and went into the left arm. He was engaged in a large business involving a good deal of work and worry, and as his private circumstances were good, I advised him to give up his business, which he did in May 1901, as his private affairs were sufficient to give him an interest without worrying or fatiguing him. From this time his condition improved, although he continued to lead a moderately active life till 1907, when, at the age of 70, he began to have a series of anginal attacks in bed. He would feel quite well during the day and was able to walk about, taking the hills somewhat leisurely, and on going to bed he slept soundly till about 5 a.m., when he would be awakened by a gripping sensation seizing his left chest over the heart, and a feeling of weight pressing under his left breast, with a cramp-like sensation in his legs. At this time I could detect nothing wrong with the heart, except that the dullness extended a little beyond the left nipple line.

I gave him directions as to his food, and suggested he should take some nourishment during the night, with the result that the attacks disappeared. They returned, however, in a couple of months' time, and in spite of various remedies, they continued to recur at periods, but not so severely. I then detected for the first time a systolic mitral murmur. In a communication from him on March 29, 1910, he wrote, ' I am very well in health, as I spend all my time in the open air, but the feeling I had in the night has not left me, though I am much better than I was.' In 1913, aged 76, he is still moderately active, though the attacks of pain tend to recur.

CASE 16.—*Angina pectoris due to senile changes.*

Male. Born 1842. Consulted me on December 11, 1908, complaining of attacks of pain which came into the chest when walking. The attacks began two years previously. He had led a very strenuous, busy life, and was a total abstainer and non-smoker. In February 1908 he had a very violent attack, and after this he rested for three months, and went to Nauheim for the cure. Latterly the tendency to pain had recurred, and the attacks were sometimes very frequent and severe, coming on always if he walked after a meal. The pain was severe and was situated across the middle of the chest, and he had to stop walking as soon as it appeared. At times the pain came on after a hard day's work and amyl nitrite would cut it short. He was a pale, thin, but healthy-looking man. The radial artery was thickened, and the blood-pressure was 140 mm. Hg. Nothing abnormal could be detected on examination of the heart and aorta, save for the presence of ventricular extra-systoles, which occurred after every 12 to 20 beats.

He was given directions to manage his life, to diminish his work, to rest after meals, which were to be taken small in quantity and often, and as he was sleepless at times, a course of bromide of ammonium from time to time was suggested. If the pain subsided, he was to resume his golf, at first moderately, then more energetically, if he felt he could play without causing any feeling of distress.

He followed this line of treatment and has been practically free from attacks ever since (1913), and he is now 71 years of age.

CASE 17.—*Angina pectoris due to senile changes. Post-mortem report.*

Female. Born 1828. Had known the patient for many years, a spare, active, hard-working woman, who had enjoyed excellent health all her life and reared a large family of healthy children. In 1902, at the age of 74, she began to be troubled with pain across her chest on exertion, and these pains occurred with such frequency and violence that I advised her to lie in bed for a few weeks. This she did, and was afterwards able to go about with comparative comfort for a couple of years, when the pain recurred, sometimes with considerable severity. Still she managed to go quietly about her household duties till August 1905, when she began to lose strength. On the 21st she felt poorly and had a cough with some expectoration ; next day she got up, but feeling sickly, got back to bed and vomited. After this she was seized with a pain of great violence across the chest, and the chest felt tightly gripped so that she could scarcely breathe. The pain also struck into both shoulders and arms. The pain gradually subsided after ten minutes, and the constricting sensation of the chest gradually passed off. I saw her shortly after, and found her somewhat collapsed, the pulse rapid and soft. There was slight hyperalgesia of the tissues of the front of the chest, and the right breast was tender.

The breathing was somewhat laboured. In spite of remedies the exhaustion became greater, the breathing more laboured, and she died on August 26, 1905, aged 77.

Dr. Keith examined the heart. There was great dilatation of the auricles and compression of the ventricle. The ventricular muscle was very friable. The orifices and valves were normal. The coronary arteries showed much atheroma with calcareous patches, yet not so great as to severely cripple the circulation in the heart. The right coronary artery was more affected than the left.

CASE 18.—*Angina pectoris due to senile changes. Sudden death.*

Female. Born 1830. She was the mother of four children and had worked hard all her life. At the age of 58 she began to be rather short of breath. She consulted me in April 1892, because she felt smothered in bed, and after a hard day's work a severe pain would strike under the left breast and into the left shoulder. The attacks of pain were very severe at times, but always associated with some extra or long-continued effort. The tissues of the left breast were tender on pressure, and so also was the first dorsal vertebra. The pulse was full and regular, 78 per minute. The heart was normal in size, and there was a systolic murmur (probably aortic) at the base.

She rested for some months and got quite well—the pain and tenderness entirely disappearing, but she remained very short of breath on exertion. She lived a quieter life, doing gradually less and less household work. In her seventy-sixth year she became weaker, but was able to do a little housework. I was sent for to see her one day, as she felt weaker than usual. I went to her cottage, and as there was no one downstairs, I mounted the stair. As I did so, her granddaughter, who had been attending to her, came out of the bedroom, and I passed her on the stairs and entered the bedroom to find the patient dead. When I called the granddaughter, she was horror-stricken, as her grandmother had just spoken to her when I was on the stair.

CASE 19.—*Angina pectoris due to senile changes.*

Ironmoulder. His work entailed much hard labour. I had known him as a hard-working, temperate-living man for twenty years. At the age of 60 he began to notice that he was very short of breath on going uphill and after a heavy day's work. He suffered from pain when walking. The suffering usually began with shortness of breath, and if he stopped, no pain would arise; but if he persisted in walking, the pain became so severe that he was compelled to stand still for a minute or two, when the pain passed off. The pain was always felt across the lower third of the chest, extending equally to the right and left, but never spreading farther. After a severe attack of the pain he passed a large quantity of pale urine. I examined him several times, but, save for a large radial pulse with a thickened arterial wall, I could detect nothing amiss. The chest was large and the lungs so voluminous that I could not make out the size of the heart. The pain became so easily provoked that he gave up work at the age of 61 years. After a time the pain was less easily provoked, but he could not walk up a hill without resting several times. Otherwise he enjoyed good health until he had an attack of enteritis and died at the age of 73.

CASE 20.—*Angina pectoris due to senile changes. Post-mortem report.*

Female. This patient was under my care for fifteen years. She had led an active life until she was 62 years of age, when she became ill with some obscure non-febrile condition, during which her chief complaint was great exhaustion. She had slight pain under the left breast, but nothing could be detected on physical examination. After some weeks she gradually recovered and resumed her daily routine. She consulted me again five years later, complaining of pain of great severity which struck across her left breast and between the shoulder-blades on the slightest exertion. Her face was pale and distressed-looking. The pulse was soft and regular. The heart was enlarged slightly to the left, and there was a systolic murmur at the base and apex and up into the carotids. There was an area of hyperalgesia of the skin over the left chest

APPENDIX 395

from the third to the sixth ribs, and from the left border of the sternum to the anterior axillary line. There was also tenderness on pressure over the left sterno-mastoid and trapezius muscles, and the third, fourth, and fifth dorsal vertebrae were tender on pressure. After this the pains became so easily provoked that the slightest exertion induced them, so that she was compelled to rest in bed. After three months' complete rest she gradually improved, and was able to get about in a quiet way, the pain occurring if she attempted much exertion. The hyperalgesia persisted and she led a restricted life for three years, until she gradually became weaker and died at the age of 71. Dr. R. T. Williamson examined the heart and reported that there was well-marked calcification along the margin of the aortic valves. There were a few calcified patches of atheroma in the aorta immediately above each aortic cusp and around the orifices of the coronary arteries. Both coronary arteries were very atheromatous and presented numerous calcareous patches in their walls. The right coronary artery for about 2 inches was almost completely calcified. The heart-muscle appeared but little affected.

CASE 21.—*Angina pectoris due to senile changes.*

Weaver. A small pale man. He consulted me in May 1896, feeling easily tired, but he continued at his work until August 1902, then 62 years of age, when he began to suffer from attacks of pain across the lower part of the chest. This came on at first occasionally after meals, and he got rid of it by belching up a lot of air. On September 5, 1902, while at his work, the pain came on with such severity that he was compelled to leave work. The pain began with a gripping sensation referred to the upper part of the epigastrium. This was followed by a severe pain which struck across his chest and down his arms on the inner side of the upper arm and ulnar side of the forearm to the wrist. The pain was very severe for twenty minutes, then passed off leaving him very weak. An examination failed to reveal any abnormality. He was ordered to rest for a few weeks, and while resting the pain disappeared, and he resumed his work and continued it until January 1904. Up to this time he had no pain unless he walked fast after meals. He could always walk better three hours after meals. But from January 1904 the pain became more easily provoked, at times with the slightest exertion, as taking his clothes off and getting into bed. The pain would be so bad that he would get up and sit by the fireside. The slightest walk at times would provoke an attack which would last for twenty minutes. I watched him carefully for three years, and repeated examination failed to reveal any abnormal sign. His blood-pressure at this time used to vary, being sometimes as low as 130, and sometimes reaching 200 mm. Hg. The attacks varied in the ease with which they were provoked, but I failed to find any evidence of their greater liability during the time when the blood-pressure was raised. During 1907 changes were evidently going on in the neighbourhood of the aortic orifice. On March 22 I first noticed the first sound was faint, and on the 27th of the same month there was a slight aortic systolic murmur. On April 14 the murmur was indistinct, and on May 14 the aortic systolic murmur was marked. During this period the rate and rhythm of the heart was steadily about 60 per minute. The blood-pressure varied from 130 to 200 mm. Hg., and the attacks of pain were easily provoked. I tried many remedies to give him relief, but the best was 5–10 grains of chloral, taken as soon as the attack came on; this he found gave him ease in about 10 minutes, and, taken at night when suffering and repeated once, would give him a good night.

From 1907 until 1910 he was able to go about in a quiet manner, liable to attacks of pain on walking uphill. He died on March 9, 1911, aged 70. For a year previous to his death he had become weaker, and during the latter months of his life dropsy set in and he died of heart failure.

CASE 22. *Angina pectoris, great exhaustion, death. Post-mortem report.*

Male. Born 1851. He worked as a mule-spinner, lived a temperate life, and denies having had syphilis. In 1904 he began to have a dull pain across his shoulders, which was relieved by rubbing.

In 1905 he began to suffer from a slight pain in his arm and across his chest after walking up four flights of stairs to his work in the early morning. This got gradually worse, and he consulted me on September 18, 1905, then 54 years of age. His complaint then was of the pain coming on only after exertion, as mounting a high stair. He was a spare man and pale. His radial pulse was large and the artery thickened; the blood-pressure was 150 mm. Hg. There was a faint apex beat and the heart's dullness extended 2 inches outside the left nipple. There was also a slight dullness over the manubrium sterni. The aorta could be felt in the episternal notch, and there was tracheal tugging. The sounds were clear save for a faint murmur, diastolic in time, heard best at the bottom of the sternum and also slightly at the apex. An examination by the X-rays showed a diffuse dilatation of the aorta.

Until his death, in February 1906, the patient had numerous attacks, in one of which I saw him. I also made many notes of the symptoms and of the conditions producing the attacks. At first the pain occurred only after exertion, as going up a hill or upstairs, or walking against a cold wind, or excitement, as being engaged in a political discussion. It started in the little finger, passed up the ulnar border of the forearm to the inside of the upper arm and back of the shoulders and across the chest, and settled at the bottom of the breast-bone, where it persisted for some minutes. The pain sometimes struck into the right arm and sometimes up to the left side of the neck and behind the ear. There was never any sensation of tightness across the chest and he could breathe quite easily, nor was there any hyperalgesia of the tissues of the chest. At first there was no sense of impending death and no increased flow of saliva, though at times he passed a large quantity of urine after an attack. For some months his condition varied; sometimes he felt well and able to undertake a good deal of effort without pain, and again, without any apparent cause, the liability to pain increased, but only on exertion. During all these months no change could be detected in his condition, and the blood-pressure was remarkably uniform, whether he were well or suffering. On several occasions I tested him for the goose-skin reflex and autonomic sensation, i. e. the chilly sensation which accompanies the appearance of the goose-skin, and I obtained a curious result. In some individuals when the skin under the left breast is stimulated, as by giving a brisk rub with a piece of flannel, a wave of goose-skin spreads up the chest and into the arm, accompanied by the chilly sensation. There is usually also a dilatation of the pupil. On trying this experiment on the patient, his face lighted up and he said in a tone of surprise, 'That cold feeling is exactly where I feel the pain,' and he described with his right hand the inside of the arm, the ulnar side of the forearm, and the little finger. He also repeatedly said he felt the same chilly sensation in his left cheek.

The onset and distribution of the pain varied as time went on. In January 1906 the pain became more readily induced, and struck with such suddenness that it seemed to appear in the left arm and in the chest at the same moment. Also the pain became violent across both shoulders at times. The pain did not extend into the forearm and fingers, but remained fixed across the chest from nipple to nipple and in the upper arm. When he was asked if there were any difference in the character of the pain in the chest and arms, he replied that he did not think so, except that if anything the arm pain was the more severe. The pain at this time was described as 'awful', and he felt as if he would die sometimes when it was very bad. When the pain was on he used to be very fidgety, and could not keep still, but latterly he used to remain motionless and sometimes dare not move because he felt the pain might come on. He had had for years occasional attacks of spasms or cramp in the muscles at the small of his back. In February 1906 he kept very quiet, as he felt that very slight movement might induce an attack, and on the first of that month, when going to bed, he was seized with one of these spasms in his back, and the pain seemed to start the pain in his chest and arms, and for a quarter of an hour he had the most severe attack of pain he ever had, and during this attack the saliva dribbled out of his mouth and he felt as if he would die and he wanted to die. His blood-pressure on February 2, 1906, was 150 mm. Hg.

After this the pain came on so readily that he was forced to stay at home. Even getting into bed would induce an attack. At this time the pain, after striking into the chest and arm, seemed to settle in the upper part of the epigastrium, and gave rise to a sense of fullness, and then he endeavoured to belch wind and swallowed air to assist him in this.

In a note made on February 12 I state that the previous day, when feeding himself, an attack of pain came on at 3 p.m. which lasted till 7 p.m., when he lost consciousness. The pain shifted about all the time, from his epigastrium to his chest and arm. He recovered consciousness shortly afterwards, and the pain continued less severely for some hours. When I saw him he was taking some food, but was feeding himself entirely with his right arm, keeping his left resting across his breast. Inquiring as to the reason of this, he told me he dared not move his left arm, as when he did so he always induced an attack of pain. His blood-pressure was then 95 mm. Hg., and the pulse very small.

The following night the attack of pain was induced by the slightest movement, and during a severe attack he lost consciousness and died.

The heart was removed and sent to Dr. Keith, who reported that the left ventricle had been hypertrophied but is now dilated, especially the apical two-thirds. There are no areas of fibrosis, but the muscle-fibres are small and very brown. The aorta is dilated. There is a considerable degree of endarteritis of the coronary artery, leading to a reduction of its lumen, at parts to half the normal. The aorta is also affected, especially at the origin of the coronary arteries, which instead of measuring 3–4 mm. in diameter measure only 1·5 mm. The mitral valve is slightly thickened and shortened, probably from the same affection as the arteries. The mitral orifice is slightly dilated, and also the aortic orifice. The septum is stretched and shows perforation. The sino-auricular node is large and contains much fibrous tissue. Tænia terminalis hypertrophied.

CASE 23.—*Angina pectoris.*

Male. Born 1858. Consulted me on March 14, 1904, complaining of a pain which came across the chest when walking. This did not trouble him at work, but only when walking. He had been conscious of this for some months, but lately the pain has been more severe and the attacks more easily provoked. He had been a temperate liver, but his work necessitated his lifting very heavy weights (a tackler in a weaving shed).

He described the pain as coming only if he were walking ; if he stopped as soon as it appeared, it would pass off gradually, but if he persisted in walking the pain increased, until the severity of it compelled him to stop. After five minutes or so the pain would disappear. The pain started on the lower third of the chest in front, then it radiated up the chest and along into the inner side of the upper arm and the ulnar side of the forearm to the wrist. It also extended to a less degree into the same region of the right arm. The pain also passed up into the throat. During the time the pain was on the mouth filled with saliva, and as soon as the pain subsided he passed a large quantity of pale urine. After the pain had subsided he could walk a great distance with comfort. Sometimes the pain remained fixed for a time in the fleshy part of the arm. The above description was got from the patient after he had carefully observed the nature of the attacks. When he first described them to me they were vague, but after I had told him to note carefully all the phenomena connected with the attacks, his description became clear and precise. The attacks were always induced by walking after meals. He could lift heavy weights and cycle long distances without any pain.

With instructions as to his food (the meals to be small and frequent and to rest after them), and diminution of his exertion, he improved greatly, and after six months the attacks were only occasionally induced and were much slighter.

After this I lost sight of him, but on inquiry I find that he continued in fair health and was able to follow his work until 1911, when he met with an accident, falling off a tramcar and fracturing the bone of his left leg below the ankle. From this he never recovered, and he died on March 10, 1912, the cause of death being certified as ' heart disease and caries of the bone of the left ankle and general break-down '.

CASE 24.—*Angina pectoris, Cheyne-Stokes respiration, pulsus alternans. Post-mortem report.*

Male. Born 1863. I attended this patient first in 1880 for an attack of small-pox. He made a good recovery and continued in good health until 1905, when he began to notice he was getting rather short of breath on exertion. He was a stout man and had been a schoolmaster, but for the past few years he had been engaged as cashier and clerk to a cattle-dealing firm. There was no history of syphilis and he was a temperate liver. In the early part of 1906 he began to experience pain in the chest on walking, slight at first, but in a few months' time it would come on when walking and increase in severity until it compelled him to stop, when it passed off in a few moments. He rested for a couple of months and regained a great deal of strength, so that he was able to go about in a quiet way without distress. In the early part of 1907 the pain returned and became much more easily provoked, so that he was compelled to keep the house. In February he began to suffer from Cheyne-Stokes respiration and attacks of severe dyspnœa, coming on when asleep (probably arising from the apnœic stage of the Cheyne-Stokes breathing). Notes taken on March 10 state that the heart was only slightly enlarged, extending on the left to the middle line, and the sounds were clear. The pulse increased in rate, 110 per minute, and showed marked pulsus alternans especially after an extra systole. There was no albumen in the urine, no dropsy, no enlargement of the liver. He died a week later at the age of 46.

Professor Keith's report on the heart stated that it was similar to Case 35, except that the ventricle was hypertrophied and the arteries more sclerosed. The whole heart was slightly increased in size. The valves were quite healthy, except that the mitral was slightly thickened. There was intense endarteritis, especially of the left coronary artery, the lumen of which was much diminished. The anterior interventricular artery was occluded. The apical half of the left ventricular muscle was much fibrosed, the subendocardial and the subpericardial fibres being least affected. There was some fibrosis of the tænia terminalis.

CASE 25.—*Angina pectoris, post-mortem report.*

Male. Aged 52. He consulted me on March 11, 1903, for a pain in his chest and arms, which had suddenly seized him an hour before. He was a foreman engineer and had led a temperate healthy life. For some months before his present illness he had been feeling weak, easily tired on exertion, but he continued his very active life in spite of that. He had been at his work for an hour when he was seized with the pain, which was at first of great severity. It began over the lower part of the sternum and struck up into both arms and his fingers tingled. I saw him an hour later. The pain had abated, but was still present. He was a short, powerfully built man, and his face was greyish-white in colour. The pulse was full and regular, 64 beats per minute. The heart was normal in size and the sounds were low and soft. At the base and mid-sternum there was a systolic murmur.

I first gave him an inhalation of nitrite of amyl, which increased the rate of the heart and softened the pulse, but gave him no relief. Then he had an injection of morphia, and afterwards the pain gradually passed off. After a week's rest he got about and gradually resumed his work. He had to avoid any strenuous effort, as he became at times very short of breath and the pain would tend to return. He remained fairly well until January 17, 1905, when he had another attack while sitting at tea in the evening after his day's work. He was feeling quite well, when a curious tingling sensation began in his chest, a vague sort of painful feeling in his arm. This passed off, and ten minutes later the pain started with great severity across the middle of the chest, passed into the left chest and up into the left side of the head and neck, and into the left arm. While the pain continued he broke into a profuse perspiration. Whisky and hot water gave him a little ease and the pain suddenly subsided after half an hour. He was very weak after the attack, but he felt better on the 22nd. On the 23rd he was seized with a slight attack when walking out. That evening he had a severe attack, which began about seven o'clock and persisted with varying severity till I saw him at half-past nine. His face was grey and pinched, and beads of perspiration stood out on it. The pulse was rapid and hard. I gave him amyl of nitrite to inhale, but the relief was slight and transient. I tried chloroform, but he could not bear the sense of suffocation, so I gave him an injection of half a grain of morphia, from which he got relief after a few minutes. From this time the attacks of pain were so readily induced that he was obliged to keep in bed and obtain relief by the use of chloral and morphia. Gradually he became weaker and was unable to rest in bed, and had to sit up and go to sleep with his head resting on a table. Swelling of the legs and Cheyne-Stokes respiration set in. Towards the end of March he began to expectorate small clots of blood. The pulse had been persistently increased in rate, up to 120 per minute, until he died on June 1, 1905, at the age of 54. The heart was large and full of blood, the lungs were congested and had numerous infarcts. There were also infarcts in the kidneys. The veins and venules of the heart were distended. The arteries of the heart and aorta showed a slight thickening of the intima, but the muscle-coat was hypertrophied. There was a remarkable thickening of the base of the mitral cusp, but no stenosis. The tricuspid orifice was dilated. The interauricular septum was so stretched that the foramen ovale had been reopened. The right ventricle was hypertrophied and dilated, the left dilated and atrophied. There was a considerable degree of degeneration of the muscle-fibres and a slight degree of fibrosis.

CASE 26.—*Angina pectoris. Death during an attack.*

Male. Aged 51. Consulted me on May 3, 1912, complaining of pain coming on with great severity when he exerted himself. The patient was an active, healthy-looking man, but very nervous. He led a strenuous business life. For many years he had suffered from dyspepsia. Two years before seeing me he suffered from pain in the chest and down the left arm on exertion, especially after a meal. Latterly these attacks became so easily provoked that he could not go up a flight of stairs, or walk 100 yards without being pulled up by an attack. Physical examination revealed no abnormality, and eighteen months before he had been insured for a large sum as a healthy man. I urged immediate rest, but in vain. A month later I was called to see him in the early morning. He had had a big dinner, and was roused out of sleep at 2 a.m. by severe pain. He had one attack after another and sometimes lost consciousness. I saw him in two attacks—the pulse became feeble and imperceptible while he was in the pain, and he died during one of these attacks.

CASE 27.—*Angina pectoris with the pulsus alternans. An attack described. Death.*

Male. Aged 59. Complained of shortness of breath on slight exertion, consciousness of the heart intermitting, and of attacks of pain, sometimes of great severity, across the chest.

He had scarlet fever when young and rheumatic fever several times between the ages of 20 and 30. This left him when he went to live in the tropics at the age of 31, where he stayed for seventeen years. He had yellow fever once, dysentery several times, and lumbago frequently. At the age of 46 he began to suffer from slight pain in the chest, chiefly on exertion. This would disappear for a time and return. At the age of 57 he had a series of very violent attacks of pain in the chest after a period of very hard physical labour and mental worry and anxiety. This left him very exhausted, and the attacks were provoked by the slightest exertion. After a long rest he gradually regained strength, so that he was able to go about quietly, though any little excitement or exertion would speedily provoke an attack.

He consulted me when he was 59 years of age ; he was a pleasant-featured, healthy-looking man. walked quietly, and seemed careful to avoid much exertion. The breathlessness was not only easily provoked, but he would waken at night with a sense of suffocation, so that he had to sit up in bed and try and get more air. He described the attacks as being due to a difficulty in controlling his breathing, and related his sensations thus : ' I sometimes have distressing attacks, when the inspirations are nearly swamped by spasmodic expirations. No sooner do I begin to draw in a breath than the muscles which cause expiration convulsively take charge, so that breathing consists of very short hurried attempts to draw in air and very long convulsions forcing it out.' His attacks of pain he describes as coming on after exertion and sometimes during the night, especially if he had been busy or excited during the day (a description of a typical attack is given below).

Except for his heart trouble he was healthy. The radial artery was thickened, the pulse-rate 64, with occasional extra-systoles ; the blood-pressure 165 mm. Hg. The heart's dullness extended 2 inches beyond the nipple line on the left, and there was a harsh mitral murmur. The murmur due to the extra-systole was louder than the murmur at the normal systole. There was no albumen in the urine. The radial tracings showed pulsus alternans sometimes after an extra-systole. He had had much treatment, and although he was much better when he was quiet and could get good nights' sleep, his affairs necessitated his attending to them. I gave him some general directions as to his food, which was to be taken small in quantity and thoroughly masticated, and suggested his taking 5 grains of chloral at night on those days when he was over-tired or excited ; inhalation of oxygen for the breathlessness in the night. Following these directions he obtained considerable relief for a time. A year later he had a slight attack of pneumonia, from which he recovered. On visiting him one day during his convalescence, he was talking in a somewhat excited manner, when he was seized with an attack of pain.

The pain began with a slight aching in the left forearm on the inner side and passed up the arm to the armpit, then across the chest, with a disagreeable gripping sensation. This was immediately followed by pain along the jaws, like a bad toothache. The pain in the arm and chest became less severe, while the pain in the jaw was very distressing. After three or four minutes the pain eased, then returned in half a minute as severely as before, but was limited to the jaw, the left side of the neck, and the throat. The throat pain was associated with a feeling of tightness which added to the distress. Half an ounce of brandy gave no relief, and he then took five grains of chloral, and after three or four minutes the pain gradually eased and he lay back in a semi-sleepy state. The duration of the attack was about ten minutes. During the attack the face, which immediately before had been bright and humorous in expression, became drawn and still, though there was no apparent change in colour. I noted his pulse during the whole attack and took tracings ; it did not alter perceptibly in rate, rhythm, or size. During a brief period at the beginning, extra-systoles were frequently present, but as the attack continued they became fewer. After the first few minutes the skin became moist, and this increased until at the expiration of the attack his whole body was moist with perspiration. He talked quietly and sensibly, and told me the region to which the pain was constantly shifting and its varying severity. He disliked the use of nitro-glycerine and amyl nitrite, though they usually gave relief, as they induced a severe headache afterwards.

He rallied after this attack and was able to get about for a few months, but the attacks became more and more easily provoked till he was forced to keep his bed, and he died from gradually increasing weakness of the heart at the age of 61.

CASE 28.—*Angina pectoris, cardiac aneurysm, rupture of the heart. Sudden death.*

Born 1843. The patient was a sober, industrious man, and had led an active life. He had fair health, though suffering at times from rheumatic-like pains in his back. In September

1891, then 58 years of age, after his midday meal he was hurrying along the street, when he was seized with a choking sensation and a pain which started over his left breast, striking up both sides of his neck. He was forced to stand still for twenty minutes until the pain had subsided. Similar attacks occurred during the following month, and he consulted me on October 28, 1891. He described the pains as always starting over the left breast, and radiating sometimes into the left armpit and down the left arm, and sometimes into the neck. He felt when the pain was on as if he were going to die. On examination I found the patient was healthy-looking and well nourished and with a ruddy complexion. The pulse was regular and of good strength, and the arteries slightly thickened. The heart was of normal size, the dullness extending 3½ inches to the left of the middle line. The sounds were clear and free from murmurs. The tissues in front of the left chest were tender on pressure. There was also some tenderness on the skin and deeper tissues of the left chest behind, and the second dorsal vertebra was tender on pressure. There was also marked tenderness on pressing over the second left rib in the middle line.

On October 20, while walking, the patient had a very severe attack, the pain striking into the left chest and into the jaw. When the pain was bad the mouth filled with saliva. When I examined him the following day I found the hyperalgesia in the region already referred to very much increased.

After resting the attacks diminished in severity, until, in December 1891, he was able to walk 200 yards with comfort. If he walked further, or if he attempted to walk quickly, the pain would pull him up. The pain latterly had struck into the left arm and extended to the little finger.

On December 30, 1891, while sitting at his desk, he died suddenly. On post-mortem examination the heart was found to have ruptured, the pericardial sac being full of blood. There was a small aneurysm, the size of a marble, in the wall of the left ventricle, where the ventricular cavity was separated from the pericardial sac by a thin wall consisting only of pericardium and endocardium. In this thin wall there was a narrow slit. The coronary artery was very atheromatous. The external anterior thoracic nerve was found to be lying under the place, over the second rib, that had been so tender to pressure during life.

CASE 29. *Angina pectoris. Post-mortem report.*

A man, aged 52 years, who had been under observation at frequent intervals for four years. His chief and almost only complaint during that time had been of a pain induced by exertion. At times the pain had been so easily excited that he had had to keep quiet in bed for several days, and then he would be comparatively free for some time. He was a pale thin man, whose countenance had the drawn lines expressive of great suffering. I had many times made a careful examination of his heart, but could detect no abnormality.

The pain was described invariably as arising in the left chest and extending to the armpit, down the inside of the arm, and the ulnar border of the forearm to the wrist, whence it extended across the palm to the thumb, leaving the fingers unaffected, but causing great aching in the thumb (Fig. 10). On February 8, 1894, he again consulted me, complaining, in addition to the constant recurrence of the foregoing pain, of a soreness and tenderness of the scalp. The nature and extent of this I could not well determine. In the month of March this soreness of the scalp had developed into attacks of headache, readily induced by exertion, but also coming on when quite still. This headache started always at the left eyebrow, and might remain fixed there, but usually spread to the back of the head, including both sides. There was no sensory abnormality of the skin, but there was tenderness on pressure over the supraorbital nerves. This headache became so violent that the patient had to keep to his bed, and finally he became comatose, developed Cheyne-Stokes respiration, and died on March 27.

At the post-mortem examination the heart was found very flabby, and the walls of both ventricles were soft and friable. There was well-marked atheroma of the coronary arteries.

In many places the arteries and their branches were calcified. Microscopic examination of the cardiac muscle (left ventricle) revealed fatty degeneration.

CASE 30.—*Angina pectoris ; sudden death.*

Born 1859. The patient had enjoyed good health and worked hard up till 1906. He had been a hard drinker for some years up to 1893, when he became a total abstainer, and he continued his abstemious habits till his death. He consulted me on August 13, 1907. For over twelve months he had been troubled with a sense of discomfort in the chest on exertion, and latterly he had been having attacks of very severe pain coming on during exertion. He described the pain as striking just under the right breast and passing upwards to the right arm, when the pain would be felt very severely in the 'flesh' of the upper arm, on the inner side ; sometimes the pain would pass down to the ring and little fingers, and sometimes it would strike into his neck. While the pain lasted he would often feel the chest held tight, so that he had to stretch his arm to release the tightness and take a big breath. Sometimes this feeling of tightness would come on first, and would be followed later by the pain. After the pain subsided he would eructate a quantity of air and pass a large quantity of pale urine (I saw him once immediately after an attack and examined the urine, which had a specific gravity of 1003 ; he passed a large quantity). The patient was stout, with a somewhat flabby complexion. The pulse was large, full, and regular, 70 per minute. The blood-pressure was 120 mm. Hg. The heart's dullness extended 2 inches to the left beyond the nipple line. There was also some dullness over the second and third left interspaces near the sternum. There was pulsation in the episternal notch and slight tracheal tugging. Examination with the X-rays revealed the heart to be enlarged to the left, and there was some enlargement in the region of the aorta. There was an aortic systolic murmur ; the other sounds of the heart were free from murmurs.

On scratching under the right breast the peculiar sensations (autonomic sensations) started, which passed into and down the arm in the exact situation in which the pain was felt.

During the four months this patient was under my care the attacks of pain varied much in frequency. After resting for a few days he was usually able to go about for a week or two with fair comfort. After a restful holiday of three weeks at the seaside in October, he returned greatly improved and able to walk a considerable distance in comfort. When, however, he attempted to walk quietly up a hill, the pain would return with great severity. The pain was always felt worse in the right side, sometimes striking from the right breast to the right shoulder-blade, and directly down the right arm. During these four months I made numerous observations on his blood-pressure, and found it vary from 120 mm. to 170 mm. As a rule he was better and would be able to walk faster when his blood-pressure was high. Thus after three weeks' rest at the seaside, and when he was freer from pain than at any other time he was under my care, his blood-pressure was 170 mm. Hg.

My last observation was made on November 8, 1907, and was to the effect that he felt quite well when resting, but walking readily induced the pain. I did not see him again, but I saw in the newspaper that in August 1908 he had been found dead in bed and a coroner's inquest had been held on his body.

CASE 31.—*Angina pectoris, with severe pain in the left arm ; post-mortem report.*

Female. Aged 60. Complained of pain in her chest, radiating into the left arm, and persisting in the left forearm with great severity. It was easily induced by exertion, and one day when coming to see me she had hurried. While I was examining her the pain seized her with great violence ; she described it as being situated almost entirely in the left forearm, which she pressed across her chest. I took tracings of her radial and jugular pulses. The heart's rate was increased, but the radial pulse was of a good size (Fig. 193). I gave her amyl nitrite and it relieved the pain at once. The patient died three months after from heart failure, and Dr. R. T. Williamson examined the heart for me and found marked atheroma and calcification of the coronary arteries and extensive fibrous changes in the muscle of the left ventricle.

CASE 32.—*Angina pectoris, with irregularity of the heart of obscure origin. Freedom from attacks for nearly three years.*

Male. Aged 68 at his death. Consulted me on November 17, 1899, because of pain over his chest on exertion. He was a millwright by trade—a big powerful fellow. As he was in com-

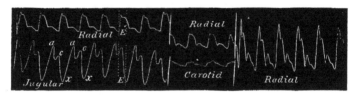

FIG. 193. Taken during an attack of angina pectoris—the radial pulse is seen to be of good size (Case 31).

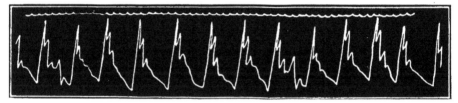

FIG. 194. Large irregular pulse during an attack of angina pectoris (Case 32).

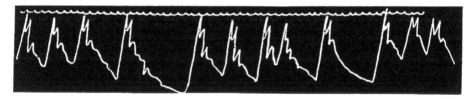

FIG. 195. The same as Fig. 194 (Case 32).

fortable circumstances I advised him to give up hard manual work. He followed this advice, and was free from pain until July 8, 1902, when he was seized with violent pains on going up a hill. He came home and went to bed, when the pain returned, and I saw him during an attack of agonizing severity which lasted over ten minutes. While amyl nitrite was being fetched, I took tracings of his pulse (Fig. 194 and 195). The amyl nitrite gave him a little ease, and the pain gradually subsided. During the attack the character of the pulse did not alter, and there was no sign of contracted arteries. The heart was irregular, due mainly to extra-systoles, sometimes interpolated as in Figs. 194 and 195. He had repeated attacks, and died in one on July 10, 1902.

CASE 33.—*Angina pectoris with frequent extra-systoles. Sudden death.*

Male, 43 years of age. Consulted me on September 13, 1900. Had good health until a year before, when he began to be short of breath on exertion. Shortly after this he suffered from a pain that shot into his left arm when he exerted himself. Four days before coming to me the pain struck with great severity into his chest and down the inside of the left arm, and lasted for half an hour. He had been a heavy drinker. On the 19th he called again upon me; was seized with the pain, which held him for some minutes, and I got tracings of the jugular and radial pulses while the pain was present. The pulse increased in rate and became irregular

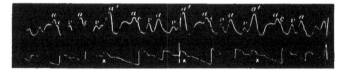

FIG. 196. Shows extra-systoles occurring during an attack of angina pectoris (Case 33).

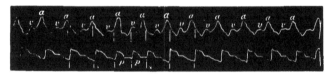

FIG. 197. Shows an interpolated extra-systole during an attack of angina pectoris. The first radial beat *P* is an interpolated extra-systole (Case 33).

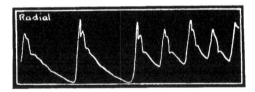

FIG. 198. Tracing of radial pulse showing the appearance of the pulsus alternans after a long pause during an attack of angina pectoris (Case 34).

(Fig. 196 and 197). These irregularities are due to ventricular extra-systoles; in Fig. 197 the extra-systole is interpolated between two normal beats.

The patient improved under treatment, and I did not see him again after the end of September. He dropped dead in January 1901, while watching a football match.

CASE 34.—*Angina pectoris with obscure irregular action of the heart during attacks. Death.*

Female. Aged 68. Had been under my care for five years, suffering from cirrhotic kidney. Her pulse was always hard and regular. On February 28, 1900, she was seized with an attack of angina pectoris. These attacks kept recurring, though she lay in bed. I saw her in an attack on the 30th; her face was blanched and shrunk, and damp with perspiration. The pulse became very irregular, as in Fig. 198. Relief was only obtained by large doses of opium, vaso-dilators having no effect (amyl nitrite, whisky and hot water). Next day she was better and her pulse quite regular. She died in the following week during an attack of angina pectoris.

CASE 35.—*Angina pectoris, with Cheyne-Stokes breathing, pulsus alternans. Post-mortem report.*

Male. Aged 57. Consulted me on May 1, 1905, complaining of weakness on exertion, a sense of great exhaustion and trembling of the legs. He first noticed the breathlessness three years before on hurrying up a hill, when he had a severe attack. He felt fairly well until six months after, since which time the breathlessness was very easily provoked.

He had been a lifelong abstainer, and had led a steady, regular life. In his younger days his work entailed severe bodily effort, but for the last twenty years his occupation as mill manager had not demanded much exertion. Twenty years before he had an attack of 'inflammation of the kidneys'. He was a powerfully built man; face greyish in colour, pulse rapid (86 per minute) and hard, the artery large and leathery in consistence. Heart was enlarged, dull to the nipple line. The sounds were clear and distinct ; the urine contained a large quantity of albumen. Blood-pressure, 210 mm. Hg. He was directed to take his food in small quantities, and to chew it thoroughly ; to have his bowels freely opened ; and he was put upon iodide of potassium. He improved wonderfully for a time, all the albumen disappearing from the urine,

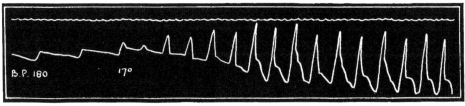

FIG. 199. Tracing taken from the radial artery after the air-bag connected with the manometer had obliterated the pulse at a pressure of 190 mm. Hg. The air was allowed to escape gradually, and when the pressure fell to 180 mm. Hg. the sphygmograph received the stronger beats, and the smaller beats came through when the pressure fell to 170 mm. Hg. When the pressure in the air-bag was exhausted the pulse tracing showed rhythmical variation in the size of the waves—that is, the pulsus alternans (Case 35).

but he began to relapse. Abstinence from meat was tried and seemed to do him good, but only for a short time. The blood-pressure records were very confusing, sometimes falling to 145 and rising to 210, and this independent of drug or diet. There was no corresponding improvement in his condition with the fall of blood-pressure. When it was low he felt depressed, and sometimes felt very well when it was high. His pulse was usually alternating in rhythm, and this peculiarity was more marked when the pressure was high. When the pulsus alternans had disappeared with lowered blood-pressure, it could easily be brought back by running up a flight of stairs. The difference in pressure between the beats was about 20 mm. Hg. —that is to say, if the radial pulse was obliterated by raising the pressure in the cuff to 200 mm. Hg., and the air allowed to escape from the cuff, the large beats would be felt coming through at 190 mm. Hg., while the smaller would not be felt till the pressure in the cuff had fallen to 170 mm. Hg. (see Fig. 199).

Notwithstanding the alternating rhythm, the pulse-rate was practically regular (Fig. 200). In May 1906 extra-systoles began to appear, and they gave a peculiar character to the tracing. Thus, in Fig. 200 the tracing shows a perfectly regular rate with small and large beat alternating, except in the centre, where there are two small beats in succession. On measuring the tracing it will be found that the second of the two smaller beats (r') occurs a little too early. The jugular tracing shows that the auricular wave (a) is perfectly regular, therefore r' is a ventricular extra-systole and after it there is a longer pause than normal, so that the beat after the pause is large, and the succeeding beat smaller than the other beats.

This increase of the alternating character of the rhythm is seen in Fig. 201. Here there are two extra-systoles, one as in Fig. 200 after the small beat and the other after a large beat, and here also the character of the alternating rhythm is more marked after the extra-systole.

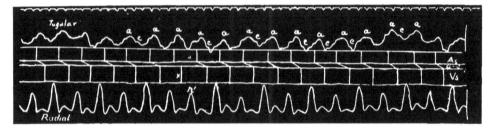

Fig. 200. Typical pulsus alternans with ventricular extra-systole r'. In the diagram it is shown to occur prematurely (downstroke ×) and independently of the auricular stimulus. After the extra-systole there is a longer pause, and the alternating character of the pulse becomes more marked (Case 35).

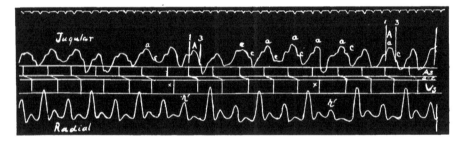

Fig. 201. Here there are two extra-systoles (r' r'), one after the small heat and the other after the large beat of the alternating rhythm (Case 35).

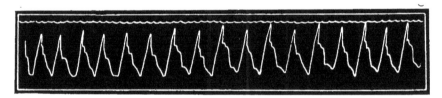

Fig. 202. Large alternating pulse during an attack of angina pectoris. B.P. 190 (Case 35).

The patient also began to have attacks of angina pectoris. His condition fluctuated very much. During a period when he was worse than usual he called to see me, walking up a steep hill on the way. He began to feel a tightness across his chest which developed into a severe pain. I examined him and took a tracing of his pulse (Fig. 202). I took his blood-pressure and found it 190 mm. Hg. His pulse did not alter in character during his suffering, and the height of the waves showed that there was no contraction of the artery, nor did it differ in character from the pulse tracing taken when he was free from pain. I gave him amyl nitrite to inhale, the pulse quickened (Fig. 203), and the amyl nitrite gave him instant relief. Fifteen minutes after he was quite free from pain, his blood-pressure had risen to 200 mm. Hg., and the alternating character became more marked. He became restless and disturbed at night, and the attacks of pain became more frequent, until he was put upon bromide of ammonium, when he began to sleep better, and the angina disappeared. Towards the end of 1906, Cheyne-Stokes respiration appeared, his nights became very restless, and he could only be relieved by opium and chloral. During the apnœic stage he would wake up in great distress, suffering from intense breathlessness, and would breathe heavily for ten minutes. In January dropsy set in, the heart dilated, and his blood-pressure fell permanently to 150 mm. Hg. and under. The urine became scanty. Various preparations of digitalis and other drugs were tried with little good results, and the patient died in March 1907. Permission was only given to examine the heart, and the following is the report of the post-mortem appearance :

' *Musculature.*—Hypertrophied, but the apical half of ventricle is fibrosed and dilated ; large pre-mortem clot adherent to the anterior wall of the left ventricle. Thickness of wall at base, 18–22 mm.; over the fibrosed area, 6–8 mm. The musculature at the mouth of the superior vena cava is hypertrophied. Tænia terminalis is hypertrophied, and under the microscope shows many fibres atrophied and fibrosed.

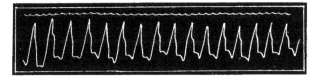

FIG. 203.   Under amyl nitrite (Case 35).

' *Valves and orifices.*—Mitral cusps thickened ; tricuspid, pulmonary, and aortic healthy. Auriculo-ventricular orifices smaller than normal, due to tonus or contraction of the musculature of the base.

' *Arteries.*—Patches of atheroma in aorta, especially at orifices of coronary arteries. Intense endarteritis of left coronary artery, diameter 6 mm., lumen 2·5 mm. ; the interior is especially thickened. The right coronary artery is not so much affected. All the arteries of the heart above 1·5 mm. in diameter are affected if they lie *outside* the musculature of the heart ; if surrounded and supported by the musculature, less affected. The anterior interventricular artery was most affected, while the artery to the auriculo-ventricular bundle from the right coronary was more like a needle-prick.

' Sino-auricular node, less musculature (more fibrosed) than in health, still not marked. The auriculo-ventricular bundle is normal in size, and its fibres and cells are normal.'

CASE 36.—*Angina pectoris, with pain in chest, arms, throat, and behind the head.   Partial recovery, with recurrence and sudden death seven years after first onset.*

Basketmaker.   At the age of 60 he noticed a slight pain on exertion, but paid no attention to it at first.   It gradually became worse and increased in severity until he consulted me at the age of 62.   The pain only appeared when walking, and especially after meals.   He had to rest every 60 or 70 yards, so that in walking to his work he used to take 20 minutes, whereas formerly 7½ minutes had been ample time.   After noting a number of attacks he described the pain as striking up his breast-bone, into his throat, and very severely behind the ears. When he described the position to me, he grasped with the fingers of each hand both mastoid processes.   Sometimes the pain would also strike into both arms, down the inside to the elbows. There was usually hyperalgesia of the skin and subcutaneous tissues around the left breast, while the sterno-mastoid and trapezius muscles were tender on pressure. The heart revealed no abnormality. The first sound was muffled and the second sounds slightly accentuated.

For a time he seemed to improve under treatment, but he relapsed, and he gave up work and went quietly about. He rested for two years, when he felt much better and resumed work again. He followed his work for three years, towards the end of which time the pain began to return, and he dropped dead at the age of 67.

CASE 37.—*Angina pectoris. Syphilitic aortitis. Improvement under treatment.*

Male. Aged 35. Consulted me on October 1, 1912, complaining of severe pain which struck across the chest, chiefly on the right side. It started first ten months before, and he thought it was due to indigestion and consulted a doctor, who after some weeks detected some change in the heart and said it was the heart which was troubling him. Since that time the pain had been very easily provoked, so that a very slight exertion would at times bring it on. In very bad attacks the pain lasted for a few hours, at first felt only across the chest, then spreading down the left arm and up into the throat. He had been resting for some weeks.

The patient was pale and thin. The pulse was collapsing, and the apex beat large and diffuse in the fifth interspace and outside the nipple line. There were murmurs, systolic and diastolic in time, heard loudest over the aortic area. A Wassermann test gave a positive reaction.

He was recommended complete rest and anti-syphilitic treatment (salvarsan injections). This was done, and he gradually improved so that he put on flesh and the size of the heart diminished, though the murmurs persisted, and in six months' time all the pain had gone and he was able to play a game of golf without distress.

CASE 38.—*Angina pectoris. Syphilitic aortitis. Partial recovery.*

Female. Aged 43. Engaged as a medical missionary in India. She was in fair health until March 1906, when she was inoculated for the plague, and her heart became irregular. She auscultated it then, and the sounds were clear and free from murmurs. In September 1906 she became ill, feeling tired, exhausted, and sleepless, and giddy in stooping. She auscultated her heart and detected a diastolic aortic murmur. The apex beat was in the sixth space and just outside the nipple line. She rested, but difficulty in breathing arose, not only on exertion but sometimes in bed. In October she began to suffer from attacks of pain referred over the middle of the sternum.

She rested for eight months and then resumed her work, but her health failing, she came to this country in the early part of 1909 and consulted Sir Clifford Allbutt, who recognized the condition as being first aortic supra-sigmoid syphilis, followed later by invasion and partial destruction of the aortic valves. He sought for a history of syphilis, and brought out the fact that in 1897 she had an ulcer on her finger, which healed with difficulty, and was followed by a sore throat and rash. Under his direction she was put through a course of anti-syphilitic treatment, though the Wassermann reaction taken on the occasion was negative. She consulted me in July 1909. She was pale but well nourished. The pulse was rapid, 90 when she lay quiet, large, and collapsing. The heart's apex was in the fifth space and slightly in the sixth, and extended out well beyond the left nipple line. The impact was distinct but not very large. I had some difficulty at first in differentiating the heart-sounds. The first sound was of a rumbling character, but ended abruptly both at the apex and at the base. The second sound at the base was followed by a short diastolic murmur, heard also over the bottom of the sternum.

She had taken very careful notes of her symptoms. From these notes and her description I obtained the following facts: The pain was at first confined to the chest, but after 1907 it extended into the arms and especially the left forearm and hand on the ulnar side, and sometimes limited to the left inner condyle. In 1908 and 1909 the pain in addition extended up into the neck and along the lower jaw. The most frequent time of occurrence was in the early morning between 2 and 7 a.m. Frequently the pain would arise in connexion with a dream in which she was hurrying to catch a train. Emotion and physical exertion would always induce an attack of pain, and sometimes on beginning to eat. The blood-pressure was always raised above the normal level during the attacks of pain, and the pulse slightly increased in rate, and the artery was small and hard. Immediate relief was always obtained by the administration of $\frac{1}{100}$ or $\frac{1}{50}$ grain of trinitrin. She had kept a chart of the blood-pressure and pulse-rate during a number of attacks, and there was always a rise during the attacks.

At the time I saw her she was having soamin injections once a week. In September she noticed after an injection, a swelling had appeared at the site of the injection, which persisted till she had the injection on the following week. Following on this second injection, she became irritable and confused, and paralysis of both legs followed, and she was very ill for a week; then she gradually recovered, and by the middle of December all nervous symptoms had disappeared. The heart condition had improved, in so far as the pain was less easily provoked and less severe, though the physical signs remained. Feeling better, she determined to return to her work in India. In a letter dated March 1913 she described herself as much better and able to do her work, though her capacity was restricted.

CASE 39.—*Angina pectoris. Aortic valvular disease.*

Female. Born 1850. She had several attacks of rheumatism from her 18th to her 20th year, and the doctor told her it 'had got to her heart'. She married at the age of 28, and had one child when she was 30 years of age. She continued to have slight attacks of rheumatism, but was in fair health till the age of 38, when she began to have attacks of palpitation. At the age of 40 she had a severe attack of pain in her chest, which continued for some time until she fell on the floor unconscious. She kept her bed for some time, but when she began to move about the pain would return with agonizing severity. I saw her eight months after the attacks began, in April 1891, when she was under my care in the Victoria Hospital, Burnley. My notes taken at that time state that the attacks of pain were very frequent, sometimes so severe that when she was about her household duties she would fall unconscious, and was found several times by her neighbours lying unconscious. She described the attacks as beginning with a sensation of beat all over the body, then immediately after, a pain of great severity would strike into her left breast and be felt round to the back over the left shoulder-blade and down the inner side of the left arm and ulnar side of the forearm to the little and ring fingers. The attacks usually passed off in a few seconds and left her greatly exhausted, and with a feeling of great soreness in the places where the pain was felt. When at her worst she would have as many as sixteen attacks in one day, and they would be induced by the slightest exertion, such as talking. She felt during the attack that if it continued, she would die, and she lost consciousness frequently.

In the many examinations I made during the year (1891) she was under my care, I always found marked hyperalgesia of the skin and breast of the left side and of the left sterno-mastoid muscle, and great tenderness on pressure of the upper dorsal spine. There was also a good deal of tenderness of the skin and deeper structures of the chest-wall on the left side, the area being somewhat ill defined.

The heart was slightly enlarged, dull to the left nipple line, and there was a rough systolic murmur heard in the aortic area and in the carotids, while the aortic second sound was markedly accentuated. The radial tracing showed an anacrotic wave. The patient was healthy-looking, and well nourished, but evidently very neurotic. While in bed the attacks of pain did not recur. After resting two months she went home much improved, but returned to the hospital in September as bad as ever. She was kept in bed for three months and then sent home, and I heard nothing of her for eleven years. In November 1903, when visiting the workhouse infirmary, I found her there. She stated that after leaving the Victoria Hospital in 1892 she rested for two years, and was practically free from the attacks and was fairly well for three years, after which the pain returned as badly as before. Her doctor gave her injections of morphia, and this not only gave her relief, but seemed to ward off attacks. So much benefit did she imagine she experienced from the morphia that she began to use it herself, and so numerous were the injections that when she showed me her arm it was simply covered with cicatrices from the shoulder to the wrist, the result of the numerous hypodermic injections of morphia. In later years her ankle- and knee-joints had become somewhat stiff and deformed from rheumatism, so that she was scarcely able to walk, and, being helpless, she was removed to the workhouse.

Her description of her later attacks agreed exactly with those given twelve years before, and a re-examination of the chest showed that the heart was still of the same size, the aortic murmur still present, and also now a systolic murmur mitral. There was still the marked hyperalgesia in the left chest and sterno-mastoid muscles. She died in 1905.

CASE 40.—*Angina pectoris, syphilitic origin. Blocking of coronary arteries. Degeneration of heart muscle. Post-mortem report.*

Male. Aged 35. Consulted me on April 15, 1912, on the recommendation of Dr. Hartigan, who could find no lesion of the heart. The complaint was one of great pain which struck in the lower part of the chest over the sternum, and into the left arm, which felt powerless after the pain had subsided. The patient was a carman and had led a strenuous life. There was a positive Wassermann reaction. In January, when doing some heavy bodily labour, the pain seized him and lasted for nearly a quarter of an hour. Since then the tendency for the pain to recur had become so great that it came on if he walked 100 yards.

The patient was a healthy-looking man, the hands were blue and cold. The pulse was quiet and regular, and the blood-pressure 130 mm. Hg. The heart was not enlarged, and the sounds were clear and free from murmurs. In fact, the only abnormality I could detect was the shock due to the ventricular systole, which could be felt over his chest. The urine was normal.

As I suspected some serious affection of the heart muscle, I sent him for rest and observation to the Mount Vernon Hospital. While there he had several attacks of severe pain when at rest, and they were becoming easily provoked. The pain was always in the same situation as first mentioned. On June 4 he had a series of attacks, and when walking about to get relief he fell down and died in a few minutes.

The heart was removed and sent to Professor Woodhead, and the following is an abstract of his report:

' On examining this heart the most marked changes were in the aorta immediately above the aortic ring. It is extremely difficult to find the orifices of the coronary arteries; the right is almost closed by the thickened aortic intima, the left is very much constricted. On the distal side of the constricted orifice there appears to be little or no alteration of the lumen or thickening of the intima. In the aorta above the coronary vessels are large patches of considerable size, and raised one-sixteenth of an inch above the surface, in which the intima is greatly thickened. Most of the patches are somewhat grey and gelatinous-looking, only here and there are they becoming opaque or yellow. There is some thickening of the muscular wall of the left ventricle. Marked mottling of the inner surface probably indicates fatty degeneration of the heart muscle. There may be some slight thickening,' but much less mottling of the muscular wall in the right ventricle; there is marked thickening of the endo-cardium of the left auricle, but none of the right.

' Under the microscope the swollen patches in the aorta appear to be the result of (a) absorption of fluid by the fibrous tissue, (b) accumulation of cells, very like lymphocytes, with here and there a few polymorphonuclear leucocytes around the vasa vasorum, and in little patches of the deeper layers of the intima, in the muscular tissue, and in the adventitia; (c) proliferating connective tissue-cells. These collections of cells are very like small gummatous masses, in which, however, there appears to be no degeneration.

'In the wall of the aorta around the orifice of each coronary vessel is well-defined thickening of the various coats, in which similar cellular masses are distributed. Most of the vasa vasorum are filled with blood. Near the orifice of the right coronary artery there is a great thickening of the intima, evidently the result of a subacute inflammatory process. Some infiltration of the muscular coat around the smaller vessels, great thickening of the connective tissue-fibres, and marked increase in the number of cells between the fibrous tissue and around the blood-vessel of the adventitia.

'There is a similar change taking place around the left coronary vessel. Microscopical examination of the left ventricular wall shows in certain areas, especially towards the apex, a considerable increase in the amount of interfascicular fibrous tissue. In these areas there has evidently been considerable wasting and absorption of the muscular tissue. In some of the patches corresponding to the grey mottled areas seen in the papillary muscles, the muscle-cells themselves are large, swollen, and homogeneous-looking; others stained with hæmatin Van Giesen have a reddish-brown colour as compared with the rather yellower brown of healthy muscle.

'Many of these muscle-cells are highly vacuolated, the vacuolations in some cells occupying almost the whole section of the fibre, in others forming a sort of "court" around the nucleus. Patches of opaque homogeneous muscle in a condition of hyaline or vitreous degeneration may be seen scattered over the section. In other areas, again, the vacuolated muscle-cells contain large droplets of fat well brought out by Soudan III.

'In other areas the muscle-fibre is simply undergoing a fatty degeneration, small granules of fat being seen in the muscle-fibres, the striation in the latter being much less marked than usual.

'The atrophied muscle-fibres often lie enclosed in reticular spaces formed by bundles of coarse connective tissue which stand out as pink homogeneous bands.

'There can be little doubt that the degenerative changes taking place in the muscle-wall, especially of the wall of the left ventricle, are the direct result of the cutting off of the blood-supply through closure of the coronary arteries, the process being assisted by the special poison developed, plus accumulated waste-products. The heart muscle, of course, would act much less effectively under these conditions, and the degenerative changes must have led to heart failure.'

CASE 41.—*Aortic aneurysm—angina pectoris—pain, mainly on the right side. Post-mortem report.*

Female. Born 1840. The patient came under my care in 1882, suffering from pleurisy with effusion. I also detected evidence of an aneurysm on the right side of the chest at the level of the third and fourth ribs near the sternum. Her husband was a syphilitic, and her three children showed evidence of congenital syphilis. The aneurysm increased in size till it was perceptible to the sight, bulging at the place mentioned, and pulsated so largely that I easily obtained numerous tracings from it. Until her death in 1894 the swelling increased at various times, and she used to spend some weeks at a time in bed, when the swelling subsided. In August 1889 she began to complain of attacks of pain coming on with exertion. The pain at first was slight, but increased in severity until she was compelled to rest. The pain started in the right breast, and passed down the inside of the right arm to the elbow. There was no hyperalgesia of the skin or deeper structures. The apex heat was large and in the sixth space, 2 inches outside the nipple line. The aneurysmal swelling was seen protruding and pulsating at the level of the third to the fifth ribs on the right side, inside the nipple line. The sounds of the heart were soft and somewhat muffled, but there were no murmurs.

The attacks of pain subsided on resting, but tended to recur when she was much exhausted. She led a somewhat restricted though useful life till March 1894, when she became slightly feverish. Her pulse showed frequent extra-systoles, and on March 24 the pulse showed the irregularity characteristic of the pulsus alternans after an extra-systole, and she died two days later.

At the post-mortem examination there was a quantity of pus between the ribs and the sac of the aneurysm. The pericardium was adherent, the mitral orifice was narrowed, admitting only one finger; the tricuspid orifice admitted four fingers. There was marked thickening of the lower part of the mitral cusp. Tricuspid and pulmonary valves were normal. Very slight alteration was present in the aortic valves. There was extensive atheroma of the aorta. In the ascending arch of the aorta on the convex right border about $\frac{7}{8}$ inch above the aortic valves was a circular opening about the size of a penny, which formed the communication between the aorta and a large aneurysmal sac. The sac was distended with clots up to this opening. There was slight atheroma of the coronary arteries.

CASE 42. *Aortic disease. Attacks of angina pectoris. Post-mortem report.*

Male. Admitted to Mount Vernon Hospital on July 5, 1910. Was 35 years of age and married.

History.—He had been a soldier, and up to three years before did heavy work as a labourer, but for the twelve months preceding admission had been unable to work. The patient had had rheumatic fever at 15, and was then told that his heart was affected. He had had two slight subsequent attacks. Twelve years before he had had a chancre and was treated for ten days. There had been no secondary manifestations. He had had diphtheria eleven years before. For the preceding five years he had been subject to attacks of pain in the chest, of a severe gnawing kind, accompanied by painful gripping of the chest, dyspnoea, faintness, fear, palpitation, throbbing, and sometimes nausea. During the attack he perspired freely. The pain passed off very gradually. The attacks occurred frequently, sometimes every hour. They came on even when he lay in bed, and, to obtain ease, he often slept after an attack kneeling on a pillow and resting his chest on the edge of the bed.

State on admission. Examination.—When free from pain the patient usually lay very quietly in bed, avoiding all movement. When he had to move for any purpose, he did so with deliberation, evidently in fear that some untoward act might provoke an attack. When spoken to, he replied in a quiet unemotional manner. During the attacks of pain he resorted to various devices to find an easy position, and was frequently found leaning on a chair or kneeling by his bedside. His face was pale and drawn, his body fairly well nourished. The rate of the pulse varied between 70 and 90 beats per minute. The radial pulse was large and collapsing. The ulnar artery was also large, and there was visible pulsation of the subclavian and carotid arteries. After rubbing the forehead, capillary pulsation was seen. The apex beat of the heart was displaced downwards and to the left, and extended 2 inches beyond the nipple line. Its area was increased, and it was thrusting in character. At the aortic area loud systolic and diastolic murmurs were heard. There was also a murmur, systolic in time but of different character, over the apex.

Site of the pain.—The following is the patient's own account of his attacks, checked by observations made during them. He stated that the pain commenced in the region of the lower end of the sternum, spreading across to the left breast, then up the left side of the chest, down the inner side of the upper arm (left) to the ulnar side of the arm and hand. In severe attacks the pain was felt along the left jaw, and sometimes also along the right jaw and down the right arm. When the pain was felt along the lower jaw it was worst opposite two decayed and tender teeth, one in either jaw. When the pain started it rapidly reached its worst. In addition to the pain in the chest there was a sense of pressure, which the patient described as similar to the sensation felt when the manometer bag compressed the arm. After the attack passed off, the throat was tender, and there was pain on swallowing for some hours.

Appearance of the patient during an attack.—The patient was pale and somewhat sallow, but when the attacks came on he became still paler and slightly cyanosed. He breathed deeply and frequently and occasionally held his breath in inspiration. He moved uneasily if lying down, and as the pain increased he got up, preferring to stand, leaning over a chair and pressing his chest firmly against the chair-back. Perspiration usually broke out and his forehead became damp. When in bed or leaning over the chair, the shock of each ventricular contraction gave a movement to his trunk and to the bed or chair on which he was resting.

Duration of the attacks.—The attacks were often slight and would pass off in a few minutes, but some lasted for a few hours. While suffering from those lasting the longer time, the patient usually changed his position, generally ending by kneeling with his head resting on the bed, in which position he would wait till the attack passed off, spending the remainder of the night asleep in this position.

Frequency of the attacks.—The attacks varied in frequency; sometimes he would have as many as twelve in the day, six during the daytime and six during the night. At other times they would be less frequent, but there was rarely a day that he did not experience three or four attacks.

Causes inducing the attacks.—Most of the attacks came on from no apparent cause; thus when lying quietly in bed asleep or awake the attack might come on, and would often be of the most severe kind. Exertion, such as walking, would induce them, and any cause of mental excitement, for example interrogation or a physical examination, was sufficient to start them. So provocative was this last circumstance, that we desisted from examining him until the treatment had subdued the attacks.

The pulse and blood-pressure.—Usually the pulse-rate varied from 76 to 90 beats per minute, but during an attack the radial artery became small and contracted and the rate increased to 136 beats per minute, gradually falling as the attack passed off. Coincident with the increase in the pulse-rate there was a rise in the blood-pressure. When free from pain the blood-pressure fluctuated from 118 to 138 mm. Hg. When the attacks came on, and the rate increased, there was a coincident rise in the blood-pressure and in the pulse-rate, the blood-pressure rising in severe attacks as high as 240 mm. Hg., and in one attack over 300 mm. Hg. As the pain subsided the blood-pressure fell. During an attack the coincident changes in the pain and blood-pressure occurred, whether the subsidence of the attack came about spontaneously or by the use of remedies.

The effects of remedies in an attack.—The following account of one attack presents a typical picture of the more salient events, and the effects of remedies. On July 10, 1910, as we entered the ward, the patient was lying in bed, and his blood-pressure was at once taken. He was a little startled, and the blood-pressure was found to be 160. He was left alone for a few minutes, while an examination was made of some of the other patients. On returning to his bed the blood-pressure was still found to be 160. Expecting an attack to supervene, the instrument was kept applied and the pressure taken at intervals of one or two minutes. The pain began in the manner already described, and as it increased in severity the blood-pressure gradually rose to 220, when nitrite of amyl was inhaled. The face became flushed, but relief was not marked until a second capsule of nitrite (each capsule contained 5 minims) was inhaled. The pain ceased and the blood-pressure fell to 154 mm. Hg. Immediately after the cessation of the inhalation, the pain began to return, slight at first, but gradually becoming more severe. At the same time the blood-pressure began to rise, till in $3\frac{1}{2}$ minutes it rose from 164 to 220 mm. Hg. Chloroform was then administered and rapidly pushed till he was partly unconscious; the same result followed, the blood-pressure fell, and the pain disappeared. When the chloroform inhalation ceased the blood-pressure rose, and the pain returned. This attack was subsequently relieved by an injection of morphia. The alterations in blood-pressure are shown in the accompanying chart, from the records taken during the attack described (Fig. 204). Hypodermic injections of morphia gave relief, and the following is an observation typical of the results after ⅓ grain of morphia.

Dose.	Hour.	Blood-Pressure.	Pulse-Rate.	Sensations.
	11.55	172	124	Pain moderate.
Morphine	11.58			
⅓ gr.	12.2	188		Pain worse.
	12.7	202	120	Pain severe.
	12.10	184	116	Pain a little better.
	12.15	172	120	Pain still lessening.
	12.30	154	116	Pain same. Patient lying more quietly.
	12.35	164	116	Pain easier, pupils moderately contracted.
	12.40	164	120	Eructations of gas, which gave relief. 'Pain is still there.'
	12.55		80	Pain disappeared.

Progress and treatment.—It was manifest from the first that the exhaustion of the patient's heart was so extreme that it was vain to expect a restoration of the heart's strength. Moreover he had been under treatment for years, and a few days before being admitted to the Mount Vernon Hospital he had been discharged from a hospital where he had lain for several weeks unrelieved. Various means were employed to give relief during the attacks, while other measures were adopted to prevent their recurrence. For the relief during attacks all remedies that acted speedily were very transient in their effect, and immediately the patient recovered from their effects the pain returned, as is shown in the observation of July 10 (Fig. 204). At the suggestion of Professor Cushny, a mixture of nitrous oxide gas and oxygen was inhaled. This produced a transient loss of consciousness, and the pain returned with the return of consciousness. The only remedies that were effective were morphia and chloral, and these had to be pushed until their soporific effects were produced. In searching for the cause of the attacks we recognized that the nervous system was implicated, as shown by the excitability of the vaso-constrictor mechanism and the readiness with which the pain and rise in blood-pressure were provoked. It was resolved, therefore, to direct the treatment mainly to the nervous condition, and for this purpose bromide of ammonium was prescribed. On July 11 the patient was given 20 grains three times a day, and this was continued till the 27th, when the dose was increased to 30 grains thrice daily. No definite effect was detected for the first ten days after beginning the bromide, but then he became slightly drowsy, although the attacks continued to occur. After the dose had been increased, he became more languid and drowsy, and the attacks became greatly modified, becoming much rarer (one to three a day), and so slight that the patient said they were not worth complaining about. He stated further that he had not had such ease for many years as he had for a few days at this time. On August 1, as he was very drowsy and free from attacks, the medicine was stopped, and resumed on the following day in doses of 7½ grains thrice daily. He gradually came out of the stupor and the attacks began to recur, though they were not so frequent as before taking the bromide. On account of the recurrence the dose was increased on the 5th to 15 grains thrice daily, but this had little effect, the attacks recurring with their old severity. On the 10th the dose was increased to 30 grains thrice daily and continued till the 18th, when the dose was reduced to 25 grains. During this time the attacks recurred, but they were not severe. On the 18th the patient became violent and delirious, and was soothed only by the administration of morphia or hyoscine. He became weaker, his pulse-rate increased to 140, and he became unconscious and died on August 22.

A post-mortem examination was made, and the heart sent to Professor Woodhead for examination. The following is a summary of his report:

The heart was enormously dilated, weighing 34 oz. The left ventricle was dilated, the thickness of the wall being from 2·5 centimetres to 1·3 centimetres. The cusps of the aortic valves thickened at the margin and retracted. The right ventricle was slightly dilated, the thickness of the wall being from 0·85 to 0·65 centimetres. Both auricles much dilated. The mitral and tricuspid valves slightly thickened at their margins, and both orifices dilated. The aorta somewhat thickened by patches of early atheroma. The right coronary artery slightly narrowed, the left patent and large. There was wonderfully little change in these vessels.

Microscopic examination shows that there was some increase in the size of the muscle-fibres of the left ventricle. In some places dense masses of fibrous tissue, with atrophy of the muscle-fibres, were detected.

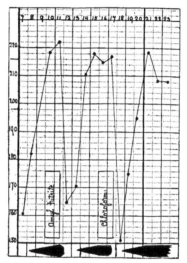

Fig. 204. Chart showing the rise of arterial pressure during an attack of angina pectoris, and the effect of amyl nitrite and choloroform on the pressure. The figures in the left border represent mm. Hg. and the figures on the top represent minutes. The observation began at 11 7 a.m.
The wedge-shaped figures represent the pain, the increase in width representing an increase in pain and the space between the figures a cessation of pain.

CASE 43.—*Auricular fibrillation.*

Male. This patient first consulted me on November 25, 1900, his age being then 51, complaining of shortness of breath on exertion. He had felt well until the previous year, when he had attacks of shortness of breath and a choking sensation which passed off. During the last few months the shortness of breath had come on with the slightest exertion and his legs had begun to swell.

There was no history of rheumatism or other infectious complaint.

He was a healthy-looking muscular man. The pulse was continuously irregular, and tracings taken at this time showed the irregularity to be characteristic of auricular fibrillation. The heart was slightly enlarged, being dull to the nipple line. He was put to bed for a few weeks and given digitalis, and he improved remarkably. I did not see him after September 2, 1901, until March 20, 1905. In the meantime he had worked out a method of treating himself by making a decoction of foxglove leaves. When his legs swelled so that he could not lace his boots comfortably, he found he was short of breath, and he took his decoction for a few days till the swelling disappeared. On this date I noted that the heart had not altered, the pulse was still irregular and the jugular veins were very full. From this date I saw him at frequent intervals till 1909. My last examination of him was on January 22, 1909, when he was on his second honeymoon. He looked well save for a slight yellow tinge in his face. The heart's dullness extended 1 inch beyond the left nipple line. There were no murmurs. The heart was still irregular and an electrocardiogram showed the characteristic signs of auricular fibrillation. I heard from him on March 26, 1913, when he wrote saying he was getting along very well: ' the more I walk out the less dropsy I have in my legs. I still keep my foxglove leaf by, and I am positive I could not live without it.'

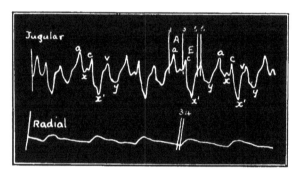

FIG. 205. Shows a regular rhythm and an auricular venous pulse and wide *a–c* interval (space *A*). Taken 1892 (Case 44).

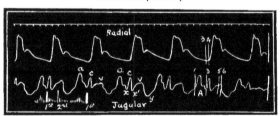

FIG. 205 A. Shows a regular rhythm and an auricular venous pulse and wide *a–c* interval (space *A*). Taken 1903 (Case 44).

CASE 44.—*Old rheumatic affection of the heart, with long-continued impairment of the auriculo-ventricular bundle, with a delay between the As and Vs. Sudden inception of a slow and irregular action of the heart (auricular fibrillation), with disappearance of all evidences of auricular contraction, at first transient, later permanent.*

Male. Born 1851. I attended him for an attack of rheumatic fever in 1883. He was left with a damaged mitral valve, but remained in fair health till 1897, when he had serious heart failure. From this also he made a good recovery, and his heart remained perfectly regular till 1904. I have taken tracings of his apex, radial pulse, and jugular pulse at frequent intervals since 1892. His heart was invariably regular except for a short period in 1897, the irregularity being due to dropping out of ventricular systoles (mild heart-block, see Fig. 155). His jugular pulse was always of the auricular form, a peculiarity in this case being a persistent increase in the *a–c* interval. Tracings of the jugular and radial pulses, taken in 1892, are given in Fig. 205 ; in 1903 in Fig. 205 A. Jugular and apex tracings are represented in Fig. 206. The rhythm is regular, and the auricular wave, a, is well marked in both apex and jugular tracings. There was a long diminuendo murmur after the second sound, and a well-marked presystolic murmur separated by a brief interval from the first sound (shading in Fig. 205). In the numerous tracings of the apex beat I have taken up to April 19, 1904, there was always a well-marked auricular wave, a, preceding the large wave. When he visited me on the last-named date I found his heart continuously irregular, and on taking tracings of the jugular pulse I found it of the ventricular type (Fig. 122 and 206); the presystolic murmur had gone, and there was at the time only a diastolic murmur. The wave due to the auricular systole had disappeared from the apex tracing. Here, again, with the appearance of the ventricular venous pulse and continuous irregularity, all evidences of the contraction of the right and left auricles had disappeared. When this patient called to see me in the

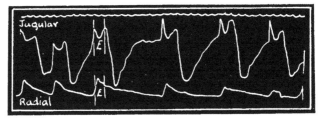

FIG. 206. Shows a slow irregular rhythm with the ventricular form of the venous pulse (Case 44, April 19, 1904).

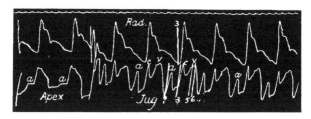

FIG. 207. Shows a regular rhythm and the presence of the auricular wave in the apex and jugular tracings (Case 44, April 26, 1904).

following week I found his heart perfectly regular, the auricular wave present in the venous pulse, the presystolic murmur and the auricular wave in the apex tracing also present (Fig. 207). These conditions continued until November 1904, when his heart again became irregular, and all evidence of auricular systole again disappeared. From that date up to the present (1913) the heart has remained in this state, and on the numerous occasions when I have taken long tracings I have never yet found the heart regular. Electrocardiograms, taken in 1910, showed the features characteristic of auricular fibrillation.

CASE 45.—*Auricular fibrillation with an efficient heart.*

Male. Aged 60. Consulted me first on June 19, 1907, complaining of being short of breath on exertion and of fluttering of the heart at times. He had led a strenuous business life, was a temperate liver, and gave no history of any form of infection. He was a spare lean man, with cold hands and a slightly dilated stomach. The heart was irregular in its action, and the venous pulse was of the ventricular form. The heart was not increased in size and there were no murmurs. I advised him to take a pleasant, restful holiday, and he went to Norway, and reported himself on August 21 as feeling remarkably well. The heart's condition was the same. I saw him again in July 1909 ; he was still in good health, attending to his business, and playing occasionally two rounds of golf in one day. The heart had not altered, and an electro-cardiogram confirmed the diagnosis of auricular fibrillation. In March 1913 (66 years of age), he still leads an active useful life.

CASE 46.—*Auricular fibrillation, with a rheumatic history. Mitral stenosis. Heart fairly efficient under digitalis.*

Male. Had rheumatic fever, at the age of 31, in 1888. I attended him for inflammation of the lungs in 1891, from which he made a good recovery. A note made at the time on the state of the heart stated that the dullness extended to the right of the sternum; the apex beat was in the nipple line, 4½ inches from the mid-sternal line. The first sound was clear and the second slightly reduplicated. After this time he kept well and did not consult me again until January 11, 1906, when he complained of being very short of breath and the spitting of a little blood. The pulse was continuously irregular, and the jugular pulse was of the ventricular form (auricular fibrillation). The heart's dullness was difficult to percuss, but the left border was just inside the nipple line. There was a diastolic murmur at the apex filling up the whole pause between the second and first sounds, when the heart was rapid, but falling short of the first sound when there was a long pause. The rate was about 100. He was put on tincture of digitalis, and his heart quietened down and in a week he felt much better. He went on well until January 25, 1907, when he walked some distance against a strong cold wind and felt 'smothered', and for a few weeks he felt breathless. From this he recovered and was able to go quietly, under the influence of digitalis taken when required, about his business, a grocer. From a report in 1913, I learn that he is still keeping fairly well and able to get about in a quiet way.

CASE 47.—*Auricular fibrillation. Good effect of digitalis.*

Male. Aged 58. This patient was first seen in September 1909, complaining of pain over the left chest of varying intensity and of great shortness of breath and weakness. He had had rheumatic fever at 17, influenza at 46. He was conscious of his heart beating irregularly in 1902, and had been under treatment more or less ever since, and a great variety of drugs and methods had been tried ; but in spite of this he had steadily got worse during the last few months. The patient was tall and spare, his face slightly livid, the breathing very distressed, so that he had to lie propped up in bed. The legs were slightly swollen and the liver was a little enlarged. The radial pulse was rapid, 110 per minute, and fibrillation of the auricles was present. The jugular venous pulse was noted, and a tracing showing the ventricular form of venous pulse was obtained. The heart was enlarged and the dullness extended 1 inch beyond the nipple line on the left.

I gave a diagnosis of ' nodal rhythm ' (auricular fibrillation), and said that the patient would probably improve on digitalis. The doctor in attendance said that digitalis had been tried and was ineffective, and I found that it had been given in small doses, and I suggested giving doses of 1 drachm of the tincture a day till a reaction was obtained (p. 232). The doctor reported to me later that, after 5 drachms, the patient had responded remarkably to the digitalis and all the distressing symptoms had disappeared, and he found that he could keep the pulse-rate moderate with small doses. I saw the patient again in May 1910. The pulse was still irregular and the dullness extended to the nipple line. He was rather breathless and had not been taking the digitalis. I strongly insisted upon the necessity for keeping the heart always under its influence by such doses as were found effective. I saw him again in March 1911. He found he could get about quietly by taking doses of 5–10 drops of the tincture, and if the heart got faster he increased the dose until it slowed.

In 1913, I hear that he is still going about quietly under this régime.

CASE 48.—*Aortic, mitral, and tricuspid disease. Angina pectoris. Auricular fibrillation. Death.*

Female. Born 1849. This patient came under my care in 1880, suffering from all the symptoms of gastric ulcer. She had had rheumatic fever at the age of 22. When I first saw her there was a slight increase in the size of the heart and a presystolic murmur. I attended her for two attacks of rheumatic fever in 1883 and 1884, and at various times for symptoms of gastric ulcer. She was very poor and lived a laborious and anxious life, having three children dependent upon her. In 1891 she consulted me for a severe pain which struck into her left chest and spread into the left arm and down the arm to the little finger. The attacks of pain were sometimes so severe that she felt as if she would die. There was marked hyperalgesia of the skin and deeper tissues of the whole left chest, and also of the left sterno-mastoid and trapezius muscles. The heart was increased in size, the dullness extending to the left 5 inches and the apex beat being in the sixth interspace. There was a presystolic and systolic murmur heard at the apex. She had also much pain after food, and referred it to a limited area in the middle of the epigastrium. She came to me again in September 1892, suffering from weakness and shortness of breath. In addition to the heart symptoms described she had a slightly enlarged liver which pulsated, and tracings showed it to be of the auricular type, and from this I inferred that she had tricuspid stenosis.

After a period of rest in hospital she improved and was able to go about her work. In January 1894 she again consulted me, and I took her into the hospital. She complained of pain in the chest and arms again, on the slightest exertion, and also of being sick and vomiting, and the recurrence of the pain in the epigastrium. There was extensive hyperalgesia of the chest and upper part of the abdomen, but it was too indefinite to map out with any certainty. For the first time in the numerous examinations I had made, I now detected a diastolic aortic murmur.

The patient improved to a slight extent, and was able to get about, though liable to attacks of pain in her chest and arms on exertion, until 1898, when she had a severe attack of heart failure, with dropsy, enlarged liver, and rapid irregular pulse. She recovered to a certain extent, but the pulse remained irregular and the liver pulse, which had hitherto been of the auricular form, now showed no signs of the auricle, and was of the ventricular form (see Figs. 119, 120, 121). The presystolic murmur disappeared, and she presented the symptoms which we now recognize as being characteristic of auricular fibrillation. Before this attack the heart had invariably been regular, with the exception of an occasional ventricular extra-systole.

This patient lived until 1899, and in the numerous tracings taken up to her death the rhythm was never again found regular, nor was there present either the presystolic murmur or the wave in the liver pulse due to the auricle. Here, again, the irregularity in the action of the heart was coincident with the disappearance of all signs of auricular systole, namely, the disappearance of the auricular wave from the liver pulse, showing the cessation of the action of the right auricle, and the disappearance of the presystolic murmur, showing the cessation of the action of the left auricle.

The report of the post-mortem examination of the heart is as follows: ' Extreme stenosis of mitral and tricuspid orifices ; great dilatation of auricles, with atrophy of the musculature. There is a large nodular mass of endocardial thickening showing calcareous masses in its centre and active inflammatory proliferation at its periphery, on the endocardium, under the aortic orifice, and situated in the pars membranacei septi right over the auriculo-ventricular bundle. At one point the inflammatory extension has invaded and involved a great part of the bundle. The stretching of the bundle is extreme, and there is cell proliferation which Professor Keith regards as due to changes in the walls of the small vessels.

' There is extreme atrophy of the upper part of the interventricular septum. It measures only 4 mm. instead of 14–18. The sub-endocardial tissue is thickened, and in parts the Purkinje system is fibrosed and atrophied.'

CASE 49.—*Sudden inception of auricular fibrillation shown by the disappearance of the auricular wave from the jugular pulse, and of the presystolic mitral murmur, with the appearance of permanent irregularity in the heart's action, and ventricular form of the venous pulse. Post-mortem report.*

Female. Born 1864. I first saw this patient in 1895, she being then 31 years of age. There was a history of acute rheumatism in her youth, and she had marked mitral stenosis. She became pregnant in 1896, and I watched her during the pregnancy and puerperium. She had a long illness from gastric ulcer in 1899. During these years I made frequent observations on her heart. It was invariably regular, and the jugular pulse always showed a well-marked wave due to the systole of the right auricle. There was at first a presystolic mitral murmur

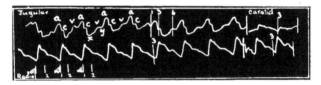

FIG. 208. Simultaneous tracings of the jugular and radial pulses in the first part, of the carotid and radial in the latter part. The jugular tracing shows the form characteristic of the auricular venous pulse where the wave, *a*, due to the auricle precedes the carotid wave, *c* (downstroke 3). The shading underneath represents the time of the presystolic murmur (Case 49, November 5, 1895).

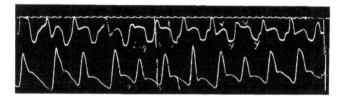

FIG 209. The jugular pulse is now of the ventricular form—no auricular wave precedes the downstroke 3, and the rhythm is irregular (Case 49, March 19, 1904).

of the crescendo type, and latterly a long murmur following the second sound and running up to the crescendo presystolic murmur. The position of the presystolic murmur in the cardiac cycle is diagrammatically represented in the shading under the radial tracing in Fig. 208. This perfect regularity of the heart's action continued until she suffered from an attack of heart failure in 1900. Coincident with this failure the heart's action became irregular, and the jugular pulse showed no sign of a wave due to the auricular systole at the normal period of the cardiac cycle (Fig. 209) The crescendo presystolic murmur had disappeared, while the diastolic portion persisted, as shown by the shading under the apex tracing in Fig. 211.

From this date until she died, in February 1907, these altered conditions persisted, Fig. 210 being a simultaneous tracing of the jugular pulse and radial taken in December 1906, and Fig. 211 of the jugular and apex beat taken February 1907, shortly before she died.

The following is an abbreviated report on the post-mortem examination of the heart:

'Valves: Great stenosis of the mitral valves; tricuspid valves shallow and incompetent; pulmonary and aortic valves normal. Coronary arteries healthy; coronary veins dilated to twice their normal diameter. Superior and inferior venæ cavæ much dilated. The sino-auricular node is normal, but the auricular wall below it is atrophied and fibrous. The tænia terminalis is hypertrophied. The auriculo-ventricular bundle has partly assumed the characters of the ordinary muscular fibres, and has been stretched, and the auriculo-ventricular node is flattened by the great interauricular pressure. The central fibrous body is marked (fibrous and contracted), and the artery perforating it is atheromatous. The apical half or two-thirds of the left ventricle shows extensive fibrosis. The fibrotic process approaches and incorporates

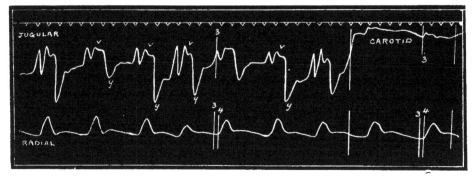

FIG. 210. The jugular pulse is of the ventricular form (Case 49, December 1906).

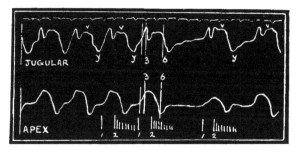

FIG. 211. The jugular pulse shows the same features as in Fig. 210 (Case 49, February 1907).

the musculature along a sharply defined line. In the fibrotic tissue are nodules characteristic of rheumatic conditions. Since the fibrotic process is most marked at the base of the musculi papillares, it is possible that it may have spread from the mitral valves.'

CASE 50.—*Aortic valvular disease (rheumatic origin). Angina pectoris. Auricular fibrillation.*

Female. Born 1840. Suffered from rheumatic fever at the age of 20. She married and had one son born in 1875. In 1892 she came under my care. She was then thin and spare, with an anxious expression of countenance. She complained of being very short of breath on exertion and of feeling ' done up '. The radial pulse was large and full and collapsing (typical Corrigan). On rubbing the forehead capillary pulsation was visible in reddened patches of skin. The heart's dullness extended to the nipple line, the sounds were clear and distinct, and there was a diastolic aortic murmur. The heart's action was frequently irregular, due to occurrence of ventricular extra-systoles. Under suitable treatment she regained a good deal of strength and was able to lead a fairly active life, but there were recurring periods of great weakness and prostration. After an attack of influenza, in 1893, a small area over the third rib in the nipple line became tender on pressure. As years passed on this tender area became more extensive during the period when the heart weakness was most marked. In 1898 she began to have slight attacks of pain across the upper part of the chest, and from this time onwards I frequently found extensive areas of hyperalgesia, especially affecting the left breast, the left pectoralis major, sterno-mastoid, and trapezius muscles. In later years I desisted from testing for hyperalgesia because the patient said that for hours afterwards she suffered from intolerable aching in the places I had pinched. At times when she was feeling well and able to go about actively this hyperalgesia would completely disappear. About 1900 she began to notice that during her weak periods exertion brought on a pain which started in the left breast and passed into the left arm. In 1903, after some sleepless nights, she had periods of exhaustion, when a continual aching would persist under the left breast and arm, increasing to attacks of great violence on the least exertion. The pain would be referred to the chest and arm, and was accompanied by a sensation as if the chest were being gripped. There was also a sense of great exhaustion, and of impending death. The mouth very often was dry, and she passed a large quantity of clear urine after the attack had subsided. At this time the heart's dullness extended 1 inch outside the nipple line. When fairly well the diastolic murmur was loud and heard all over the chest; there was in addition a systolic murmur heard at the apex following the first sound and running up to the second. During the times when she was liable to the attacks of angina pectoris the sounds became remarkably modified, faint, and indistinct. Also at these times the hyperalgesia was more marked. From 1904 onwards she could only walk about quietly on the level with comfort; the slightest hurrying or walking uphill brought on the attacks of pain. She also had periods of sleeplessness, and after a few disturbed nights she would become so profoundly exhausted that the effort of dressing caused attacks of angina pectoris. Under full doses of bromide of ammonium she slept soundly, and the attacks diminished in frequency and severity. She afterwards found that when she felt sleepless, if she took the bromide she obtained comfortable sleep, and was able to ward off the attacks of heart depression and accompanying pain. During 1904 and afterwards her husband noticed that when she slept soundly the breathing would stop, then gradually increase, then gradually diminish till it stopped, the cessation lasting sometimes 20 seconds (Cheyne-Stokes respiration). The heart's rhythm would sometimes be interrupted by ventricular extra-systoles, but for long periods none would be present. During the periods when she experienced great heart weakness no change in the rate or rhythm of the heart could be detected. In July 1906 she suddenly became very breathless and the heart's action very rapid. I did not see her till a few days after this had started, and I found the heart very rapid, 120 beats a minute, and very irregular, the venous pulse now showing the characteristic ventricular form ; in other words, auricular fibrillation had set in. After a couple of months the heart's action slowed to about 90, still irregular, and with the ventricular form of venous pulse. She was unable to leave her bed and suffered little pain, except occasionally after a restless night, when on the following day she would suffer from pain under the left breast. Small doses of chloral (5 gr.) would induce sleep and relieve the pain.

The heart's action continued irregular, and in January 1907 she became gradually weaker, and died in February at the age of 67, seven months after the onset of auricular fibrillation. It is noteworthy that the heart did not increase in size with the onset of the irregularity, nor was there any dropsy of the legs or trunk, although there were towards the end numerous fine crepitations at the base of the lungs.

CASE 51.—*History of many years of extra-systoles, sometimes becoming very frequent. Transient attacks of auricular fibrillation, slight at first, becoming more prolonged till it became permanent. Died five months after permanent establishment of fibrillation. Post-mortem report.*

Female. Born 1846. I had known and attended her for slight ailments at intervals since 1880. In 1892 I obtained tracings of her pulse, which showed extra-systoles. These occurred sometimes at rare, sometimes at frequent intervals (Fig. 99). They were usually ventricular in origin, but occasionally nodal and auricular. I also noted in 1892 that there was a gallop rhythm of the heart when it was regular. In 1900 she began to have attacks of ' palpitation ' of short duration, and I obtained tracings of the radial and jugular during one of these attacks, and they showed a transition of the venous pulse to the ventricular form during the attack. On October 13, 1903, she felt weak and exhausted, and had a distressing fluttering sensation within her chest, and I found the heart's action extremely irregular. The attack lasted four or five hours. The tracings taken during the attack were of the same character as Fig. 212. On October 19 she was again seized with a similar attack, which lasted a whole day, and the tracings in Fig. 212 convey a very good idea of the character of the heart's

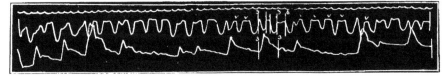

FIG. 212. Characteristic irregularity on the sudden inception of auricular fibrillation ; the jugular pulse is of the ventricular form (Case 51).

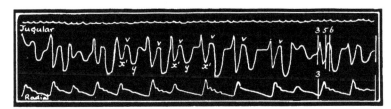

FIG. 213. The rhythm is still irregular and the jugular pulse is of the ventricular type (Case 51).

irregularity. The next day the heart was quite regular and the jugular pulse a typical example of the auricular form.

On October 27 the heart again became very irregular. This attack continued without intermission until November 1. On October 29 the heart's action became much slower, but the irregularity still persisted, and the character of the jugular pulse showed a curious change (Fig. 213), viz. during the ventricular systole (the period between the perpendicular lines 3 and 6) there are two waves, while there is no wave at the normal time of the auricular wave. The heart suddenly reverted to the normal rhythm, and became regular with a typical auricular venous pulse (Fig. 99).

The attacks gradually lessened in frequency and duration until June 12, 1904, when, after a long walk in the country, she was seized with an attack which lasted for a fortnight. A few days before the attack finally subsided the heart became normal in its rhythm for a few hours. On October 16, 1904, this abnormal rhythm again started, and continued, with great dilatation of the heart, dropsy, ascites, and hydrothorax, until her death on March 17, 1905. In this case drugs of the digitalis group did little to delay the progress of heart failure, although pushed to their full extent.

In this patient the remarkable changes described on p. 252 were seen most typically. A few hours after an attack the heart dilated, the liver enlarged, the face became swollen and livid. Immediately the normal rhythm was restored, the patient at once felt relief, and in a few hours all the abnormal symptoms disappeared.

As this patient lived close to my house I saw her very frequently, and had the opportunity of watching the attacks begin and finish. Once when taking a tracing the attack started, and on several occasions the attacks ceased while I was watching her. I have accumulated a great number of tracings taken at all stages (Fig. 214).

Report of the post-mortem examination of the heart:

'*Arteries.*—Left coronary chiefly affected; lumen narrowed. Anterior interseptal artery which supplies the auriculo-ventricular bundle closed completely; right coronary affected, but to a less degree.

'*Orifices and Valves.*—Valves not diseased. Mitral orifice dilated, tricuspid dilated, inferior caval dilated, aortic normal.

'*Musculature.*—Tænia terminalis hypertrophied. Auriculo-ventricular bundle large; the fibres have the appearance of being stretched, having lost their stellate reticular form; applied closely, and rather longer than usual. The right and left septal divisions are normal in appearance. The interauricular septum is stretched. The apical two-thirds of the left ventricle shows large patches of fibrosis, and the trabeculæ with the Purkinje system are stretched, and certainly not healthy—fibrosis and atrophy—result of endarteritis.'

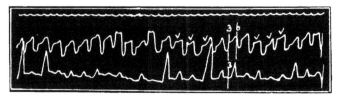

FIG. 214.   Shows the character of the irregularity (auricular fibrillation) persistent one month before death (Case 51).

CASE 52.—*Disappearance of large auricular waves from the venous pulse with the onset of auricular fibrillation. Post-mortem report.*

Female. Born 1850. Enjoyed good health till 1900, when she began to be short of breath. I saw her first in November 1902. She was then very weak, and had to lie in bed propped up; the legs and abdomen were swollen and the urine scanty; the pulse was small, weak, and regular, and there was a large pulsation in the veins of the neck. The heart's dullness extended 2 inches to the right of the mid-sternal line, and 1 inch to the left of the nipple line. The sounds were clear and free from murmur.

Under treatment she improved very much, the pulse becoming slower, but she had several relapses, until the final breakdown in November 1904. I took a large number of tracings at different times up till November 1904, and the rhythm was invariably regular, and the jugular pulse of the auricular type. On one occasion after digitalis she developed a pulsus alternans. The breakdown at the last-mentioned date was the most severe she ever had, the legs and abdomen being enormously swollen and the pleural cavities containing a large quantity of fluid. The pulse was now continuously irregular, and the venous pulse had completely changed its character, being of the ventricular form. She died in December 1904, two months after I had detected the presence of auricular fibrillation.

The report on the post-mortem examination of the heart is as follows :

'Greater part of auricle has been left behind in subject.

'The right ventricle is of quite average length and atrophied; left ventricle is of quite average length and dilated and atrophied.

'*Arteries.*—Show patches of thickening and dilatation, but nowhere is lumen so reduced as to greatly impede circulation. Aorta shows patches of atheroma.

'*Orifices and valves.*—Valves healthy; mitral orifice 29 mm. diam., tricuspid 30 mm., both dilated.

'*Musculature.*—There is atrophy and perivascular fibrosis; this is extensive in basal part of left ventricle, especially at upper border of interventricular septum, but elsewhere fibrotic changes not marked.

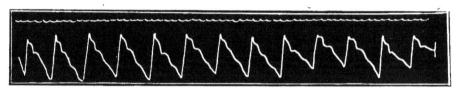

FIG. 215. Regular pulse between attacks of auricular fibrillation (Case 53).

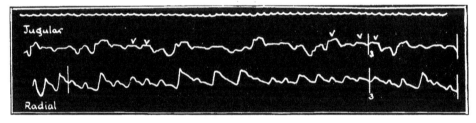

FIG. 216. Permanent inception of auricular fibrillation, leading to a fatal issue in three weeks (Case 53).

'*Auriculo-ventricular system.*—The network at beginning of bundle is normal in size and form, although certain cells which seem inflammatory in nature are present. The bundle, on the other hand, is stretched and small; the fibres show no reticular structure, and in parts show fibrosis. The Purkinje system is overlaid by a very thick fibrous endocardium. There is a marked degree of stretching of the apical half of the left ventricle, and the trabeculæ are thin and atrophied ; on section, some of the Purkinje fibres are seen to be undergoing fibrous changes.'

CASE 53.—*Sudden inception of auricular fibrillation, with persistent rapid heart action, dilatation of the heart, dropsy, death in three weeks.*

Female. Aged 65. I had attended her for various ailments (rheumatism, bronchitis, &c.) during a period of over twenty years, and her heart had invariably been quite regular. On June 20, 1904, she returned from the seaside to her home and sent for me. She had been taken ill a few days before, her chief complaint being shortness of breath. When I saw her she was propped up in bed, and breathing rapidly and laboriously. Her pulse was extremely rapid and irregular, but I did not have my polygraph with me. Next day when I called to see her, I found her greatly improved, out of bed, and free from distress. Her pulse was full, regular, and not rapid (Fig. 215). The following day, however, she was again very bad, and Fig. 216, taken on June 23, gives a good idea of her pulse, which was rapid. The irregularity was characteristic of fibrillation. I tried all sorts of remedies to slow the heart—digitalis and opium, adrenalin, trinitrin, &c., but all without avail. The heart dilated, dropsy set in and became very extensive, and she died three weeks after the permanent establishment of auricular fibrillation.

CASE 54.—*Large auricular waves in the jugular and liver pulsation. Presystolic mitral and tricuspid murmurs. Attacks of angina pectoris. Sudden disappearance of all signs of auricular contraction, with the appearance of continuous irregularity in the heart's action. Sudden death.*

Female. Born 1862. Came under my care in 1891. She suffered from shortness of breath on exertion. She had erysipelas in the face in 1883 and 1885, and since then she had been short

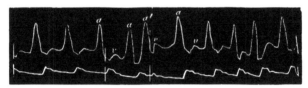

FIG. 217. Simultaneous tracings of the jugular and radial pulses, showing a large wave (*a′*) due to an extra-systole of the auricle (Case 54).

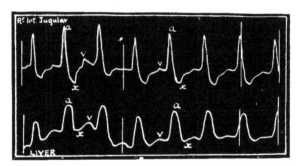

FIG. 218. Simultaneous tracings of jugular and liver pulses. *a*, auricular wave ; *v*, ventricular wave ; *x*, auricular depression (Case 54).

of breath, and with a tendency to swelling in the legs. The pulse was small, quick, and usually regular, but I occasionally detected an extra-systole, which Fig. 217 shows to be auricular in origin. There was a large pulsating swelling on either side of the neck near the sternal end of the clavicle, but no distinct pulsation in the veins above these swellings. When compared with the carotid pulse there were seen to be two distinct movements, the one larger than the other, and the larger movement could be observed to precede that of the carotid pulse (Fig. 49). The liver could be felt pulsating just below the ribs, and the liver pulse was of the same character as the jugular (Fig. 218).

The area of cardiac dullness was increased, extending transversely $1\frac{1}{2}$ inches to the right beyond the middle line. There was always present a long murmur, presystolic in time, heard best at the apex ; another, shorter and rougher, of a different character, but corresponding in time, was heard best over the middle of the sternum. The latter murmur was occasionally absent at first, but ultimately became a constant phenomenon. There was also a murmur, systolic in time, heard at the apex. At the base the second sound was reduplicated. No murmur was heard in the carotids, but there was a distinct sound heard over the pulsating swelling in the neck synchronous with the pulsation and preceding the first sound of the heart. This sound could also be heard under the clavicle and over Poupart's ligament, i.e. over the valves of the subclavian and femoral veins. The jugular and subclavian valves being competent, the jugular bulb became distended into a ball-like protrusion over the inner end of the clavicles, and the pulsation was conspicuous at the distance of 10 yards. In May 1893 she came to me complaining of a disagreeable smarting pain in the left axilla. I examined her and found the skin in the axilla and adjacent regions of the thorax to be extremely hyperæsthetic (Fig. 8). A few days later she began to suffer from attacks of pain in the left breast and down the inside of the left arm, and on examination I found that the hyperæsthesia had extended (Fig. 7). These attacks of pain became so severe on the slightest exertion that she was forced to lay up. From this time, she had at different periods suffered from severe attacks of pain, and I occasionally found that when she was very ill the hyperæsthesia embraced nearly the whole of the left chest and the inside of the left arm, and also a portion of the front of the right chest. The left sterno-mastoid and trapezius also became very sensitive. She improved, and when I again examined her on May 25, 1894, she complained of a disagreeable pain located

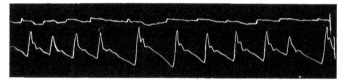

Fɪɢ. 219. Simultaneous tracings of a slight movement in the neck and of the radial pulse. The rhythm is now continuously irregular, with a tendency to long pauses. The tracing from the neck was taken from the same situation which gave the jugular pulse in the two preceding figures, and demonstrates the absence of any wave due to the auricle (Case 54. 1895).

on the inner side of the right forearm. I examined the place and found it to be extremely hyperæsthetic (Fig. 7).

The patient became gradually weaker and had severe attacks of angina pectoris on the slightest exertion. At 3 a.m., October 9, 1895, she awoke and was conscious that the beating in her neck had ceased. She called my attention to this next morning, and on examination I found that there was now no pulsation in the jugular bulb. Thus Fig. 210 was taken from her on October 9, 1895, and the receiver was held over the place where the jugular tracings, Fig. 49 and 217, were obtained, and it will be observed that there is a complete absence of the auricular wave which is so marked in these tracings. In Fig. 219 there is only a faint movement due to the carotid, and possibly at the beginning of this tracing a slight ventricular venous pulse can be detected. Careful examination showed that the liver pulse had entirely disappeared, as well as the mitral and tricuspid presystolic murmurs.

On October 13, 1895, four days after the onset of the fibrillation, on getting out of bed, she fell and died.

Before removing the heart at the post-mortem examination I injected water forcibly into the superior vena cava, and the water could not pass beyond the jugular valves, but distended greatly the jugular bulb. The report on post-mortem examination of the heart is as follows: 'Marked tricuspid and mitral stenosis. There is dilatation of the apex of the left ventricle, pre-mortem clot in apex of right auricle. The series of sections of auriculo-ventricular bundle is good, and shows that in this heart the node at the commencement of the main bundle and the septal divisions were uncommonly well developed. Main bundle healthy. There are signs of great venous back-pressure in the capillaries and veins. The arteries in the neighbourhood of the bundle are not thickened.'

CASE 55.—*Auricular flutter.*

Male. Born 1863. The patient had enjoyed good health until the year 1901, when, while serving in the South African War, he had had a mild attack of typhoid fever. After recovering from the fever he noticed his heart occasionally becoming rapid and irregular, giving rise to a disagreeable sensation of fluttering in the chest. These attacks came on frequently on waking up in the morning, and for some months they were almost a daily occurrence. They became less frequent during 1902 and 1903, but increased in frequency in 1904. After this they occurred with great frequency, and in 1905 he consulted a physician for fainting attacks. He had had a good deal of pain at times in the chest, which resembled attacks of angina pectoris. The pulse at this time was very frequent and irregular. In 1906 he became very weak and greatly distressed by the heart's action, and he went into the Edinburgh Hospital under the care of Dr. Gibson. After two months' rest and treatment the heart's action became regular and he felt much stronger. From that date until November 1909 he felt on the whole fairly well and able to attend to his duties, though he had occasional slight attacks of rapid irregular action of the heart. From November 1909 the attacks became increasingly frequent until April 1910, when the heart remained persistently rapid and irregular. It was in this condition when he consulted me in May 1910.

When I saw the patient at my house on May 1, he walked in a slow, deliberate manner, with an aspect of great distress and apprehension. He had to stop every few steps, and I felt inclined to think that there was a good deal of nervous apprehension. I found the pulse rapid, 150 per minute, soft and irregular, and at that time I did not realize the cause of his great fear. Seeing, however, that he was very ill, I took him under my care in the Mount Vernon Hospital, and the following is a brief summary of the very numerous observations we made.

The patient lay in bed with his shoulders raised. His face was slightly livid and had an anxious expression. He was well nourished and otherwise healthy looking. His pulse was small, soft, and regular except for occasional pauses ; its rate was 140. The blood-pressure was 100 mm. Hg. The heart's dullness lay 0 and 4¼ inches to right and left of the mid-sternal line. The sounds of the heart were like the tic-tac of the foetal heart, and were free from murmurs. The patient was afraid to exert himself, fearing the heart would go off with a rapidity and violence such as frightened him.

Treatment and progress.—The patient at first felt greatly exhausted, the heart persistently beating at a rate between 130 and 150 per minute, with occasional short periods of irregularity at a lower speed. For the first five or six weeks he had attacks during which the heart's rate became enormously increased. These were sometimes provoked by a very slight exertion, such as by standing up for a few moments or by having the bowels moved. A few of these attacks were observed, and the pulse-rate graphically recorded, and a speed of between 290 and 300 beats per minute was attained, the highest rate of the human heart I have ever seen graphically recorded (Fig. 140). It was utterly impossible to count the heart's rate either from the pulse or by auscultation of the heart. These attacks lasted for half an hour to an hour, and during this time the patient was in great distress. They grew less frequent, and finally disappeared after various remedies had been tried. The pulse-rate still continued to be rapid though it became irregular more frequently. The attacks of extreme rapidity occurred chiefly during the night, when he was awakened by disagreeable dreams.

On June 22 he was put on ammonium bromide, 20 grains three times daily, and this was continued till July 22. Shortly after beginning the medicine, his nights were more composed and the violent and rapid attacks gradually diminished, till after a couple of weeks they ceased entirely. On July 22 he was put on tincture of digitalis, 20 minims three times daily. At this time his pulse-rate was always between 140 and 150 beats per minute (Fig. 220), with occasional pauses. No effect was produced till the 27th, when 5 drachms of the tincture had been taken and he suffered from nausea. The pulse fell to 55 beats per minute and became

continuously irregular (Fig. 221), with occasional paroxysms of rapid rate (140 per minute)
lasting for a few seconds. The irregularity was characteristic of auricular fibrillation and the
jugular tracing occasionally showed the fibrillary waves, when the rate was slow and irregular
(Fig. 222). On the 28th, periods of regular rhythm at about 70 beats per minute, varied with

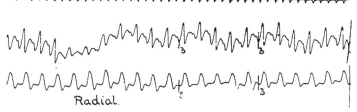

FIG. 220. Tracing of radial and jugular pulses during a period of continuous tachycardia.
Rate, 140 beats per minute. An electrocardiogram showed that the auricle was beating at
double the ventricular rate = auricle 280, ventricle 140 (Case 55).

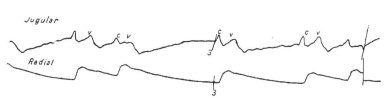

FIG. 221. Shows the irregular pulse due to auricular fibrillation (Case 55). (This and the
three following tracings are from *Heart*, vol. ii, p. 380.)

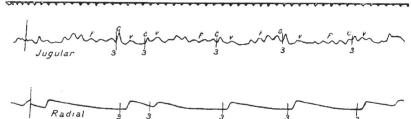

FIG. 222. Slow irregular pulse due to auricular fibrillation, showing coarse fibrillation waves (*f*)
(Case 55).

periods of fibrillation at about 50. The regular periods evidently belonged to the normal
rhythm, and an auricular wave *a* could be detected in the tracing in the neck before the carotid
(Fig. 223). The digitalis was stopped on the 28th as the patient felt sick, but was resumed on
the 30th and continued in half-doses(½ drachm per day) till August 7. From August 2 to 10
the heart beat slowly and irregularly at a rate of from 40 to 50 beats per minute, and the jugular
tracings showed occasionally marked fibrillation waves (Fig. 222). From August 17 to 24 the
heart's rhythm was very inconstant, showing periods of the normal rhythm, tachycardia,

and auricular fibrillation. After the 24th the periods of tachycardia became more frequent. On September 4 the digitalis was resumed, at first in 5-minim doses three times daily; on September 17 it was increased to 10 minims three times daily; he was kept on this quantity till October 7, when he was discharged. On September 7, three days after starting the digitalis, the attacks of tachycardia did not last so long, and from this date they gradually decreased till the 29th, when the heart became quite steady and the rhythm normal (Fig. 224). In the tracings we could detect occasional auricular extra-systoles. After his discharge we kept in touch with the patient, who continued to take his digitalis ($\frac{1}{2}$ drachm per day). He gradually regained his strength, and the attacks of tachycardia recurred at rare intervals and for only a few minutes. In 1913, I heard that he was forced to lead a very quiet life, as exertion induces the rapid heart rate.

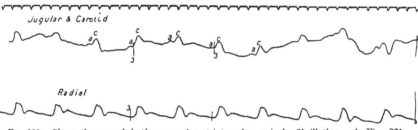

Jugular & Carotid

Radial

FIG. 223.   Shows the normal rhythm occurring at intervals; auricular fibrillation, as in Figs. 221 and 222, being present at other times (Case 55).

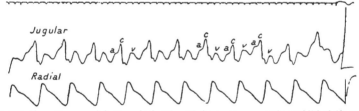

Jugular

Radial

FIG. 224. Shows the normal rhythm which ultimately became permanently established (Case 55).

CASE 56.—*Auricular flutter.   Effect of digitalis.   Recovery.*

Male. Aged 74. He was well until January 30, 1910, when he noticed his heart was beating very irregularly, and after this he felt weak and was easily rendered short of breath. The rapid action of the heart persisted up to the time that I saw him in May 1910, with Dr. Ford Anderson. So long as he kept quiet he felt no distress, but he felt weak and disinclined to take any exertion. He lay in bed, slightly propped up, his face and lips being of a dusky hue. The veins of the neck were distended and beat rapidly. The radial pulse was regular, 150 per minute. The heart's dullness extended to the nipple line and there were no murmurs. There were no other signs of heart failure.

On considering the patient's condition and his lack of response to treatment, Dr. Anderson and I thought it might be worth a trial to push the digitalis, and Dr. Hume Turnbull undertook to observe the result, which he has published.

Tincture of digitalis was given in doses of 20 minims three times a day and continued for six days, when the patient felt uncomfortable and the pulse was found to have fallen to 86 and was markedly irregular; the tracings showing that the irregularity was due in all probability to varying degrees of block. With the cessation of the digitalis the rapid rhythm gradually returned, until four days afterwards the heart had resumed the rapid regular rhythm. Some nine days later, that is on July 9, digitalin granules (Nativelle's), one three times a day, were prescribed. After taking thirty-three, he complained of nausea and loss of appetite, and on the 20th the pulse had fallen to 76, and the tracing taken two days later showed that auricular fibrillation had occurred. At this time he was mentally confused for a few days and somewhat delirious. On July 24 the pulse was regular and the heart's action normal, and from this time onwards he gradually regained his strength. Electrocardiograms taken by Dr. Lewis on May 10, 1910, showed the auricular rate to be 150 and the ventricular rate 300, and those taken on November 16, 1910, showed a normally acting heart.

Since that time he has continued in good health and has no trouble with his heart (1913).

CASE 57.—*Attacks of auricular flutter, at first at rare intervals, latterly persistent. Syncope. Effect of digitalis and strophanthus.*

Clergyman. Born 1860. The patient had led, on the whole, a vigorous and active life until the last few years. At the age of 15 or 16 he had had an attack of palpitation after playing a game of football. Since that time he had had one or two attacks every year until 1909, when the rapid action of the heart became continuous. In 1900 he had an attack of diphtheria which left behind extensive paralysis affecting the legs and arms. After six months he slowly recovered, but was conscious of the feeble action of the heart, and he had frequent attacks of palpitation. Notwithstanding this, he continued in charge of a large parish and worked very hard until 1906, when he had an attack of syncope. He went away for a change and rest for six months, and then took charge of a small parish. When cycling in 1909 he noticed that he was very weak, and Dr. Blackburn found his pulse going at the rate of 130 per minute, at or about which rate the pulse has continued until the date of examination.

I saw the patient with Dr. Blackburn on January 9, 1912. He was rather stout but healthy looking. His chief complaint was being easily tired and a disposition to shirk work, which troubled him, as he had always worked hard and with zest. He could walk three or four miles without distress. He was conscious of his abnormal heart action, which caused him a little uneasiness. The pulse was rapid and soft, and occasionally irregular, 140 beats per minute. Blood-pressure 115 mm. Hg. The heart's dullness extended to the nipple line and the sounds were free from murmurs.

I asked Dr. Lewis to take an electrocardiogram, and he reported that the ventricle was beating at 150 per minute and the auricle at 300 per minute. There was occasional irregularity, due to periods when the ventricle responded only to every fourth auricular contraction in place of every second.

When the patient returned home Dr. Blackburn put him on digitalin granules, one being taken four times a day. He quickly responded, and on the fourth day there was slight nausea and the pulse-rate fell to 67 and was regular. A few days later the heart again increased in rate. Although the digitalis was resumed and stopped several times, the heart could not be kept under control for long. He again consulted me on May 3, and the rate of the heart was still 150 per minute, with frequent periods of irregularity, when it beat at a slower rate. It was deemed advisable to give the digitalis another trial, and Dr. Lewis took charge of him. He was again tried with Nativelle's granules, the dose being gradually increased from one to four granules per day. He began the drug on May 5, the ventricular rate being 156 and the auricular 312 beats per minute, as revealed by the electrocardiograph. In a few days the pulse became slower and irregular, varying from 70 to 140 per minute, the ventricular rate being extremely liable to variations with the slightest exertion. The auricular rate kept constant until May 28, when the drug was stopped ; the patient suffering from nausea and retching.

Thirty-six granules had been taken altogether in the twenty-three days, and the rate of the auricles kept high, although the ventricular rate fell as low as 74 per minute. After a few days rest tincture of strophanthus was tried and continued for fourteen days, during which the patient took altogether 15 drachms 15 minims. The result was very similar to that obtained with the digitalin, and as it had induced diarrhœa, it was stopped. The patient was distinctly better, due probably to the rest and to the slower ventricular rate.

CASE 58.—*Auricular flutter, provoked by exertion.*

Male. Born 1859. He complained of being pulled up on walking by a sense of exhaustion. He could walk quietly for three or four miles, but if he hurried or walked against the wind, exhaustion was easily induced. Up till 1908 he had led a vigorous life and done a good deal of mountain climbing. In 1908, after a long cycle ride, he felt strangely done up, and from this date he experienced the sense of exhaustion on exertion. He had been to Nauheim four times, and though he experienced no trouble when he rested, as soon as he began to exert himself the exhaustion set in. He knew his heart was irregular for long periods while he was leading an active life, and that as soon as he rested the heart became quite regular.

The patient was sent to me by Dr. Linnell on April 11, 1911. He was rather stout and healthy looking. The pulse was small, soft, and continuously irregular (Fig. 139). The heart's dullness extended to the nipple line and the sounds were clear and free from murmurs.

I asked Dr. Lewis to take an electrocardiogram, and he reported that the auricle was beating regularly at 260 per minute, while the ventricular rate varied from 90 to 130. As a rule, the ventricle responded to each alternate auricular contraction; 2:1 and 4:1 periods occurring from time to time.

I saw the patient again on October 1, 1912; he had been going on much the same, that is, long periods when the heart gave him no trouble, followed by periods of heart irregularity and easy exhaustion. Such periods always stopped after a few days' rest. He had again been to Nauheim for a cure, and while resting the heart returned to its normal action, but after he left the irregularity and exhaustion returned as soon as he began to walk energetically. On this visit his heart was perfectly normal and the jugular pulse was of the normal auricular type.

CASE 59.—*Paroxysmal tachycardia due to auricular flutter.*

Male. Born 1858. Up till the age of 19 the patient was healthy and played vigorous games, but at this age he became disagreeably conscious of intermission of the heart's action. The intermittent action would persist for periods of a month, and was usually worse at breakfast, and also in the night, when he would have to get up, expecting to die. He was very dyspeptic, and constipated from this time until he was 32 years of age. He began big game hunting in 1891, and since that time he had led a vigorous, strenuous life, and had had a great deal of financial worry and domestic sorrow.

He had never had syphilis, but had malaria in 1891, and an operation for piles in 1911, during which he took gas and ether without trouble.

He had been liable to ' heart attacks ' since 1877, which had become somewhat altered of late years. The attacks might come on quite unexpectedly, and without any assignable cause, and might last for an hour or for several days. (The attack in which I found him had lasted ten days.) The rate suddenly increased from 67 per minute to 130–140; he was conscious of this acceleration, but it did not cripple him much, and he usually continued his avocation. He said he purposely walked hard for several hours during an attack and actually felt better after it. During these attacks Dr. Stainthorpe had frequently felt the heart intermittent, the intermission occurring after two or three beats or after ten or twelve. When the heart was quiet the size and sounds were normal, but it increased slightly in size during an attack. Various forms of treatment had been tried, including two visits to Nauheim, but all with no result. I saw him on February 20, 1912. He was a healthy-looking man, but of a spare habit.

He complained chiefly of the disagreeable consciousness of the heart's action and a certain degree of lassitude when the heart was so rapid. The pulse was quite regular, 110 per minute. From the electrocardiograms taken by Dr. Lewis the ventricular rate was 114 per minute, and the auricular 228. The heart was dull to the nipple line, but no other abnormality could be detected. On February 23 I persuaded him to undergo a course of treatment. He rested in bed and was given three granules of Nativelle's digitalin per day. In thirty-six hours the pulse-rate had fallen to 70 per minute; then he was given two granules per day till the 26th, when the pulse was 68 (ten granules altogether). Dr. Stainthorpe wrote to me on March 5 saying the pulse had kept under 76 per minute without digitalis and the patient had lost all his distress and felt much better.

On December 22, 1912, Dr. Stainthorpe wrote to me that the patient had enjoyed good health, though he had occasionally mild attacks of his old trouble, which now only last for a few hours.

CASE 60.—*Auricular flutter. Angina pectoris. Effect of digitalis.*

Male. Born 1850. He had enjoyed fair health until the middle of 1910, when he noticed he was gradually becoming readily short of breath. In January 1912 he had a severe attack of influenza, followed a few weeks later by an attack of gout and bronchitis. When he recovered from these attacks he was very easily exhausted and readily rendered breathless. Dr. Willey wrote to me saying that an increase in the rate of the heart had persisted since his illness, and he was confident it was not present before. The patient had had much business worry during the last few years.

He was sent to me by Dr. Willey on March 19, 1912. He was a big stout man with a florid complexion. He complained chiefly of breathlessness and exhaustion on slight exertion. His pulse was small, regular, and 130 beats per minute. There was marked pulsation in the jugular veins similar to Fig. 220. The heart's dullness was increased, extending 1 inch beyond the nipple line. The systolic blood-pressure was 160 mm. Hg. I sent the patient to Dr. Lewis to get an electrocardiogram, and he reported that the auricle was beating at double the rate of the ventricle. As the condition seemed a recent one, I recommended that he should have a period of rest. This was done, and he again consulted me on May 23, 1912. He stated that the breathlessness and exhaustion were still easily produced, and, in addition, he had attacks of pain striking into the chest on exertion, on one occasion with such violence that he fell on his knees ; the pain lasted only for a few seconds. On four occasions he lost consciousness ; he dropped suddenly down in the street and at once recovered himself ; at another time when at breakfast he suddenly lost consciousness for ten minutes. An examination revealed the same condition as before, that is, a persistent tachycardia of 130 beats per minute, and the peculiar venous pulse, and enlargement of the heart. I was anxious to see the effect of digitalis; Dr. Lewis looked after him, and he has published the result of his observations. I give a summary of his report. The auricular rate was fairly constant, about 270 per minute, while the ventricle was always beating at half this rate. The tincture of digitalis was started on May 24, and continued until the 31st. No effect was perceived until the 30th, when the pulse-rate varied from 114 to 137 per minute, while the auricular rate was 274. This was due to the fact that the response of the ventricle to the auricle varied, sometimes there being one ventricular response to every two auricular beats, or sometimes there being only one to every four auricular beats. On May 31, seven days after starting the digitalis, and after the patient had taken altogether 4 drachms 55 minims, vomiting set in and the pulse-rate fell to 94 per minute, and was very irregular, while the auricular rate continued at 278. The irregularity was due to the varying responses of the ventricle to the auricular beats. The digitalis was stopped for a few days, the pulse remaining irregular. While the rapid auricular rate (260 to 268 per minute) persisted the patient was put on tincture of strophanthus, on June 4. This treatment was continued till June 20, and the patient had taken 15 drachms 15 minims of the

F f

drug. It never affected the auricular rate, though the ventricular rate was markedly affected, being irregular and varying at times from 80 to 130 beats per minute, due to the varying response of the ventricle to the auricular beats. After the stopping of the drug the rhythm of the ventricle became regular, about 130 beats per minute, while the auricle continued to beat at double the rate of the ventricle.

CASE 61.—*Paroxysmal tachycardia due to auricular flutter and auricular fibrillation.*

Male. Aged 61. In July 1912 he had an attack of influenza and pneumonia, and the heart was found to be rapid and irregular. Early in December he saw Dr. Grenier, who found him complaining of a sensation of constriction in the præcordial region. The pulse was 144, with a disorderly rhythm. He was put to bed, and in a few days œdema of the legs and of the base of both lungs set in. Some days later the heart quietened down under digitalis. The heart had been better since, though he had had occasional attacks of tachycardia. In one attack, January 13, 1913, he felt very faint and almost lost consciousness.

I saw him on February 1, 1913, and found him an active, healthy-looking man. The pulse was regular, 80 beats per minute; the blood-pressure was 175 mm. Hg. The heart's dullness extended ½ inch beyond the nipple line and the sounds were clear.

I saw him again two days later. He said he felt quite well and was not conscious of anything amiss with the heart. The pulse was beating rapidly, 155 beats per minute, quite regularly for short periods, then very irregularly. I took a long tracing, and found remarkable variation in the pulse, sometimes rapid and irregular (auricular fibrillation) and sometimes rapid and regular (auricular flutter), and then for a short time the rhythm would be quite normal (Fig. 142 and 144). An electrocardiogram taken by Dr. Lewis during the rapid regular period shows the auricle beating at a rate of 308 and the ventricle at 154 per minute, while the first two leads were taken, but a few minutes later, when the third lead was taken, the heart had reverted to the normal rhythm, one auricular beat to one ventricular beat at the rate of 90 beats per minute (Fig. 143). A later electrocardiogram taken during the irregular period showed auricular fibrillation. When I last saw this patient he was feeling well; the heart was quite normal in its action, though he was conscious of his heart beating irregularly for several hours at a time. I saw him in one such attack and found the auricle was fibrillating.

CASE 62.—*Auricular flutter.*

Male. Aged 62. Consulted me on October 22, 1912. Complained of breathlessness on exertion and swelling of the ankles at night. The breathlessness was noticed first when playing golf in August. He said that he had giddy attacks during the last two years; one bad attack lasted for a minute, when everything went round. His doctor said he had had a large and irregular heart for ten years. He was a big pale man. The pulse was rapid, 90 per minute, and occasionally irregular (Fig. 133). There was a large diffuse apex outside the nipple line. The sounds were muffled. The tracings of the radial pulse showed alternation following the extra-systoles, and it is to be noted that the apex beat is just as large and full with a small radial beat as with a large one, in contrast with the apex beat due to an extra-systole (Fig. 149). The jugular tracing (Fig. 133) shows three waves to one pulse-beat, so that the auricle was beating three times as fast as the ventricle. This agrees with the electrocardiogram taken by Dr. Lewis. When there was a pause in the ventricle the rapid auricular beats come out very clearly, as shown in Fig. 129 and 134, the former being taken at a different time by Dr. J. Hay.

He again consulted me in March 1913. He had been having a long, restful holiday, and was feeling better and fit for work. The heart's action was quite normal, one auricular beat preceding each ventricular beat, the pulse-rate being 75 per minute. Otherwise the heart was in much the same condition as before.

CASE 63.—*Auricular flutter. Cheyne-Stokes respiration. Death.*

Male. Born 1855. He led an active and strenuous life till the end of December 1909. At this time he had an attack of influenza, during which he worked at high pressure, but seemed none the worse for it and continued his strenuous life. In January 1910 while shaving he noticed that he was breathless and that his cheeks were very blue. He lay down and felt that his heart was beating very rapidly, about 180 per minute. After resting he got up and resumed his work, but in a few days he became so weak and breathless that he had to stay in bed. A few days later he felt better, though the heart-rate persisted at over 140. A tracing taken on January 21, 1910, showed a pulse-rate of 170. At the end of January he went away for ten days' rest, and returned on February 6, and though he resumed work he was weak and breathless. I saw him on February 13. He was able to be up, but was very breathless on going upstairs. The pulse was very irregular, about 75 per minute. The tracing from the neck showed numerous small waves, which I now recognize as characteristic of auricular flutter. The heart's dullness extended to the left nipple line, and the sounds were free from murmurs. Save for the breathlessness on exertion there was no sign of heart failure. Two days later an electro-cardiogram was taken which showed a regular ventricular rhythm with a rate of 145 per minute, the auricular rate being 290 per minute—exactly double.

After this date the patient continued at work, and on February 18 he had a very busy and worrying day, and had to run to catch a train. On the 19th he felt ill and his temperature was 100° F. On the 20th the temperature was normal, and the pulse was small and very irregular and many beats imperceptible. The heart-beats were 180 per minute and very irregular. There was marked pulsation in the epigastrium ; the heart's dullness extended ¾ inch outside the nipple line ; the veins of the neck were full and engorged. During the night the breathing was difficult and Cheyne-Stokes in character. In the morning of the 22nd, the pulse-rate was 180, and in the evening it fell to 104. For the next few days the pulse remained very rapid, and the condition of the patient became worse, with orthopnœa, Cheyne-Stokes respiration, and partial loss of consciousness. On February 26 the heart suddenly reverted to the normal rhythm, falling to between 60 and 70 beats per minute, and all the symptoms of heart failure speedily passed off. After this he felt very well, and kept so until he had a return of the tachycardia on March 8. This continued for a few days, then suddenly disappeared. From this date he gradually improved and went for a month's holiday. He returned to work and kept fairly well till the summer of 1912, when he again became conscious that the heart was acting abnormally, but he still pursued his strenuous life and went for a holiday in August, but had to return home and go to bed. When I saw him in September the rate of the heart was rapid, about 117, and irregular and characteristic waves of auricular flutter were found in the jugular tracing. He was slightly livid and lay propped up in bed. At times he had Cheyne-Stokes respiration, and the heart dullness extended to 2 inches outside the nipple line.

He had been taking digitalis and the dose was increased, with the result that the ventricle became slower, and he gained some strength and made a partial recovery, but the auricular flutter persisted ; the heart always tended to increase in rate, but was kept in check by the digitalis, till his death occurred unexpectedly in January 1913.

CASE 64.—*Auricular flutter, the result of an acute infection.*

Male. Aged 47. Seen with Dr. Williams on December 4, 1912. The patient had scarlet fever in childhood, which left him slightly deaf. He had had good health and led a temperate life. He was quite well up to November 28, 1912, and on that day he played a game of golf and enjoyed it. That evening there was a slight rise in his temperature and he coughed up some blood-stained sputum. He was rather breathless and dusky on the next day. On December 2 he had an attack of great breathlessness and the pulse became rapid, irregular, and at times

F f 2

scarcely perceptible. From the breathlessness he recovered in an hour. When I saw him on the 4th he lay propped up in bed, the face of a dusky tinge, the breathing slightly laboured and becoming markedly so in turning over. The heart's dullness extended to the nipple line, the action was irregular and the sounds muffled. Above each clavicle the jugular bulb was seen beating so forcibly as to be perceptible to the touch, and giving rise to a short sharp sound. A tracing showed the jugular pulse to be occasionally irregular, and each large wave in the jugular occurred immediately before a radial pulse-beat (Fig. 225). There was impaired resonance of the bases of both lungs and a few fine crepitations.

He improved in his general condition from this date, though his pulse was very irregular at times. In a few days albumen appeared in the urine, and the quantity of urine passed gradually diminished. Still he seemed to be mending, and on January 16 he was able to get up, but was very short of breath, and the heart's action continued very irregular.

From this date he gradually became worse, Cheyne-Stokes respiration developed, the urine became scanty and dropsy appeared, extending gradually up the legs to the abdomen. The

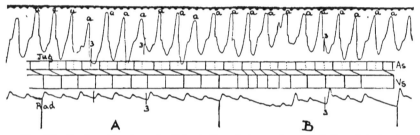

Fig. 225. Tracing of jugular and radial pulsations during an abnormal rhythm of the heart—probably auricular flutter. The intercalated diagram suggests the explanation, that in addition to the large wave, a, in the jugular, there was another auricular wave which occurred during the ventricular diastole (see Fig. 132). The irregularity in the radial tracing is probably due to the ventricle responding to each auricular beat for a short period. The periods A and B, though of the same duration, include the same number of auricular beats, but include a different number of ventricular systoles, which Lewis has shown to be characteristic of auricular flutter (Case 64).

heart's dullness increased in size and a mitral murmur developed, and the rhythm continued irregular. The Cheyne-Stokes respiration was very marked, and during the apnœic stage I obtained tracings from the jugular pulse, showing two well-marked waves to one ventricular beat (Fig. 132). He gradually sank and died on April 2, 1913.

CASE 65.—*Syphilitic aortitis and myocarditis, aortic regurgitation. Auricular flutter.*

Female. Aged 39. Admitted to hospital on September 22, 1912, complaining of shortness of breath, pain in the abdomen, and swelling of the legs. This had been present for three and a half months, when she first noticed shortness of breath, and during the last six weeks her legs had swollen. There was no history of rheumatic fever, but a Wassermann reaction was positive.

On admission there was slight dyspnœa, œdema of the legs, and cyanosis of the lips. The apex beat was in the sixth space, 6¼ inches from the mid-line. The limits of the heart's dullness were 1 and 6¼ inches to the right and left of the mid-line, in the fourth space. There were systolic and diastolic aortic murmurs audible over all the præcordium. There were crepitations at the base of both lungs. The liver extended 1 inch below the costal margin in the right mid-clavicular line. The urine was acid, 1020, and albumen was present.

On rest in bed she showed improvement which lasted for seven days. Then she had attacks of dyspnœa, associated with perspiration and with pain over the præcordium. The liver increased in size, and there was tenderness over the liver. She was placed on the tincture of digitalis on October 16, 1912, 1 drachm per day; on the 23rd the digitalis was discontinued because of nausea and vomiting. There was slight improvement in the general condition and a decrease in the amount of œdema, but no slowing of pulse-rate or increase of blood-pressure.

On November 18, 1912, the administration of digitalis was again commenced; on the 25th, during its administration, the character of the jugular pulse became altered, and showed the presence of auricular flutter. Her general condition gradually became worse, there was more œdema and ascites. She left the hospital on December 4, and died ten days later at home. The auricles were in a state of flutter when she left the hospital. After the onset of auricular flutter the general symptoms became worse, but no change was found in the area of cardiac dullness, or the character of the murmurs, but the pulse became irregular (Fig. 226).

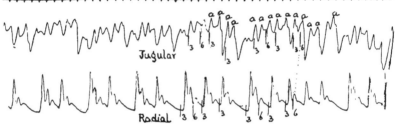

Fig. 226. Shows an irregular radial pulse, and a jugular pulse with numerous auricular waves (Case 65).

CASE 66.—*Myocardial disease affecting the auriculo-ventricular bundle. Pulsus alternans. Cardiac asthma. Auricular flutter as a terminal condition.*

Male. Aged 63. Consulted me first on April 27, 1910. The patient felt quite well until November 1909, when he was troubled with a cough and shortness of breath. In the last few months he had been troubled with attacks of great breathlessness occurring about 3 a.m. These attacks were very severe and lasted for about half an hour. The attacks were accompanied by coughing and some phlegm. The patient was a big, powerful-looking man. The pulse was large and the arterial wall thickened; the blood-pressure was 125 mm. Hg. There was an occasional extra-systole, followed by the pulsus alternans for a few beats. The heart was enlarged and the apex beat was 2 inches outside the nipple line. The first sound was reduplicated. A tracing of the jugular pulse shows an increased a–c interval (Fig. 152), and electrocardiograms taken by Dr. Lewis showed an increase in the P–R interval, and the electric changes characteristic of damage to the right branch of the bundle, that is, the left ventricle started contracting before the right.

The patient denied a history of syphilis, but certain scars in the leg had a suspicious appearance. There was a slight trace of albumen in the urine. The patient improved under treatment and kept fairly well until July 1912, when he had an attack of gout which weakened him. I had seen him from time to time during the interval and detected little change. I saw him on April 5, 1912, and he felt weak, but could play a game of golf with comfort. In January 1913 he went abroad and was taken seriously ill, with great weakness and breathlessness. I saw him on March 2. He lay propped up in bed in a slight stupor, with marked Cheyne-Stokes respiration, and the pulse was very rapid, varying in rhythm, periods of regularity varying with periods of irregularity. Slight waves in the jugular pulse, indicative of auricular flutter, were present at this time.

The patient's condition did not improve, and he gradually sank and died in May 1913.

CASE 67.—*Auricular flutter. Attacks of loss of consciousness. Death.*

Male. Born 1833. He enjoyed good health until 1901, when he began to have attacks of loss of consciousness. In one of these attacks he fell, and was found to have dislocated his shoulder. As a rule the attacks came on quite suddenly ; he would fall and immediately recover, but would feel dazed and weak and be conscious of a feeble action of the heart. As a rule the attacks readily passed off. In 1906 he partook of a hasty lunch, and then hurried half a mile to catch a train. After getting into the train he became unconscious, and at the next station he was carried to a hotel, where he lay unconscious for several hours and with a pulse so small that the doctor in attendance thought he was dead on several occasions. He recovered and had a few much slighter attacks since. He was conscious at times of his heart running away, but he kept quiet and it passed off after a few minutes or a few hours.

When I saw him with Dr. Ford Anderson on February 21, 1911, he was a tall, spare man, with a blue nose and cold fingers. The pulse was occasionally interrupted by extra-systoles. The heart's dullness was not increased to the right, but extended to the nipple line on the left. The apex beat was somewhat diffuse and forcible. There was no murmur, but the first sound at the apex was soft, and when he lay down it was inaudible.

I saw him again on August 2, 1912. He was suffering from great prostration, due to an attack which had come on thirteen days previously and had continued till I saw him. He was very pale and distressed looking, and lay propped up in bed ; the pulse was barely perceptible and so rapid as to be uncountable. The deep jugular veins were full and pulsated largely. From the tracing the rate was just over 200 per minute, and I had the greatest difficulty in getting a record of the radial pulse, while a record was easily obtained from the jugular. The heart's dullness was at this time outside the nipple line, there were no murmurs; the first sound was scarcely audible and the second sound was markedly accentuated. There was no dropsy or enlargement of the liver. The patient was put on digitalin granules, one being given every six hours. This was continued for three days, when the pulse-rate fell to 100 per minute. The patient became very restless and his mind wandered. The digitalin was stopped. After this various remedies were tried, but none seemed to have a definite effect. The pulse-rate for the next month varied markedly in rate, being 180 beats per minute, and sometimes falling as low as 74 ; sometimes quite regular, at other times irregular. As I did not seen him after August 2 I am not able to say whether the abnormal action was continuous all that time, but from the account of the rate and rhythm given by Dr. Ford Anderson I should think it was fairly persistent, it may be with intervals of the normal rhythm. The patient's general condition varied much ; he was at times fairly comfortable, but often suffered from severe prostration. Slight excitement or exertion would often induce an attack of very rapid heart action. He gradually became weaker and died.

CASE 68.—*Attacks of paroxysmal tachycardia, probably due to auricular flutter.*

Male. Aged 27. Consulted me on March 7, 1910, complaining of sudden attacks of palpitation. The patient had scarlet fever followed by rheumatic fever in 1887, and he had another attack of rheumatic fever in 1902. It was shortly before this attack that he had his first attack of palpitation. The patient was spare, with cold hands and blue fingers. The lips were cyanotic, and his face became very blue on exertion or during an attack of palpitation. The pulse was regular, 64 per minute, and the jugular pulse was of the normal auricular type. The heart was not enlarged, and the first sound was muffled when he stood up.

The attacks of palpitation of which he complained were at first of only a few minutes' duration, and occurred infrequently. During the last few years they had occurred every few weeks and lasted from half an hour to six hours, and one attack, seven years before, lasted a week. The attacks begin suddenly, and he feels weak and disinclined for exertion while they are on, though he can walk quietly without distress. Violent exertion will bring them on, and also when the stomach feels upset they are readily provoked. As a rule if he takes ipecacuanha wine the attacks will cease a few minutes after he is sick and vomits. He had gone through a great variety of treatments, including a rest cure, but nothing has seemed to prevent the attacks.

At my request he kept a diary for nearly a year, and the following account gives an idea of his experiences for a month:

May 10. Palpitation came on at 10 p.m. Took Ipec. about 10.10 p.m., sick, no effect. Ipec. again at 11.15 p.m., sick, and attack stopped at midnight.

May 17. Woke with palpitation at 5.15 a.m. Took Ipec. twice, sick, and attack stopped at 6.30 a.m.

May 22. Palpitation came on when called at 7 a.m. Took Ipec., no result. Had breakfast, took Ipec. again, no result. Finally after having taken four lots of Ipec. the doctor gave me some soup, sick again, and attack stopped at 11 a.m.

May 29. Palpitation came on at 7 a.m. Took Ipec., sick, and attack stopped at 7.40 a.m.

The patient went on in fair health, interrupted occasionally by the attacks of tachycardia till the middle of January 1911, when he had an attack of rheumatic fever. The temperature was not high and only a few joints were affected. On the 19th he started an attack of paroxysmal tachycardia which continued till the date of my visit to him on the 24th. He had on several occasions taken ipecacuanha and vomited, but this had failed to stop the attack. When I saw him he was sitting up in a chair, unable to lie down, the breathing laboured; the face, lips, hands, and feet were deeply cyanosed. The radial pulse was frequent and scarcely perceptible (see Fig. 135). The heart's beat was forcible, particularly under the left nipple, and this impulse could be felt as far out as the anterior axillary line. The sounds were clear and distinct. The veins of the neck were full and pulsated (Fig. 135). The liver was 2 inches below the ribs and pulsated (Fig. 136). He was desirous of trying the ipecacuanha again, but his medical attendant was afraid that he was so exhausted that he would not be able to stand the strain of vomiting. As he felt that he would get relief, and as I had nothing better to offer, I consented to his taking the ipecacuanha again. In half an hour he vomited, and the heart at once reverted to the normal and he experienced great relief. After this he gradually improved, but the attacks kept recurring with exhausting frequency. I saw him again on February 17, 1911, when he was in an attack which had been going on for several hours. He said he could stop the attack by swallowing and belching air, and this he did, but what happened is shown in the tracing, Fig. 131; he probably induced a slight degree of heart-block, so that the ventricle responded less readily to the auricular beats (assuming that it was a case of auricular flutter). After a few minutes it started off at the rapid rate. He was conscious of the temporary character of the altered rhythm, and recognized that it was different from the normal action of the heart. He repeated the experiment and got a similar response. From this date he gradually improved, and for the last two years he has been able to follow his profession, though liable to be crippled at intervals by a short attack.

CASE 69.—*Digitalis effect in auricular flutter (?), producing auricular fibrillation and the normal rhythm.*

Female. Aged 16. Seen first on March 21, 1903. Had had rheumatic fever, and for some years had suffered from breathlessness and palpitation on exertion. This had increased, and there was slight œdema of the legs. There was marked pulsation of the veins of the neck of the auricular type (Fig. 227). The pulse was small, regular, 86 per minute. There was great heaving of the left chest with the movements of the greatly enlarged heart. The apex beat was large and diffuse, and felt in the sixth interspace and in the anterior axillary line. There was a loud, rough systolic murmur heard over the whole heart and round to the back, but loudest at the apex. With rest and digitalis she rapidly improved. She broke down again, and a note on January 9, 1904, states that the abdomen was greatly swollen, the liver enlarged, the legs œdematous, and the urine scant. The radial pulse was small, soft, and rapid, 126 per minute, while the jugular pulse was of the ventricular type. Under digitalin granules she again improved, but in February the granules were stopped, and she speedily broke down again. On March 10, 1904, the condition was similar to that described on January 9, the radial and jugular pulse-tracings being shown in Fig. 227 A.

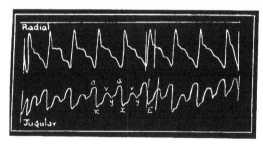

FIG. 227. This and the seven following tracings are from the same patient. Here the pulse is regular, and the jugular pulse is of the auricular type (Case 69, March 1903).

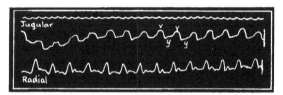

FIG. 227 A. The jugular pulse is now of the ventricular type (Case 69, March 10, 1904).

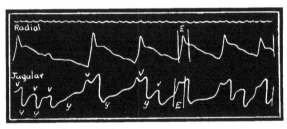

FIG. 227 B. The jugular pulse is still of the ventricular type, but under the action of digitalin the radial has become slow and irregular (Case 69, March 18, 1904).

She was prescribed digitalin granules, one per day. They speedily took effect, and on March 18 the pulse had become slow and irregular (Fig. 227 B). The urine had greatly increased in quantity, the abdomen and liver had diminished in size, and all signs of dropsy had gone. The digitalin was continued till March 28, one granule being taken every second day, and she continued in fair health, the pulse still slow and irregular, as shown by Fig. 228, which was taken on March 26.

The digitalin was stopped on March 28. Four days after stopping it the pulse had increased to 85 per minute, though she felt still fairly well. On April 5—that is, eight days after stopping the digitalin—the rate of the heart had increased to 120 beats per minute, the pulse had become small and weak, and the jugular distension had increased (Fig. 229). The other signs of heart failure were beginning to show themselves. She was again put on digitalin, one granule per day. On April 9 the pulse was still 120 per minute. On April 11 it was 130, on April 14 it had again become slow and irregular (Fig. 230).

The digitalin was again stopped, but as the pulse began to increase in rate, on April 17, one granule per day was prescribed. The patient continued in fair health, but as the pulse did not slow down satisfactorily, on May 1 I doubled the dose. I did not take any further

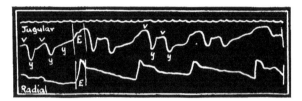

Fig. 228. Shows the characteristic effect of digitalis being maintained. (March 26, 1904.) The jugular tracing shows the nature of the arrhythmia, and the coupled beats resemble the tracings in Fig. 189 and 192, &c. (Case 69).

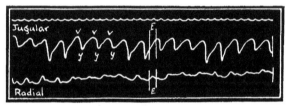

Fig. 229. Eight days after stopping the digitalin, failure again set in, the pulse here being 120 per minute, and the jugular pulse being still of the ventricular type (Case 69, April 5, 1904).

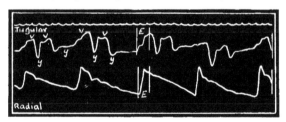

Fig. 230. Nine days after beginning the digitalin the characteristic effect is reproduced (Case 69, April 14, 1904).

tracings till May 14, contenting myself with watching for the slowing of the pulse. Finding it did not yield as before to the increased doses of digitalin, I took tracings on this day, and found a perfectly regular radial pulse, while the jugular pulse had completely changed character, being now of the auricular type—that is, the auricle had again resumed its normal action and the heart chambers contracted in their normal sequence. Occasionally, for a short period, it would show a slight alternating rhythm, as in Fig. 231.

The digitalin was stopped, and the patient continued in fair health for some months. The jugular pulse continued of the auricular type, and the pulse was quite regular until her death in December 1905, except during a short period shortly to be described. On December 18, 1904, she was again beginning to get œdema of the legs, and the abdomen began to swell, and she was very breathless. The pulse was small, soft, and rapid, 110 per minute, and the jugular pulse was still of the auricular type. She was prescribed one granule of the digitalin per day. No improvement had taken place by December 27, when she was ordered to take two granules per day. By January 2, 1905, the rate had fallen to 80, as a rule quite regular, but occasionally an extra-systole of ventricular origin would occur (Fig. 232). Sometimes for a period these ventricular extra-systoles would appear after every second beat. The digitalin was stopped, and the arrhythmia disappeared. (It is now recognized that a rapid

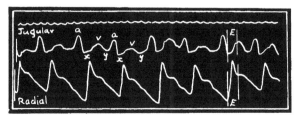

Fig. 231. With continued use of digitalin the normal rhythm of the heart returned, as shown by the fact that here the jugular pulse is of the auricular type (Case 69, May 15, 1904).

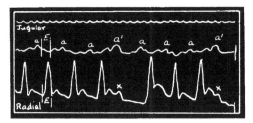

Fig. 232. Shows a jugular pulse of the auricular type with the occasional occurrence of a ventricular extra-systole. The auricular waves (a and a') occur at regular intervals, while the small waves ($\times$) in the radial occur prematurely. The larger size of a' is due to the fact that when the auricle contracts the ventricle is already in systole, and therefore cannot receive the auricular contents, which are thus sent back into the veins, producing this larger wave (Case 69, January 2, 1905).

regular pulse is not characteristic of auricular fibrillation, so that I infer that the heart failure, with rapid regular rhythm, was due to some other abnormal action, probably auricular flutter, which passed into fibrillation as in Case 55.)

CASE 70.—*Frequent attacks of paroxysmal tachycardia, with no serious effects, in old age.*

Male. Born 1827. Has suffered from frequent attacks of rapid action of the heart, accompanied by a feeling of great prostration since he was 76 years of age. During the attacks he feels very exhausted, and lies in bed ; they last from half an hour to twelve hours. He may be free from them for weeks, at other times he has several in one week. I have seen him in consultation during these attacks and also when quite free from them. In the latter condition he is a hale man, considering his years, and takes an active part in his business ; his heart shows no abnormality, and his pulse is slow and regular (Fig. 233). During the attack he lies very still in bed his face is pale and slightly drawn. He does not care to make much exertion, but has no actual suffering. The pulse sometimes attains a rate of 200 per minute at the beginning of the attack. It was always several hours after an attack had begun before I saw him, and the pulse was usually between 150 and 170 beats per minute. Fig. 233 is a tracing of his jugular and radial pulses while free from the attack; there was very slight pulsation in the neck, and I had some difficulty in getting a tracing. Its character, however, clearly shows it to be of the auricular form. Fig. 234 shows the radial and jugular pulses during an attack. I had considerable difficulty in getting satisfactory tracings, as the patient was in bed in a position not conducive to taking a good tracing, but in all those I took the characters were the same as in Fig. 234.

When last I heard of him (1908), at the age of 81, he was in fair health, and still liable to these attacks.

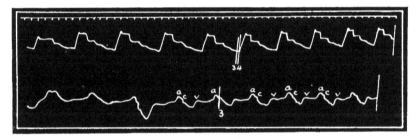

FIG. 233. Tracings from a man aged 78, when free from an attack of paroxysmal tachycardia (Case 70).

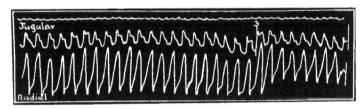

FIG. 234. From the same patient that gave Fig. 233, during an attack of paroxysmal tachycardia. Note slight pulsus alternans in the radial tracing (Case 70).

CASE 71.—*Frequent attacks of paroxysmal tachycardia without serious symptoms.*

Female. Aged 35. Eight months pregnant with her second child. For several years she suffered from breathlessness, and was conscious that her heart beat ' very queerly '. She was under my care for only a few weeks, and I saw her during several attacks of paroxysmal tachycardia. After she left me I heard that she had had an easy confinement, and some years later was in fair health, though still at times prostrate on account of her heart. The periods of abnormal rhythm were of varying duration, the attacks not being continuous, but interrupted frequently by normal beats. At other times the heart would only show frequent extra-systoles. When the heart was irregular the venous pulse was always large, while when the heart was regular it was scarcely perceptible, and it was with difficulty that I got the faint tracing of it in Fig. 235. The waves in the jugular, though slight, are recognizable, and the jugular pulse is of the auricular type. In Fig. 236 the heart is acting irregularly. The radial pulse shows three long pauses at × × ×. The auricular waves, a and a', in the venous pulse occur at regular intervals. During each long pause in the radial there is a large wave, a', due to the auricle, and larger than the other auricular waves, for the reason already given, namely, because at the period at which the auricle contracted the ventricle was in systole, and hence a larger wave was sent back into the veins. It will be noted that after the large auricular wave, a', there

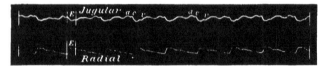

Fig. 235. Simultaneous tracings of the jugular and radial pulses. The jugular pulse is of the auricular form. These and the following five tracings are from the same patient (Case 71).

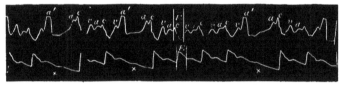

Fig. 236. Simultaneous tracings of the jugular and radial pulses during irregular action of the heart. The auricle preserves its rhythm, there being a arge wave, a', during the premature contraction of the ventricles (Case 71).

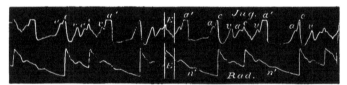

Fig. 237. Shows the same as Fig. 236 (Case 71).

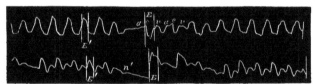

Fig. 238. Simultaneous tracings of the jugular and radial pulses, showing two normal radial beats in the centre of the tracing. Corresponding to the ventricular systole, E, there is a fall in the jugular pulse when the radial beat is normal, and a rise, E', when it is of abnormal origin (Case 71).

is never a ventricular wave. This tracing exemplifies the form of irregularity due to premature stimulation of the ventricles alone (ventricular extra-systole).

In Fig. 237 a very similar irregular condition is present, the difference being that every third arterial beat here is missed, and is represented in the radial tracing by the notch n'. In these three tracings (Fig. 235, 236, and 237) the period E, representing the time when the semilunar valves are open, shows in the jugular pulse a great fall. In Fig. 238 the radial tracing shows two normal beats in the centre of the tracing, all the others being of abnormal origin. The beat preceding the full beats shows only a notch, n', as in Fig. 236. The venous pulse at the time of the normal radial beats shows the same features as are present with the normal radial beats in the three preceding tracings, namely, a small auricular wave, *a*, the carotid wave *c*, the auricular depression during the period *E*, and the ventricular wave *v*. But when the venous pulse corresponding to the abnormal beats is considered, a remarkable change is found. There is but one large wave and one large fall, and the period when this wave occurs is during the ventricular systole *E'*, in striking contrast to the large depression at the time with the normal radial beats shown in the three preceding tracings. A similar condition is seen in Fig. 239, where there is a continuous variation from the normal rhythm to the abnormal. In Fig. 240, with the exception of one normal beat preceded by a long pause, the jugular pulse is of the ventricular form. The transition from one form of jugular pulse to the other is well brought out in Fig. 239.

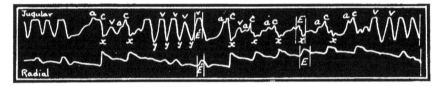

FIG. 239. Shows an alternation of the normal and abnormal rhythms (Case 71).

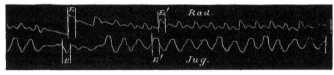

FIG. 240. There is only one normal beat (*E*), all the other beats being of abnormal origin (Case 71).

CASE 72.—*Attacks of paroxysmal tachycardia, slight at first, but becoming permanent and causing death. Post-mortem report.*

Male, born 1860. This patient first consulted me in January 1900. He had an attack of rheumatic fever at 14 years of age. In 1896, after walking for twenty minutes at a rapid pace, he felt extremely weak and exhausted. After this he was always short of breath on exertion. A year later, immediately after throwing a cricket-ball, he felt the heart flutter for a few seconds. Ten minutes after this the heart ' fluttered and beat quickly for six or seven hours '. He had had an attack of this kind every two or three weeks since. These attacks lasted from a few minutes to thirty hours. At first he could sometimes stop the attack by bending down and taking a deep breath, but this was ineffective at this time. Sometimes he passed a large quantity of clear urine in the course of an attack. During an attack, if in bed, he felt exhausted and limp, if walking he was easily tired, and if he had to work for some hours he felt swollen round the waist and very sore over the upper part of his abdomen, and felt pain, sometimes very severe, across the back under the shoulder-blades. During the night the sleep was disturbed. The pulse during these attacks had varied under my observation from 170 to 220 beats per minute. When the heart was acting quietly a short presystolic murmur at the apex and also a soft diastolic murmur over the middle of the sternum could occasionally be detected. It often happened that these murmurs could not be perceived. On producing slight redness by rubbing the forehead, the capillary pulsation could be readily seen. Occasionally the pulse-rate fell to 48 beats per minute. During the attack, irregularity of the pulse had been detected, due to the pulsus alternans (Fig. 241). The patient (who was a very intelligent man) stated that sometimes when the attack of rapid heart-action ceased the heart gave three or four violent beats at intervals longer than the usual pulse-rate. The patient died on November 21, 1900. During the last four months the pulse-rate continued rapid for days together, during which time he would lie prostrate and exhausted. Sleep could only be got by large doses of morphia. During the last two weeks of his life the heart acted slowly only at rare and brief intervals. Signs of heart failure quickly supervened—the face swollen and livid, and general œdema.

It is only necessary here to call attention to the pulsation in the liver and in the veins, which became of the ventricular form during an attack (Fig. 63 and 69).

Report of post-mortem examination of the heart :

' Coronary artery healthy ; coronary sinus and veins dilated, but not markedly so.

' Left auricle greatly dilated and interauricular septum greatly stretched.

' Mitral orifice = a linear chink 18 × 3mm. Anterior cusp of mitral valve and chordæ tendineæ are the site of a warty hard vegetation, the size of a hazel-nut.

' Tricuspid valves healthy, but orifice dilated.

' Myocardium = partial fibrosis in areas. Everywhere the small vessels and capillaries are dilated and the nuclei in their walls dividing, and in the neighbourhood of capillaries are plasma cells. This is markedly the case with the upper part of the auriculo-ventricular bundle and lower part of node.

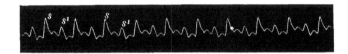

FIG. 241. Pulsus alternans during an attack of paroxysmal tachycardia, sixty-six hours from its commencement (Case 72).

' The sino-auricular node is very well marked, but appears in parts to be more fibrous than usual, and the vessels show the proliferation of cells seen elsewhere in the heart.

' The pathological process which has affected the mitral valves spread up to the central fibrous body, and where the bundle perforates this there are signs of cellular changes in the margin of the bundle. In some sections of the auriculo-ventricular bundle lower down, nearer the ventricles, there are seen in it small areas from which the muscular tissue seems to have disappeared. There are thus distinct evidences of cellular changes in the bundle.'

CASE 73.—*Pulsus alternans. Death.*

Male. Aged 73. Consulted me on January 19, 1911. He was quite well until two years before, when he had some domestic anxiety. A year previously, after an attack of influenza, his heart dilated and became irregular, and since then he had been gradually getting weaker and more breathless. Within the last few months traces of albumen had appeared in the urine. He complained of attacks of constriction across the chest at night when he was in bed. The pulse was large, full, and irregular, due to the frequent occurrence of extra-systoles. In the tracing there was a slight pulsus alternans after the extra-systole (Fig. 242). The heart was dull 1 inch beyond the nipple line, and the apex had a jolting character. The sounds were soft and faint.

Six weeks later dropsy appeared in his legs, followed by ascites and hydrothorax, and he died two months after I saw him.

CASE 74.—*Pulsus alternans. Death.*

Male. Aged 50. Consulted me on August 6, 1911. He considered himself in good health nine months before, when he began to find that he was short of breath and his doctor found his heart-rate sometimes as high as 120 or 130 beats per minute. Of late he had been disturbed at night with attacks of 'asthma' (probably Cheyne-Stokes respiration), and he was very short of breath on slight exertion. The pulse was large and one could perceive that every second beat varied, a large beat alternating with a small one, and the tracing showed a distinct pulsus alternans (Fig. 145). The blood-pressure was 200 for the big beats and 180 for the small. The heart's dullness extended 2 inches beyond the nipple line; the sounds were muffled, but free from murmurs.

He was ordered complete rest for three weeks, and I saw him again on September 16, He was feeling very much better and the attacks of dyspnœa had disappeared, and he could walk quietly without distress.

He returned to work and went on well for three weeks, when he began to take liberties with himself and was again seized with great breathlessness and compelled to stay in bed. He died suddenly two days later.

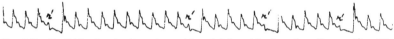

FIG. 242.   Radial tracing showing extra-systoles, *r'*, followed by the pulsus alternans (Case 73).

CASE 75.—*Pulsus alternans.   Cheyne-Stokes breathing.   Death.*

Male.   Aged 62.   Consulted me on March 10, 1911.   He had lived abroad and had been quite healthy until this time, when he suffered from breathless attacks in the night.   He admitted that he had been rather breathless on exertion for the last five years, but thought little of it, and had not consulted a doctor.   His account of his breathlessness was that he went to sleep and woke suddenly feeling as if he was being suffocated.   He breathed heavily for a few minutes, then raised himself up in bed and tried to sleep again.   Sometimes he could not walk 100 yards without getting breathless, and at other times he could walk a mile in comfort.   He used to sleep well, but lately his sleep had been broken by breathless attacks.   During the last year several times on exertion he had suffered from pain, sometimes very severe, striking into the chest and left arm.

He was a healthy-looking man, well nourished.   The pulse was regular, but a tracing showed well-marked pulsus alternans.   The blood-pressure was 200 mm. Hg.   The heart was dull 1 inch outside the nipple line, the sounds were muffled, and there was a slight trace of albumen in the urine.   Suspecting the tendency to Cheyne-Stokes respiration while taking a tracing of his pulse, I requested him to go to sleep, and when he became quiet and half asleep he developed well-marked Cheyne-Stokes respiration.

Some months later dropsy set in, and he died in January 1912.

CASE 76.—*Cardiac asthma.   Pulsus alternans.   Post-mortem report.*

Male.   Aged 72.   I had known the patient for over twenty-five years as a steady, sober, and industrious man.   He worked at his occupation as an engineer up to within a year of his death—though in later years he did not do much laborious work.   He had a slight attack of hemiplegia in December 1906.   He consulted me in June 1907, because he passed blood in his urine.   Except for being rather short of breath, he felt fairly well.   He looked a hale old man.   His radial arteries were large and tortuous, pulse full, seemingly regular.   His heart's dullness extended to the nipple line.   The sounds of the heart were clear except for a musical murmur, systolic in time, heard over the whole heart region, but loudest in the aortic area. It varied distinctly in loudness, a loud murmur alternating with one less loud. When I took a radial tracing it showed a well-marked pulsus alternans. He visited me several times. The urine became quite clear, but the heart's condition continued, and extra-systoles were sometimes very frequent, and the pulsus alternans gave to the pulse the appearance of extreme irregularity.

Early in August he complained greatly of attacks of bad breathing in the night. He would go to sleep quite quietly and then awake suddenly with a sense of suffocation, and sit up in bed breathing heavily. After half an hour he would feel easier, but could not lie down, and had to be propped up in bed. These attacks occurred on several occasions, until they disappeared in September, when his legs began to swell, and he expectorated quantities of blood-stained mucus and small clots of blood. His heart's dullness extended 2 inches beyond the nipple line ; the veins of the arm became full. Venesection was tried, but with little good result, and he died in October.

An analysis of the tracings taken showed that the irregularity which looked so hopelessly confused was due to the mixture of the pulsus alternans with extra-systoles.

Report of the post-mortem examination of the heart :

' The mitral and tricuspid valves show no pathological changes. The aortic valves are slightly thickened and adherent. The auricles are not markedly dilated ; the coronary sinus is filled with post-mortem clot. The ventricles are not dilated, except at the apical part of the left. Both coronary arteries show a thickening of their coats, with dilatation, the left more than the right, and the anterior interventricular branch of the left most affected. At the apex of the left ventricle is an area showing intense fibrosis with deposits of premature clot, but microscopic sections show the Purkinje and inner muscle-layer healthy.

' The auriculo-ventricular node and bundle show a fibrosis, not intense, and also a stretching of the bundle, as if the pars membranacea had been stretched. There is no sign of cellular change in the bundle or node, except the predominance of the fibrous tissue over the muscle-tissue—the muscle-fibres, instead of reticulating, being stretched and parallel.'

CASE 77.—*Heart-block occurring at an early age.*

Aged 24. Consulted me in February 1913, because the pulse was always slow. He felt very well and played strenuous games, such as tennis, but when playing hard he got slightly dizzy and mentally confused, and is perhaps more short-winded than other young men. He fainted several times at the age of 17. He had an attack of whooping-cough at the age of 2, and became reduced to a skeleton. He slowly recovered, and the first note made in regard to the pulse was at the age of 5, when a physician found it beating at the rate of 43 per minute. After this date his pulse was always found slow, and he saw a physician at the age of 19, when the rate was still 43. Notwithstanding this he had led an active life. The patient is tall and spare, but healthy-looking. The pulse is regular at 42 per minute. A tracing of the jugular and radial pulses shows that the auricular rate is 87 per minute. The ventricle is evidently contracting independently of the auricle, that is to say, complete heart-block is present (Fig. 165). The heart is enlarged, the dullness extending 1½ inches beyond the left nipple line. There is a rough systolic murmur heard all over the heart, and I cannot be sure at what region it is heard loudest. I made him run rapidly up and down a flight of stairs and he became slightly breathless and giddy, but the pulse-rate was not accelerated, and I detected a few long pauses, one of which I caught (Fig. 243).

CASE 78.—*Heart-block, at first partial, later complete. Loss of consciousness and convulsions occurring with the onset of complete block.*

Male. Aged 56. Consulted me on May 21, 1910, complaining of getting easily tired, especially in the legs below the knees, and of being breathless on the slightest exertion. He was quite well and led an active life till early in 1909, when he observed that he was getting weak and breathless. In January 1909 he felt so weak that he feared he might collapse, and consulted a physician, who diagnosed neurasthenia and heart strain. At this time his heart's action was sometimes slow and the physician said he had bradycardia. He was sent for a long sea voyage, and returned feeling better, but the rate was still slow and he underwent a course of treatment for three months with some slight improvement.

The patient was big and stout, but healthy looking. The pulse was slow and regular, 30 beats per minute. The heart was enlarged, the dullness extending to the left slightly beyond the nipple line. The sounds were clear. A tracing taken of the jugular pulse showed that there were two auricular waves to one radial or carotid beat (Fig. 244). The auricular

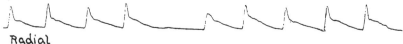

Radial

FIG. 243. Tracing of the radial showing a long pause after exertion (Case 77).

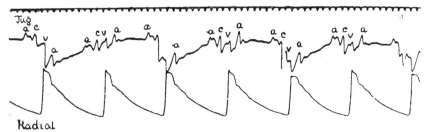

Radial

FIG. 244. Shows a 2 : 1 heart-block (Case 78).

beat following the ventricular was slightly premature. The interpretation of the jugular curve was confirmed by the electrocardiogram. While I was taking a long tracing the patient developed slight Cheyne-Stokes respiration.

Massive doses of oxygen restored the normal rhythm for brief periods, and increased the frequency of the ventricular beats (3 : 2 rhythm) for short periods. During the normal rhythm there was always a wide a–c interval.

On June 26 the patient fell unconscious and recovered after ten minutes. From this date till he died, on July 15, the heart was always slow, and he had frequent attacks of loss of consciousness, sometimes lasting for half an hour, during which time he would have convulsions. The pulse-rate then would be from 4 to 10 beats per minute. During the conscious periods he was very weak and the pulse-rate about 25 per minute, and the auricular rate 90 per minute, the heart-block being complete (Fig. 164). He died during an attack of loss of consciousness with convulsions.

CASE 79.—*Sudden inception of auricular fibrillation and heart-block, lasting for about three weeks. Angina pectoris.*

Male. Born 1852. A stout, healthy-looking individual. I had known him for about twenty-eight years, and had attended him at various times for trivial complaints, and in 1903 for an attack of erysipelas of the face. He had enjoyed good health, was getting fat and somewhat short of breath. On November 9 he was hurrying from the train to a football match a mile distant from the station. As he approached the football field he was seized with pain across the middle of the chest, but as it was not severe he pushed on till he arrived at the field. He sat down, but the pain increased, striking into both arms, and his hands went white and cold. He felt as if he wanted to breathe deeply but could not. He endured the suffering for twenty minutes, and as it became worse, and he felt as if he would die, he was assisted off the field, put into a cab, and driven to the station. He was given some brandy, which made him sick. The pain gradually diminished, and he returned home by train ; as he was better he walked home (about a quarter of a mile), but felt sick and short of breath. He went to bed, and one of my colleagues saw him and found his pulse between 30 and 40 beats per minute. I saw him next morning. He felt very weak ; the pain was nearly gone, though it had kept recurring through the night. He had some pain if he took a deep breath. The pulse-rate was 52 ; the

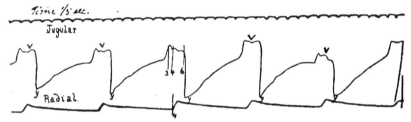

FIG. 245. Simultaneous tracings of the jugular and radial pulses. The jugular pulse is of the ventricular form. Pulse-rate, 40 per minute (Case 79, November 24, 1907).

heart's dullness extended from mid-sternum to 2 inches beyond the nipple line ; apex beat faint in the fifth interspace ; sounds clear and free from murmur. The superficial jugular vein was very full, but did not pulsate. The deep jugular was large, filling up during ventricular systole, and collapsing suddenly at the beginning of ventricular diastole. There was no sign of an auricular wave preceding the ventricular systole. The patient was kept in bed, and his condition did not undergo much change for the next fortnight, except that the pain gradually grew less till it finally disappeared and he was able to sit up. The pulse-rate varied, sometimes falling as low as 30, but never rising above 52. On November 24 a long tracing was taken with the ink polygraph, and the rate showed great uniformity ; the rhythm was also quite regular. Fig. 245 is a small portion of the tracing taken on that day, and represents the same features as were present on November 10 ; the rate was 40 per minute, the rhythm regular, and the venous pulse of the ventricular form. When I next examined him, on November 29, his pulse had increased in rate, with occasional intermissions. I had the greatest difficulty in getting a tracing of the jugular pulse ; he had a very short fat neck. But imperfect as the tracings were, they showed a return of the auricular wave a to its normal period before c. From this date he gradually improved, and has been able to get about, though he is perhaps a little shorter of breath than before his attack. Tracings were taken from him in December 1908, and on May 11, 1909. The venous pulse was the same on both occasions, and showed an auricular wave, a, preceding the carotid wave, c, while the rate was 68 per minute ; the rhythm was regular. In 1913 he was in good health and had no return of the attacks.

CASE 80.—*Auricular fibrillation and heart-block associated with mitral stenosis. Occasional attacks of syncope and convulsions (Adams-Stokes syndrome).*

Male. Born 1865. When a soldier in India he had dysentery at the age of 20, syphilis at the age of 22. He had malarial fever in America at the age of 27. In 1894 he had the first attack of syncope. After lying up for a week he went out, and in hurrying to avoid a cab he fell unconscious on the pavement, but quickly recovered. He consulted a doctor, who said his heart was affected. Two years later he was laid up with shortness of breath and swelling of the legs, and was treated for 'mitral disease'. He partially recovered, and had frequent attacks of weakness until the final break-down occurred in 1905. He had been feeling ill for

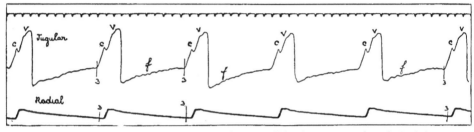

FIG. 246. Simultaneous tracings of the jugular and radial pulses. The jugular pulse is of the ventricular form, and the rate about 28 per minute. (Note auricular fibrillation waves *f, f*.)

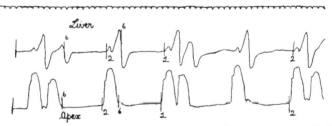

FIG. 247. Tracings of the liver pulse and apex beat in heart-block with auricular fibrillation showing the coupled beat (Case 80).

some years, but had worked hard, and had kept himself going on brandy, bovril, eggs, &c. He says his pulse was slow in 1903, and that it has remained so ever since.

In 1904 he began to have mild 'fits' in which he lost consciousness and was slightly convulsed. From November 1905 to April 1906, he had a great number of fits, some severe with convulsions and cyanosis, others slight without convulsions. He had no attacks for a year, but he had a very severe one in April 1907, and since then only three mild attacks. He had lived a life of hard work with frequent bouts of drinking.

The patient was tall, spare, and intelligent-looking. The face was usually ruddy, with a faint duskiness. He walked slowly and carefully, and his gait was slightly ataxic; if he hurried or got excited he became giddy. He had a somewhat violent temper, and when in a passion his face became dusky and cyanosed. When lying down there was a large pulsation, seen in the deep jugular on both sides, heaving in the lower part of the neck, as in Fig. 246. It was very slow and synchronous with the apex beat. The liver was slightly enlarged and pulsated (Fig. 247).

The radial pulse was slow and deliberate, usually about 30 per minute, and quite regular. At times two beats were close together, and were followed by a long pause. These coupled beats might appear at rare intervals or alternate with a single beat, or they might appear continuously for a short period. The apex beat was large and diffuse in the sixth interspace, and in the anterior axillary line. The heart dullness extended 1 inch to the right of the middle line and 8 inches to the left.

There was a rough blowing systolic murmur, heard best at the apex and propagated towards the axilla. The second sound was clear and well struck and followed by a soft murmur. This diastolic murmur was heard only over a limited space at the apex, and was not always perceptible. It was, as a rule, faint and faded away.

A large number of tracings were taken from this patient at different times, and they always presented the same features, the only difference being that sometimes the coupled beats were more frequent or were entirely absent. The jugular tracing always showed one large wave occupying the whole time of ventricular systole, occasionally with fibrillation wave during diastole (Fig. 246).

On July 6, 1911, he began to have a series of attacks of loss of consciousness and slight convulsions, which occurred at varying intervals till his death on July 8. Dr. Silberberg took careful note of his condition during his latter days. The heart-rate at times varied slightly in rate and rhythm. In place of the usual slow rhythm, a series of beats, probably of the same nature and origin as the extra-systoles, would follow one another for varying periods, so that the ventricular rate sometimes attained a speed of 60 per minute. At the end of such a period the ventricle would stand still before it again took on its own rhythm, and it was during this period that the loss of consciousness and slight convulsions occurred. The following is from Dr. Silberberg's account of the case: ' The attacks of unconsciousness and the mild convulsions commenced at 5 o'clock on the morning of July 6, 1911. They ceased at 9 a.m. but returned at 11 a.m., and continued at short intervals till 1 p.m. Between 1 p.m. and 2.30 p.m. he was free from them. From this hour until death occurred (the morning of the 8th) there was a similar repetition of relapse and recovery.

' The attacks were of varying duration, lasting for a few seconds to twenty or thirty seconds. They were accompanied, one and all, by a lapse of the ventricular beats, readily observed at the prominent apex beat. The onset of unconsciousness was gradual, and the patient was aware of the impending attack, being conscious that his heart had temporarily ceased to beat. He became restless, he groaned, and uttered words of complaint. In a few seconds he could not be roused ; the eyes rolled upwards and deviated to the right, the pupils dilated fully, and the corneal reflex was lost. Cyanosis of the face, already present, deepened to lividity ; the breathing became stertorous and air was sucked in vigorously, his cheeks sinking deeply between his edentulous gums. Much flatus was passed. After twenty seconds of unconsciousness, epileptiform manifestations appeared ; the convulsions started in the face, the arms became rigid, and spasmodic flexor movements appeared. The lower limbs showed no convulsive movements. A single beat of the heart, during the fit, lightened the degree of unconsciousness, two or three beats brought him to a dazed condition, and after a few more beats he rapidly recovered, conversing rationally, though necessarily showing exhaustion. The first beat of the recovery was usually a weak one, the ensuing beats were more forcible. During the periods of comparative lucidity he complained of aching and sore feelings all over, more especially in the limbs. He was too feeble and exhausted to move. Pain, relieved by eructation, was present over the upper abdomen. On several occasions he vomited a pint or more of greenish fluid, an incident which seemed to afford relief.'

Dr. Lewis has published an account of some of the features of this case when he was under his care. The post-mortem was carried out by Dr. Lewis and the heart sent to Dr. Cohn for microscopic examination. The following is a summary of the account which has been published :

'The medulla oblongata showed no gross lesion. The vagus nerves were normal, but parallel with each nerve there was a small one containing a hæmorrhage. The heart was hypertrophied in all its cavities. There was an aneurysm in the right upper portion of the left ventricle. There was partial sclerosis of the septum ventriculorum and complete sclerosis of the septum membranaceum. The myocardium contained numerous scars. There was practically no acute inflammation. The sino-auricular node was in part destroyed, being replaced by connective tissue. The main stem of the auriculo-ventricular bundle was divided from the auriculo-ventricular node by sclerotic tissue ; and the distal end of the main stem, its point of division, and the upper parts of both branches were destroyed by the same process. The arteries of the heart showed hypertrophy of the media, degeneration of their muscle-fibres, and hyperplasia of the intima, causing either partial (the more common lesion) or complete obliteration of the lumina. The aorta showed athero-sclerosis. The liver showed chronic congestion, as did also the spleen, pancreas, and kidneys.'

CASE 81.—*Inception of auricular fibrillation, the heart's rate at first not infrequent, but becoming slow with attacks of unconsciousness and epileptic fits. Death during an attack. Post-mortem report.*

Male. Born 1838. I had known this patient intimately since 1894. He was a healthy, vigorous man up till 1907. He was a very heavy smoker, and for a great many years he smoked two ounces of tobacco and half a dozen cigars a day. I had occasion to examine him in 1906, and found his heart normal in rate and rhythm, though for some years he had been rather short of breath. I again examined him in February 1907, and found that his heart was continuously irregular, with the disorderly rhythm characteristic of the auricular fibrillation. He was not conscious of the change, but there was a further increase in his breathlessness. He was still able to attend to business, and to play a game of golf. He lived some distance from me, and I did not see him again until October 11, 1907, when I was asked to see him with his medical attendant, Dr. O'Connor, to whom I am indebted for an excellent account of his many seizures. The history given was that his pulse had become very slow for some months, and that latterly he had been seized at times with attacks of unconsciousness. The pulse-rate on such occasions was found below 30 beats per minute. He was very weak and faint when I saw him, the pulse varying in rate from 30 to 40 beats per minute, and irregular, with long pauses at times. During the long pauses there was often a small premature beat in the jugular (see v', Fig. 248). The heart's dullness extended 1½ inches beyond the left nipple, and there was a soft blowing murmur at the apex. There was a small amount of albumen in the urine. The attacks of unconsciousness continued, and I saw him again in November, when the heart's condition was much the same. After this the pulse-rate increased, the attacks disappeared, and he went to Torquay in June 1908, where he had a slight recurrence of his attacks of loss of consciousness. From this he recovered, and continued well till August 4, when after some effort he was seized with great breathlessness, and the attacks of unconsciousness recurred. These increased in number and severity, and for two whole days he was unconscious and deeply cyanosed. For some hours he passed from one epileptic seizure to another as if affected with uræmic convulsions. He also developed Cheyne-Stokes respiration. The pulse during these convulsive attacks was not perceptible. The severity of the attacks gradually lessened, and in the month of September his pulse-rate rose to 50 or 60 beats per minute. In October he had a number of very transient fainting attacks. Dr. O'Connor described the attacks as resembling *petit mal*. Thus, while the doctor was talking to him, the patient's face would suddenly become pale, and consciousness would be lost for a brief period. During these attacks no pulse could be felt at the radial.

I saw him again on December 18, 1908. He was able to go about, and had been free from attacks for a few weeks. The pulse was rather slow, about 60 per minute, and irregular. The heart's dullness extended 1¼ inches beyond the left nipple, the sounds were clear, with a faint doubling of the first sound. There was no dropsy, and the urine was free from albumen.

On May 5, 1909, he was seen by Dr. John Hay, who took a long tracing with the ink polygraph. The rhythm was of the disorderly kind, characteristic of auricular fibrillation, and the jugular pulse was of the ventricular form. In August 1909 the heart's action became very infrequent, and he was seized with attacks of loss of consciousness and epileptic convulsions, and he died in one of these attacks.

The heart was sent to Dr. A. E. Cohn, who made a thorough examination of it, and he has published an account of his findings. Great increase of the connective tissue of the sino-auricular node was found. There was also present interstitial myocardial lesions of the auricles and ventricle, but more especially of the right auricle, but there was only slight increase of connective tissue scattered through the auriculo-ventricular node and branches.

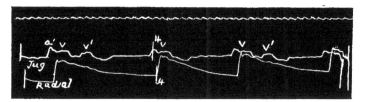

Fig. 248. Simultaneous tracings of the jugular and radial pulses. The jugular pulse is of the ventricular form. During the long pauses in the radial pulse, there are small premature beats, v', in the jugular. The pulse-rate varied from 25 to 30 beats per minute. The patient was just recovering from a series of syncopal and epileptic attacks (Case 81, October 11, 1907).

CASE 82.—*Myocardial degeneration, probably alcoholic.*

Male. Born 1843. I had attended this patient for an attack of erysipelas in 1880, following on a wound on the head. He made a good recovery and led a healthy active life until 1890, when he began to drink heavily at intervals. He would be quite an abstainer for many months, and then he would drink heavily for a few weeks. After 1900 these outbreaks occurred three or four times a year. During his drinking bouts his heart became rapid in its action and dilated, and it was generally because of the extreme prostration that he stopped drinking for a time. When he ceased drinking, in a few weeks' time his heart would be quite normal, and there was no limitation in the heart's power. After rather a long bout in 1907 he pulled himself together, and ceased to take alcohol except in limited quantities.

In May 1909, then aged 66, he consulted me, as he was feeling the heart thumping at times, though he was able to go about his affairs. He was taking no exercise and was getting stout. The pulse was hard, the blood-pressure 210, and there were frequent extra-systoles followed occasionally by a very slight pulsus alternans. The heart's dullness extended to the left as far as the nipple line and the sounds were clear. There was no albumen in the urine.

On March 29, 1910, he was feeling fairly well, he could walk about in comfort. The pulsus alternans was well marked, and the blood-pressure for the large beats was 180. On October 18, 1910, he reported himself as doing well, though rather short of breath.

About the middle of February 1911 he felt slight distress at times across the chest, but the breathing was easier, and there was only slight pulsus alternans. In April of this year he reported that he was feeling weakly and had been so for a fortnight, and that he had a dragging sensation over the heart. He was sleeping badly and felt squeamish and sickly about 3 a.m. He had wakened up early in the morning, feeling breathless. The heart's dullness was 1 inch outside the left nipple line. Six weeks later he was seized with an attack of intense dyspnœa during the night, which lasted four or five hours, and during which he went very blue and was scarcely conscious. He recovered from this and went on fairly well. I saw him on June 17 ; he had been troubled at night with the breathing, though there were no very bad attacks. There was an account from his doctor of an attack of distress (not with bad breathing) when his pulse-rate was nearly 200 per minute. He had also had Cheyne-Stokes respiration. He was lying comfortably in bed when I saw him. The pulse was rather frequent, 110 per minute, and I could detect the pulsus alternans very slightly and for short periods. The heart's dullness now extended 2 inches beyond the nipple line, and the apex was diffuse and rather forcible.

After this the patient gradually went downhill, with attacks of dyspnœa during the night, and he died on August 19, 1911.

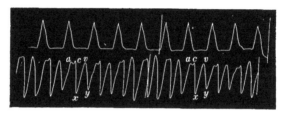

FIG. 249. Simultaneous tracings of radial and jugular pulses, to show the large jugular pulse while the heart was poisoned (Case 83).

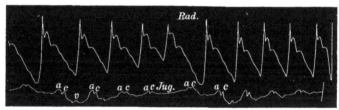

FIG. 250. Taken 10 days after Fig. 249, to show the difference in the character of the radial and jugular pulses in recovery (Case 83).

CASE 83.—*Poisoned heart from arsenic and beer.*

Aged 37. I had this patient under observation for two years, generally for some discomfort after a drinking bout. I saw him on May 15, 1902, complaining of pain across the chest and difficulty in breathing. He had been drinking rather heavily of late and consuming a good deal of beer. He had been for a walk into the country on the morning of the day I saw him, and had taken rather a hilly road and had been seized with the pain and distress in breathing. When I saw him he was in bed with his shoulders raised, tossing from side to side, because of the pain in his chest, which was not then severe, but sufficient to prevent his lying down in comfort. His eyes were slightly jaundiced, and the radial pulse was large, full, and compressible, 130 beats per minute. The apex beat was diffuse and in the middle line, and the dullness extended 2 inches beyond the nipple line on the left and ½ inch to the right of the middle line. There was a loud, blowing systolic murmur heard loudest over the third left costal cartilage. The veins of the neck were full and pulsated largely, the waves ascending as high as the angle of the jaw. The neck was long and the veins stood out, and there were two waves (*a* and *v*) to each beat of the radial pulse, the neck thus presenting the appearance of a continuous movement (Fig. 249). The liver was slightly enlarged, and the subcutaneous tissues covering it (skin and muscle) were very tender on pressure.

With rest and sedatives and abstinence from alcohol, the heart symptoms gradually subsided, the rate became slow, the pulsation in the veins of the neck disappeared, and ten days after the patient was much improved (Fig. 250). The dullness decreased, the heart's apex was inside the nipple line, and the systolic murmur was almost gone.

After this the patient's progress was uninterrupted, and he went on well for several months till he began drinking again, and nine months after he had another attack of heart failure, which followed a very similar course and was again followed by recovery on abstaining from alcohol. At this time it was discovered that the beer was contaminated with arsenic, and this individual stopped the beer-drinking. A year later he developed delirium tremens. He had not been drinking beer but whisky and brandy. This time there was no dilatation of the heart nor pulsation in the veins of the neck, though the pulse was rapid. The patient died from exhaustion.

CASE 84.—*Poisoned heart from streptococcal infection.*

Aged 53. The patient was sent to me by Sir A. Wright on April 14, 1911, because of the condition of his heart. On walking across my consulting-room, the patient was very breathless, and had to sit a few minutes before he had breath to speak. He complained of pain across the chest and breathlessness on the slightest exertion. He was very strong and well up till two years ago, when he had a double pneumonia, and since that time he has been extremely weak and breathless and has been getting gradually worse. Sir A. Wright reported that he had still a streptococcal infection of the lungs which he proposed to treat by vaccines. The patient's face had a jaundice tinge and was slightly livid. The pulse was large and soft, 70 per minute. The heart was dull 1 inch beyond the nipple line on the left. The sounds were clear, and the jugular veins were full and pulsated largely.

The picture presented by the patient so strikingly resembled that of Case 83 that I concluded that the patient's heart was being poisoned, as in that case, by the toxins of some microbic infection, so that I sent him back to Sir A. Wright with this view, and suggested that his treatment by vaccines would be far more likely to be successful than anything I could suggest. The vaccine treatment was employed with the most successful results, so much so that by October the patient had improved so greatly that he was able to go shooting. Two years later I heard that he was leading an active life, and free from any heart trouble.

CASE 85.—*Muscular rheumatism and a myocardial affection. Partial heart-block.*

Male. Aged 60. In May 1909 the patient suffered from some obscure rheumatic pains in the back and right shoulder. One day he was turning the handle to start his motor car, when he was seized with a severe pain in his back. From this time on he suffered from pain and stiffness in the back and muscles of the limbs, which persisted in spite of treatment, including a visit to Harrogate. There was also some swelling of the ankles, and his big toe became tender and swollen. While at Harrogate his heart became slow and irregular, and he was seen by Dr. Wardrop Griffith in July. Dr. Griffith found the pulse-rate between 28 and 30 beats per minute, and on taking a tracing of his radial and jugular pulse he found that the slow rate was due to partial heart-block, the ventricle responding sometimes to every two auricular beats and sometimes to every three. After a few days the rate increased.

I saw the patient on July 23, when there was still a good deal of muscular pain. The heart was normal in size, the sounds faint but free from murmurs, the rate 75 per minute and quite regular. The jugular tracing revealed a wide *a–c* interval, two-fifths of a second (the normal being one-fifth). From this date till the end of the year 1909 he continued to suffer from the muscular pain, and his heart varied in its rate and rhythm.

In a letter written to me by his doctor on November 28, he said he was recovering from his seventh attack of slow heart-rate. At times his heart-rate would reach 110 beats per minute, and would be followed by a period during which the heart-rate would be 40 per minute and under. As a rule the rate would be from 64 to 72 per minute. After January 1910 the pain diminished and finally disappeared, and the heart rhythm has been regular, about 70 per minute. Since then frequent observations have been made up to 1912, and the pulse has always been regular and the patient had quite recovered.

CASE 86.—*Subacute affection of the heart-muscle with heart-block and angina pectoris.*

Female. Born 1851. She was healthy and active, and the mother of eight children. When about 40 years of age (1891), she began to have attacks of palpitation and shortness of breath. At the age of 42 I made the following note : ' heart easily excited, and gets palpitation on going upstairs, and becomes short of breath. The dullness extends 4 inches to the left of the middle line, and there is a large apex beat in the 5th interspace. A systolic murmur is heard at the apex and is propagated into the axilla.'

Apart from the attacks of palpitation and breathlessness, she continued to live an active life, passing through the catamenial period and getting stout. In 1904, at the age of 53, she consulted me, complaining of great shortness of breath and violent throbbing in the neck and in the upper part of the chest in the middle. The pulse was between 90 and 100 beats per minute, large and forcible. There was marked pulsation in the carotids, but no jugular pulsation. There was a faint apex beat in the fifth interspace, and the heart's dullness extended 5 inches to the left of the mid-line. There was a rough murmur, systolic in time, at the apex and at the base. Notwithstanding rest and various remedies she did not improve, and in June she visited Nauheim and underwent a six weeks' cure, baths, exercise, &c., followed by a visit to Switzerland, after which she returned home distinctly worse. She had lost a good deal of flesh, and was unable to undertake effort because of the palpitation and the breathlessness. The distressing throbbing in the neck and upper part of the chest still persisted. In September she became very ill; the temperature began to rise a few degrees, and she developed a severe attack of erythema nodosum in her legs. After a fortnight the fever subsided and the erythema nodosum cleared away. The pulse still continued rapid, and I tried once more the effect of digitalis. She had had it repeatedly before, but it did the heart no good and caused sickness. This time, however, it affected the heart. She began on September 18 with three granules of Nativelle's digitalin, and continued this until the 29th, when she became conscious of the heart missing a beat, with big throbs after the pause. Graphic records of the pulse showed that the intermission was due to heart-block, the stimulus from the auricle failing to reach the ventricle. The drug was stopped on October 4, and the irregularity completely disappeared. The heart became much quieter, the rate being 72 per minute and the dullness extended to the left for 4 inches.

The patient continued in fair health till February 1905, when she developed another attack of erythema nodosum. This subsided in two weeks' time, but before it had quite gone the heart's action again became irregular, due to partial heart-block, this time spontaneously, as she had been taking no digitalis. The heart-block was at times only occasional, but at other times the ventricle responded only to every alternate auricular contraction (2 : 1 rhythm). After some weeks this again disappeared. At this time the heart's dullness was within the nipple line, and the systolic murmur still persisted. From my notes I see that I was in doubt whether the murmur was aortic in origin or only mitral, as it was not propagated into the carotid.

From this date she gradually regained a certain amount of strength, the throbbing in the neck became much less distressing, and she began to put on flesh. In the early part of 1906 she began to experience attacks of pain in the left chest and arm. These were slight at first, but became more severe, till she again consulted me on June 24, 1906. The pain at this time would sometimes only occur in the arm and remain there, with a severe ' aching ', of a somewhat

indefinite character. At other times the pain would start in the chest in front and strike round
the left side to the left shoulder-blade and radiate in an ill-defined manner into the left arm.
The pain would come on at rest, and was usually worst on first waking in the morning.

On examining the heart I found it dull to the nipple line, a systolic murmur being heard
at all the areas, but loudest at the aortic area, propagated up to the clavicle and into the carotids.
The aortic second sound was accentuated. The heart was regular and the blood-pressure
170 mm. Hg. After taking more rest the pain gradually disappeared, but tended to recur
when she was tired or exerted herself too much. In later years the pulse slowed down, and
on examining her in January 1909, I found the pulse-rate was 52 per minute before she got
up from bed, but at that time she could not walk far without inducing the pain in the left
chest and arm, so that she was compelled to rest. If she persisted the pain became intolerable.
In February 1909 she had another violent attack of erythema nodosum, from which she made
a good recovery. The liability to pain in the chest always came on after a period when she had
been more than usually active, so that she takes more rest, and apart from this, she is remarkably well. For the last four years she has remained in good health (1913); the tendency to
attacks of pain is still present when she exerts herself beyond a certain limit.

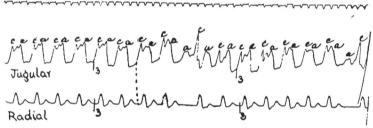

FIG. 251.   Shows partial heart-block—the wide *a–c* interval and occasional dropping out of
a ventricular beat (Case 87).

CASE 87.—*Subacute rheumatic affection of the myocardium.*

Male.   Aged 38.   He complained of shortness of breath on exertion, and of being conscious that his heart was irregular at times, and easily provoked to rapid action on exertion.   He had noticed this first in November 1910, and it has persisted, getting gradually
worse, and was very distressing at times.   He was in good health until May 1910, when he
suffered from slight pain in the right shoulder and elbow, with some grating in the joints on
movement.   He first thought that the pain was due to playing tennis.

I examined the patient on March 15, 1911, when the pain still persisted in his right shoulder,
but he now recognized it as 'rheumatic'.   He was pale and the pulse was soft, rapid (104 per
minute), with frequent intermissions.   The heart's impulse was slight, the dullness extended
on the left to the nipple line, the first sound at the apex was slightly muffled.

An examination of the tracing of the jugular pulse showed that there was a delay between
the auricular and ventricular contractions, and that the intermission in the pulse was due
to the ventricle occasionally failing to respond to an auricular systole (Fig. 251).

Dr. Lewis took an electrocardiogram and found a marked delay between auricular and
ventricular systoles.

The patient was advised to rest, and on examination on the 18th, he showed a perfectly
regular pulse, 75 per minute.   The tracings from the neck still showed an increase in the *a–c*
interval.   On April 1 he felt much better; the pulse was still regular at 65 per minute, and the
a–c interval was of normal duration (⅕ second).   The patient was advised to continue his

work, but to avoid all unnecessary exertion and to rest as much as possible. This he did, and in a few months he felt quite well, and all signs of heart trouble had entirely disappeared. In 1913 he reports that he is quite well.

CASE 88.—*Subacute rheumatic affection of the myocardium.*

Female. Aged 53. She complained of attacks of great prostration, during which she was conscious of her heart beating and thumping in an irregular manner.

She had been in fair health until 1908, when she had a very bad attack of lumbago and sciatica. She was treated at Buxton and Matlock, and returned home in the middle of July, somewhat relieved, but still a good deal crippled.

Shortly after this time she began to be troubled with attacks of breathlessness and palpitation. This continued until August 19, 1908, when she was put to bed and remained there till I saw her on January 14, 1909. Her husband (a doctor) noted at times that her pulse varied in rate and rhythm, sometimes rapid and irregular, at other times very slow.

At times the patient complained of great distress, feeling as if she were about to lose consciousness, and she felt her heart beating in an abnormal fashion. This happened when the heart was increased in rate as well as when it was slow. During the latter part of December she had several attacks of breathlessness which came on without any cause, lasting for ten to fifteen minutes. On January 10 she suffered a great deal from thumping of the heart and fluttering, with breathlessness, and later in the day she lost consciousness for a brief time, and she felt very chilly.

When I was called in to see her on January 14, 1909, she was laid in bed, propped up and feeling greatly distressed in breathing if she lay lower down. She described the attacks of throbbing of the heart, which she also felt in the neck, and which gave rise to a sense of suffocation. The pulse was perfectly regular when I saw her, about 75 per minute. The heart's dullness extended on the left to the nipple line. There was no apex beat to be detected; the sounds were soft; the first sound was somewhat impure, both at the apex and base. There was scarcely any pulsation in the veins of the neck, so that I could only get a very imperfect tracing, but it showed distinct evidences of a wide *a-c* interval.

From this date she continued to have occasional attacks of heart trouble, sometimes going for many days in perfect comfort; at other times the heart would become very slow and irregular in its action. From the doctor's account I cannot be certain that it was due to partial heart-block, but I gather that in all probability this was the case.

Towards the end of 1909 she began to improve, and the heart condition ceased to trouble her, and at the end of the year the symptoms disappeared, with the exception of the weakness. She wrote to me in December, saying that she had kept very well, and had only occasionally slight attacks of breathlessness, but that she was suffering from rheumatism in her feet and ankles.

During 1910 she gradually lost the rheumatic symptoms and steadily improved, and she is now able (1913) to resume her ordinary life, with practically no discomfort. Her heart shows no abnormal sign.

CASE 89.—*Subacute rheumatic affection of the myocardium.*

Male. Aged 40. He complained of breathlessness on walking a short distance and also a sense of exhaustion. If he persisted on walking further he suffered a pain under his left breast, which disappeared in a few minutes after resting. These symptoms appeared in 1910, and became very readily provoked, and he was compelled to give up his work and rest. After a few weeks' rest he went on a voyage for three months and seemed to get all right. He kept well till July 1911, when he had a slight paralytic seizure, affecting the left side, which quickly passed off, but there had lately been a return of this weakness.

Five years before he was examined for life insurance and he was passed as a first-class life; there was no cardiac murmur.

He had suffered of late years on several occasions from attacks of lumbago, and had had typhoid and malarial fevers. There was no specific history. There was no albumen in the urine.

The patient was a big, powerfully-built man and looked healthy. The pulse was soft, regular, 70 beats per minute. Blood-pressure 150 mm. Hg. The heart's impact was slight, and the dullness extended to the left nipple line. There was a rough systolic murmur with a slight musical quality at the apex. A tracing of the jugular pulse showed a slight but distinct increase in the a–c interval and an electrocardiogram, taken by Dr. Lewis, showed also an increase of the period between the auricular and ventricular systoles, and, in addition, the electrocardiogram showed those deflexions characteristic of hypertrophy of the left ventricle.

The patient again consulted me in December 1912, having just returned from a trip to South Africa, and feeling very much better. The only symptom he complained of was a tendency for the feet to swell after a long and hard day's work. He was suffering at the time from lumbago. The heart condition was unaltered, there still being a slight increase in the a–c interval. I again saw him in May 1913, and he was much better.

CASE 90.—*Normal rhythm. Mitral and aortic disease. Digitalis produced heart-block, extra-systoles, and pulsus alternans, and increased the flow of urine, but had no effect on the auricular rate.*

Male. Aged 16. Admitted to hospital complaining of shortness of breath and pain in the left chest, and swelling of the legs and abdomen.

The patient had been well up till 5 years of age, when he began to be short of breath. From this age until admission he had been five times in hospitals. There was no history of rheumatism or sore throat. For some weeks before admission his breathing had been getting worse and his legs had begun to swell.

State on admission. The patient lay propped up in bed ; the breathing was laboured. The face was pale, puffy, and rather distressed looking. The radial pulse was large, collapsing, and regular. The apex beat was large and diffuse outside the nipple line in the fifth and sixth interspaces. There was a rough systolic murmur at the apex and at the aortic area there was a faint diastolic murmur. Both bases of the lungs behind were dull, and there were numerous fine crepitations with deep breathing. The jugular veins were full and pulsating. The liver extended 3 inches below the costal margin and pulsated. Both the liver and jugular pulsations were of the ventricular form as a rule, but occasionally there was a small auricular wave in each. There was some fluid in the abdominal cavity, and the legs and thighs were swollen. There was a slight trace of albumen in the urine.

Treatment and progress. The patient was very ill on admission. On the day after admission, he vomited and expectorated some blood-stained sputum. On October 23 he was found in a state of collapse; the pulse was small, rapid (140–50) and regular, the extremities were cold, the face pallid, the ears blue. He was very restless, the alæ nasi were working, the breathing was distressed. After an inhalation of oxygen and a hypodermic injection of digitalin he rallied. Some hours after he had another attack and again rallied in half an hour. On the following day he was put on tincture of digitalis, 20 minims three times a day, and he gradually improved, the urine increasing and the ascites and dropsy disappearing. The digitalis was continued till November 9, when he had taken 15 drachms. On November 7 his pulse became slower and irregular as a result of partial heart-block, the auricular contractions being unaffected. He vomited on November 7 and 9, and the drug was stopped on the latter date. The patient's general condition was much improved and he felt brighter and better, though the heart's rate and size were not much affected. During this period his temperature was always slightly raised. After a week's cessation of the digitalis it seemed as if the heart was increasing in size, so he was again put on tincture of digitalis, 20 minims three times a day, and this was continued till the 24th, when he had had 9 drachms. On the 21st his radial pulse-rate fell to 100 and became irregular, owing to partial heart-block ; an examination of the jugular tracing showed no change in the auricular rate and rhythm (Fig. 252 and 253).

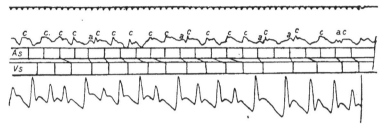

Fig. 252.—Shows an irregular pulse produced by digitalis. The tracing from the neck is a mixture of the jugular and carotid pulse, and most of the auricular waves are not distinct. The intercalated diagram explains the relation of the auricular to the ventricular rhythm, and shows the irregularity is due to partial heart-block (Case 90). (Fig. 252–5 are from *Heart*, vol. ii, p. 361.)

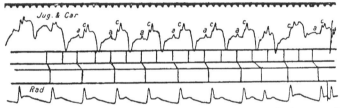

Fig. 253. The interpretation as shown in the diagram represents a 2 : 1 rhythm except in one instance (Case 90).

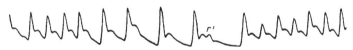

Fig. 254. Tracing of the radial pulse showing an extra-systole (*r′*) followed by the pulsus alternans. The long pause before the extra-systole was due to heart-block (Case 90).

There were also occasional extra-systoles and the pulsus alternans (Fig. 254). Early in the morning of the 25th he vomited and the drug was stopped. From this date he continued to feel very well and comfortable, though there was only a slight improvement in the heart's condition. The liver dullness varied much from time to time without any coincident change in the heart.

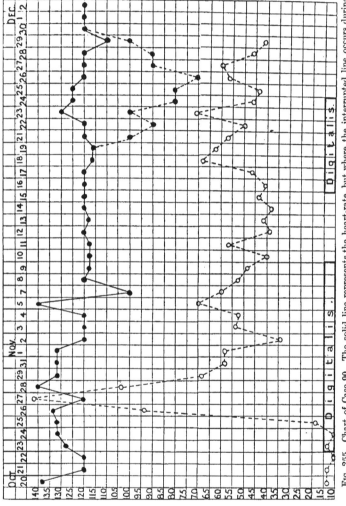

Fig. 255. Chart of Case 90. The solid line represents the heart-rate, but where the interrupted line occurs during a period of partial heart-block, the solid line represents the auricular rate and the interrupted line the ventricular rate The interrupted line with circles represents the amount of urine.

Date.	Drug.	Pulse-Rate.	Blood-Pressure.	Size.	Urine.	Remarks.
Oct.						
20		138		2½–5¾	14	
21		120			14	Vomited and expectorated blood-streaked phlegm.
22		120			10	Vomited several times. Feels much better to-day. Coughing less, breathing easier.
23		128			14	Collapse.
24	Digit. ʒⅰ p.d.	132			5	Better. Still restless, has terrifying dreams. Vomiting.
25		132			19	No vomiting, feels easier.
26		134	120	1¼–5	94	Very much better, dyspnœa gone, can lie down and move about in bed quite comfortably.
27		120	132		141	Feels very well.
28		140	126		104	
29		132	120		68	
30					56	
31		132	130	1¼–4¾	58	
Nov.						
1		132	130		34	
2		120	132		54	Feels well, looks pale. Lungs clear.
3		120	120	1¼–5	53	Feels well.
4		120	114		70	Feels well.
5		140	130		60	Feels well.
7		100	130		53	Feels well, vomited twice to-day. Pulse irregular (partial block).
8		120	124		49	Feels well, pulse regular, no more vomiting.
9	ʒxv Digit. stopped	118			57	Vomited twice this morning. Pulse irregular.
10		118	128		40	Feels well, no nausea, pulse regular.
11		118	118		44	Feels well, liver 3 inches below ribs.
12		120	128		34	Feels well.
13		118	116		42	
14		120	130		39	Feels well.
15		120	118	2¾–6¼	44	Feels well.
16	Digit.	120	118		42	Feels well.
17	ʒⅰ p.d.	120	120		47	Feels well.
18		116	122	2–6	68	Slight headache last night.
19		116	118		63	No headache.
21		A120* V100	112	1¾–6	57	Feels well.
22		A120 V 90	120		50	Feels well, pulse irregular, partial block.
23		A130 V100	120		71	Feels well.
24	ʒix Digit. stopped	A125 V 80	134		46	Feels well.
25		A125 V 80	134	1½–5½	44	Vomited twice this morning.
26		A120 V 70	134		51	Feels very well.
27		A120 V 90				
28		A120 V 90	108	1½–5	60	Feels well.
29		A110 V100	120		64	Feels well.
30		A120 V120	130		46	Feels well.
Dec.						
1		120	126		41	Feels well.
2		120	114			

* A and V. The auricular and ventricular rates respectively, counted from the graphic records (see Chart, Fig. 255).

CASE 91.—*Partial heart-block, produced by digitalis and by swallowing.*

Male. Aged 25. Consulted me for a stiffness and swelling in sundry joints, wrists, ankle, and knee, on May 4, 1906. The heart was rapid in its action, 120 per minute ; slightly enlarged, with systolic mitral and tricuspid murmurs. There was marked pulsation in the neck, of which Fig. 256 is a tracing. The movement due to the carotid was always large, and forms a marked feature (wave *c* in all the tracings). In the course of the next fortnight there gradually developed double aortic murmurs. By May 23, under treatment, he had gradually improved, the rate of the heart falling to 90 beats per minute.

As the *a–c* interval, space *A*, in Fig. 256, showed a delay in the function of conductivity, I reasoned that the carditis had probably affected the auriculo-ventricular fibres, and had

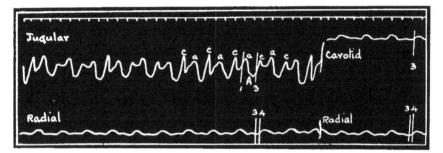

Fig. 256. The jugular tracing shows a wide *a–c* interval (space *A*) (Case 91, before digitalis).

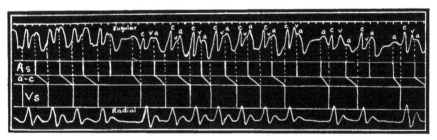

Fig. 257. After taking nineteen digitalin granules the pulse became irregular, which the intercalated diagram shows to be due to dropping out of the ventricular systoles—a mild form of heart-block (Case 91).

depressed the function of conductivity. I administered digitalin granules, one to be taken three times a day.

I kept him under observation, but could detect no change in the heart's action until May 30, after he had taken nineteen granules. On this date I found the pulse at times very irregular. Fig. 257 is a tracing, showing the nature of the irregularity. Between the jugular and radial pulses I have intercalated a diagram illustrating the events in the tracing from the neck. It will be noticed that before a ventricular beat drops out there is a gradual lengthening of the *a–c* interval, and that the dropping out of the ventricular systole is manifestly due to an increased depression of the conductivity of the fibres joining *a* and *v*—that is to say, the stimulus from the auricle is blocked before it reaches the ventricle. I stopped the digitalin, and a few days later all signs of irregularity had disappeared. The patient himself was conscious when his heart was irregular, and I remarked to him that the irregularity had gone ; he replied, ' I can bring it back.' I asked him how he could do so, and he said, ' By swallowing.' I asked him to swallow, and he did so, and immediately I detected long pauses in his pulse, while, on auscultation of the heart, no sounds were heard during the pauses. I took a large number of tracings for an hour and a half, during which time he swallowed forty or fifty times, and the alteration in the pulse-rate never failed to appear. The characteristic changes are seen in Fig. 258 and 259. After swallowing there are each time three regular beats, then the pulse slows in the manner shown in the tracings. After two or three slow beats the rate of the heart increased for six or seven beats, then gradually slowed in the manner shown in the latter part of the tracings. Occasionally during the secondary slowing one ventricular systole would drop out, as is shown in Fig. 259. In Fig. 259 I have intercalated a diagram which shows the nature of the arrhythmia, and it can there be seen that the long pauses in these tracings are preceded by an increase of the a–c interval, just as happened when the patient was under the influence of digitalis (Fig. 257), and that the dropping of the ventricular systole was due to a block of the stimulus from auricle to ventricle. The numbers given under the radial tracings

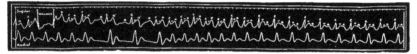

FIG. 258. Shows a reflex effect of the vagus due to swallowing. After the act of swallowing the pulse became very slow, because of the dropping out of the ventricular systoles (see diagram in Fig. 259). After this the heart's rate increased slightly, then became slow again (Case 91).

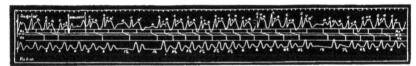

FIG. 259. Shows the same as Fig. 258, except that during the second period of slowing after swallowing there is a long pause due to the dropping out of a ventricular systole.

in Fig. 259 represent tenths of seconds, and from these numbers the manner in which the rate of the pulse varies can better be realized.

The susceptibility of the heart to the act of swallowing continued for a week, then entirely disappeared. There is no doubt it arose through reflex stimulation of the vagus induced by the act of swallowing. The analogy between the effects of digitalis and of reflex stimulation of the inhibition by swallowing appears worthy of note, as it indicates that the action of the drug here is exerted through its effects on the inhibitory centre, and not through the changes it induces in the heart-muscle directly. Digitalis, as is generally known, affects the vagus centre and also the myocardium, and it is often difficult to determine which is the factor in its therapeutic effects.

CASE 92.—*Mitral stenosis. Digitalis produced slowing of the whole heart, extra-systoles, and temporary auricular fibrillation.*

Female. Aged 28. Consulted me on April 24, 1907, complaining of swelling of the abdomen, shortness of breath, and palpitation. She began to feel ill in November of the previous year;

she had rheumatic fever fifteen years previously. The face was dusky, the breathing laboured, the legs and abdomen swollen. She passed a small amount of urine. There was rapid pulsation in the veins of the neck—two to each radial pulse (Fig. 260)—the pulse was small and regular, blood-pressure 100 mm. Hg. A thrill systolic in time could be felt over the upper part of the chest. The movement of the heart farthest to the left was 3 inches beyond the nipple, and showed an indrawing during ventricular systole (giving rise to an inverted cardiogram). The heart's dullness extended half an inch to the right of the sternum. At the apex there was heard a presystolic murmur, a diastolic murmur, and a reduplicated second sound. At the base there was a loud, rough murmur systolic in time, heard also over the carotid. There was also a slight diastolic murmur at the aortic area. Over the heart's dullness inside the nipple there was another murmur systolic in time, and while listening one could imagine that two hearts were working, a series of sounds being heard immediately under the stethoscope, while another series of sounds could be heard faintly and seemingly at a distance.

Sometimes when the heart was regular but slow, a confusing change took place. During the diastole of the heart there was a sudden increase in the intensity of the diastolic murmur, in

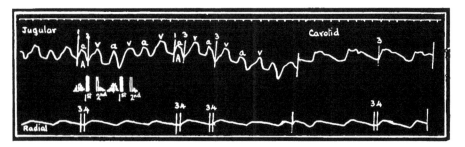

Fig. 260. Shows two pulsations in the jugular tracing (a and v) to one radial pulse. The a–c interval (space A) is increased. The shading shows the sounds of the heart and the murmurs present at the apex, viz. a presystolic murmur separated by a brief interval from the first sound, a reduplicated second sound followed by a diastolic murmur. These features of the jugular pulse and sounds and murmurs were always present when the patient was not under the influence of digitalis until the final establishment of auricular fibrillation (Case 92).

fact a mid-diastolic murmur followed after a pause by the first sound. When I drew the position of the murmur under a tracing I found it corresponded to the position of the auricular wave in the jugular tracing (Fig. 260), and no doubt it was due to the auricular systole. When the heart became very slow, because of the digitalis, the longer rest gave the auriculo-ventricular fibres time to recover and the murmur was heard nearer and nearer the first sound, and sometimes it ceased to be heard. This only happened when the heart became very slow and the auricular wave in the jugular approached quite close to the carotid, as in Fig. 261 and 262. The patient was put on the digitalis, squills, and calomel pill, one taken three times a day. On May 1, after taking eighteen pills, she was passing more urine. She felt much better on the 8th—the swelling had gone from the abdomen and the legs were less in size. On the 15th the swelling had all gone, she had a little diarrhœa and felt sickly, but breathed easier and was able to walk better. The heart was slow and irregular. On examination there was only one wave visible in the jugular, and when recorded it was found synchronous with the carotid pulse (Fig. 263). There was no presystolic murmur, but only a long diastolic murmur at the apex. The tracing shows the jugular pulse to be of the ventricular type; *auricular fibrillation had occurred.* The pills were stopped, but the heart was still irregular on the 19th. On the 26th it was regular and the jugular pulse double waved, as in Fig. 260. She felt better, but the legs and abdomen were swelling again. Digitalin granules were prescribed, one three times a day. On the 31st the pulse became irregular, and tracings taken on this day and on June 2 showed that it was due to the slowing of the whole heart. On June 4 the heart had again taken on auricular fibrillation, which persisted until the 17th, when the auricular contractions appeared and the heart showed frequent pauses. She was taking one granule of digitalin per day until the 23rd, when it was stopped, and on the 28th the heart was found rapid and regular and the pulsation in the veins double waved, as in Fig. 260. Up till November 4 these reactions due to digitalis continued to appear ; sometimes auricular fibrillation would appear and sometimes the long pauses as in Fig. 261, and occasionally extra-systoles (Fig. 264). A few days after stopping the digitalin the heart invariably became regular. On November 6, after digitalin treatment had ceased, auricular fibrillation started spontaneously, the heart beating rapidly, but it could be slowed by digitalis or strophanthus.

Interpretation of tracings. The tracings showing auricular fibrillation call for no special description, as they resemble the tracings of the ventricular venous pulse so fully described elsewhere. The only point which seems novel is that when it began under the influence of digitalis it was a slow rhythm resembling in some respects the cases of nodal bradycardia.

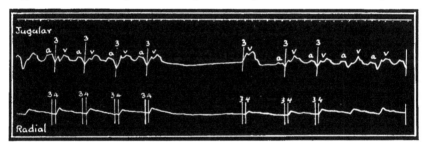

FIG. 261. Shows the temporary arrest of the whole heart from digitalis (Case 92). The first beat after the long pause is an escaped ventricular beat, there being no auricular beat preceding it.

On the other hand, when it started independently of digitalin the heart's action was rapid, as is usually the case.

In Fig. 261 there is a long pause in which the whole heart stands still ; during these pauses no sound could be heard and the tracings show the auricles arrested as well as the ventricle—differing thus from heart-block. It will be observed that after the long pause the radial beats were at first small, then gradually increased in size, but as the pulse was small and soft the ink polygraph did not show the beats well ; I therefore took several tracings with the Dudgeon sphygmograph with the same result. Here the gradual increase of the radial pulse after the long pause is very evident. The pauses lasted sometimes from three to four seconds, but sometimes they lasted nineteen-fifths of a second. This standstill of the whole heart is probably due to vagus stimulation. The staircase phenomenon after the pause has been shown experimentally to occur after a vagus standstill of the whole heart, and, according to Gaskell, arises in two ways : (1) From exhaustion of contractility—the vagus stimulation depresses all the functions and their restoration is gradual, that of restoration of contractility being shown by a gradual increase in the strength of the beat. (2) From depression of conductivity, the stimulus for contraction not spreading throughout the whole heart, but reaching at first a limited number of fibres, and gradually reaching more and more until they all respond. The staircase phenomena in this case may possibly be due to the filling of the empty artery.

The pauses were not always long, and the heart would beat slowly for a short period.

When this happened, the relation of the auricular systole to the ventricular underwent
an interesting change. As I have already remarked, the *a–c* interval was always increased
in this patient, but digitalis did not interfere with the conduction of the stimulus from

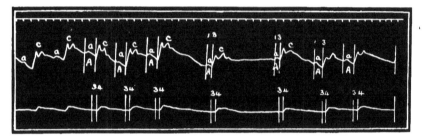

FIG. 262. The upper tracing was taken high up in the neck and shows a slight auricular wave (*a*)
preceding the carotid pulse (*c*). After a long pause the *a–c* interval (space *A*) is much diminished
(Case 92).

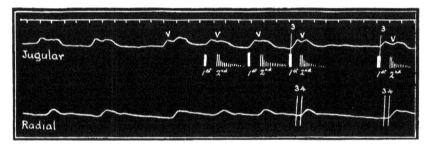

FIG. 263. Shows the inception of auricular fibrillation after digitalis. Compare the jugular pulse
and the murmurs with Fig. 260 (Case 92).

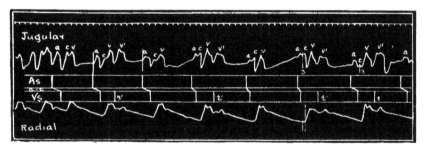

FIG. 264. Extra-systoles, *r'*, probably of ventricular origin, due to digitalis. The waves *v'* are
due to the extra-systole. There are occasional long pauses when no extra-systole occurred,
followed by a shortening of the *a–c* interval (Case 92).

auricle to ventricle. When the heart acted slowly the auriculo-ventricular fibres obtained
a long rest, with the result that the *a–c* interval gradually diminished. Fig. 262 shows the
carotid and radial pulses. The carotid is taken from under the right jaw, but the wave (*a*) due

to the auricular systole is present in the tracing. When the heart was beating at the more rapid rate, the a–c interval (spaces A) was nearly two-fifths in duration, whereas when beating at the slower rate it became less than one-fifth in duration. This was brought out particularly well in some tracings, where the auricular wave, a, gradually approaches the carotid and ventricular wave till it is not discernible as a distinct wave (Fig. 261). It was during periods such as this that I made out the change in the relation of the presystolic murmur to the first sound and its apparent cessation.

Another phase that occasionally occurred during the irregular period was the appearance of extra-systoles. Fig. 264 is a characteristic example, and shows that the extra-systoles are probably of ventricular origin, though the pauses following the extra-systoles are of varying duration, due to the influence of the digitalis on the sinus.

This case, as I have said, is an exception to the general rule that when there is a delayed a–c interval, digitalis increases it and produces blocking.

Records of blood-pressure showed generally a fall (100 mm. Hg.) when there was much dropsy, and a rise with slowing of the heart to 135 or 140 mm. Hg. Sometimes, however, the pressure was 130 with dropsy, and no increase occurred with its disappearance and the coincident improvement of the patient's condition after taking digitalis.

The patient died in March 1908.

INDEX

PAGE

ABDOMINAL AORTA
    tracing of 165
    pulse of, compared with the liver
      pulse 165, 166
ABDOMINAL VEINS
    stasis in 98
ABNORMAL RHYTHMS . . 25
A–C INTERVAL
    cases showing great increase of . 263,
              416, 464, 466
    definition of . xxi, 149, 151, 153, 262
    increased 263, 266
    in cases of extra-systole . . 193
      significance of . . . 193
      variations in duration of . 193
ACCELERATOR NERVES . . 41
ACCUMULATION
    of blood in abdominal veins . . 98
ACONITE 384
ACUTE ŒDEMA
    of the lungs in heart failure . . 56
ADAMS-STOKES DISEASE . . 261
ADAMS-STOKES SYNDROME . 49
    in nodal bradycardia . . 262
    See also HEART-BLOCK . . 261
ADHERENT PERICARDIUM . . 343
    inverted cardiogram in . 126
    liver pulse in 345
ADHESIVE MEDIASTINO-PERI-
    CARDITIS 343
    ætiology 343
    Broadbent's sign of . . 343
    prognosis of 345
    symptoms . . . 343
    Talbot and Cooper on . . 344
    treatment of . . . 345
ADRENALIN 97
AFFERENT NERVES
    See NERVES OF THE HEART . . 41
AGENTS INFLUENCING
    the vaso-motor system . . 97
AIR, BELCHING OF
    after an attack of angina pectoris . 91
AIR HUNGER 51

PAGE

AIR SUCTION . . . 78
    in angina pectoris . . 78, 79
    in paroxysmal tachycardia . . 243
ALBUMINURIA
    in dilatation of the heart . . 309
ALCOHOLIC HEART . . . 22
    dilatation of 307
    rate in 172
ALIMENTARY TOXINS
    and the heart 291
ALTERATION IN POINT OF ORIGIN
    OF CARDIAC CYCLE . . . 181
AMYL NITRITE
    action of 381
    in angina pectoris . . 85, 382
ANACROTIC PULSE
    in aortic stenosis . . . 339
ANATOMY OF THE HEART . . 32
ANEURYSM
    pulsation of the neck in . . 146
ANGINA PECTORIS
    active lesions in . . . 83
    air suction in . . . 78, 79
    amyl nitrite in . . . 85
    aortic aneurysm with . . 71
    aortic lesions in . . . 83
    aortic regurgitation with . 71, 83
    aortic stenosis with . . 71, 83
    aortic valvular disease with . 71, 83
    arterial pressure in . . 71, 79
    arterial pressure during attacks of . 79
    association with exhaustion of heart
      muscles 72
    atheroma of coronary arteries with 71
    belching of air during an attack of 78
    bodily exertion causing . 77, 80
    bromide of ammonium in . . 84
    cardio-sclerosis with . . 77, 395, 397
    cause of attacks after a meal . 99
    character of the attacks . . 77
    chloral in 85
    chloroform in . . . 86
    cold causing 99
    conditions inducing an attack of 71, 77
    conditions predisposing to an attack
      of 71, 72
    conductivity in cases of . . 62

PAGE

ANGINA PECTORIS (continued)—
constriction of chest in . . . 78
contraction of intercostal muscles
in 70
coronary arteries in . . . 72
danger in slight attacks of . . 83
death during an attack of 397, 399, 402,
404, 410
definition of term . . . 72
dilatation absent in severe . . 301
disease of the coronary arteries
with . 394, 395, 397, 398, 401, 403,
407, 411
duration of the attacks of . . 77
effect of dilatation in . . . 85
excitability in cases of . . 89, 90
excitement causing . . . 71
exhausted heart muscle and exhausted nervous system with 72, 73
exhaustion of contractility causing 72, 73
exhaustion of left ventricle causing 72
extra-systoles during an attack of 79,
404, 423
feeling of impending dissolution in 79
food in 85
full stomach a cause of . . 77
herpes zoster compared with . 65
hyperalgesia after an attack of 68, 80
hyperalgesic areas in . . 69, 80
impaired nourishment of the heart
muscle causing . . . 77
improvement of condition of heart
in 84
increase of urine in attack of . . 80
in mediastino-pericarditis . . 344
irritable focus in spinal cord causing
recurrence of 77
mental excitement causing . 71, 77
mechanism of production of symptoms of 76
merely a group of symptoms . . 72
method of investigation in a case of 82
micturition after an attack of . 78
nitro-glycerine in . . . 86
in mitral stenosis . . 334, 426
over-exertion causing . 73, 386, 389, 391
pain in 78
persistence of pain after an attack
of 79
pathology of heart with . 71, 72
increased peripheral resistance causing 71
pain or viscero-sensory reflex . 69
perspiration during an attack of . 78
position assumed during an attack
of 78
prognosis in . . . 80, 81, 260
' pseudo-angina ', a bad term . 81
the pulse in (illustrative cases) . 79
pulsus alternans with . 81, 259, 260
a reflex protective phenomenon . 62
region of pain in 65

PAGE

ANGINA PECTORIS (continued)—
resemblance of, to intermittent
claudication 72
rest in 84
saliva increased in . . . 78
sense of impending death during
an attack of 79
a sign of impaired contractility . 72
site of pain during an attack of . 78
state of arteries during an attack
of 79
state of heart during an attack of . 79
stimulation of skin a cause of . 77
suction of air during an attack of 78, 79
summation of stimuli causing . 72
susceptibility of nervous system
in 81
a symptom of exhausted contractility 73
a symptom of exhausted heart
muscle 72
symptoms after an attack of . 79
symptoms during an attack of . 78
tendency to recurrent attacks of . 80
tonicity with 72
treatment by ammonium bromide . 84
treatment by chloral . . . 85
treatment during an attack of . 85
treatment of condition inducing . 84
trinitrin in 86
unconsciousness during . . 78
urine, increased secretion after . 78
urine increased in . . . 79
vagal reflexes in . . . 69
valvular disease with . . . 89
vaso-dilators in . . . 85
vaso-motor 99
viscero-motor reflex in . . . 69

ANIMALS
insensitiveness of viscera in . . 59

ANTIARIN
action on tonicity . . . 30

AORTA
aneurysm of, with angina pectoris . 400
in the fixation of the heart . . 39
tracings of abdominal . . . 165

AORTIC DISEASE
ætiology of 337

AORTIC REGURGITATION . . 339
angina pectoris in . . . 339
arteries visible in . . 131, 339
capillary pulsation in . . . 339
in endocarditis 282
facial aspect in 340
movement of liver in . . . 340
murmur characteristic of . . 339
pulse in 132, 339
symptoms of heart failure due to . 341

PAGE

AORTIC STENOSIS . . . 338
  angina pectoris with . . . 339
  murmur characteristic of . . 338
  pulse in 339
  symptoms of 338

AORTIC VALVE DISEASE . . 337
  angina pectoris in . . . 341
  congenital 338
  hypertrophy of the left ventricle in 338
  after rheumatism . . . 338
  from sclerotic changes . . . 340

AORTIC VALVES
  rupture of 338

APERIENTS 385

APEX BEAT 116
  alteration of, due to retraction of
    lung 127
  in aortic regurgitation . . . 340
  auricular wave in . . . 120
  definition of 116
  due to extra-systoles . . . 190
  due to right ventricle . . 124, 125
  how to record 105
  in auricular fibrillation . 219, 222
  period of contraction . . . 118
  period of filling of the ventricles . 120
  period of relaxation of ventricular
    muscle 119
  period of ventricular outflow . 119
  and the retraction of the lung . 118
  interpretation of a tracing of, due
    to left ventricle . . . 117
  showing coupled beats . . . 375
  systolic plateau in tracings of . 119
  time of opening of auriculo-ventri-
    cular valves 120
  variation in position of . . . 116

APEX OF HEART
  arrangement of muscle-fibres at . 39
  movement of 116

APOPLEXY
  pulmonary 55

APPEARANCE OF THE PATIENT . 44

AREAS
  of pain in affections of the heart . 65
  of pain in hyperalgesia . . . 65

ARM
  pain in, during an attack of angina
    pectoris . . . 66, 67, 68, 78
  development of 63
  nerve-supply of 63
  reason for heart pain felt in . . 69

ARTERIAL DEGENERATION
  and high blood-pressure . . 139
  and cardio-sclerosis . 140, 308, 317

ARTERIAL DEGENERATION (continued)—
  blood-pressure in . . . 316
  chloral in 320
  blood-pressure of doubtful value in
    prognosis 318
  bromide of ammonium in . . 320
  definition of . . . xxi, 314
  early symptoms of . . . 316
  and extra-systoles . . . 316
  and heart failure . . . 317
  heart in 317
  and auricular fibrillation . . 317
  and obliteration of the capillaries . 314
  oxygen in 320
  prognosis in 318
  iodide of potassium in . . . 320
  recognition of 319
  sleep in 320
  subjective pneumonia in . . 317
  superficial arteries in . . . 316
  symptoms of 314
  treatment 318
  treatment in mild cases . . 319
  conditions causing . . . 314

ARTERIAL PRESSURE
  in angina pectoris . . 71, 79
  during attacks of angina pectoris . 79
  in cardiac asthma . . . 53
  effect of capillary obliteration on . 315
  cause of 137
  in Cheyne-Stokes respiration 54, 55
  with exhaustion of contractility . 79
  difficulties in obtaining . . 139
  digital examination of . . . 139
  effect of digitalis on . . . 359
  diminished . . . 143, 144
  effect of dilatation of the heart on . 141
  graphic records of . . . 142
  heart failure with increased . . 141
  causes of increased . . . 140
  method of measuring . . . 136
  increased by diminution of capil-
    lary field 314
  action of nitrites on . . . 143
  with the pulsus alternans . . 260
  resistance of arterial walls in
    estimating 140
  significance of a fall of . . . 144
  treatment of high . . . 143
  in valvular disease . . . 79

ARTERIAL PULSE
  examination of 129
  inspection of the arteries . . 131
  nature of movements of . . 129
  superiority of digital examination . 129

ARTERIAL WALLS
  condition of 131
  in estimating arterial pressure . 139

PAGE

ARTERIES
digital examination of . . 129, 131
function of elastic coats of . . 137
hypertrophy of muscular coat of . 139
inspection of 131
in surgical operations how recognized 130
state of, during an attack of angina
pectoris 79
visible movements of . . . 131

ARTERIOLES
dilatation of, in exophthalmic
goitre 131
dilatation of, in aortic regurgitation 131

ARTERIO-SCLEROSIS
causation of 314

ARTERY
nature of movements of tortuous 130, 131
size of the 132
supplying auriculo-ventricular bundle, condition of, in auricular
fibrillation 217
changes in radial due to fever . 279

ARTIFICIAL WAVES
in tracings 136

ASTHMA, CARDIAC . . . 53
arterial pressure with . . . 53
associated symptoms . . . 53
in cardio-sclerosis . . . 53
conditions giving rise to . . 54
pulse in 53
sleep with 53
signs of 53
treatment of 54

ATHEROMA OF CORONARY ARTERIES
angina pectoris in . . . 71

ATROPINE 384
in heart-block 384

ATTACKS
of breathlessness in heart failure . 53

AUDITORY NERVE
stimulation of 59

AURICLE
electrocardiogram of . . . 110
hypertrophy of right, in tricuspid
stenosis 337
starting-place of the heart's contraction 35

AURICULAR DEPRESSION
in a jugular pulse . . . 149

AURICULAR DIASTOLE
effect of, on the jugular pulse . 149

AURICULAR EXTRA-SYSTOLES . 195

AURICULAR FIBRILLATION . 181
a grave complication of . . 341
and angina pectoris . . . 228
associated with mitral disease . 340

PAGE

AURICULAR FIBRILLATION (continued)—
character of the pulse . . . 228
clinical characteristics . . . 227
common in middle-aged . . 340
condition of auriculo-ventricular
bundle in 217
continuous laboured breathing in . 52
doubtful result of . . . 230
earthy countenance in . . . 340
effect on the heart's efficiency . 225
electrocardiogram of . . . 110
end very varied 341
heart failure in 227
history associated with rheumatic
fever 227
in pneumonia 281
marked effect of digitalis in . 225
pain, area in 68
patients' sensations . . . 227
prognosis in 229
pulmonary haemorrhages in . . 56
Sutherland on, in rheumatic fever . 281
symptoms of heart failure . . 228
treatment, general . . . 232
treatment in chronic cases . . 234
transient attacks of . . . 231

AURICULAR FLUTTER
a common clinical condition . . 237
and digitalis 248
Cheyne-Stokes respiration . . 240
conditions giving rise to . . 238
definition of . . . xxi, 236
explanation of tracings . . 241
jugular pulse in 240
loss of consciousness in . . 49
MacWilliam's work on . . 237
prognosis in 249
pulsus alternans in . . . 246
radial pulse in 245
relation to auricular fibrillation . 247
relation to paroxysmal tachycardia 247
symptomatology 238
treatment of 249

AURICULAR HYPERTROPHY
with ventricular jugular pulse,
significance of 158

AURICULAR LIVER PULSE . . 162
case of 426

AURICULAR MOVEMENTS . . 120

AURICULAR MUSCLE
atrophy of 158

AURICULAR PRESSURE CURVE . 148

AURICULAR SYSTOLE
disappearance from normal place
in cardiac cycle . 157, 158, 220, 221
effect of, on radial pulse . . 269
murmurs due to . . . 323, 331

PAGE

AURICULAR VENOUS PULSE
See JUGULAR PULSE . . . 145

AURICULAR WAVES . . . 120
in apex tracings, cause of . 120, 125
in apex tracings, time of . . 120
in apex tracings in heart-block . 265, 269, 273
in a jugular pulse, cause of . 149, 156
in the ventricular jugular pulse . 157

AURICULO-VENTRICULAR BUNDLE 32
arterial supply of . . . 35
in cardio-sclerosis . . . 318
in arrhythmia 264
relation of, to central fibrous body 264
impaired in cases with extra-
systole 192
function of fibres of . . 35, 185
healthy in heart-block . . . 270
affected in influenza . . . 280
lesions of 184
involved in mitral stenosis . . 330
position of 32
isolation of 32
association with auricular fibrillation 276
in paroxysmal tachycardia . . 258
pathology of, illustrative cases . 397
in diphtheria 280
in puerperal fever . . . 280
in rheumatic fever . . 280, 281
in septic poisoning . . . 280
starting-place of heart's contraction 34

AURICULO-VENTRICULAR NODE
constitution of 34
function of 35, 37
position of 34
in cases of auricular fibrillation . 276
in paroxysmal tachycardia . . 258
starting the heart's contraction . 34
structure of 35

AURICULO-VENTRICULAR SEPTUM
action of muscles on . . . 39

AURICULO-VENTRICULAR VALVES
opening of 120

AUTONOMIC NERVOUS SYSTEM
insensitiveness of structures supplied by 58

BACK PRESSURE
theory of 5

BATHS
in treatment 364
Nauheim 365

BEAT OF THE HEART
effects of exhaustion . . . 14

BED
lying in, effect of on heart . 52, 307

PAGE

BELLOWS MURMUR . . . 339

BILIARY COLIC. See COLIC.

BLEEDING
character of, in capillary ob
litera-
tion 315

BLOCKED AURICULAR EXTRA-
SYSTOLES 203

BLOOD ANTISEPTICS . . . 289

BLOOD-PRESSURE
See ARTERIAL PRESSURE.

BODILY COMFORT
in treatment 353

BODILY EXERTION
a cause of angina pectoris . 71, 73

BOWEL
insensitiveness of . . . 58
resection of, in conscious subject . 58

BRADYCARDIA
classes of 177
causes of 178
normal bradycardia . . . 177
extreme cases of 178
definition of 177
loose employment of term . . 177
due to vagus stimulation . . 177

BRAIN
diagram showing relation to sensory nerve 60

BRANDY
during an attack of angina pectoris 85

BREASTS
hyperalgesia of 88

BREATHING
inability to stop 52
laboured, with dilatation of the
heart 52
laboured, on exertion . . . 53
laboured, in heart failure . . 52
laboured, a sign of exhaustion of
the heart 53
exercises in œdema of the lungs 309, 312
rapid, a sign of heart failure . . 52

BREATHLESSNESS . . . 51
attacks of 53
sudden attack of, in aortic regurgitation 341
in heart failure 51
cause of 51
due to infarct in lungs . . . 56
treatment of 263
See also ASTHMA, CARDIAC.

BRIGHT'S DISEASE
mitral regurgitation in . . . 335
pericarditis in 282

PAGE

BROADBENT AND THE PULSE 129, 131

BROADBENT'S SIGN
in mediastino-pericarditis . . 343

BROMIDE OF AMMONIUM . . 94
in angina pectoris . . 84
in exophthalmic goitre . . 174

BROMIDES 382
in cardio-sclerosis . . . 320

CALOMEL 312

CAPILLARY FIELD, DIMINUTION
OF 314
a factor in raising arterial pressure 315
effect of, on the heart . . . 315
in cardio-sclerosis . . . 314
effects of 315
effect of, on blood-pressure . . 315
evidences of 316

CAPILLARY PULSATION
in aortic regurgitation . . . 339

CARDIAC ASPIRATION . . 120
due to ventricular systole . . 122
causing movements of the liver . 122

CARDIAC ASTHMA . . . 53
pulsus alternans in . . . 53

CARDIAC CYCLE
diagram of events in a . . . 148

CARDIAC EXHAUSTION
and susceptibility to nerve stimulation 73

CARDIAC NEURASTHENIA . . 89

CARDIAC NEUROSIS . . . 89

CARDIAC RESPONSE
in cardio-sclerosis . . . 317
limitation of, a sign of heart failure 12
and prognosis 349
field of 45

CARDIOGRAM
nature of a 148
inverted 126, 127

CARDIO-MOTOR CENTRES . . 40

CARDIO-SCLEROSIS
aetiology 313
and aneurysm 400
and angina pectoris . . . 83
and arterial degeneration . . 315
auricular fibrillation in . . 317
with auricular fibrillation, effect of
digitalis in 250
auriculo-ventricular bundle in . 317
blood-pressure in . . . 316
cardiac asthma in . . . 317
change in symptoms with dilatation 317
condition of arteries in . . 316
Cheyne-Stokes respiration in . 317

PAGE

CARDIO-SCLEROSIS (continued)—
exhaustion of conductivity in . 317
exhaustion of contractility in . 317
definition of . . . xxii, 313
diet in 319
dilatation of the heart in . . 318
disease of the kidneys with . . 317
effect of digitalis in . . . 312
extra-systoles in 317
extreme, without dilatation . . 317
heart-block due to . . . 317
illustrative cases . 399, 407, 437
irregularities in 317
mitral regurgitation in . . 317
murmurs in 317
paroxysmal tachycardia in . . 250
pathology of 314
primitive cardiac tissue in . . 270
prognosis in 318
progress of 314
pulsus alternans with . . . 317
reason for variety of symptoms in . 318
reserve force in 317
of rheumatic origin . . . 313
sensory phenomena in . . . 319
significance of cardiac asthma in . 318
symptoms of 315
diversity of symptoms in . . 316
and syphilis 314
treatment of 318
visceroo-motor reflex in . . 61

CARDITIS
produced by febrile affections . 277,
283, 285, 287

CAROTID ARTERY
relation of, to jugular vein . . 146

CAROTID PULSE
movement due to . . . 153
as a standard 152

CAROTID WAVE
in the jugular pulse . . . 153

CASES ILLUSTRATING
effect of ammonium bromide in
angina pectoris . 392, 393, 414
pathology of cardio-sclerosis 446, 447
effect of digitalis on the heart . 418,
430-1, 433
heart-block . . . 448-53
relation of heart-block to auricular
fibrillation 451
heart's power of recovery . . 430
effects of digitalis on auricular
fibrillation . . 418, 430-1, 433
the inception of auricular fibrillation 420,
423, 425
bradycardia in auricular fibrillation 454
the pathology of auricular fibrillation 453
paroxysmal tachycardia . 438, 442-6

PAGE

CASES ILLUSTRATING (continued)—
   significance of the pulsus alternans
          446–8
   character of the pulse in angina pec-
    toris   412, 413, 414
   severe heart affection in pneumonia 280

CAUSES OF MYOCARDIAL AFFEC-
  TIONS   2

CAUSES OF CONFUSED DIAGNOSIS   3

CAUSES OF VARIATION
   of pressure in the auricles and
    jugular veins .   .   .   149
   Frey's explanation of .   .   149

CELLULAR FOCI
   in heart muscle, in rheumatic fever 284

CENTRAL FIBROUS BODY
   function of   .   .   .   39
   position of.   .   .   .   39
   relation of, to auriculo-ventricular
    bundle   39

CEREBRAL ANÆMIA .   .   24
   in heart-block   .   .   .   272

CEREBRAL EMBOLISM
   in mitral stenosis   .   .   334

CEREBRAL FUNCTIONS
   effects of failing heart on .   50

CEREBRO-SPINAL NERVOUS SYS-
  TEM   60

CERVICAL FASCIA
   in the fixation of the heart .   39

CERVICAL NERVES   .   .   63

CHEST, CONSTRICTION OF .   47
   in angina pectoris   .   69, 73
   during an attack of angina pectoris 73
   a viscero-motor reflex .   .   69

CHEST-WALL
   and movements of the heart .   114
   hyperalgesia of, in dilatation of the
    heart   .   .   .   73, 302

CHEYNE-STOKES RESPIRATION .   54
   artificial production of   .   55
   arterial pressure in   .   .   54
   with Bright's disease .   .   55
   in cardio-sclerosis   .   .   55
   condition of heart in .   .   55
   conditions simulating .   .   55
   consciousness during apnœic stage 55
   effect of dilatation of the heart on 306
   in heart-block   .   .   .   274
   John Hunter's description of .   55
   mental condition in   .   .   55
   prognosis in   .   .   .   54
   during sleep   .   .   .   53
   suffering due to .   .   .   54
   talking during apnœic stage .   55

PAGE

CHEYNE-STOKES RESPIRATION
  (continued)—
   treatment of   .   .   .   54
   twitching of muscles in   .   54

CHILDREN
   periodic respiration in .   .   55
   heart irregularity in   .   186, 187

CHLORAL   357
   in angina pectoris   .   .   86
   in cardio-sclerosis (senile heart) . 320

CHRISTIAN SCIENTISTS AND X
  DISEASE   102

CICATRIZATION OF THE HEART
   after rheumatic fever .   .   284

CIRCULATION
   object of the   .   .   .   10
   purpose of the .   .   .   10

CLASSIFICATION OF SYMPTOMS
   in visceral disease   .   .   57

CLIFFORD ALLBUTT AND ARTERIO-
  SCLEROSIS   314

COLD
   effect of, on the heart's rate .   178

COLD AIR
   exposure to, a cause of angina
    pectoris   99

COLD BATHS
   in exophthalmic goitre   .   173

COLD HANDS
   in the X disease .   .   .   101

COLIC, BILIARY
   hyperalgesia in .   .   .   61
   situation of pain in   .   .   62

COLIC, RENAL
   situation of pain in   .   .   62

COMPARISON OF AURICULAR
  PRESSURE
   with the jugular pulse .   .   146

COMPENSATION   .   .   .   6

COMPENSATORY PAUSE
   cause of, in extra-systole   .   193

COMPLAINTS, CHIEF   .   .   46

COMPLETE HEART-BLOCK .   269

COMPRESSION OF CHEST
   sense of   47

CONDUCTIVITY   .   .   .   29
   affections of   .   .   .   261
   cause of depressed   .   .   271
   depression of, in febrile affections
    of the heart   .   .   .   283
   depressed in rheumatic hearts . 270
   depression of, increased by digitalis 271
   method of recognizing depression of 261
   significance of depression of .   271

PAGE

CONDUCTIVITY (continued)—
prognosis in depression of . . 274
influence of rest upon . . . 264
irregularity due to depression of . 266
manner in which depression of is
produced in mitral stenosis . 332

CONGENITAL AFFECTIONS OF THE
HEART
ætiology 343
prognosis 345
symptoms 343
treatment 345

CONGENITAL DEFECTS OF AORTIC
VALVES 338

CONSCIOUSNESS
loss of 48
during apnœic stage of Cheyne-
Stokes respiration . . . 55

CONSCIOUSNESS OF THE HEART'S
ACTION 47

CONSCIOUS SUBJECT
resection of bowel in . . . 58

CONSTIPATION
in heart failure 358

CONSTRICTION OF CHEST. See CHEST.

CONTINUOUS INCREASED FRE-
QUENOY
causes of valvular disease . . 171
myocarditis 171
constant over-exertion . . 172
'soldier's heart' 172
alcohol 172
auricular fibrillation . . . 172
pregnancy 172
toxic conditions 172
neurotic cases 172
exophthalmic goitre . . . 173

CONTINUOUS LABOURED BREATH-
ING IN HEART FAILURE . . 52

CONTRACTILITY 29
angina pectoris due to exhaustion
of 72
arterial pressure with exhaustion of 317
effect of digitalis on . . . 248
conditions inducing exhaustion of . 8
exhaustion of, due to degeneration
of muscle 11
exhaustion of, due to dilatation . 301
exhaustion of, due to imperfect
nutrition 30
exhaustion of, due to increased rate 170
exhaustion of, due to obstruction to
the heart's work . . . 315
effect of rest on exhausted . . 358
exhaustion of, in pneumonia . 287
exhaustion of, the cause of angina
pectoris 72

PAGE

CONTRACTILITY (continued)—
necessity for recognizing exhaustion of 14
prognosis of exhaustion of . . 310
pulsus alternans, a symptom of
exhaustion of 256
reserve force of 15
reflex symptoms of exhaustion of . 25
symptoms of exhaustion of, in
rheumatic hearts . . . 284
symptoms of exhaustion of, in
cardio-sclerosis . . . 318
symptoms of exhaustion of . 16, 21

CONVALESCENCE
after febrile affections of the heart 290

COR BOVINUM . . . 338

CORONARY ARTERIES
in cases of angina pectoris . 394, 395,
397, 398, 401, 403, 407, 411
heart-block in sclerosis of . . 270

CORONARY SINUS
heart's contraction starting at . 38
how regurgitation into is prevented 38

CORRIGAN'S PULSE . . . 339

CUTANEOUS DISTRIBUTION
of cervical and upper nerves . 63

CYANOSIS
in congenital heart affections . 346
oxygen in . . . 346, 357
in paroxysmal tachycardia . . 253

DEATH
during an attack of angina pectoris 78
due to digitalis 236
due to heart-block . . . 274
sense of impending, during an
attack of angina pectoris . . 79
during paroxysmal tachycardia . 253

DEFINITIONS
apex beat 116
a–c interval xxi
arterial degeneration . . . xxi
auricular fibrillation . . . xxi
auricular flutter xxi
auricular venous pulse . . xxi
auriculo-ventricular bundle . . xxi
auriculo-ventricular node . . xxi
cardiac asthma 54
cardio-sclerosis xxii
carditis . . . 306, 314
conductivity xxii
contractility xxii
extra-systole xxii
heart-block xxii
hyperalgesia xxii
myogenic theory . . . xxii
nodal rhythm xxii
palpitation xxii

PAGE

DEFINITIONS (continued)—
paroxysmal tachycardia . . xxii
pulsus alternans xxii
pulsus bigeminus . . . xxii
sino-auricular node . . . xxiii
sphygmogram 134
tonicity . . . . xxiii, 301
ventricular rhythm . . xxiii, 261
ventricular venous pulse . . xxiii
viscero-motor reflex . . . xxiii
viscero-sensory reflex . . . xxiii

DEGENERATION OF HEART MUSCLE
See SENILE HEART. . . . 313

DELUSIONS 50

DEPRESSION OF TONICITY OF
THE HEART 301

DEPRESSOR NERVE . . . 41

DESIRE TO BREATHE . . . 51

DEVELOPMENT
of arms 63
of the heart 32

DIABETES
pericarditis in 282

DIAGRAM
showing relation of brain, spinal
cord, and skin to a sensory nerve 60

DIAPHRAGM
in the fixation of the heart . . 39

DIASTOLIC MURMUR . . . 331

DIASTOLIC NOTCH
in a sphygmogram . . . 135

DIASTOLIC PERIOD
in a sphygmogram . . . 135

DIASTOLIC WAVE
cause of 135
in the jugular pulse . . . 154

DICROTIC WAVE
cause of 135

DIET
in cardio-sclerosis . . . 319
in treatment . . . 360, 361

DIGESTIVE TUBE
nature of symptoms produced by . 58

DIGITAL EXAMINATION
of the arteries . . . 131
of the arterial pressure . . 138
of the arterial pulse . . . 129

DIGITALIS 232
and blood-pressure . . 233, 377
in cardio-sclerosis . . . 377
causing heart-block . . . 373
causing intermittent pulse . . 275
causing pulsus alternans . . 373
conditions in which it is useful . 377

DIGITALIS (continued)—
conditions in which it is useless . 379
effect on conductivity . . . 377
increasing depression of conductivity 377
effect on contractility . . . 377
danger in administration of . . 235
extra-systoles due to . . . 191
effect on dilatation of the heart . 311
action of different preparations . 378
effect on dropsy . . . 312, 378
effect on enlargement of the liver . 311
action of, on the human heart 30, 377
illustrative cases, showing effects of 430,
431, 433
effect on auricular fibrillation . 231
susceptibility of auricular fibrillation to 232
effect on auricular fibrillation due
to cardio-sclerosis . . . 317
in practice 376
use of, in prognosis . . . 311
effect on rate 377
reason for uncertain action of . 379
reason for contradictory effects of . 379
significance of coupled beats produced by 375
and slow respiration . . . 55
sudden death due to . . . 379
action on tonicity . . . 377
in the treatment of dilatation . 373
method of use 233
hypodermic injections of digitalin
unsatisfactory . . . 379
preparation and administration of . 378
Nativelle's granules of digitalin . 378
method of administration . . 234
digitalis does not raise the blood-
pressure 377
importance of slowing the heart's
action 377
special efficacy in cases of auricular fibrillation 377

DIGITALIS, SQUILLS AND CALOMEL
in cardiac dropsy . . . 312

DILATATION OF THE HEART . 300
in febrile affections . . . 284
albuminuria in 309
alcoholic . . . 301, 307
dropsy in . . . 307, 308
effect on angina pectoris . . 306
effect on arterial pressure . . 306
laboured breathing in . . . 52
effect on cardiac asthma . . 306
in cardio-sclerosis . . . 318
cause of 300
effect on Cheyne-Stokes respiration 306
of no importance in young healthy
hearts 310
a rare condition 310

PAGE

DILATATION OF THE HEART
(continued)—
diuretin, theocin-sodium acetate in   312
consequences of   305
exhaustion of contractility due to .   12
effect of digitalis on   .   .   .   312
effects of   305
evidence of   302
and functional murmurs   .   .   304
causing epigastric pulsation .   .   123
due to fever   284
effect of, on the jugular pulse   .   160
enlarged liver in   308
manner of production of   .   300, 301
manner in which symptoms are
produced   305
and mitral regurgitation   .   334, 335
and mitral stenosis   .   .   .   333
localised oedema in   .   .   .   307
treatment   311
with auricular fibrillation   .   .   230
its significance in auricular fibrillation   231
œdema of the lungs in .   .   .   308
in paroxysmal tachycardia   .   .   306
significance of   307
the position of the heart in   .   302
value of auscultation of bases of
lungs in   308
hypostatic pneumonia in   .   .   309
prognosis in   310
reflex symptoms produced by   .   305
in rheumatic fever   .   .   .   284
signs of   302
bearing of, on treatment   .   .   306
urinary symptoms in .   .   .   309
in myocardial degeneration .   .   306

DILATATION OF LEFT VENTRICLE
in mitral stenosis   .   .   .   333

DIMINISHED FREQUENCY
of the heart's action   .   .   .   177

DIPHTHERIA
the condition of the heart in   277, 287
fatal syncope in   287

DIPLOCOCCUS RHEUMATICUS   .   283

DISAPPEARANCE OF PRESYSTOLIC
MURMUR   332

DISEASE OF HEART MUSCLE,
NATURE OF,
shown by irregularities   .   .   306

DISPLACEMENT OF THE CHAMBERS
OF THE HEART
in dilatation   .   .   .   302, 303

DISSOCIATION OF PLACES
in starting the heart's contraction   33, 34

DIURESIS IN HEART FAILURE
cause of profuse   310

PAGE

DIURETIN
in dilatation of the heart   .   .   312

DIZZINESS
in heart failure   48

DOG
irregular heart-action in   .   .   185

DORSAL NERVES
peculiar field supplied by upper   .   63

DOUBLE AORTIC MURMUR .   .   339
Corrigan's water-hammer pulse in.   339
capillary pulsation in .   .   .   339
bellows murmur in   .   .   .   339

DROPSY
in arms and face   .   .   .   307
effect of digitalis in   .   .   .   312
dilatation of the heart causing   .   308
a sign of dilatation of the heart   .   307
manner of onset of   .   .   .   307
in cases of auricular fibrillation   .   307
in paroxysmal tachycardia   .   .   252
in rheumatic heart cases   .   .   307
the secretion of urine with   .   307
significance of   307
treatment of   311

DRUGS
in treatment   370

DYSPNŒA. See BREATHLESSNESS   .   51

E

meaning of period   .   .   114, 152

EFFECT OF PRESSURE ON ABDO-
MEN   98

EINTHOVEN ON PULSUS ALTER-
NANS   258

EINTHOVEN'S STRING GALVANO-
METER   108

ELECTRIC CHANGES
due to heart-beat   .   .   .   108
in muscular tissue   .   .   .   108

ELECTROCARDIOGRAM   .   .   110
of the auricle   108
of the ventricle   108
the normal   108
of heart-block   111
of the nodal rhythm .   .   .   99
of extra-systoles   110

ELECTROCARDIOGRAPH   .   .   108

EMBRYOCARDIA
loose employment of term   .   .   88

ENDOCARDITIS
in acute fevers   277
malignant   284
misleading term   278
symptoms of   282

ENEMATA   358

PAGE

ENLARGEMENT AND PULSATION
OF THE LIVER 161

ENLARGEMENT OF THE LIVER . 308
  signs of 162
  conditions causing . . . 163
  jaundice in 164
  differential diagnosis of . . 165
  and pulsation 166
  prognosis of 166
  treatment of 167

EPIGASTRIC PULSATION
  causes of 123
  in fevers 278
  in pernicious anaemia . . . 123
  in typhoid fever 123
  and the shock of ventricular systole 127
  time of 123

EPILEPTIC ATTACKS . . . 49
  due to heart-block . . . 272

ERLANGER—EXPERIMENTAL
HEART-BLOCK 268

ERYSIPELAS
  the heart in 277

ERYTHROL TETRANITRATE . 382

ESCAPED VENTRICULAR BEATS
AND NODAL BEATS . . . 204

ESSENTIAL FACTOR IN HEART
FAILURE 5, 351

ESSENTIAL PRINCIPLE IN TREAT-
MENT 351

EVENTS IN A CARDIAC CYCLE 134, 147

EXAGGERATED SENSORY PHE-
NOMENA
  'Heart tonics' in . . . 94
  bromide of ammonium in . . 94
  sea-bathing in 94
  treatment of . . . 92, 93
  prognosis in 92
  air suction in 91
  characteristics of . . . 90
  in heart failure 89
  with pathological heart changes . 90

EXAGGERATION OF REFLEX
SYMPTOMS
  in nervous people . . . 89

EXAMINATION OF THE ARTERIAL
PULSE 129

EXAMINATION OF THE PA-
TIENT 43

EXCITABILITY OF THE HEART . 29
  and angina pectoris . . . 71

EXCITEMENT
  a cause of angina pectoris . . 71

PAGE

EXERCISES
  rules for employment of . . 363
  special 363
  value of different forms of . . 362
  breathing 312

EXHAUSTED HEART MUSCLE
  the cause of angina pectoris . . 71

EXHAUSTING DISEASES
  heart-rate increased in . . 176

EXHAUSTION
  evidences of 16
  value of estimating degrees of . 16
  sense of in heart failure . . 46
  effects of on individual heart-beats 14
  restoration of the exhausted heart 17
  signs of 21

EXOPHTHALMIC GOITRE . . 173
  arteries visible in . . . 173
  peripheral circulation in . . 174
  cause of increased frequency in . 173
  characters of the pulse tracing in . 173

EXPECTORATION
  blood-stained, in dilatation of the
  heart 306

EXPERIMENTAL STIMULATION
OF VAGUS NERVE . . . 185

EXTRA-SYSTOLES
  electrocardiogram of . 110, 181, 189
  extra-systoles, definition of . xxii, 188
  extra-systoles, classification of . 192
  extra-systoles, in angina pectoris . 79
  extra-systoles and variations of the
  a–c interval 196
  extra-systoles, different forms of . 191
  extra-systoles in acute affections . 281
  extra-systoles, frequency of occurrence when at rest . . . 199
  extra-systoles in arterial degeneration 317
  extra-systoles, auricular . . 195
  extra-systoles and the auriculo-
  ventricular bundle . . . 198
  extra-systoles, bromide of ammonium in 201
  extra-systole with cardiac asthma 53
  extra-systole with cardio-sclerosis . 316
  extra-systole cause of compensatory pause 193
  extra-systole, character of the
  irregularity 188
  extra-systoles, conditions inducing 198
  extra-systole due to digitalis 191, 199
  extra-systole due to indiscretions
  in food 199
  extra-systole due to indiscretions in
  alcohol 199
  extra-systole due to indiscretions in
  tobacco 199
  extra-systoles, aetiology . . 198

PAGE

EXTRA-SYSTOLES (continued)—
extra-systole, relationship to heart-
block 270
extra-systole, nodal . . . 197
extra-systole, effect on mind . 199
extra-systoles and auricular fibrillation 200
extra-systoles, place of origin of
ventricular 193
extra-systoles and the primitive cardiac tube . . . 192, 197
extra-systole, prognosis of . 199, 208
extra-systoles and pulsus alternans 259
extra-systoles distinct from the
pulsus alternans . . . 259
extra-systoles, sensations produced
by 199
extra-systoles, sounds due to . 190
extra-systoles, treatment of . . 201
extra-systole, ventricular form of . 192
extra-systoles, varieties of . . 191
extra-systoles in the X disease . 101
extra-systoles, transient loss of
consciousness with . . . 49
extra-systoles, prognosis entirely
favourable 201
extra-systoles, not in themselves a
sign of disease . . . 200
extra-systoles, interpolated . . 193
extra-systoles, recognition by auscultation 190

FACIAL ASPECT 44
in aortic regurgitation . . . 340
during an attack of angina pectoris 78
PAINTING 48
FATTY DEGENERATION OF THE
HEART 313, 315
in acute febrile affection . . 289
pulsus alternans in . . . 256
FEBRILE AFFECTIONS OF THE
HEART
convalescence after . . . 290
symptoms in 279
treatment of 289
auriculo-ventricular bundle affected in 280
unsatisfactory result of vaccines . 289
FEVER
dilatation of the heart in . . 278
effect of, on the heart . . . 279
heart symptoms in . . . 279
pulse-rate in 278
varying reaction on heart of . 278
rapid dilatation of the heart in . 281
due to damage of the auriculo-ventricular bundle . . . 280
and the heart 22
symptoms in myocarditis during . 279
manner of affection of the heart in 277

PAGE

FEVER (continued)—
irregular pulse in . . . 280
symptoms in endocarditis during . 282
symptoms in pericarditis during . 282
FINGERS
clubbing of 346
FIXATION OF THE HEART . . 302
FOCUS, IRRITABLE, IN THE
SPINAL CORD . . . 61, 76
due to angina pectoris . 69, 76
a cause of the tendency to recurrent
attacks of angina pectoris . 73
symptoms of 73
FRACTURED TIBIA
pulmonary infarct from . . 56
FUNCTION OF TONICITY OF THE
HEART 301
FUNCTIONAL
pathology of the heart . . 2
impairment of the heart . . 8
evidences 8
FUNCTIONS OF THE HEART
MUSCLE-FIBRES . . . 28
FUNCTIONS OF THE PRIMITIVE
CARDIAC TUBE . . . 261

GALVANOMETER
in abnormal rhythms . . . 109
GANGLION CELLS . . . 41
their function . . . 41, 42
GASKELL'S BRIDGE
experiment 33
GIDDINESS 48
GRAPHIC RECORDS
of arterial pressure . . . 139
of heart movements . . . 116
of the jugular pulse . . 146, 149
use of 116
GRAVE CONDITIONS
due to auricular fibrillation 229, 230, 236
GRIPPING OF CHEST
in angina pectoris . . 69, 78

HÆMOPTYSIS
in mitral stenosis . . . 333
HÆMORRHAGE
from the lungs in heart failure . 55
HALDANE AND POULTON
on Cheyne Stokes respiration . 54
HALLER'S OBSERVATION
on the insensitiveness of the viscera 59
HALLUCINATIONS
in failing heart 50
HARVEY'S OBSERVATION
on the insensitiveness of the heart 58

PAGE

HEAD AND CAMPBELL
on causation of herpes zoster . 65

HEALTHY PEOPLE
sinus irregularity in . . . 186

HEART
ganglion cells of 41
afferent fibres of . . . 41
acceleration fibres of . . . 41
vagus stimulation of . . . 41
nerve supply of 39
movements of, in contraction . 38
co-ordination of 30
functions of 30
development of the . . . 32
functional anatomy of. . . 38
the febrile 278
restoration of the exhausted . 17
specialized muscle nerve, tissue of 32
acute febrile affections of the . 279
in ague 279
in an attack of angina pectoris . 79
apex, arrangement of muscle fibres
at 39
auriculo-ventricular bundle in acute
affections of 280
auriculo-ventricular bundle in rheumatic affections of . . . 280
relationship to sensory nerves . 63
pain areas in affections of . . 65
areas of hyperalgesia in affections of 65
sensory phenomena in over-exertion of normal . . . 73
tone of 300

HEART ABNORMALITIES
mental state induced by . . 101

HEART'S ACTION WITH AURICU-
LAR FIBRILLATION . . . 225

HEART-BLOCK . . . 181, 261
in acute affections . . . 270
apex beat in . . . 266, 268
auricular waves in apex tracings in
cases of 120
auriculo-ventricular bundle found
healthy in 270
due to cardio-sclerosis . . . 317
produced by swallowing . . 465
cases illustrating relation of, to
auricular fibrillation 276, 450, 454
depression of conductivity without
arrhythmia 262
arrhythmia in 264
post-mortem changes in . . 270
prognosis with syncopal attacks . 275
patient's sensations in an attack . 274
prolonged standstill of ventricle . 273
atropine in 275
complete 269
Hering and Erlanger on . . 266

PAGE

HEART-BLOCK (continued)—
effect of auricular contraction on
radial pulse 269
raised beats due to depression of
conductivity in . . . 266
significance of milder forms . . 271
methods of recognizing depression
of conductivity . . . 261
independent ventricular rhythm
due to 267
Cheyne-Stokes respiration in . 274
definition of . . . xxii, 261
due to digitalis 271
cases of, produced by digitalis . 271
electro-cardiogram of . . . 111
and epileptiform attacks . . 272
aetiology 269
relationship to extra-systole . . 270
inexcitability of ventricle in . . 274
relationship to auricular fibrillation 276
prognosis in 275
due to septic poisoning . . 281
symptoms in a case of . . . 273
symptoms associated with . . 271
and syncopal attacks . . . 272
producing slow pulse-rate . 271-3
vagus stimulation producing . 271
treatment of 275
loss of consciousness in . . 50

HEART CHANGES
with increased rate . . . 169

HEART, CONDITION OF
in Cheyne-Stokes respiration . 54

HEART, CONGENITAL AFFECTION
OF 346

HEART'S CONTRACTION
electrical changes due to . . 108
normal starting-point of . 33, 36
starting in the primitive cardiac
tube 33
starting-places of . . . 181
starting in the auricle . . . 181
starting in the sinus venosus . 181

HEART, DEVELOPMENT OF THE . 32

HEART DILATATION
in acute febrile affections . . 281
and blood-pressure . . . 79
and epigastric pulsation . . 123
laboured breathing in . . . 52
and mitral regurgitation . . 334

HEART IN DIPHTHERIA . 277, 287

HEART, EMBARRASSMENT OF . 13
by pericardial effusion . . . 283

HEART IN ERYSIPELAS . . 277

HEART EXHAUSTION
laboured breathing in . . . 24
from obstruction to its work . 315

PAGE

HEART EXHAUSTION (continued)—
from want of exercise . . . 363
from want of rest . . . 77
consciousness of heart's action in
heart failure 24
Cheyne-Stokes respiration in . 25

HEART FAILURE
and arterial degeneration . . 141
and valve lesions . . . 2
constipation in 358
essential factor in . . 3, 351
with a fractured leg . . . 308
jaundice in 164
means exhaustion of reserve force 5,
8, 11
mitral stenosis induces . . 330
mitral regurgitation . . . 334
muscle exhaustion in . . . 334
nature of symptoms in . . 3
and auricular fibrillation . 225–8
cause of recovery from . . 15
due to valve defects . . . 329
wasting in 308
what is it ? 5
transient loss of consciousness in . 49
cerebral symptoms in . . . 48
giddiness in 48
back-pressure theory, evil of . . 7
essential symptoms of . . . 3
how it begins 12
memory in 24
earliest symptoms of impending, in
the aged 308
production of symptoms of . . 23
origin of views of causation of . 6
objective signs of . . . 26
pathological changes in . . 7
reserve force, relation between
exhaustion and restoration of . 12
reflex symptoms in heart failure . 25
patient's chief complaints . . 46
breathlessness in . . 46, 51, 53
sense of exhaustion in . . . 46
pain in 47
hyperalgesia of skin in . 47, 74
loss of consciousness in . . 48
sense of suffocation in . . . 52
inability to stop breathing in . 52
rapid breathing in . . . 52
continuous laboured breathing in . 52
laboured breathing on exertion in . 53
slow respiration in . . . 55
hæmorrhage from the lungs in . 55
acute œdema of lungs in . . 56
reflex phenomena in . . . 57
vagal reflexes in 68
sensory disorders as a result of . 71
sensory disturbances in . . 74
sterno-mastoid, hypersensitiveness
in 75
trapezius, hypersensitiveness in . 75

PAGE

HEART FAILURE (continued)—
pectoralis major, hypersensitiveness
in 75
and increased blood-pressure . 141
remedial measures in . . . 357

HEART, FEBRILE 278

HEART, FEBRILE AFFECTIONS
OF THE 277

HEART, FIXATION OF . . 211, 302

HEART, FUNCTIONAL ANATOMY
OF 38

HEART IN INFLUENZA . . 287

HEART, INSENSITIVENESS OF
THE 58

HEART IRREGULARITY
classification 181
significance of 180
during attacks of angina pectoris . 79
due to auricular flutter . . 182
due to failure of conduction . . 182
due to depression of conductivity . 266
consciousness of 47
meaning of term ' auricular fibrillation ' . . . . xxi, 216
in myocarditis . . . 279–81
significance of in pneumonia . 287
due to respiration . . . 184
during slow respiration . . 55
reveals the pathology of the heart 180,
279
sensation produced by . . . 47
arising at the sinus . . . 183
arising at the sinus, character of . 183
arising at the sinus, ætiology of . 183
arising at the sinus, prognosis of . 186
arising at the sinus, symptoms of . 185
arising at the sinus, symptoms associated with 186
arising at the sinus, due to vagus
stimulation 186
in X disease 101

HEART MOVEMENTS
graphic records of . . . 116

HEART MUSCLE
angina pectoris in exhaustion of 71, 72
angina pectoris in degeneration of . 71
characteristics of function of fibres
of 28
classification of functions of fibres of 28
conditions exhausting reserve force
of 12
co-ordination of functions of . 28
development of 28
estimation of reserve force of . 15
function of conductivity . . 29
function of contractility . . 29
function of excitability . . 29
function of stimulus production . 28

PAGE

HEART MUSCLE (*continued*)—
function of tonicity . . . 29
unequal endowment of functions of
fibres 28
unequal exhaustion of functions of
fibres 31
impaired nourishment of, a cause
of angina pectoris . . . 72
importance of 10
meaning of 11
involved in mitral stenosis . . 330
recovery of 290
reserve force of 11
rest force 11
sclerotic changes in . 313, 316, 330
the two forces of 11

HEART MUSCLE-FIBRES
characteristics of . . . 30
functions of 30

HEART, NATURE OF SYMPTOMS
PRODUCED BY 45

HEART OVERSTRAIN . . . 172

HEART, PERCEPTIBLE MOVE-
MENTS OF 116

HEART IN PNEUMONIA . . 285

HEART, POSITION OF, IN THE
CHEST 112

HEART-RATE
in alcoholics 172
cause of increased . . . 175
effect of cold on 178
continuously increased . . 171
exhaustion of contractility due to
increased 14
difficulties in reckoning increased 169
effect of digitalis on . . . 224
increased on exertion . . . 171
increased in exhausting diseases . 170
in exophthalmic goitre . . 173
increased frequency of . . 168
meaning of increased . . . 169
in myocardial affections . . 171
increased in neurotic people . . 172
the normal . . . 168, 169
in palpitation 174
in pregnancy 172
in tuberculosis 176
in valvular disease . . . 171

HEART REACTION
to the nature of the fever . . 277

HEART, RELATIONSHIP TO SEN-
SORY NERVES . . . 63

HEART IN RHEUMATIC FEVER 283, 284

HEART, RUPTURE OF . . 141, 301

HEART IN SEPTIC INFECTION 287, 288

PAGE

HEART, THE SOLDIER'S . . 172

HEART SOUNDS
during an attack of angina pectoris 79
in depressed conductivity . . 262
due to extra-systoles . . 190, 191
with pulsus alternans . . . 255
with pulsus bigeminus . . 191
with sinus irregularity . . 185
in septic infections . . . 288

HEART'S STRENGTH
standard of measurement of . . 4

HEART IN TYPHOID FEVER . 277

HEART, VENTRICULAR RHYTHM
in heart-block 267

HEMIPLEGIA
in acute febrile affections . . 282

HENDERSON
and aortic disease . . . 325

HERPES ZOSTER
eruption of, in arm . . . 65
pain of simulating angina pectoris . 89
Head and Campbell on causation of 65

HIBERNATING ANIMAL
and periodic respiration . . 55

HIGH BLOOD-PRESSURE
not a disease 139

HILL AND ROWLANDS
and arterial pressure . . . 138

HILTON
on pain and protection . . 62

HIS'S BUNDLE. *See* AURICULO-VEN-
TRICULAR BUNDLE . . . 34–8

HOFFMANN
on pulsus alternans . . . 258

HOLLOW MUSCULAR ORGANS
resemblance of symptoms in . . 57

HOT DRINKS
during an attack of angina pectoris 85

HUNTER, JOHN 51
his description of a curious attack 51
his description of Cheyne-Stokes
respiration 55

HYDROTHERAPY . . . 178, 364–9

HYPERALGESIA
after an attack of angina pectoris 79, 80
in acute dilatation of the heart and
liver 68
in angina pectoris . . . 69
of breasts 47, 74
definition of xxii
due to exhausted contractility . 75
due to dilatation of the heart . 68
in enlargement of the liver . . 68
extensive in neurotic people . . 74
with auricular fibrillation . . 74

PAGE

HYPERALGESIA (continued)—
of skin and muscles in gastric ulcer   61
with valvular disease .   .   .   74
in visceral disease   .   .   65

HYPERPIESIS   .   .   .   140

HYPERTROPHIED HEART
is always an impaired heart .   .   296

HYPERTROPHY
of muscular coat of arteries .   .   315
of left ventricle in aortic valve
disease   340
of right auricle in tricuspid stenosis   337

HYSTERIA
heart pain in   .   .   .   89

INABILITY
to stop breathing in heart failure   52

INADEQUACY
of usual methods to estimate the
heart's efficiency   .   .   .   4

INCREASED ARTERIAL PRESSURE   139
treatment of   .   .   .   143
fertility of nitrites in   .   .   143
effect on the heart of   .   .   140
prognosis of   .   .   .   141

INCREASED FREQUENCY
of the heart's action   .   .   168
due to mental excitement   .   169
classification of cases of   .   169
the result of a call on the heart's
energy   170
after wasting diseases—typhoid,
anæmias, myocarditis   .   170
prognosis of   .   .   .   176
main cause of   .   .   .   175
irregular paroxysms of   .   174

INCREASED PERIPHERAL RE-
SISTANCE
a cause of angina pectoris   .   72

INFANTS AND THE SINUS IR-
REGULARITY   .   .   .   186

INFAROT, PULMONARY   .   59

INFARCTS DURING ACUTE AFFEC-
TIONS OF THE HEART   .   282

INFECTIVE ENDOCARDITIS   .   287
prognosis of   .   .   .   288
heart in   .   .   .   287
treatment of   .   .   .   289
organisms of   .   .   .   287

INFLUENZA, AURICULO-VENTRI-
CULAR BUNDLE AFFECTED IN   280

INK POLYGRAPH .   .   .   105

INQUIRY INTO NAUHEIM TREAT-
MENT   365

INSENSITIVENESS OF THE
BOWEL   .   .   .   58

PAGE

INSENSITIVENESS OF THE VIS-
CERA TO ORDINARY STIMULI .   57

INSPECTION OF THE ARTERIES .   131

INSPECTION OF THE JUGULAR
PULSE   .   .   .   145

INSPIRATION, EFFECT OF, ON
ABDOMINAL VEINS .   .   101

INSPIRATORY SWELLING OF
JUGULAR VEINS   .   .   101

INSTRUMENTAL METHODS
of examination   .   .   .   104
sphygmograph .   .   .   104
polygraph   105
ink polygraph   .   .   .   105
electrocardiograph   .   .   108
Einthoven's string galvanometer .   108
galvanometer in abnormal rhythms   109

INSURANCE COMPANIES
heart's efficiency.   .   .   18

INTERCOSTAL MUSCLES
spasm of   70

INTERMITTENT CLAUDICATION .   72

INTERMITTENT PULSE
due to depression of conductivity   .   .   .   266, 271
due to depressed conductivity in
febrile affections   .   280, 284
due to exhausted contractility   .   256
produced by digitalis   .   .   373
due to extra-systoles   190, 191, 198, 200
in pneumonia   .   .   .   287
sensations with   .   .   .   47

INTERPOLATED EXTRA-SYSTOLE   193

INTERPRETATION OF THE JUGU-
LAR PULSE   .   .   147, 151

INTERPRETATION OF A SPHYG-
MOGRAM   134

INTERPRETATION OF A TRACING
OF THE APEX BEAT .   .   117

INTERSYSTOLIC PERIOD
(a–c interval)   .   .   .   262

INTERVAL, PRESPHYGMIC .   .   262

INVERTED CARDIOGRAMS
significance of   .   .   .   126

INVERTED SPHYGMOGRAM .   130, 131

IODIDE OF POTASSIUM   .   .   382

IRREGULAR ACTION OF THE
HEART   .   .   .   180
classification of .   .   .   182
auricular flutter .   .   .   182
significance of   .   .   .   180
classification of sinus irregularities   181
recent advance in knowledge of   .   180

PAGE

IRREGULAR PAROXYSMS OF IN-
CREASED FREQUENCY . . 174
causes of 174
failure of conduction of auriculo-
ventricular bundle . . . 182
pulsus alternans 182
IRREGULARITY
nature of disease shown by . . 180
See also HEART IRREGULARITY.
IRREGULARITY CHARACTERISTIC
OF AURICULAR FIBRILLATION 219
IRRITABLE FOCUS IN SPINAL
CORD 61, 80
IRRITABLE HEART AFTER RHEU-
MATIC FEVER 284

JAUNDICE
with dilatation of the heart . . 164
with heart failure . . . 164
the pulse-rate with . . . 178
JUGULAR PULSE 145
anomalous forms of . . . 159
auricular wave in the . . . 149
auricular depression in the . . 149
ventricular wave in the . . 150
ventricular depression in the . 153
the carotid wave in the . . 153
causes of 157
carotid wave of 153
changes due to variation in rate of
heart 154
compared with auricular pressure . 148
conditions giving rise to a . . 159
a diastolic wave in the . . 154
effect of dilatation of the heart on
the 305
in auricular flutter . . . 240
effect of opening the tricuspid valves
on the 150
with extra-systoles . . 190–3
factors producing the . . . 149
graphic records of the . . . 149
how to record the . . . 146
inspection of the . . . 145
interpretation of the . . 151, 155
methods of analysing a tracing . 154
methods of reading . . . 146
meaning of the ventricular form of
the 157
in mediastino-pericarditis . . 344
recognition of events in . . 146
with auricular fibrillation . . 220
notch on ventricular wave . . 153
significance of ventricular form of
the 137
standard for interpreting a . . 151
time of opening of tricuspid valves
in the 150
in extra-systole 194

PAGE

JUGULAR PULSE (*continued*)—
in tricuspid disease . . . 150
with tricuspid regurgitation . . 150
what it shows . . . 145, 146
variations of, due to heart's rate . 155
ventricular form of the . . 156
in pregnancy 160
with auricular flutter . . . 240
JUGULAR VALVE SOUND . . 337
JUGULAR VEINS
inspiratory swelling of . . . 101
relation of, to carotid and subclavian arteries . . . 145
thrills produced by compression of 220

KEITH
and ruptured heart . . . 301
researches of 34
KEITH AND CHAUVEAU
work of 39
KENT, STANLEY
work of 34
KIDNEY DISEASE AND CARDIO-
SCLEROSIS 317
'KNOTEN' OF TAWARA . . xxi
See AURICULO-VENTRICULAR NODE.

LABOURED BREATHING
on exertion in heart failure . . 53
LACTIC ACID
action on tonicity . . . 30
LEG, FRACTURE OF
and heart failure . 52, 56, 308
LEWIS
and electrocardiograms . . 110
LIFE INSURANCE
and the prognosis of symptoms . 347
LISTER
and the pulse 130
LIVER
pain due to the . . . 46, 47
LIVER ENLARGEMENT
a cardinal symptom of heart failure 308
effect of digitalis on . . . 311
in dilatation of the heart . . 308
with auricular fibrillation . . 228
pain and tenderness in . . 228
with paroxysmal tachycardia . 252
signs of 162
treatment 167
prognosis of 166
and pulsation 166
conditions causing . . . 163
differential diagnosis of . . 165
conditions causing . . . 163
jaundice in 164

PAGE

LIVER MOVEMENTS
different forms of   .   .   . 165
in aortic regurgitation .   .   . 340
due to cardiac aspiration   .   . 122

LIVER PULSATION   .   .   . 162
coupled beats in 375
differential diagnosis of   .   . 165
distinct from liver movement   . 162
forms of   162
how to record   .   .   . 106, 107
with auricular fibrillation   .   . 164
prognosis of   166
with paroxysmal tachycardia   . 252
in tricuspid stenosis   .   . 164, 337

LUNG, RETRACTION OF   .   . 127

LUNGS
acute suffocative œdema of .   . 56
apoplexy of   56
bleeding from 55
displacement of, with dilatation of
the heart   .   .   . 303, 304
infarct into   56
in the fixation of the heart .   . 39

LUNGS, ŒDEMA OF   .   .   . 308
in the elderly   56
factors in the production of .   . 309
first sign of   308
how produced   50
method of examining for   .   . 308
in mitral stenosis   .   .   . 56
prognostic significance of   .   . 308
symptoms of   308
in typhoid fever 56

MALIGNANT ENDOCARDITIS   . 287

MAREY
and the pulse   130

MARTIN'S
modification of Riva-Rocci sphygmo-
manometer   142

MASSAGE
in treatment   364

MECHANISM OF THE PRODUC-
TION OF PAIN 59

MEDIASTINO-PERICARDITIS
angina pectoris in   .   .   . 343
ætiology of   343
jugular pulse in 344
liver pulse in   344
prognosis in   345
symptoms of   343
treatment of   345

MEMORY 50, 178

MENTAL EXCITEMENT
a cause of angina pectoris   .   . 77

PAGE

MENTAL FACTOR
in treatment   352

MENTAL STATE
in Cheyne-Stokes respiration   . 54
induced by heart abnormalities   . 93
in the X disease   102
induced by physician's warnings   . 93
induced by visceral disease   .   . 92

MESENTERY, INSENSITIVENESS OF 58

METHOD OF DESCRIBING HEART
AFFECTIONS   1

MICTURITION—INCREASED
after an attack of angina pectoris .   . 80

MID-DIASTOLIC MURMUR   .   . 331

MITRAL MURMURS
due to acute endocarditis   .   . 288
due to dilatation 305
See also MURMURS.

MITRAL REGURGITATION   .   . 334
muscle failure—an important feature in   335
in cardio-sclerosis   .   . 316, 335
causes of 334
conditions inducing heart failure in 334
with dilatation of the heart .   . 305
murmurs due to 334

MITRAL STENOSIS
angina pectoris in   .   .   . 333
causes of 330
complications of   .   .   . 333
cerebral embolism in .   .   . 333
conditions inducing heart failure in 330
dilatation of left ventricle in   . 333
delayed conductivity with   .   . 330
hæmoptysis in   333
involvement of auriculo-ventricular
bundle in   330
heart failure in   333
moderate 330
murmurs due to 330
meaning of disappearance of presystolic murmur of .   .   . 332
not an acute condition   .   . 330
auricular fibrillation in   . 330, 333
paroxysmal tachycardia in   .   . 333
post-mortem changes in   .   . 333
progress of   332
a progressive lesion   .   .   . 332
sclerosis of muscle with   .   . 330
symptoms in   332

MOUTH
becoming dry in angina pectoris   . 91

MOVEMENTS DUE TO CAROTID
PULSE   130

MOVEMENTS OF THE HEART   . 116

PAGE

MOVEMENTS OF RESPIRATION
effect of, on the pulmonary circulation 309
MOVEMENTS IN TREATMENT, SPECIAL 363
MULTIPLE
auricular extra-systoles . . 206
ventricular extra-systoles . . 207
extra-systoles 208
extra-systoles, cause of . . 208
extra-systoles, prognosis of . . 208
MURMURS
due to aortic incompetence . . 339
due to aortic stenosis . . . 338
auricular systolic 331
cause of functional . . . 323
in cardio-sclerosis 316
diastolic 331
diastolic, due to mitral stenosis . 331
due to endocarditis . . . 282
meaning of, in acute conditions . 282
due to mitral stenosis . . . 330
due to patent ductus arteriosus . 346
due to pericarditis . . . 282
presystolic, character of . . 331
presystolic, disappearance of, in auricular fibrillation . . . 331
presystolic, how produced . . 331
presystolic, meaning of disappearance of 332
presystolic, position of in cardiac cycle 331
presystolic, separation of, from first sound 331
presystolic tricuspid . . . 337
presystolic, varying relation to first sound 331
significance of musical . . 282
systolic, due to mitral regurgitation 334
systolic, due to mitral stenosis . 331
tricuspid systolic . . . 337
MUSCARIN
action on tonicity . . . 30
MUSCLE EXHAUSTION
a factor in heart failure . . 334
MUSCLE FAILURE
symptoms in . . . 306, 307
MUSCLES, ABDOMINAL
reflex stimulation of . . . 61
MUSCLES, CONTRACTED IN GASTRIC ULCER 62
MUSCLES, INTERCOSTAL . .
contraction of, in angina pectoris . 70
MUSCLE, STERNO-MASTOID
hyperalgesia of 91
MUSCLES, THEIR PRIMITIVE FUNCTION 61

PAGE

MUSCLE STIMULATION
in visceral disease . . . 61
MUSCLES, TONICITY OF . . 301
MUSCLES, TWITCHING OF
in Cheyne-Stokes respiration . 54
MUSCLE, TRAPEZIUS
hyperalgesia of 91
MUSCULAR HYPERALGESIA
consequence of, in liver enlargement 161
MUSCULAR ORGANS
resemblance of symptoms in hollow 57
MUSCULAR RHEUMATISM
and angina pectoris . . . 70
MUSICAL MURMURS
significance of . . .
MUSKENS
on pulsus alternans . . . 258
MYOCARDITIS 171
causes of 2
heart-rate in 171
in acute fevers 279
in rheumatic fever . . 283–5
irregular action of the heart in . 296
symptoms of 297
MYOCARDIUM 295
introduction 295
evidences of impairment of . . 296
rate of the heart . . . 296
rhythm 296
size of heart 296
dilatation of the heart . . . 297
acute affections of . . . 297
subacute affections of . . . 297
heart-block in ditto . . . 298
recovery in 298
prognosis of myocardial disease . 298
wide a–c interval in . . . 298
'senile changes' in the heart . 299
MYOGENIC DOCTRINE . . . 27
definition of theory . . . xxii

NAUHEIM BATHS 365
NECK
pain in, during an attack of angina pectoris 68
NERVES
diagram showing stimulation of, in visceral disease . . . 60
optic, stimulation of . . 57, 59
peculiar field supplied by upper dorsal 64
sensory, stimulation of . . 59
sensory, relationship of, to heart . 63
stimulation of trunk of . . 59
sympathetic, diagram showing relation to viscera and sensory nerve 60

PAGE

NERVES OF THE HEART
accelerator 41
afferent 41
depressor 41
effect of, on the functions of muscle-
fibres 28
effects of, on the heart muscle . 40
in auriculo-ventricular bundle . 35
influence on the heart's rhythm . 181
inhibitory 40
action of sympathetic . . . 40
origin of sympathetic . . . 40
action of vagus 40
vagus, effect of stimulation of, on
depressed functions . . . 40
See also VAGUS.

NERVOUS SYSTEM
reaction of visceral disease on . 87
hypersensitiveness of . . . 87
valvular disease with exhausted . 90

NEURASTHENIA
cardiac 101
and sinus irregularity . . . 186

NEUROGENY 27

NEUROSES, CARDIAC . . . 88

NEUROTIC PATIENTS
treatment of 353

NITRITE OF AMYL . . . 381
during an attack of angina pectoris 85

NITRITES 381

NITRITES AND HIGH BLOOD-PRES-
SURE 382

NITRO-GLYCERINE . . . 382

NODAL BRADYCARDIA
auricular fibrillation . . 177, 228

NODAL EXTRA-SYSTOLES . . 197

NORMAL
rate of the heart 168
average at different ages . . 168
increased by exertion . . . 169
auricular systole and ventricular
extra-systole together . . 194

NORMAL VENOUS PULSE . . 152
See JUGULAR PULSE.

NOTHNAGEL
on angina pectoris . . . 99

NOURISHMENT OF HEART MUSCLE
angina pectoris due to impaired 71, 72

NUTRITION
exhaustion of contractility due to
imperfect 284

OBJECT OF THE PHYSICIAN'S
EXAMINATION 1

OBSCURE CASES
prognosis in 349

PAGE

ŒDEMA. See DROPSY . . . 307

ŒDEMA OF THE LUNGS . . 56
See LUNGS, ŒDEMA OF.

ŒDEMA, PULMONARY. See LUNGS 56

OPENING OF TRICUSPID VALVES
point in tracings . . . 150

OPIATES
to be avoided 383

OPIUM 383
in angina pectoris . . . 86
in cardio-sclerosis . . . 320

OPPRESSION OF THE CHEST .
in the elderly 175

OPTIC NERVE
stimulation of . . . 57, 59

ORIGIN OF MISTAKEN DIAGNOSES 278

ORTHODIAGRAPH
use of 114

OSLER, SIR WILLIAM
and infective endocarditis . . 288

OVER-EXERTION
causing angina pectoris . . 77
sensory phenomena in normal heart 73

OVERSTRAINED HEART . . 172

OXYGEN 383
in angina pectoris . . 86, 383
in cardiac asthma . . 86, 383
in treatment 383

PACEMAKER OF THE HEART . 35

PAIN
absence of, in pericarditis . . 282
in angina pectoris, region of . 78
persisting after an attack of angina
pectoris 78
of biliary colic, situation of . 62
due to exhausted contractility . 72
function of 62
in gastric ulcer 61
of heart affections, reasons for, in
arm 64
of heart affections, situation of . 65
of herpes zoster, simulating angina
pectoris 89
over the liver 47
in enlargement of the liver . 162, 308
mechanism of its production . 57
due to peristalsis of the bowel . 58
radiation of 47
of renal colic, situation of . 62
significance of 47
situation of 47
caused by spasm of hollow muscles 57
vague notion of position of . 45
why it is referred . . . 62

PAGE

PALPITATION 48
  definition of . . . xxii, 174
  causes of 174
  heart-rate in 174
  and paroxysmal tachycardia, dis-
    tinction between . . . 174
  sensation during . . . 174
  sign of exhausted contractility . 298
PARALYSIS OF THE AURICLE
  evidences of 156
PAROXYSMAL TACHYCARDIA . 251
  of auricular origin . . . 251
  auriculo-ventricular node affected
    in cases of 218
  in cardio-sclerosis . . . 317
  acute heart failure in . . . 252
  and arterial degeneration . . 317
  cases illustrating 432, 434, 438, 442–6
  conditions producing . . . 256
  different forms of . . . 255
  definition of . . . xxii, 251
  dilatation of the heart with . . 252
  liver enlargement in . . . 252
  liver pulsation during . . . 252
  meaning of the term . . xxii, 251
  in mitral stenosis . . . 333
  and palpitation, distinction between . 174
  pathology of . . 217, 238, 333
  primitive cardiac tissue in . . 209
  prognosis in 253
  pulsus alternans due to . . 255
  symptoms of 251
  sudden relief on cessation of . 252–3
  sudden changes due to . 252, 253
  treatment of 253
PATENT DUCTUS ARTERIOSUS
  murmurs of 346
PATENT FORAMEN OVALE . . 346
PATHOLOGY OF HEART
  in angina pectoris . . 71–3
  in cardio-sclerosis . . . 330
  in auricular fibrillation 217, 238, 270, 333
  in paroxysmal tachycardia 217, 238, 333
  shown by irregularity . 180, 181
PATHOLOGICAL VENOUS PULSE 156
  See VENTRICULAR JUGULAR PULSE.
PATIENT
  position assumed by . . . 44
  preliminary examination of . . 44
  respiration of 44
  sensations of 44
  sensations of, a guide to condition
    of reserve force . . . 45
  necessity for precision in state-
    ments of 44
PATIENT'S ASPECT . . . 44
PATIENT'S CONSCIOUSNESS
  of the heart's action . . . 47

PAGE

PATIENT'S GAIT 44
PATIENT'S HISTORY . . . 44
PATIENT'S SENSATIONS . . 44
PATIENT'S STATEMENTS
  importance of 43
PECTINATE FIBRES OF AURICLES
  their function and position . . 39
PECTORALIS MAJOR
  hypersensitiveness of, in heart failure 75
PENIS
  ram's-horn 312
PERICARDIAL ADHESIONS
  after rheumatic fever . . . 284
PERICARDIAL EFFUSION .
  embarrassing the heart . . 283
  simulating dilatation . . 282, 283
  symptoms of 283
PERICARDIAL SAC
  in the fixation of the heart . 38, 302
PERCUSSION WAVE . . . 134
PERICARDITIS
  in acute fevers 282
  a misleading term . . . 283
  a painless affection . . . 282
  symptoms of 282
  See also MEDIASTINO-PERICARDITIS 343
PERICARDIUM
  adherent 343
  insensitiveness of . . . 58
  in rheumatic fever . . . 283
PERIODIC RESPIRATION . . 55
PERIPHERAL RESISTANCE
  effect of increased . . . 315
PERISTALSIS
  of the bowel, pain caused by . 58
PERITONEAL ADHESIONS
  insensitiveness of . . 58, 343
PERNICIOUS ANÆMIA
  epigastric pulsation in . . . 123
  jugular pulse in 159
  heart-rate in 170
PERSPIRATION
  during an attack of angina pectoris 78
PETIT MAL 48, 49, 272
PHYSICAL SIGNS
  significance of 23
PHYSIOLOGICAL VENOUS PULSE
  See AURICULAR JUGULAR PULSE . 146
PILO-MOTOR REFLEX . . . 67
  auricular fibrillation in . . 281
  asthenic pulse in . . . 286

PAGE

PILO-MOTOR REFLEX (continued)—
prognosis of irregularities of the
pulse in 287
missed pulse beats in fatal cases of 280

PLATEAU, SYSTOLIC
in apex tracing . . . 117, 119

PNEUMONIA
case illustrating severe heart affection in 285
the heart in 285
hypostatic 308
irregular heart in . . . 286
auricular fibrillation in . . 217
pericarditis in 282
the pulse in 287
pulsus alternans in . . . 256

POISEUILLE
and the pulse 130

POISONED HEARTS
symptoms subjective . . . 292
increased rate 292
dilatation 292
venous engorgement . . . 292
associated symptoms . . . 293
prognosis 293
treatment 293

POLYGRAPH 105
the clinical 105
the ink 105

POSITION OF THE HEART
Waterston's work on . . . 112

POSITION OF THE HEART IN
DILATATION 302

POST-MORTEM RECORDS OF CASES
of angina pectoris   394, 395, 397, 398,
399, 401, 405, 411, 412, 415
of cardio-sclerosis . 448, 453, 454
of auricular fibrillation   419, 420, 424,
427, 454
of paroxysmal tachycardia . . 446
of pulsus alternans . . 398, 405
heart-block 453

POSTSPHYGMIC PERIOD . . 148

POWER OF RECOVERY
a basis for prognosis . . . 348

POYNTON AND PAINE
on rheumatic fever . . . 283

PREDICROTIC WAVE . . . 134

PREGNANCY
jugular pulse in 160
heart-rate increased in . . 172
slow pulse-rate in . . . 178
and œdema of the lungs . . 308

PRESPHYGMIC INTERVAL 118, 125, 262

PRESPHYGMIC PERIOD . . 148

PAGE

PRESSURE. See ARTERIAL PRESSURE.

PRESYSTOLIC MURMUR
varying position of in cardiac cycle   331
varying relation to first sound . 331
disappearance of . . . 332
See also MURMURS.

PRESYSTOLIC THRILL. . . 331
the first sign of mitral stenosis . 331

PRICE
on auricular fibrillation in diphtheria 281

PRIMARY WAVE
in a sphygmogram . . . 134

PRIMITIVE CARDIAC TISSUE
in cardio-sclerosis . . . 316
cases illustrating pathology of   270, 446,
448, 453, 454
and extra-systoles . . . 192
functions of 32
in the mammalian heart . . 34
affected in auricular fibrillation . 217
the starting-place of the heart's
contraction in the . . 35, 38

PRIMITIVE CARDIAC TUBE . 32
functions of 32

PRINCIPLES OF TREATMENT . 355

PROGNOSIS 347
in angina pectoris . . . 80
basis for 348
in cardio-sclerosis . . . 318
in cases with exaggerated sensory
symptoms 92
in Cheyne-Stokes respiration . 55
in depression of conductivity . 274
in congenital affection of the heart 346
in exhaustion of contractility . 298
dangers of ignorance in giving a . 347
in dilatation of the heart . . 310
use of digitalis in . . . 311
of extra-systoles . . . 199
effect of a gloomy . . 348, 356
the field of cardiac response in 348, 349
in heart-block 274
and life insurance . . . 347
in liver enlargement . . . 311
importance of 347
in increased heart-rate . . 176
in mediastino-pericarditis . . 345
in auricular fibrillation with increased rate . . . 229–32
in obscure cases . . . 349
in paroxysmal tachycardia . . 253
of the pulsus alternans . . 259
the reserve force in . . 348, 349
responsibility of giving a . . 347
of sinus irregularities . . 186
patients with obscure symptoms . 349

PAGE

PROGNOSIS (continued)—
in syncope 349
in typhoid fever 288
in valvular affections . . . 341
responsibility of the medical profession 347
PROGRESSIVE NATURE . .
of valvular sclerosis . . . 332
PROTECTION
the function of contracted muscles 61
the function of pain . . . 62
PROTECTIVE MECHANISM
angina pectoris a . . . 72
in gastric ulcer 62
in joint disease 62
reflex 57
PSEUDO-ANGINA PECTORIS .
a useless and misleading term . 88
PUERPERAL FEVER
auriculo-ventricular bundle affected
in 280
the heart in 288
PULMONARY ARTERY
tracings from . . . 118, 119
PULMONARY CIRCULATION
effect of respiratory movements on 309
PULMONARY STASIS. See LUNGS . 56
PULMONARY VEINS
heart's contraction starting at 32, 33
PULSATION
of the liver 162
causes of epigastric . . . 123
PULSATION, CAPILLARY
in aortic regurgitation . . . 339
PULSE
anacrotic 339
in aortic incompetence . . 339
in aortic stenosis . . . 339
in angina pectoris . . . 79
character of irregularity in auricular fibrillation 218
causes of unequal radial . . 133
Corrigan's 339
digital examination of arterial 129, 131
effect of auricular contraction on
radial 269
liver 162
how to record liver . . . 107
condition of the walls . . . 132
size of the artery . . . 132
character of 132
comparison of both radial pulses . 133
definition of a sphygmogram . 134
errors in results of . . . 134
in puerperal fever . . . 288
intermission due to depressed conductivity . . 262, 269, 273
intermission due to extra-systoles 190,
194, 197

PAGE

PULSE (continued)—
nature of movements of arterial . 130
not due to expansion of the artery 130
in palpitation 174
in pneumonia 287
rate, classification of diminished . 177
rate, slow, due to heart-block . 273
rate of 132
rate, slow, due to true bradycardia 178
size of 133
rate, reckoning of the . . . 132
rate during syncopal attacks . 273
impact of 133
rhythm of the 133
slow, due to feeble contraction of
ventricle 177
water-hammer 339
wave, impact of the . . . 133
wave, size of 133
what is it ? . . . 129, 130
value of a sphygmogram . . 133

PULSE, VENOUS. See JUGULAR PULSE 146

PULSUS ALTERNANS . . . 257
in acute affections of the heart . 280
in angina pectoris . . 259, 260
and arterial pressure . . . 141
with cardiac asthma . . . 53
in cardio-sclerosis . 316, 317, 318
causation of 258
conditions giving rise to the . . 256
definition of . . . xxii, 255
differential diagnosis of . . 258
due to digitalis 373
distinct from extra-systoles . . 259
distinct from pulsus bigeminus . 258
Einthoven on 258
gravity of prognosis in . . . 260
with extra-systoles . . 257, 317
field of response with . . 259
frequency of 256
heart sounds with . . . 257
Hoffmann on 258
how produced 258
with paroxysmal tachycardia 255, 259
in pneumonia 256
Muskens on 258
prognosis of 259
significance of . . 259, 260, 318
significance of, in cardio-sclerosis 317,
318
treatment of 260
a symptom of exhausted contractility 258
Windle on 257

PULSUS BIGEMINUS
definition of . . . xxii, 189
heart sounds in 190
distinct from pulsus alternans . 258
due to extra-systoles . . . 181
multiple extra-systoles . . 181

PAGE

PULSUS BISFERIENS
in aortic stenosis . . . 339
PULSUS CELER 169
PULSUS PARADOXUS
in mediastino-pericarditis . . 344
PULSUS TARDUS 177
PURKINJE FIBRES . . . 35
PURPOSE OF VISCERAL REFLEXES 61
PYÆMIA
heart in 288

RADIAL PULSE
as a standard 130
causes of unequal . . . 133
RAPID BREATHING
in heart failure 52
RARE FORMS
of cardiac irregularity . . . 203
REACTION
of visceral disease on the nervous
system 87
RECURRENT ATTACKS
of angina pectoris . . . 80
REFLEX PHENOMENA
in heart failure 57
REFLEX PROTECTIVE PHENOMENA
in visceral disease . . . 57
REFLEX SYMPTOMS
during an attack of angina pectoris 78
cause of exaltation of . . . 62
in dilatation of the heart . . 305
due to exhaustion of contractility . 296
in enlargement of the liver . . 161
exaggerated in neurotic people . 87
REFLEX, VISCERO-MOTOR . . 61
REFLEX, VISCERO-SENSORY . 59
in angina pectoris . . . 69
REFLEXES, VISCERAL, PURPOSE
OF 61
REGURGITATION
into coronary sinus, how prevented 38
into veins, how prevented . . 39
RELATIVE IMPORTANCE
of symptoms 3
RENAL COLIC 62
RESECTION OF BOWEL
in conscious subject . . . 58
RESERVE FORCE . . . 12
estimation of amount of . . 15
conditions exhausting the . 12, 21
of the function of contractility . 31
in prognosis . . . 348, 349

PAGE

RESERVE FORCE (continued)—
restored by training . . . 349
increased heart-rate with exhaustion of 13
importance of exhaustion of . . 14
exhaustion and restoration of . 15
signs of exhaustion of . . . 21
See also HEART MUSCLE . . 15
RESPIRATION
effect of movements of, in the pulmonary circulation . . . 309
causing irregular heart action . 183
slow, due to digitalis . . . 55
slow, inducing irregular action of
the heart 55
slow, and vagus stimulation . . 55
RESPIRATORY SYMPTOMS . . 51
RESPONSE, FIELD OF
in heart-block 274
the standard of heart's strength 11, 15
RESPONSIBILITY
which should be taken . . . 347
REST 290
effect of, on depressed conductivity 275
importance of, in exhausted contractility 358
in treatment 359
want of, a cause of exhaustion of
the heart 358
want of, a cause of angina pectoris 77
RESTLESSNESS
treatment of 382
RETRACTION OF STRUCTURES
during ventricular systole . . 120
RETROGRADE EXTRA-SYSTOLE . 195
RHEUMATIC AFFECTION OF THE
HEART
causing auricular fibrillation 212, 238, 284
RHEUMATIC FEVER
affection of auriculo-ventricular
bundle in . . 217, 284, 330
auricular fibrillation . . . 217
cellular foci in heart muscle in . 284
dilatation of the heart in . . 284
extra-systoles in a fatal case of . 281
heart in 283
heart symptoms in . . . 284
irritable heart after . . . 284
salicylates in 289
mitral stenosis due to . . . 330
myocarditis in 284
pericardial adhesions after . . 284
pericarditis in 282
symptoms of heart affections in . 284
slow cicatrization in heart after . 284
Paynton and Paine on . . 283

PAGE

RHEUMATIC HEART
exhaustion of contractility in . 284
RHEUMATIC HEART CASES
dropsy in 307
RHEUMATIC HEART WITH AURI-
CULAR FIBRILLATION
effect of digitalis on . . . 232
RHEUMATISM, MUSCULAR
contraction of intercostal muscles in 70
RHYTHMICAL CONTRACTION OF
THE HEART
cause of 28
RIBS
resection of, in adhesive medias-
tino-pericarditis . . . 345
RIGHT VENTRICLE
and epigastric pulsation . . 123
RIGHT VENTRICLE CAUSING THE
APEX BEAT 124
ROY AND ADAMI
work of 41
RUPTURE OF AORTIC VALVES . 338
RUPTURE OF THE HEART . . 141
with arterial degeneration . . 141
RUSSELL
and arterial pressure . . . 138

SACRO-SPINALIS MUSCLES . . 162
tenderness of, in liver enlargement . 162
SALICYLATE OF SODA
in rheumatic fever . . . 289
SALIVA, INCREASED SECRETION OF
in angina pectoris . . . 78
SALT
in angina pectoris . . . 85
in dropsy 360
SALVARSAN
and enlargement of the liver . . 161
SCHOOLBOYS
and the sinus irregularity . . 186
SCLEROSIS OF MUSCLE
with mitral stenosis . . . 330
SCLEROSIS OF VALVES AND
HEART MUSCLE
association of 330
SCLEROTIC CHANGES
progressive nature of . . . 316
SEA-BATHING . . . 94, 364
SEDATIVES 382
SEGMENTATION OF THE BODY
cause of 63
SENILE HEART 313
œdema of the lungs with . . 317
symptoms caused by the . . 315
introduction 313

PAGE

SENSATIONS OF PATIENTS
during an attack of heart-block
syncope 272, 274
SENSE OF EXHAUSTION . . 46
cause of 97
SENSE OF IMPENDING DEATH
in angina pectoris . . . 79
in palpitation 175
SENSE OF SUFFOCATION
in heart failure 52
SENSITIVENESS
to vaso-motor stimulation . . 97
SENSORY DISORDERS
as a result of heart failure . . 71
SENSORY DISTURBANCES
in weakened hearts . . . 74
SENSORY PHENOMENA
in cardio-sclerosis . . 90, 317
in nervous people . . . 91
SEPTIC INFECTIONS
auriculo-ventricular bundle affected
in 280
the heart in 287
heart-block in 280
SEPTUM, AURICULO-VENTRICULAR
action of muscles on . . . 39
SHERRINGTON
on visceral reflexes . . . 61
SHOCK DUE TO VENTRICULAR
SYSTOLE 127
SINO-AURICULAR BLOCK . . 203
SINO-AURICULAR NODE
constitution of 34
definition of term . . . xxiii
functions of 35
position of 34
the starting-place of the heart's
contraction 35
SINUS IRREGULARITIES . . 183
character of 183
in healthy people . . . 186
and the X disease . . . 186
youthful type of irregularity . 183
ætiology 183
vagus, origin of . . . 183
often respiratory in origin . 184
symptoms of 185
associated symptoms of . . 186
diagnostic significance of . . 186
— Deane 186
— Lewis 186
— Nicholson 186
— Watson Williams . . . 186
significance after toxic fevers . 187
no treatment required . . . 187

PAGE

SINUS VENOSUS 32
   formation of 32
   in the mammalian heart . . 34
   starting-place of the heart's contraction 35
SKIN, ATTENUATION OF
   due to obliteration of capillaries . 314
SKIN, HYPERALGESIC
   after an attack of angina pectoris . 80
SLEEP
   angina pectoris induced by want of 320
   with cardiac asthma . . . 53
   Cheyne-Stokes respiration during . 54
   importance of, in treatment . . 382
   necessity for, in cardio-sclerosis . 320
   necessity for inquiry into . . 44
SLEEPLESSNESS
   inducing angina pectoris . . 320
SLOW BREATHING . . . 55
SLOW PULSES
   classification of 138
SLOW RESPIRATION
   in heart failure 55
SLOWING OF THE WHOLE HEART
   by digitalis . . . 373, 377
SOLDIER'S HEART . . . 172
SOLDIERS
   sinus irregularity in healthy . . 186
SOUNDS AND MURMURS OF THE
   HEART 321
   introduction 321
   functional 321
   organic 321
   valve lesions of little significance
   of themselves 321
   attitude of the profession towards . 322
   variation in sounds . . . 322
   altered first sounds . . . 323
   altered second sounds . . . 323
   functional murmurs, cause of . 323
   quantity of blood which causes a
   murmur 324
   functional and organic differentiation of 325
   functional murmurs, significance of 326
   bogey of regurgitation . . . 327
   organic murmurs, significance of . 327
SOUNDS OF THE HEART
   in cardio-sclerosis . . . 317
   due to extra-systoles . . 190, 198
   in auricular fibrillation . . 222, 223
   in sinus irregularity . . . 185
SOUTHEY'S TUBES
   in the treatment of dropsy . . 312
SPAS
   treatment at 365
   cause of efficacy of treatment at . 367

PAGE

SPASM OF HOLLOW MUSCLES
   a cause of pain 57
SPHYGMIC PERIOD . . . 148
SPHYGMOGRAM
   definition of 134
   errors in results of . . . 134
   diastolic notch in a . . . 135
   diastolic period in a . . . 135
   diastolic wave in a . . . 135
   events of the cardiac revolution 134, 147
   instrumental defects in a . . 136
   interpretation of a . . . 134
   inverted 130, 131
   the primary wave in a . . . 134
   systolic period in a . . . 134
   tidal wave in a 134
   the value of a 133
SPHYGMOGRAPH, THE . . . 104
SPINAL CORD
   diagram showing relation to sensory
   nerve 60
   effect of reflex stimulation on . 76
   irritable focus in . . . 61, 73
   irritable, in visceral disease . . 61
SPIRITUS ÆTHERIS NITROSI . 382
SQUILLS 381
STANDARDS
   for recognizing events in a cardiac
   revolution 114
STANDPOINT
   from which this book is written . 4
STANDSTILL OF HEART
   due to digitalis 379
   in auricular fibrillation . . 218
   in sinus irregularity . . . 185
   in vagus stimulation . . . 465
STANNIUS' LIGATURES . 34, 272
   resemblance of, to heart-block . 272
   experiments 34
STARTING-PLACE
   of heart's contraction . . . 35
   of auricular fibrillation . . 216
STASIS, PULMONARY. *See* LUNGS 56
STEELL
   and enlargement of the liver . 161
   and aortic stenosis . . . 339
STERNO-MASTOID . . . 75
   hypersensitiveness of, in heart
   failure 302
STIMULANTS
   danger in the use of . . . 95
STIMULATION OF THE SKIN
   CAUSING ANGINA PECTORIS . 77
STIMULUS PRODUCTION . . 28
   and angina pectoris . . . 76

PAGE

STROPHANTHONE
use of 235

STROPHANTHUS 379
no distinction in action . . 380
half as active as digitalis . . 380
not to be added to water . . 380
hypodermically of no value . . 380

STRYCHNINE
of little use in treatment . 354, 385

SUFFOCATION, SENSATION OF 52, 53
in Cheyne-Stokes respiration . 54
a symptom of exhausted contractility 302

SUFFOCATIVE ŒDEMA OF LUNGS 56

SUGGESTION IN TREATMENT . 92

SULPHONAL 320, 383

SURGICAL OPERATIONS
how arteries recognized in . . 130

SUTHERLAND
on Cheyne-Stokes respiration . 54

SWALLOWING
effect of, on conductivity . . 465
stimulates the vagus . . . 465
effect of, on the heart . . . 184

SYMPATHETIC FIBRES
in sino-auricular node . . . 35

SYMPATHETIC NERVES
See NERVES OF THE HEART . . 41

SYMPTOMS
classification of, in visceral disease 57
due to changes in organs . . 57
nature of, produced by hollow
muscular organs . . . 57
of heart affection, confusing and
contradictory 2
due to impaired function of organs 57
due to nerve reflexes . . . 57
relative importance of . . . 3
respiratory 51
definition of term . . . 23
discrimination of significance of . 20

SYNCOPE 48
due to digitalis 271
fatal in diphtheria . . . 287
due to heart-block . . . 273
pulse-rate during . . . 272
prognosis in . . . 275, 349
with sinus irregularity . . . 186

SYPHILIS AND CARDIO-SCLERO-
SIS 314

SYPHILITIC GUMMATA
causing heart-block . . . 270

PAGE

SYSTOLIC PERIOD
in a cardiogram . . . 118, 119
in a phlebogram 149
in a sphygmogram . . . 135

SYSTOLIC PLATEAU . . . 119

TACHYCARDIA 168
loose employment of term . . 88
See HEART-RATE . . . 168
See PAROXYSMAL TACHYCARDIA . 251

TÆNIA TERMINALIS
contraction of, prevents regurgitation into veins . . . 39

TALBOT AND COOPER
on mediastino-pericarditis . . 34

TAWARA
bundle of . . . . xxi, 34

TEMPERATURE
relation of, to pulse-rate . . 278

TENDERNESS
in enlargement of the liver . . 162

THEOBROMINÆ SODII SALICYLAS 312

THEOCIN-SODIUM ACETATE
in dilatation of the heart . . 312

THRILL
due to aortic stenosis . . . 338
due to mitral stenosis . . . 331
due to patent ductus arteriosus . 346

TIDAL WAVE
in a sphygmogram . . . 134

TONE OF THE HEART . . . 300

TONICITY 29
and angina pectoris . . . 228
definition of xxiii
depression of 307
effect of digitalis on . . . 232
effects of drugs on . . . 30
function of 301
functional murmurs caused by depression of . . . 321, 324
importance of, in auricular fibrillation 226
symptoms of depression of . . 302

TORTUOUS ARTERY
nature of movements of . 130, 131

TRACINGS
how to take 105

TRAINING
reserve force restored by . . 349

TRANSIENT AURICULAR FIBRIL-
LATION 227, 228
See PAROXYSMAL TACHYCARDIA.

TRAPEZIUS. See MUSCLE.
hypersensitiveness of, in heart
failure 75

PAGE

TREATMENT .　　.　　.　　.　　.　　351
 of angina pectoris　　.　　.　　84–6
 of acute febrile conditions of the
  heart　　.　　.　　.　　.　　289
 of cardio-sclerosis　　.　　.　　318
 of cases with exaggerated sensory
  symptoms　　.　　.　　.　　92–5
 of Cheyne-Stokes respiration　　.　　54
 of congenital affections of the heart　346
 of exhausted contractility　　.　　311
 of dropsy　.　　.　　.　　311, 312
 bearing of dilatation on　.　　.　　310
 of dilatation of the heart　.　　311, 312
 of extra-systoles　　.　　.　　201
 of exophthalmic goitre　　.　　.　　173
 of heart failure with dropsy .　311, 312
 of high arterial pressure　　.　　143
 of heart-block after digitalis .　　.　　373
 with enlargement of the liver　.　　275
 of mediastino-pericarditis　.　　345
 of neurotic patients　.　　.　　94, 382
 of auricular fibrillation with no
  increase in rate　　.　　.　　232
 of auricular fibrillation with increased rate　　.　　.　　.　　233
 of poisoned hearts　　.　　.　　293
 of œdema of the lungs　　.　　309
 of paroxysmal tachycardia　.　　.　　253
 of cases showing the pulsus alternans　.　　.　　.　　.　　260
 of valvular affections .　　.　　342
 aperients in　.　　.　　.　　.　　358
 ammonium bromide in　.　　94, 382
 difficulty in estimating the effect of
  remedies .　　.　　.　　.　　352
 facts and definite results necessary .　370
 strychnine, caffeine, and camphor
  useless　.　　.　　.　　.　　370
 bad effects on digestive system　.　　372
 baths in　.　　.　　.　　.　　364
 bodily comfort in　　.　　.　　353
 deep breathing in　　.　　309, 312
 the condition of the bowels in　.　　358
 essential principle in　.　　.　　355
 digitalis and rest　.　　.　　.　　358
 drugs in extreme heart failure　.　　361
 diet in　.　　.　　.　　.　　360
 enemata in　.　　.　　.　　.　　358
 rules for employment of exercise in　363
 food in　.　　.　　.　　.　　360
 hypnotics in　.　　.　　.　　382
 harm of injudicious feeding in　.　　360
 massage in .　　.　　.　　.　　364
 importance of mastication in　.　　361
 milk in　.　　.　　.　　.　　361
 the mental factor in　.　　.　　353
 Nauheim .　　.　　.　　.　　365
 oxygen in .　　.　　.　　.　　383
 position assumed by patient in　.　　359
 by position　.　　.　　.　　.　　359
 rest—importance of　.　　.　　358
 sea-bathing in　.　　.　　.　　364

PAGE

TREATMENT (continued)—
 sleep in　.　　.　　.　　.　　359
 at spas　.　　.　　.　　.　　365
 cause of efficacy of spa　.　　.　　365
 by special exercises　.　　.　　363
 by special movements .　　.　　363
 by suggestion　.　　.　　92, 352
 vaso-dilators in .　　.　　.　　381
 venesection in　.　　.　　.　　364
 what to treat　.　　.　　.　　351
 best exercise is that which gives no
  discomfort　.　　.　　.　　363
 exercises in　.　　.　　.　　362
 drugs in　.　　.　　.　　.　　370
 digitalis　.　　.　　.　　.　　372
 importance of pushing digitalis　.　　373
 in less severe cases　.　　.　　361
 nervous condition of the patient .　353
 Nauheim and young patients　.　　369
 Nauheim and neurotic cases　.　　369
 results of ineffective dosage .　　354
 rest from worry .　　.　　.　　359
 'salt-free' diet .　　.　　.　　360
 walking　.　　.　　.　　.　　000
 spa treatment, cause of efficacy of　367

TRICUSPID INCOMPETENCE
 murmurs in　.　　.　　.　　.　　336

TRICUSPID REGURGITATION
 effect on the jugular pulse　.　　337
 a normal condition　.　　.　　336
 without a murmur　.　　.　　337
 and the venous pulse .　　.　　337

TRICUSPID STENOSIS .　　.　　.　　337
 cases of　.　　.　　.　　.　　337
 pulsation of liver in　.　　.　　337
 sound of jugular valves in　.　　337
 symptoms of　.　　.　　.　　337

TRICUSPID SYSTOLIC MURMUR
 position of .　　.　　.　　.　　337

TRICUSPID VALVE DISEASE
 jugular pulse in .　　.　　.　　337

TRICUSPID VALVES
 effect of opening of, on the jugular
  pulse　.　　.　　.　　.　　150

TUBE
 primitive cardiac　.　　.　　32

TUBERCULAR MENINGITIS
 periodic respiration in　.　　.　　55

TUBERCULOSIS
 heart-rate increased in　.　　.　　176

TYPHOID FEVER
 epigastric pulsation in .　　.　　123
 the heart in　.　　.　　.　　278
 heart failure in　.　　.　　.　　309
 heart-rate in　.　　.　　.　　170
 prognostic sign of œdema of the
  lungs in .　　.　　.　　.　　309
 rapid breathing in　.　　.　　52

ULCER, GASTRIC
contracted muscles in . . . 62
hyperalgesia in 62
meaning and purpose of symptoms
in 62
pain in 62
ULCERATION OF MITRAL VALVES 284
UMBILICAL REGION
cause of pain in 58
UNCONSCIOUSNESS
due to angina pectoris . . . 78
URETER
nature of symptoms produced by . 57
URINE
increased secretion of, during an
attack of angina pectoris . . 80
secretion of, in dilatation of the
heart 310
diminished secretion of, with dropsy 310
significance of diminished secretion
of 310
UTERUS
nature of symptoms produced by . 57

VAGAL REFLEXES
in heart failure 68
VAGUS NERVE
in sino-auricular node . . . 35
VAGUS SENSORY REFLEXES . 68
VAGUS STIMULATION
causing slow respiration . 55, 184
by deep breathing . . . 270
in experiment 185
in heart-block 271
by swallowing, producing heart-
block 184
by swallowing 184
producing sinus irregularities 183, 186
VALVE DEFECTS 329
associated with sclerosis of heart
muscle . . 332, 333, 339, 340
the manner of heart failure due to 329
presystolic thrill 331
heart failure symptoms show little
distinctive of valves affected . 330
murmurs present in . . . 330
VALVES
opening of auriculo-ventricular . 120
VALVULAR AFFECTIONS
and angina pectoris . 334, 339, 340
and arterial pressure . . . 141
cardiac response the only safe guide
in 341
with hyperalgesia . . . 89
and exhausted nervous system . 89
heart-rate increased in . . 171, 176

VALVULAR AFFECTIONS (continued)—
prognosis in 341
reflex symptoms exaggerated in . 89
treatment of 342
VALVULAR SCLEROSIS
progressive nature of . . 330, 333
VASO-DILATING DRUGS
in angina pectoris . . . 85
in high arterial pressure . . 143
in treatment 381
VASO-MOTOR
symptoms 96
nerves 96
functions of 96
stimulation, sensitiveness to . 97
VASO-MOTOR ANGINA PECTORIS 99
VASO-MOTOR SYSTEM
agents influencing . . . 97
suprarenal extract, action of, on . 97
pituitary extract, action of, on 97
peptone extract, action of, on . 97
nitrites, action of, on . . . 97
in aortic diseases . . . 100
VEGETATIONS IN ACUTE RHEU-
MATISM 282, 283
VEGETATIONS ON VALVES
symptoms of 282
VEINS
heart's contraction starting at the
mouths of 38
how regurgitation into is prevented 39
in the fixation of the heart . . 39
VENESECTION
indications for 364
VENOUS PULSE 145
VENTRICLE
action of pectinate fibres on . . 39
course of dilatation of left, in mitral
stenosis 304
exhaustion of the left, a cause of
angina pectoris . . . 72
filling of 120
fixation of the 39
perception of contraction of . . 117
period of contraction of . . 118
period of filling of . . . 120
period of relaxation of . . . 119
VENTRICULAR CONTRACTION .
electrocardiograms of . 108, 109
VENTRICULAR EXTRA-SYSTOLE 192
VENTRICULAR FALL
in a jugular pulse . . 149, 150
VENTRICULAR HYPERTROPHY
in aortic valve disease . . . 338
VENTRICULAR JUGULAR PULSE 156
auricular distension in . . 158
auricular wave absent in . . 157
significance of 157

PAGE

VENTRICULAR LIVER PULSE . 162

VENTRICULAR MUSCLE
action on auriculo-ventricular
septum 39
insertion of 39
relaxation of 119

VENTRICULAR OUTFLOW . . 119

VENTRICULAR PRESSURE-CURVE 148

VENTRICULAR RHYTHM . . 261
definition of . . . xxiii, 261
due to heart-block . . . 267
inexcitability of the ventricle in . 274
starting-place of 270
symptoms associated with . . 271

VENTRICULAR SYSTOLE
action of, on auricle . . . 39
retraction of structures due to . 120
shock due to . . . 125, 127

VENTRICULAR VENOUS PULSE
definition of xxiii
different forms of . . . 156

VENTRICULAR WAVE . . . 150
in a jugular pulse . . . 153

VERATRIN
action on tonicity . . . 30

VERONAL 320, 383

VISCERA
insensitiveness of . . . 58

VISCERAL DISEASES
classification of symptoms in . 57
diagram showing mechanism of reflexes in 60
effect of, on spinal cord . . 56
hyperalgesia in . . . 68, 87
mental state in 87
reaction of, on central nervous
system 87

VISCERAL REFLEXES
purpose of 61

PAGE

VISCERO-MOTOR REFLEX
definition of xxiii
in angina pectoris . . . 70
in cardio-sclerosis . . . 70
in old age 70
mechanism of 61

VISCERO-SENSORY REFLEX . 59
definition of xxiii
in angina pectoris . . . 69
mechanism of 59

WARMTH
feeling of, in exophthalmic goitre . 173

WASTING
in heart failure 308

WATER-HAMMER PULSE . . 339

WAVE, VENTRICULAR . . . 150

WENCKEBACH'S WORK . . 31

WHISKY
during an attack of angina pectoris 85

WHORL
muscle-fibres constituting . . 39

WINDLE
on pulsus alternans . . . 257

WORRY
effect of, on heart . . . 359

X DISEASE
and the sinus irregularity . . 186
slow pulse-rate in . . . 101
symptoms of the . . . 101
circulatory symptoms in . . 100
definition of 100
heart in 101
respiration in 101
Christian scientists and . . 102
cause of 102
treatment of 103

INDEX TO APPENDIX OF CLINICAL CASES

PAGE

ANGINA PECTORIS
Case 1. Result of overstrain . 386
Case 2. Result of overstrain. Recovery . . . 386
Case 3. Complete cessation for nineteen years . . 386
Case 4. With pericarditis. Recovery . . . 387
Case 5. With pericarditis and pneumonia. Post-mortem report . . 387
Case 6. From exhaustion. Recovery . . . 388
Case 7. From exhaustion. Recovery . . . 388
Case 8. 389
Case 9. 389
Case 10. With advancing changes in the heart . . 390
Case 11. 390
Case 12. Obscure action of the heart . . . 391
Case 13. From over-exertion . 391
Case 14. Remission for five years . 392
Case 15. Due to senile changes . 392
Case 16. Due to senile changes . 393
Case 17. Due to senile changes. Post-mortem report . 393
Case 18. Due to senile changes . 394
Case 19. Due to senile changes . 394
Case 20. Due to senile changes. Post-mortem report . 394
Case 21. Due to senile changes . 395
Case 22. Exhaustion. Post-mortem report . . 395
Case 23. 397
Case 24. Cheyne-Stokes respiration, pulsus alternans. Post-mortem report . 397
Case 25. Post-mortem report . 398
Case 26. Neglected . . . 399
Case 27. With pulsus alternans. Attack described . 399
Case 28. Cardiac aneurysm, rupture of the heart. Sudden death . . . 400
Case 29. Cheyne-Stokes respiration. Death . . 401
Case 30. Sudden death . . 402
Case 31. Severe pain in left arm. Post-mortem report . 402

PAGE

ANGINA PECTORIS (continued)
Case 32. Obscure irregularity. Freedom from attacks for three years . . 402
Case 33. With extra-systoles. Sudden death . . . 404
Case 34. With obscure irregular action of the heart during attacks. Death . 404
Case 35. With Cheyne-Stokes breathing and pulsus alternans. Post-mortem report . . 405
Case 36. With pain in chest, throat, and head ; partial recovery, recurrence and sudden death seven years after . . 407
Case 37. Syphilitic aortitis. Improvement under treatment . . . 408
Case 38. Syphilitic aortitis. Partial recovery . . 408
Case 39. With aortic valvular disease . . . 409
Case 40. Of syphilitic origin; blocking of coronary arteries. Post-mortem report . 410
Case 41. With aortic aneurysm— pain mainly on right side. Post-mortem report . . . 411
Case 42. With aortic disease. Post-mortem report . . 412
AURICULAR FIBRILLATION
Case 43. Effect of digitalis in . 415
Case 44. Sudden onset in old rheumatic heart. Disappearance of all evidence of auricular contraction 416
Case 45. In an efficient heart . 417
Case 46. With mitral stenosis . 418
Case 47. Good effect of digitalis . 418
Case 48. With angina pectoris and extensive valvular disease 419
Case 49. Sudden inception with permanent irregularity and ventricular form of venous pulse. Post-mortem report . . 420

PAGE

AURICULAR FIBRILLATION (continued)
Case 50. With aortic valvular disease and angina pec-
toris   .   .   . 421
Case 51 Transient attacks at first
with long-standing ex-
tra-systole. Death five
months after perma-
nent fibrillation   . 423
Case 52. Disappearance of large
auricular waves in ve-
nous pulse on estab-
lishment of   .   . 424
Case 53. Sudden inception; death
in three weeks   .   . 425
Case 54. Irregularity.   Sudden
death   .   .   . 426

AURICULAR FLUTTER
Case 55. Auricular flutter   .   . 428
Case 56. Effect of digitalis .   . 430
Case 57. Auricular flutter becom-
ing persistent. Effect
of digitalis and stro-
phanthus   .   .   . 431
Case 58. Provoked by exertion   . 432
Case 59. Paroxysmal tachycardia
due to auricular flutter 432
Case 60. Auricular flutter.   An-
gina pectoris   .   . 433
Case 61. Paroxysmal tachycardia
due to   .   .   . 434
Case 62. Auricular flutter, recovery from .   .   . 434
Case 63. Cheyne-Stokes respiration. Death   .   . 435
Case 64. Result of an acute infection 435
Case 65. With syphilitic aortitis,
aortic disease, and myo-
carditis   .   .   . 436
Case 66. As a terminal condition in
myocardial disease   . 437
Case 67. Syncopal attacks. Death 438
Case 68. Attacks of paroxysmal
tachycardia due to   . 438
Case 69. Effects of digitalis in producing auricular fibril-
lation   .   .   . 439

PAROXYSMAL TACHYCARDIA
Case 70. Frequent attacks in old
age 442

PAGE

PAROXYSMAL TACHYCARDIA
(continued)
Case 71. Without serious symp-
toms   .   .   . 443
Case 72. Becoming permanent and
causing death   .   . 445
PULSUS ALTERNANS
Case 73. Death 446
Case 74. Death 446
Case 75. Cheyne-Stokes breathing.
Death   .   .   . 447
Case 76. Cardiac asthma.   Post-
mortem report .   . 447
HEART-BLOCK
Case 77. Occurring at an early age 448
Case 78. Loss of consciousness and
convulsions   .   . 448
Case 79. Auricular fibrillation and
heart - block ; angina
pectoris   .   .   . 450
Case 80. Auricular fibrillation and
heart-block   .   . 451
AURICULAR FIBRILLATION
Case 81. With syncopal and epi-
leptiform reports   . 453
MYOCARDIAL DEGENERATION
Case 82. Probably alcoholic   . 454
POISONED HEART
Case 83. Poisoned heart   .   . 455
Case 84. Streptoccal infection   . 456
PARTIAL HEART-BLOCK
Case 85. Muscular rheumatism   . 456
MYOCARDITIS
Case 86. Subacute, with heart-
block and angina pec-
toris   .   .   . 457
Case 87. Subacute rheumatic   . 458
Case 88. Subacute rheumatic   . 459
Case 89. Subacute rheumatic   . 459
VALVULAR DISEASE
Case 90. Normal rhythm. Digitalis
produced heart-block . 460
PARTIAL HEART-BLOCK
Case 91. Produced by digitalis and
by swallowing .   . 464
MITRAL STENOSIS
Case 92. Digitalis produced slow-
ing and temporary auri-
cular fibrillation   . 465

Lightning Source UK Ltd.
Milton Keynes UK
UKHW010242220119
335963UK00012B/847/P